SANFORD GUIDE®

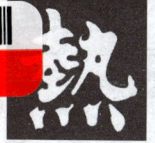

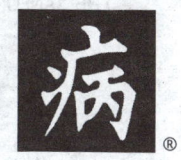

The Sanford Guide To Antimicrobial Therapy 2013

43rd Edition

THE SANFORD GUIDE TO ANTIMICROBIAL THERAPY 2013
43RD EDITION

Editors

David N. Gilbert, M.D.
Chief of Infectious Diseases and Director,
Earl A. Chiles Research Institute
Providence Portland Medical Center, Oregon

Robert C. Moellering, Jr., M.D.
Shields Warren-Mallinckrodt Professor of
Medical Research, Harvard Medical School,
Boston, Massachusetts

George M. Eliopoulos, M.D.
Chief, James L. Tullis Firm,
Beth Israel Deaconess Hospital,
Professor of Medicine,
Harvard Medical School,
Boston, Massachusetts

Henry F. Chambers, M.D.
Chief of Infectious Diseases,
San Francisco General Hospital,
Professor of Medicine,
University of California
at San Francisco

Michael S. Saag, M.D.
Director, UAB Center for AIDS Research, Professor of Medicine and Director,
Division of Infectious Diseases, University of Alabama, Birmingham

Contributing Editors

Douglas Black, Pharm. D.
Professor of Pharmacy,
University of Washington, Seattle

Brian Schwartz, M.D.
Assistant Professor
of Medicine
University of California
at San Francisco

David O. Freedman, M.D.
Director, Travelers Health Clin
Professor of Medicine,
University of Alabama, Birming

Managing Editor
Jeb C. Sanford

Emeritus
Jay P. Sanford, M.D.
1928-1996

Merle A. Sande, M.D.
1935-2007

Publisher
Antimicrobial Therapy, Inc.

The Sanford Guides are updated annually and published by:

ANTIMICROBIAL THERAPY, INC.
P.O. Box 276, 11771 Lee Highway,
Sperryville, VA 22740-0276 USA
Tel 540-987-9480 Fax 540-987-9486
Email: info@sanfordguide.com   www.sanfordguide.com

Copyright © 1969-2013 by Antimicrobial Therapy, Inc.

All rights reserved. No part of this publication may be may be reproduced, stored in a retrieval system or transmitted in any form or by any means--digital, electronic, mechanical, optical, photocopying, recording or otherwise--without prior written permission from Antimicrobial Therapy, Inc., 11771 Lee Hwy, P.O. Box 276, Sperryville, VA 22740-0276 USA

"Sanford Guide" and "Hot Disease" logo are ® registered trademarks of Antimicrobial Therapy, Inc.

Acknowledgements
Thanks to Ushuaia Solutions, SA, Argentina; Alcom Printing, Harleysville, PA and Fox Bindery, Quakertown, PA for design and production of this edition of the Sanford Guide.

Note to Readers
Since 1969, the Sanford Guide has been independently prepared and published. Decisions regarding the content of the Sanford Guide are solely those of the editors and the publisher. We welcome questions, comments and feedback concerning the Sanford Guide. All of your feedback is reviewed and taken into account in updating the content of the of the Sanford Guide.

Every effort is made to ensure the accuracy of the content of this guide. However, current full prescribing information available in the package insert for each drug should be consulted before prescribing any product. The editors and publisher are not responsible for errors or omissions or for any consequences from application of the information in this book and make no warranty, express or implied, with respect to the currency, accuracy, or completeness of the contents of this publication. Application of this information in a particular situation remains the professional responsibility of the practitioner.

Check our website for content-related notices:
http://www.sanfordguide.com

Printed in the United States of America
ISBN 978-1-930808-74-4
Pocket Edition (English)

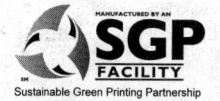

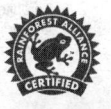

QUICK PAGE GUIDE TO THE SANFORD GUIDE*

RECOMMENDED TREATMENT—DIFFERENT SITES/MICROBES:	
BY ORGAN SYSTEM:	4 - 66
CAPD Peritonitis	213
BY ORGANISM:	
Bacteria	**67 - 69**
Highly Resistant Bacteria	**77**
CA-MRSA	**78**
Fungi	111 - 123
Mycobacteria	128 - 137
Parasites	141 - 151
Non-HIV Viruses	156 - 167
HIV/AIDS	174 - 184
Influenza	164 - 165
DURATION OF TREATMENT:	70
ANTIMICROBIAL PROPHYLAXIS:	
Pregnancy/Delivery	192
Post-Splenectomy	192
Sexual Exposure	193
Sickle Cell Disease	193
Surgical	193
Endocarditis	197
Exposure to HIV/HBV/HCV	198
Transplant Patients	201
IMMUNIZATIONS:	
Anti-tetanus	214
Rabies Post Exposure	215

ANTIMICROBIALS:

	Spectra	Adverse Effects	Dosage/S
Antibiotics	71 - 76	93 - 103	108
AG-Once Daily Dosing			109
Desensitization (Pen, TMP-SMX, ceftriaxone)			80
Pregnancy Risk Categories		81	
Antifungals	127		124 - 126
Antimycobacterials			138 - 140
Antiparasitics			152 - 155
Antivirals (Non-HIV)			168 - 172
Antiretrovirals			185 - 188

DOSE ADJUSTMENTS:	
Renal	204 - 212
Hepatic	213
Pediatric	203
DRUG INFORMATION:	
Pharmacologic Features	83
Pharmacodynamics	92
Drug-Drug Interactions	**217 - 223** (**224** ARV Drugs)
Generic/Trade Names	225
MISCELLANEOUS:	
Abbreviations	2
Parasites Causing Eosinophilia	155
Directory of Resources	216

* Adapted from materials provided by Stephanie Troy, M.D., Stanford Univ. Med. Ctr.

—TABLE OF CONTENTS—

ABBREVIATIONS 2

TABLE 1	Clinical Approach to **Initial Choice** of Antimicrobial Therapy	4
TABLE 2	Recommended Antimicrobial Agents Against **Selected Bacteria**	67
TABLE 3	Suggested **Duration** of Antibiotic Therapy in Immunocompetent Patients	70
TABLE 4	Comparison of Antibacterial Spectra	71
TABLE 5A	Treatment Options For Systemic Infection Due To Selected **Resistant Gram-Positive Bacteria**	77
5B	Treatment Options for Systemic Infection Due to Selected **Multi-Drug Resistant Gram-Negative Bacilli**	77
TABLE 6	Suggested Management of Suspected or Culture-Positive **Community-Associated Methicillin-Resistant S. aureus** Infections	78
TABLE 7	**Drug Desensitization** methods	80
TABLE 8A	**Risk Categories** of Antimicrobics in **Pregnancy**	81
8B	**Antimicrobial Dosing in Obesity**	82
TABLE 9A	Selected **Pharmacologic Features** of Antimicrobial Agents	83
9B	**Pharmacodynamics of Antibacterials**	92
9C	**Cytochrome P450 Interactions** of Antimicrobials	92
TABLE 10A	**Antibiotic Dosage and Side-Effects**	93
10B	Selected Antibacterial Agents—**Adverse Reactions**—Overview	104
10C	Antimicrobial Agents Associated with **Photosensitivity**	108
10D	Aminoglycoside Once-Daily and Multiple Daily Dosing Regimens	109
10E	Prolonged or Continuous Infusion Dosing of Selected Beta Lactams	110
TABLE 11A	Treatment of **Fungal Infections**—Antimicrobial Agents of Choice	111
11B	**Antifungal Drugs:** Dosage, Adverse Effects, Comments	124
11C	At A Glance **Summary of Suggested Antifungal Drugs Against Treatable Pathogenic Fungi**	127
TABLE 12A	Treatment of **Mycobacterial Infections**	128
12B	**Dosage** and Adverse Effects of Antimycobacterial Drugs	138
TABLE 13A	Treatment of **Parasitic Infections**	141
13B	**Dosage** and Selected Adverse Effects of Antiparasitic Drugs	152
13C	Parasites that Cause **Eosinophilia (Eosinophilia In Travelers)**	155
13D	Sources for **Hard-to-Find Antiparasitic Drugs**	155
TABLE 14A	**Antiviral Therapy**	156
14B	**Antiviral Drugs (Non-HIV)**	168
14C	At A Glance **Summary of Suggested Antiviral Agents Against Treatable Pathogenic Viruses**	173
14D	**Antiretroviral Therapy (ART) in Treatment-Naïve Adults** (HIV/AIDS)	174
14E	**Antiretroviral Drugs** and Adverse Effects	185
14F	**Hepatitis A & HBV Treatment**	189
14G	**HCV Treatment Regimens and Response**	189
TABLE 15A	Antimicrobial Prophylaxis for Selected Bacterial Infections	192
15B	**Antibiotic Prophylaxis** to **Prevent Surgical Infections** in **Adults**	193
15C	Antimicrobial Prophylaxis for the Prevention of **Bacterial Endocarditis** in Patients with Underlying Cardiac Conditions	197
15D	Management of **Exposure to HIV-1 and Hepatitis B and C**	198
15E	Prevention of Selected Opportunistic Infections in **Human Hematopoietic Cell Transplantation** (HCT) or **Solid Organ Transplantation** (SOT) in Adults With Normal Renal Function	201
TABLE 16	**Pediatric Dosages** of Selected Antibacterial Agents	203
TABLE 17A	Dosages of Antimicrobial Drugs in Adult Patients with **Renal Impairment**	204
17B	**No Dosage Adjustment** with Renal Insufficiency by Category	213
TABLE 18	Antimicrobials and **Hepatic Disease: Dosage Adjustment**	213
TABLE 19	Treatment of **CAPD Peritonitis** in Adults	213
TABLE 20A	Anti-**Tetanus** Prophylaxis, Wound Classification, Immunization	214
20B	**Rabies Postexposure Prophylaxis**	215
TABLE 21	Selected **Directory of Resources**	216
TABLE 22A	Anti-Infective **Drug-Drug Interactions**	217
22B	Drug-Drug Interactions Between **Non-Nucleoside Reverse Transcriptase Inhibitors (NNRTIs) and Protease Inhibitors**	224
TABLE 23	List of **Generic** and **Common Trade Names**	225
INDEX OF MAJOR ENTITIES		227

ABBREVIATIONS

- 3TC = lamivudine
- ABC = abacavir
- ABC% = abacavir absorbed
- ABCD = amphotericin B colloidal dispersion
- ABLC = ampho B lipid complex
- ACIP = Advisory Committee on Immunization Practices
- ADF = adefovir
- AG = aminoglycoside
- AIDS = Acquired Immune Deficiency Syndrome
- AM-CL = amoxicillin-clavulanate extended release
- AMK = amikacin
- Amox = amoxicillin
- AMP = ampicillin
- AmB = amphotericin B
- AMP-SB = ampicillin-sulbactam
- AP = antipseudomonal
- AP Pen = antipseudomonal penicillins
- APAG = antipseudomonal aminoglycoside (tobra, gent, amikacin)
- ARDS = acute respiratory distress syndrome
- ASA = aspirin
- ATS = American Thoracic Society
- ATV = atazanavir
- AUC = area under the curve
- Azithro = azithromycin
- bid = twice a day
- BL/BLI = beta-lactam/beta-lactamase inhibitor
- BSA = body surface area
- C&S = culture & sensitivity
- CAPD = continuous ambulatory peritoneal dialysis
- CARB = carbapenems (DOR, ERTA, IMP, MER)
- CDC = Centers for Disease Control
- Cefdtor = cefditoren pivoxil
- Cefpz = ceftazidime
- Ceph = cephalosporin
- CFB = ceftobiprole
- CFP = cefepime
- Chloro = chloramphenicol
- CIP = ciprofloxacin; CIP-ER = CIP extended release
- Clarithro = clarithromycin; ER = extended release
- Clav = clavulanate
- Clinda = clindamycin
- CLO = clofazimine
- Clot = clotrimazole
- CMV = cytomegalovirus
- CQ = chloroquine phosphate
- Cobi = cobicistat
- CrCl = creatinine clearance
- CrCln = CrCl normalized for body surface area (BSA)
- CRRT = continuous renal replacement therapy
- CSD = cat-scratch disease
- CSF = cerebrospinal fluid
- CXR = chest x-ray
- d4T = stavudine
- Dapto = daptomycin
- DBPCT = double-blind placebo-controlled trial
- dc = discontinue
- ddC = zalcitabine
- ddI = didanosine
- DIC = disseminated intravascular coagulation
- div = divided
- DLV = delavirdine
- Dori = doripenem
- DOT = directly observed therapy
- DRG group = B. distasonis, B. ovatus, B. thetaiotaomicron
- DRSP = drug-resistant S. pneumoniae
- DR = delayed release
- DS = double strength
- EBV = Epstein-Barr virus
- EES = erythromycin ethyl succinate
- EF2 = efavirenz
- ELV = elvitegravir
- ENT = entecavir
- ERTA = ertapenem
- ER = extended release
- Erythro = erythromycin
- ESBLs = extended spectrum β-lactamases
- ESR = erythrocyte sedimentation rate
- ESRD = endstage renal disease
- ETB = ethambutol
- Flu = fluconazole
- Flucy = flucytosine
- FOS-APV = fosamprenavir
- FQ = fluoroquinolone (CIP, Oflox, Lome, Pefflox, Levo, Gati, Moxi, Gemi)
- FTC = emtricitabine
- G = generic
- GAS = Group A Strep
- Gati = gatifloxacin
- GC = gonorrhea
- Gemi = gemifloxacin
- Gent = gentamicin
- gm = gram
- GNB = gram-negative bacilli
- Griseo = griseofulvin
- HD = hemodialysis
- HEMO = hemodialysis
- HHV = human herpesvirus
- HIV = human immunodeficiency virus
- HLR = high-level resistance
- H/O = history of
- HSCT = hematopoietic stem cell transplant
- HSV = herpes simplex virus
- IA = Injectable agent/anti-inflammatory drugs
- ICAAC = Interscience Conference on Antimicrobial Agents & Chemotherapy
- IDSA = Infectious Diseases Society of America
- IDV = indinavir
- IFN = interferon
- IMP = imipenem-cilastatin
- INH = isoniazid
- Inv = investigational
- IP = intraperitoneal
- IT = intrathecal
- Itra = itraconazole
- IVDU = intravenous drug user
- IVIG = intravenous immune globulin
- KetoG = ketoconazole
- LAB = liposomal ampho B
- LCM = lymphocytic choriomeningitis virus
- LCR = ligase chain reaction
- Levo = levofloxacin
- LP/r = lopinavir/ritonavir
- Ltra = itraconazole
- Macrolides = azithro, clarithro, dirithro, erythro, roxithro
- M. TBc = Mycobacterium tuberculosis
- mcg = microgram
- MER = meropenem
- Metro = metronidazole
- mg = milligram
- Mino = minocycline
- Moxi = moxifloxacin
- MRSA = methicillin-resistant S. aureus
- MSSA/MRSA = methicillin-sensitive/resistant S. aureus
- NB = name brand
- NAI = not FDA-approved (indication or dose)
- NF = nitrofurantoin
- NFV = nelfinavir
- NRTI = nucleoside reverse transcriptase inhibitor
- NNRTI = non-nucleoside reverse transcriptase inhibitor
- NSAIDs = non-steroidal
- NUS = not available in the U.S.
- NVP = nevirapine
- O Ceph 1, 2, 3 = oral cephalosporins—see Table 10A
- Oflox = ofloxacin
- P Ceph 1, 2, 3, 4 = parenteral cephalosporins—see Table 10A
- P Ceph 3 AP = parenteral cephalosporins with antipseudomonal activity—see Table 10A
- PCR = polymerase chain reaction
- PEP = post-exposure prophylaxis
- PI = protease inhibitor
- PIP = piperacillin
- PIP-TZ = piperacillin-tazobactam
- po = per os (by mouth)
- PQ = primaquine
- PRCT = Prospective randomized controlled trials
- PTLD = post-transplant lymphoproliferative disease

ABBREVIATIONS (2)

Pts = patients
Pyri = pyrimethamine
PZA = pyrazinamide
qid = 4 times a day
QS = quinine sulfate
Quinu-dalfo = Q-D = quinupristin-dalfopristin
R = resistant
RFB = rifabutin
RFP = rifapentine
RIF = rifampin
Rick = Rickettsia
RSV = respiratory syncytial virus
RTI = respiratory tract infection
rx = treatment
S = potential synergy in combination with penicillin,
AMP, vanco, teico

SA = Staph. aureus
SD = serum drug level after single dose
Sens = sensitive (susceptible)
SM = streptomycin
Sp = spp
SS = steady state serum level
STD = sexually transmitted disease
subcut = subcutaneous
Sulb = sulbactam
Sx = symptoms
Tazo = tazobactam
TBc = tuberculosis
TC-CL = ticarcillin-clavulanate
TDF = tenofovir
TEE = transesophageal echocardiography
Teico = teicoplanin
Telithro = telithromycin

Tetra = tetracycline
Ticar = ticarcillin
tid = 3 times a day
TMP-SMX = trimethoprim-sulfamethoxazole
TNF = tumor necrosis factor
Tobra = tobramycin
TPV = tipranavir
TST = tuberculin skin test
UTI = urinary tract infection
V = vancomycin
VISA = vancomycin intermediately resistant S. aureus
VL = viral load
Vori = voriconazole
VZV = varicella-zoster virus
WHO = World Health Organization
ZDV = zidovudine

ABBREVIATIONS OF JOURNAL TITLES

AAC: Antimicrobial Agents & Chemotherapy
Adv PID: Advances in Pediatric Infectious Diseases
AHJ: American Heart Journal
AIDS Res & Hum Retro: AIDS Research & Human Retroviruses
AJG: American Journal of Gastroenterology
AJM: American Journal of Medicine
AJRCCM: American Journal of Respiratory Critical Care Medicine
AJTMH: American Journal of Tropical Medicine & Hygiene
Am J Hith Pharm: American Journal of Health-System Pharmacy
Amer J Transpl: American Journal of Transplantation
AnEM: Annals of Emergency Medicine
AnIM: Annals of Internal Medicine
Ann Pharmacother: Annals of Pharmacotherapy
AnS: Annals of Surgery
Antivir Ther: Antiviral Therapy
ArDerm: Archives of Dermatology
ArIM: Archives of Internal Medicine
ARRD: American Review of Respiratory Disease
BMJ: British Medical Journal
BMT: Bone Marrow Transplantation
Brit J Derm: British Journal of Dermatology
Can JID: Canadian Journal of Infectious Diseases
Canad Med AJ: Canadian Medical Journal
CCM: Critical Care Medicine
CID: Clinical Infectious Diseases
CIOTTD: Current Clinical Topics in Infectious Disease
CDBSR: Cochrane Database of Systematic Reviews
Clin Micro Rev: Clinical Microbiology Reviews
CMN: Clinical Microbiology Newsletter
CMAJ: Canadian Medical Association Journal

COID: Current Opinion in Infectious Disease
Curr Med Res Opin: Current Medical Research and Opinion
Derm Ther: Dermatologic Therapy
Dermatol Clin: Dermatologic Clinics
Dig Dis Sci: Digestive Diseases and Sciences
DMID: Diagnostic Microbiology and Infectious Disease
EID: Emerging Infectious Diseases
EJCMID: European Journal of Clin. Micro. & Infectious Diseases
Eur J Neurol: European Journal of Neurology
Exp Mol Path: Experimental & Molecular Pathology
Exp Rev Anti Infect Ther: Expert Review of Anti-Infective Therapy
Gastro: Gastroenterology
Hpt: Hepatology
ICHE: Infection Control and Hospital Epidemiology
IDC No. Amer: Infectious Disease Clinics of North America
IDCP: Infectious Diseases in Clinical Practice
IJAA: International Journal of Antimicrobial Agents
Inf Med: Infections in Medicine
J AIDS & HR: Journal of AIDS and Human Retrovirology
J All Clin Immun: Journal of Allergy and Clinical Immunology
J Am Ger Soc: Journal of the American Geriatrics Society
J Chemother: Journal of Chemotherapy
Clin Micro: Journal of Clinical Microbiology
Clin Virol: Journal of Clinical Virology
J Derm Treat: Journal of Dermatological Treatment
Hpt: Journal of Hepatology
J Inf: Journal of Infection
J Med Virol: Journal of Medical Virology
J Micro Immunol Inf: Journal of Microbiology, Immunology,
  & Infection
J Ped: Journal of Pediatrics
J Viral Hep: Journal of Viral Hepatitis

JAC: Journal of Antimicrobial Chemotherapy
JACC: Journal of American College of Cardiology
JAIDS: JAIDS Journal of Acquired Immune Deficiency Syndromes
JAMA: Journal of the American Medical Association
JAVMA: Journal of the Veterinary Medicine Association
JCI: Journal of Clinical Investigation
JCM: Journal of Clinical Microbiology
JIC: Journal of Infection and Chemotherapy
JID: Journal of Infectious Diseases
JNS: Journal of Neurosurgery
JTMH: Journal of Tropical Medicine and Hygiene
Ln: Lancet
LnID: Lancet Infectious Disease
Mayo Clin Proc: Mayo Clinic Proceedings
Med Lett: Medical Letter
Med Mycol: Medical Mycology
MMWR: Morbidity & Mortality Weekly Report
NEJM: New England Journal of Medicine
Neph Dial Transpl: Nephrology Dialysis Transplantation
Ped Ann: Pediatric Annals
Peds: Pediatrics
Pharmacother: Pharmacotherapy
PIDJ: Pediatric Infectious Disease Journal
QJM: Quarterly Journal of Medicine
Scand J Inf Dis: Scandinavian Journal of Infectious Diseases
Sem Resp Inf: Seminars in Respiratory Infections
SGO: Surgery Gynecology and Obstetrics
SMJ: Southern Medical Journal
Surg Neurol: Surgical Neurology
Transpl Inf Dis: Transplant Infectious Diseases
Transpl: Transplantation
TRSM: Transactions of the Royal Society of Medicine

3

TABLE 1 – CLINICAL APPROACH TO INITIAL CHOICE OF ANTIMICROBIAL THERAPY*

Treatment based on presumed site or type of infection. In selected infections, treatment and prophylaxis based on identification of pathogens.
Regimens should be reevaluated based on pathogen isolated, antimicrobial susceptibility determination, and individual host characteristics. *Abbreviations on page 2)*

ANATOMIC SITE/DIAGNOSIS/ MODIFYING CIRCUMSTANCES	ETIOLOGIES (usual)	SUGGESTED REGIMENS*		ADJUNCT DIAGNOSTIC OR THERAPEUTIC MEASURES AND COMMENTS
		PRIMARY	**ALTERNATIVE**[1]	
ABDOMEN: See *Peritoneum, page 47; Gallbladder, page 17; and Pelvic Inflammatory Disease, page 26*				
BONE: Osteomyelitis. Microbiologic diagnosis is essential. If bone culture negative, need culture of bone. Culture of sinus tract drainage not predictive of bone culture. Review: *Ln 364:369, 2004.* For comprehensive review of antimicrobial penetration into bone; see *Clinical Pharmacokinetics 48:89, 2009.*				
Hematogenous Osteomyelitis				
Empiric therapy—Collect bone and blood cultures before empiric therapy				
Newborn (< 4 mos.) See Table 16 for dose Children (>4 mos.) – Adult: Osteo of extremity	S. aureus, Gm-neg. bacilli, Group B strep, S. aureus, Group A strep, Gm-neg. bacilli rare	MRSA possible: **Vanco+ (Ceftaz or CFP)** MRSA possible: **Vanco** Add **Ceftaz or CFP** if Gm-neg. bacilli on Gram stain. Adult doses below. Peds Doses: Table 16.	MRSA unlikely: **(Nafcillin or oxacillin) + (Ceftaz or CFP)** MRSA unlikely: **Nafcillin or oxacillin**	Table 16 for dose. Severe allergy or toxicity: **(Linezolid**[NUS] **10 mg/kg IV/po q8h) + aztreonam**). Could substitute **clindamycin** for linezolid. Severe allergy or toxicity: **Clinda** or **TMP-SMX** or **linezolid**[NUS] Adults: **ceftaz** 2 gm IV q8h. **CFP** 2 gm IV q12h. Peds dosages in Table 16. See Table 10B for adverse reactions to drugs.
Adult (>21 yrs) Vertebral osteo ± epidural abscess. Other sites. (*NEJM 355:2012, 2006*)	S. aureus most common but various other organisms. **Blood & bone cultures essential.**	MRSA possible: **Vanco** 15-30 mg/kg IV q 8-12h for trough of 15-20 mcg/ml	MRSA unlikely: **Nafcillin or oxacillin** 2 gm IV q4h	Dx: MRI early to look for epidural abscess. For comprehensive review of vertebral see *NEJM 362:11, 2010.*
Specific therapy—Culture and in vitro susceptibility results known				
	MSSA	**Nafcillin or oxacillin** 2 gm IV q4h or **cefazolin** 2 gm IV q8h.	**Vanco** 15-30 mg/kg IV q 8-12h for trough of 15-20 mcg/ml	
	MRSA—See Table 6, page 78; IDSA Guidelines *CID 52:e18-55, 2011; CID 52:285-92, 2011*	**Vanco** 15-30 mg/kg IV q 8-12h for trough of 15-20 mcg/ml	**Linezolid** 600 mg po/IV bid OR **Dapto** 6 mg/kg IV q 24h IV ± **RIF** 300-450 mg po/IV bid	**Other options if susceptible in vitro and allergy/toxicity issues (see *NEJM 362:11, 2010*):** 1) **TMP-SMX** 8-10 mg/kg/d po/IV div q8h ± **RIF** 300-450 mg bid; limited data, particularly for MRSA (see *AAC 53:2672, 2009*); 2) (**CIP** 750 mg po bid or **Levo** 750 mg po q24h) + **RIF** 300 mg po bid; 3) **Linezolid** (caution with long-term use) (*Neurology 64:926, 2005*), optic & peripheral neuropathy; 4) **Fusidic acid**[NUS] 500 mg IV q8h + **RIF** 300 mg po bid (*CID 42:394, 2006*); **Ceftriaxone** 2 gm IV q24h (*CID 54:585, 2012*)
Hemoglobinopathy: Sickle cell/thalassemia	Salmonella, other Gm-neg. bacilli	**CIP** 400 mg IV q12h	**Levo** 750 mg IV q24h	Thalassemia; transfusion and iron chelation risk factors. Because of decreasing levels of susceptibility to fluoroquinolones among Salmonella spp. and growing resistance among other gram-negative bacilli, would add a second agent (e.g., third-generation cephalosporin) until susceptibility test results available.
Contiguous Osteomyelitis Without Vascular Insufficiency				
Empiric therapy: Get cultures!				
Foot bone osteo due to nail through tennis shoe	P. aeruginosa	**CIP** 750 mg po bid or **Levo** 750 mg IV q24h	**Ceftaz** 2 gm IV q8h or **CFP** 2 gm IV q12h	See *Skin—Nail puncture, page 56.* Need debridement to remove foreign body.

* **DOSAGES SUGGESTED** are for adults (unless otherwise indicated) with clinically severe (often life-threatening) infections. Dosages also assume normal renal function, and not severe hepatic dysfunction.

[1] **ALTERNATIVE THERAPY INCLUDES** these considerations: allergy, pharmacology/pharmacokinetics, compliance, costs, local resistance profiles.

TABLE 1 (2)

ANATOMIC SITE/DIAGNOSIS/ MODIFYING CIRCUMSTANCES	ETIOLOGIES* (usual)	SUGGESTED REGIMENS* PRIMARY	ALTERNATIVE[1]	ADJUNCT DIAGNOSTIC OR THERAPEUTIC MEASURES AND COMMENTS
BONE/Contiguous Osteomyelitis Without Vascular Insufficiency/Empiric therapy *(continued)*				
Long bone, post-internal fixation of fracture	S. aureus, Gm-neg. bacilli, P. aeruginosa		Linezolid 600 mg IV/po bid[MA] + (ceftaz or CFP). See Comment	Often necessary to remove hardware after union to achieve eradication. May need revascularization. **Regimens listed are empiric.** Adjust after culture data available. If susceptible Gm-neg. bacillus, **CIP** 750 mg po bid or **Levo** 750 mg po q24h. For other S. aureus options: See Hem. Osteo. Specific Therapy, page 4.
Osteonecrosis of the jaw	Probably rare adverse reaction to bisphosphonates	Infection may be secondary to bone necrosis and loss of overlying mucosa. Treatment: minimal surgical debridement, chlorhexidine rinses, antibiotics (e.g. PIP-TZ), NEJM 355:2278, 2006. Evaluate for concomitant actinomycosis, for which specific long-term antibiotic treatment would be warranted (CID 49:1729, 2009).		
Prosthetic joint	See prosthetic joint, page 33			
Spinal implant infection	S. aureus, coag-neg staphylococci, gram-neg bacilli	Onset within 30 days: culture, treat for 3 mos (CID 55:1481, 2012)	Onset after 30 days remove implant, culture & treat	See CID 55:1481, 2012
Sternum, post-op	S. aureus, S. epidermidis, occasionally, gram-negative bacilli	Vanco 15-30 mg/kg IV q 8-12h for trough of 15-20 mcg/ml recommended for serious infections.	Linezolid 600 mg po/IV[MA] bid	Sternal debridement for cultures & removal of necrotic bone. For S. aureus options: Hem. Osteo. Specific Therapy, page 4. If setting or gram stain suggests possibility of gram-negative bacilli, add appropriate coverage based on local antimicrobial susceptibility profiles (e.g., cefepime, pip-tazo).
Contiguous Osteomyelitis With Vascular Insufficiency.				
Most pts are **diabetics** with peripheral neuropathy & infected skin ulcers (see Diabetic foot, page 16)	Polymicrobial (Gm + cocci [include MRSA (aerobic & anaerobic)] and Gm-neg bacilli (aerobic & anaerobic)]	Debride overlying ulcer & submit bone for histology & culture. Select antibiotic based on culture results & treat for 6 weeks. **No suggestions**, too many possibilities likely. If acutely ill, see suggestions, Diabetic foot, page 16. Revascularize if possible.		Diagnosis of osteo: Culture bone biopsy (gold standard). Poor concordance of culture results between swab of ulcer and bone – need bone (JAMA 299:806, 2008). Sampling by needle puncture inferior to biopsy (CID 48:888, 2009). Osteo more likely if ulcer >2 cm², positive probe (CID 48:888, 2009). Osteo more likely if ulcer >2 cm², positive probe to bone, ESR >70 & abnormal plain x-ray (JAMA 299:806, 2008). **Treatment: Revascularize if possible:** (2) Culture bone; (3) Specific antimicrobial(s). Reviews: BMJ 339:b4905, 2006; Plast Reconstr Surg 117: (7 Suppl) 212S, 2006.
Chronic Osteomyelitis: Specific therapy By definition, implies presence of dead bone. **Need valid cultures**	S. aureus, Enterobacteriaceae, P. aeruginosa	**Empiric rx not indicated.** Base systemic rx on results of culture, sensitivity testing. If acute exacerbation of chronic osteo, rx as acute hematogenous osteo. Surgical debridement important.		**Important adjuncts:** removal of orthopedic hardware, surgical debridement; vascularized muscle flaps, distraction osteogenesis (Ilizarov) techniques. Antibiotic-impregnated cement & hyperbaric oxygen adjunctive. **NOTE: RIF + (vanco or β-lactam)** effective in animal model and in a clinical trial of S. aureus chronic osteo. The contribution of rifampin-containing regimens in this setting is not clear, however (AAC 53:2672, 2009)

Abbreviations on page 2.   NOTE: All dosage recommendations are for adults (unless otherwise indicated) and assume normal renal function.

TABLE 1 (3)

ANATOMIC SITE/DIAGNOSIS/ MODIFYING CIRCUMSTANCES	ETIOLOGIES (usual)	SUGGESTED REGIMENS* PRIMARY	ALTERNATIVE[1]	ADJUNCT DIAGNOSTIC OR THERAPEUTIC MEASURES AND COMMENTS
BREAST: Mastitis—Obtain culture: need to know if MRSA present. Review with definitions: Ob & Gyn Clin No Amer 29:89, 2002. Review of breast infections: BMJ 342:d396, 2011.				
Postpartum mastitis (CID 54:71, 2012) Mastitis without abscess	S. aureus; less often S. pyogenes (Gp A or B), E. coli, bacteroides species, maybe Corynebacterium sp. & selected coagulase-neg. staphylococci (e.g., S. lugdunensis)	**NO MRSA: Outpatient:** Dicloxacillin 500 mg po qid or **cephalexin** 500 mg po qid. **Inpatient:** Nafcillin/oxacillin 2 gm IV q4h	**MRSA Possible: Outpatient:** TMP-SMX-DS tabs 1-2 po bid or, if susceptible, **clinda** 300 mg po qid. **Inpatient: Vanco** 1 gm IV q12h, (if over 100 kg, 1.5 gm IV q12h)	If no abscess, ↑ freq of nursing may hasten response; discuss age-specific risks to infant of drug exposure through breast milk with pediatrician. Corynebacterium sp. assoc. with chronic granulomatous mastitis (CID 35:1434, 2002).
Mastitis with abscess				With abscess, d/c nursing, **I & D standard**; needle aspiration reported successful (Am J Surg 182:117, 2001). Resume breast feeding from affected breast as soon as pain allows.
Non-puerperal mastitis with abscess	S. aureus; less often Bacteroides sp., peptostreptococcus, & selected coagulase-neg. staphylococci	See regimens for Postpartum mastitis, page 6.		Smoking and diabetes may be risk factors (BMJ 342:d396, 2011). **If subareolar & odoriferous**, most likely anaerobes; need to **add metro** 500 mg IV/po tid. If not subareolar, staph. Need pretreatment aerobic/anaerobic cultures. Surgical drainage for abscess.
Breast implant infection	Acute: S. aureus, S. pyogenes. TSS reported. Chronic: Look for rapidly growing Mycobacteria	Acute: **Vanco** 1 gm IV q12h; if over 100 kg, 1.5 gm q12h.	Chronic: Await culture results See Table 12A for mycobacteria treatment.	Lancet Infect Dis 5:94, 462, 2005. Coag-negative staph also common (Aesthetic Plastic Surg 31:325, 2007).
CENTRAL NERVOUS SYSTEM				
Brain abscess Primary or contiguous source In 51 pts, 30 positive by standard culture, using molecular diagnostics. 80 bacterial taxa & many polymicrobics (CID 54:202, 2012).	Streptococci (60-70%), bacteroides (20-40%), Enterobacteriaceae (23-33%), S. aureus (10-15%), S. anginosus grp. Rare: Nocardia (below), Listeria (CID 40:907, 2005). See S. aureus Comment	**P Ceph 3** [(**cefotaxime** 2 gm IV q4h or **ceftriaxone** 2 gm IV q12h) + (**metro** 7.5 mg/kg IV q12h)] Duration of rx unclear; treat until response by neuroimaging (CT/MRI)	**Pen G** 3-4 million units IV q4h + **metro** 7.5 mg/kg q6h or 15 mg/kg IV q12h	If CT scan suggests cerebritis or abscesses <2.5 cm and pt neurologically stable and conscious, start antibiotics and observe. Otherwise, surgical drainage necessary: If blood cultures or other clinical data do not yield a likely etiologic agent, aspirate even small abscesses for diagnosis if this can be done safely. Experience with Pen G (HD) + metro without ceftriaxone or nafcillin/oxacillin has been good. We use ceftriaxone because of frequency of isolation of Enterobacteriaceae. **S. aureus rare without positive blood culture; if S. aureus, use vanco until susceptibility known.** Strep. anginosus group ssp. prone to produce abscess. Ceph/metro does not cover listeria.
Post-surgical, post-traumatic	S. aureus, Enterobacteriaceae	**For MSSA: (Nafcillin or oxacillin)** 2 gm IV q4h + (**ceftriaxone or cefotaxime**)	**For MRSA: Vanco** 15-30 mg/kg IV q8-12h for trough of 15-20 mcg/ml + (**ceftriaxone or cefotaxime**)	Aspiration of abscesses usually necessary for dx & rx. If P. aeruginosa suspected, substitute (Cefepime or Ceftazidime) for (Ceftriaxone or Cefotaxime).
HIV-1 infected (AIDS)	Toxoplasma gondii	See Table 13A, page 146		

Abbreviations on page 2   NOTE: All dosage recommendations are for adults (unless otherwise indicated) and assume normal renal function.

TABLE 1 (4)

ANATOMIC SITE/DIAGNOSIS/ MODIFYING CIRCUMSTANCES	ETIOLOGIES (usual)	SUGGESTED REGIMENS* PRIMARY	SUGGESTED REGIMENS* ALTERNATIVE[1]	ADJUNCT DIAGNOSTIC OR THERAPEUTIC MEASURES AND COMMENTS
CENTRAL NERVOUS SYSTEM/Brain abscess (continued)				
Nocardia: Haematogenous abscess	N. farcinica, N. asteroides & N. brasiliensis	**TMP-SMX:** 15 mg/kg/day of TMP & 75 mg/kg/day of SMX, IV/po div in 2-4 doses + **Imipenem** 500 mg q6h IV. If multiorgan involvement some add **amikacin** 7.5 mg/kg q12h. After 3-6 wks of IV therapy, switch to po therapy. Immunocompetent pts: **TMP-SMX, minocycline** or **AM-CL** x 3+ months. Immunocompromised pts: Treat with 2 drugs for at least one year.	**Linezolid** 600 mg IV or po q12h + meropenem 2 gm q8h	Measure peak sulfonamide levels: target 100-150 mcg/mL 2 hrs dose. **Linezolid** 600 mg po bid reported effective (Ann Pharmacother 41:1694, 2007). For in vitro susceptibility testing: Wallace (+1) 903-877-7680 or U.S. CDC (+1) 404-639-3158. In vitro resistance to TMP-SMX may be increasing (Clin Infect Dis 51:1445, 2010), but whether this is associated with worse outcomes is not known. TMP-SMX remains a drug of choice for CNS nocardia infection. If sulfonamide resistant or sulfa-allergic, **amikacin** plus one of **IMP, MER, ceftriaxone** or **cefotaxime**. N. farcinica is resistant to third-generation cephalosporins, which should not be used for treatment of infection caused by this organism.
Subdural empyema: In adult 60-90% is extension of sinusitis or otitis media. Rx same as primary brain abscess. Surgical emergency: must drain. Review in LnID 7:62, 2007.				
Encephalitis/encephalopathy IDSA Guideline: CID 47:303, 2008. (For Herpes see Table 14A, page 160 and for rabies, Table 20B, page 215)	In 253 pts, etiol in 52%: H. simplex (42%), VZV (15%), M. TB (15%), Listeria (10%) (CID 49:1838, 2009). Other: arbovirus, West Nile, rabies, Lyme, Parvo B19, Cat-scratch disease, Mycoplasma, mumps, EBV, HHV-6, and others.	Start IV **acyclovir** while awaiting results of CSF PCR for H. simplex. For amebic encephalitis see Table 13A. Start **Doxy** if setting suggests R. rickettsii, Anaplasma, Ehrlichia, Mycoplasma.		Review of all etiologies: LnID 10:835, 2010. Anti-NMDAR (N-Methyl-D-Aspartate Receptor) encephalitis, autoimmune encephalitis, more common than individual viral etiologies as a cause of encephalitis in the California Encephalitis Project cohort (CID 54:899, 2012).
Meningitis, "Aseptic": Pleocytosis of up to 100s of cells, CSF glucose normal. Cultures for bacteria (see Table 14A, page 156). Ref: CID 47:783, 2008	Enteroviruses, HSV-2, LCM, HIV, other viruses, drugs (NSAIDs, metronidazole, carbamazepine, TMP-SMX, IVIG), rarely leptospirosis	For all but leptospirosis, IV fluids and analgesics. D/C drugs that may be etiologic. For lepto (**doxy** 100 mg IV/po q12h) or **Pen G** 5 million units IV q6h) or (**AP** 0.5-1 gm IV q6h). Repeat LP if suspect partially-treated bacterial meningitis. **Acyclovir** 5-10 mg/kg IV q8h sometimes given for HSV-2 meningitis (Note: this entity is distinct from HSV encephalitis where early rx is mandatory).		If available, PCR of CSF for enterovirus. HSV-2 unusual without concomitant genital herpes. For lepto, positive epidemiologic history and concomitant hepatitis, conjunctivitis, dermatitis, nephritis. For list of implicated drugs: Int Med 25:331, 2008.

Abbreviations on page 2.   NOTE: All dosage recommendations are for adults (unless otherwise indicated) and assume normal renal function.

TABLE 1 (5)

ANATOMIC SITE/DIAGNOSIS/ MODIFYING CIRCUMSTANCES	ETIOLOGIES (usual)	SUGGESTED REGIMENS* PRIMARY	ALTERNATIVE†	ADJUNCT DIAGNOSTIC OR THERAPEUTIC MEASURES AND COMMENTS
Meningitis, Bacterial, Acute: Goal is empiric therapy, then CSF exam within 30 min. If focal neurologic deficit, give empiric therapy, then head CT, then LP. (NEJM 354:44, 2006; LnID 10:32, 2010; IDSA Pract. Guid., CID 39:1267, 2004). **NOTE:** In children, treatment caused CSF cultures to turn neg. in 2 hrs with meningococci & partial response with pneumococcus in 4 hrs (Peds 108:1169, 2001. For distribution of pathogens by age group, see NEJM 364:2016, 2011.				
Empiric Therapy—CSF Gram stain is negative—Immunocompetent				
Age: Preterm to <1 mo Hearing loss is most common neurologic sequelae (LnID 10:32, 2010)	Group B strep 49%, E.coli 18%, listeria 7%, misc. Gm-neg. 10%, misc. Gm-pos. 10%	AMP 100 mg/kg IV q6h + cefotaxime 50 mg/kg IV q6h. Intraventricular treatment not recommended. Repeat CSF exam/culture 24-36 hr after start of therapy	AMP 100 mg/kg IV q6h + gentamicin 2.5 mg/kg IV q8h	Regimens active vs. Group B strep, most coliforms, & listeria. If premature infant with long nursery stay, S. aureus, enterococci, and resistant coliforms potential pathogens. **Optional empiric regimens (except for listeria): [nafcillin + (ceftazidime or cefotaxime)]. If high risk of MRSA, use vanco + cefotaxime.** Alter regimen after culture/sensitivity data available.
Age: 1 mo- 50 yrs listeria unlikely if young adult & immunocompetent (add ampicillin if suspect listeria 2 gm IV q4h)	S. pneumo, meningococci, H. influenzae now uncommon.	Adult dosage: ((Cefotaxime 2 gm IV q4-6h OR ceftriaxone 2 gm IV q12h) + dexamethasone) + vanco¹ (dexamethasone: 0.15 mg/kg IV q6h x 2-4 days. Give with, or just before, 1st dose of antibiotic to block TNF production (see Comment). See footnote² for Vanco Adult dosage and for ped. dosage	((MER 2 gm IV q8h) (Peds: 40 mg/kg IV q8h)) + IV dexamethasone + vanco¹ For severe pen. Allergy, see Comment	Value of **dexamethasone** shown in children with H. influenzae and adults with S. pneumoniae in some studies (NEJM 357:2431 & 2441, 2007; LnID 4:139, 2004). Decreases markers of inflammation in adults (CID 49:1387, 2009). In the Netherlands, adoption of dexamethasone treatment in adult pneumococcal meningitis led to reduced mortality and hearing loss compared with historical control group (Neurology 75:1533, 2010). A meta-analysis including all age groups, but mostly from developing world, showed no overall benefit in bacterial meningitis, except possibly in adults over 55 (Lancet Neurology 9:254, 2010). For severely ill patients with **β-lactam allergy**, desensitization therapy is indicated. **Empiric Therapy—positive gram stain and Specific Therapy:** for alternative agents that can be substituted to cover likely pathogens.
Age: >50 yrs or alcoholism or other debilitating assoc diseases or impaired cellular immunity	S. pneumo, listeria, Gm-neg bacilli. Note absence of meningococcus.	(AMP 2 gm IV q4h) + (ceftriaxone 2 gm IV q12h or cefotaxime 2 gm IV q4-6h) + vanco + IV dexamethasone For Vanco dose, see footnote². Dexamethasone dose: 0.15 mg/kg IV q6h x 2-4 days; 1st dose before, or concomitant with, 1st dose of antibiotic.	MER 2 gm IV q8h + vanco + IV dexamethasone For severe pen. Allergy, see Comment	For patients with severe β-lactam allergy, see below (Empiric Therapy—positive gram stain and Specific Therapy) for alternative agents that can be substituted to cover likely pathogens.
Post-neurosurgery Ventriculostomy/lumbar catheter; ventriculoperitoneal (atrial) shunt) or Penetrating trauma w/o basilar skull fracture	S. epidermidis, S. aureus, P. acnes. Facultative and aerobic gram-neg bacilli, including: P. aeruginosa & A. baumannii (may be multi-drug resistant)	Vanco 15 mg/kg IV q8h (to achieve trough level of 15-20 mcg/mL) + (Cefepime 2 gm IV q8h or Ceftaz 2 gm IV q8h)	Vanco 15 mg/kg IV q8h (to achieve trough level of 15-20 μg/mL)	• If possible, remove infected shunt or catheter. Logic for intraventricular therapy, goal is to achieve a 10-20 ratio of CSF concentration to MIC of infecting bacteria. Note potential toxicities of intraventricular doses. See CMR 23:858, 2010. • Use only preservative-free drug. Clamp/close catheter for 1 hr after 1st dose. • Timing of new V-P shunt (CID 39:1267, 2004). • Acinetobacter meningitis (LnID 9:245, 2009; JAC 61:908, 2008). • Review of nosocomial bacterial meningitis (NEJM 362: 146, 2010).
		• If severe Pen/Ceph allergy, for possible gram-neg, substitute either: Aztreonam 2 gm IV q6-8h or CIP 400 mg IV q8-12h. If IV therapy inadequate, may need intraventricular therapy: Intraventricular daily doses (CID 39:1267, 2004; CMR 23:858, 2010): Adult: Vanco 10-20 mg, Amikacin 30 mg; Tobra 5-20 mg; Gent 4-8 mg, Colistin 10 mg (or 5 mg/12h), Polymyxin B 5 mg. Peds: Gent 1-2 mg, Polymyxin B 2 mg.		
Trauma with basilar skull fracture	S. pneumoniae, H. influenzae, S. pyogenes	Vanco 15 mg/kg IV q8h (to achieve trough level of 15-20 μg/mL) + Dexamethasone 0.15 mg/kg IV q6h x 2-4 d (1st dose with or before 1st antibiotic dose)	(Ceftriaxone 2 gm IV q12h or Cefotax 2 gm IV q6h) + Dexamethasone (Adult dosage)	

¹ **Vanco adult dose:** 15 mg/kg IV q8h to achieve trough level of 15-20 μg/mL.
² **Dosage of drugs used to treat children ≥1 mo of age: Cefotaxime** 50 mg/kg per day IV q6h; **ceftriaxone** 50 mg/kg IV q12h; **vanco** 15 mg/kg IV q6h to achieve trough level of 15-20 μg/mL.

Abbreviations on page 2. NOTE: All dosage recommendations are for adults (unless otherwise indicated) and assume normal renal function.

TABLE 1 (6)

ANATOMIC SITE/DIAGNOSIS/ MODIFYING CIRCUMSTANCES	ETIOLOGIES (usual)	SUGGESTED REGIMENS* PRIMARY	SUGGESTED REGIMENS* ALTERNATIVE[1]	ADJUNCT DIAGNOSTIC OR THERAPEUTIC MEASURES AND COMMENTS
CENTRAL NERVOUS SYSTEM/Meningitis, Bacterial, Acute *(continued)*				
Empiric Therapy—Positive CSF Gram stain				
Gram-positive diplococci	S. pneumoniae	(**ceftriaxone** 2 gm IV q12h or **cefotaxime** 2 gm IV (q4–6h) + **vanco** 15 mg/kg IV q8h to achieve 15-20 μg/mL trough) + timed **dexamethasone** 0.15 mg/kg q6h IV x 2–4 days	**MER** 2 gm IV q8h or **Moxi** 400 mg IV q24h. Dexamethasone does not block penetration of vanco into CSF *(CID 44:250, 2007)*.	**Alternatives: MER** 2 gm IV q8h or **Moxi** 400 mg IV q24h. Dexamethasone does not block penetration of vanco into CSF *(CID 44:250, 2007)*.
Gram-negative diplococci	N. meningitidis	**Cefotaxime** 2 gm IV q4–6h or **ceftriaxone** 2 gm IV q12h		**Alternatives: Pen G** 4 mill. units IV q4h or **AMP** 2 gm IV q4h or **Moxi** 400 mg IV q24h or **chloro** 1 gm IV q6h
Gram-positive bacilli or coccobacilli	Listeria monocytogenes	**AMP** 2 gm IV q4h ± **gentamicin** 2 mg/kg IV loading dose then 1.7 mg/kg IV q8h		If pen-allergic, use **TMP-SMX** 5 mg/kg IV q6-8h or **MER** 2 gm IV q8h
Gram-negative bacilli	H. influenzae, coliforms, P. aeruginosa	(**Ceftazidime** or **cefepime** 2 gm IV q8h) ± **gentamicin** 2 mg/kg IV[1] dose then 1.7 mg/kg IV q8h (See Comment)		**Alternatives: CIP** 400 mg IV q8-12h; **MER** 2 gm IV q8h; **Aztreonan** 2 gm IV q6-8h. Consider adding intravenous **Gentamicin** to the β-lactam or **CIP** if gram-stain and clinical setting suggest P. aeruginosa or resistant coliforms

Specific Therapy—Positive culture of CSF with in vitro susceptibility results available. Interest in monitoring/reducing intracranial pressure: *CID 38:384, 2004*

H. influenzae	β-lactamase positive	**Ceftriaxone** 2 gm IV q12h (adult), 50 mg/kg IV q12h (peds)		**Pen. allergic: Chloro** 12.5 mg/kg IV q6h (max. 4 gm/day), **CIP** 400 mg IV q8-12h, **Aztreonam** 2 gm q6-8h
Listeria monocytogenes *(CID 43:1233, 2006)*		**AMP** 2 gm IV q4h ± **gentamicin** 2 mg/kg IV loading dose, then 1.7 mg/kg IV q8h.		**Pen. allergic: TMP-SMX** 20 mg/kg per day div q6-12h; **Alternative: MER** 2 gm IV q8h. Success reported with **linezolid** + **RIF** *(CID 40:907, 2005)* after AMP rx for brain abscess with meningitis.
N. meningitidis		**Ceftriaxone** 2 gm IV q12h x 7 days (see Comment), if β-lactam allergic, **chloro** 12.5 mg/kg (up to 1 gm) IV q6h		Rare isolates chloro-resistant. FQ-resistant isolates encountered. **Alternatives: MER** 2 gm IV q8h or **Moxi** 400 mg q24h
S. pneumoniae	Pen G MIC			
NOTES:	<0.1 mcg/mL	**Pen G** 4 million units IV q4h or **AMP** 2 gm IV q4h		**Alternatives: Ceftriaxone** 2 gm IV q12h, **chloro** 1 gm IV q6h
1. Assumes dexamethasone just prior to 1st dose & x 4 days.	0.1-1 mcg/mL	**Ceftriaxone** 2 gm IV q12h or **cefotaxime** 2 gm IV q4–6h		**Alternatives: Cefepime** 2 gm IV q8h or **MER** 2 gm IV q8h
2. If MIC ≥1, repeat CSF exam after 24-48h.	≥2 mcg/mL	**Vanco** 15 mg/kg IV q8h (15-20 μg/mL trough target) + **ceftriaxone** or **cefotaxime** as above)		**Alternatives: Moxi** 400 mg IV q24h
3. Treat for 10-14 days	Ceftriaxone MIC ≥1 mcg/mL	**Vanco** 15 mg/kg IV q8h (15-20 μg/mL trough target) + (**ceftriaxone** or **cefotaxime** as above)		If MIC to ceftriaxone >2 mcg/mL, add **RIF** 600 mg po/IV 1x/day to **vanco** + (**ceftriaxone** or **cefotaxime**).
E. coli, other coliforms, or P. aeruginosa	**Consultation advised**—need susceptibility results	(**Ceftazidime** or **cefepime** 2 gm IV q8h) ± **gentamicin**		**Alternatives: CIP** 400 mg IV q8-12h; **MER** 2 gm IV q8h. For intraventricular therapy, drug dosing, see Meningitis, Post-neurosurgery, page 9.

Prophylaxis for H. influenzae and N. meningitidis

Haemophilus influenzae type b Household and/or day care contact: residing with index case for 24 hrs in day care. Day care contact or same day care facility as index case for 5-7 days before onset		**Children: RIF** 20 mg/kg po (not to exceed 600 mg) q24h x 4 doses **Adults (non-pregnant): RIF** 600 mg q24h x 4 days		**Household:** If there is one unvaccinated contact ≤4 yrs in the household, give RIF to all those exposed (including pregnant women). **Child Care Facilities:** With 1 case, if attended by unvaccinated children ≤2 yrs, consider prophylaxis + vaccinate susceptible. If all contacts >2 yrs: no prophylaxis. If ≥2 cases in 60 days & unvaccinated children attend, prophylaxis recommended for children & personnel *(Am Acad Ped Red Book 2006, page 313)*.

Abbreviations on page 2.   NOTE: *All dosage recommendations are for adults (unless otherwise indicated) and assume normal renal function.*

TABLE 1 (7)

ANATOMIC SITE/DIAGNOSIS/ MODIFYING CIRCUMSTANCES	ETIOLOGIES* (usual)	SUGGESTED REGIMENS* PRIMARY	ALTERNATIVE[$]	ADJUNCT DIAGNOSTIC OR THERAPEUTIC MEASURES AND COMMENTS
CENTRAL NERVOUS SYSTEM/Meningitis, Bacterial, Acute/Prophylaxis for H. Influenzae and N. meningitidis *(continued)*				
Prophylaxis for Neisseria meningitidis exposure (close contact). **NOTE:** CDC reports **CIP-resistant meningococcus** from selected counties in N. Dakota & Minnesota. **Avoid CIP**. Use **ceftriaxone**, **RIF**, or single 500 mg dose of **azithro** (MMWR 57:173, 2008)		Ceftriaxone 250 mg IM x 1 dose (child <15 yrs 125 mg IM x 1)] **OR** [RIF 600 mg po q12h x 4 doses. (Children ≥1 mo 10 mg/kg po q12h x 4 doses, <1 mo 5 mg/kg q12h x 4 doses) **OR** If not CIP-resistant, **CIP** 500 mg po x 1 dose (adult)		**Spread by respiratory droplets**, not aerosols, hence close contact req. ↑ risk if close contact for at least 4 hrs during wk before illness onset (e.g., housemates, day care contacts, cellmates) or exposure to pt's nasopharyngeal secretions (e.g., kissing, mouth-to-mouth resuscitation, intubation, nasotracheal suctioning).
Meningitis, chronic Defined as symptoms + CSF pleocytosis for 24 wks	M. TBc 40%, cryptococcosis 7%, neoplastic 8%, syphilis, Whipple's disease	Treatment depends on etiology. No urgent need for empiric therapy, but when TB suspected treatment should be expeditious.		Long list of possibilities: bacteria, parasites, fungi, viruses, neoplasms, vasculitis, and other miscellaneous etiologies—see Neurol Clin 28:1061, 2010; Curr Neurol Neurosci Rep 5:429, 2005; Whipple's IJID 188:797 & 801, 2003.
Meningitis, eosinophilic IJID 8:621, 2008	Angiostrongyliasis, gnathostomiasis, baylisascaris	Corticosteroids	Not sure anthelmintic therapy works	1/3 lack peripheral eosinophilia. Need serology to confirm diagnosis. Steroid ref: IJID 8:621, 2008. Automated CSF count may not correctly identify eosinophils (CID 48: 322, 2009).
Meningitis, HIV-1 Infected (AIDS) See Table 11, Sanford Guide to HIV/AIDS Therapy	As in adults, >50 yrs: also consider cryptococci, M. tuberculosis, syphilis, HIV aseptic meningitis, Listeria monocytogenes	If HIV etiology not identified: treat as adult >50 yrs + obtain CSF/serum cryptococcal antigen (see Comments)	For crypto rx, see Table 11A, page 118	C. neoformans most common etiology in AIDS patients. H. influenzae, pneumococci, TBc, syphilis, viral, histoplasma & coccidioides also need to be considered. Obtain blood cultures. L. monocytogenes risk >60x ↑, % present as meningitis (CID 17:224, 1993).
EAR				
External otitis Chronic	Usually 2° to seborrhea	Eardrops: [(polymyxin B + neomycin + hydrocortisone qid)] + selenium sulfide shampoo		Control seborrhea with dandruff shampoo containing selenium sulfide (Selsun) or [(ketoconazole shampoo)] + (medium potency steroid solution, triamcinolone 0.1%).
Fungal	Candida species	Fluconazole 200 mg po x 1 dose & then 100 mg po		CIP po for treatment of early disease. Debridement usually required. R/O osteomyelitis: CT or MRI scan. If bone involved, treat for 4–6 wks. PIP without Tazo may be hard to find: extended infusion of PIP-TZ (4 hr infusion of 3.375 gm every 8h) may improve efficacy (CID 44:357, 2007).
"Malignant otitis externa" Risk groups: Diabetes mellitus, AIDS, chemotherapy. Ref.: Oto Clinics N Amer 41:537, 2008	Pseudomonas aeruginosa in >90%	[IMP 0.5 gm IV q6h) or MER 1 gm IV q8h) or CIP 400 mg IV q12h (or 750 mg po q12h)] or (ceftaz 2 gm IV q8h) or CFP 2 gm q12h) or PIP 3 gm IV q4–6h + tobra or TC 3 gm IV q4h + tobra) (See tobra dose Table 10D)		
"Swimmer's ear" PIDJ 22:299, 2003	Pseudomonas sp., Enterobacteriaceae, Proteus sp. (Fungi rare). Acute infection usually 2° S. aureus	Eardrops: Oflox 0.3% soln bid or [(polymyxin B + neomycin + hydrocortisone) qid] or (CIP + hydrocortisone bid) —active vs. gm-neg bacilli. For acute disease: dicloxacillin 500 mg po 4x/day. If MRSA a concern, use TMP-SMX, doxy or clinda		Rx includes gentle cleaning. Recurrences prevented (or decreased) by drying with alcohol drops (1/3 white vinegar, 2/3 rubbing alcohol) after swimming, then antibiotic drops or 2% acetic acid solution. Ointments should not be used in ear. Do not use neomycin drops if tympanic membrane punctured.

Abbreviations on page 2.   NOTE: All dosage recommendations are for adults (unless otherwise indicated) and assume normal renal function.

TABLE 1 (8)

EAR (continued)

Otitis media—Infants, children, adults

ANATOMIC SITE/DIAGNOSIS/ MODIFYING CIRCUMSTANCES	ETIOLOGIES (usual)	SUGGESTED REGIMENS* PRIMARY	SUGGESTED REGIMENS* ALTERNATIVE[1]	ADJUNCT DIAGNOSTIC OR THERAPEUTIC MEASURES AND COMMENTS
Acute otitis media—Infants, children, adults Two PRDB trials indicate efficacy of antibiotic rx if age < 36 mos & definite AOM (NEJM 364:105, 116 & 168, 2011)				
Initial empiric therapy of acute otitis media (AOM) NOTE: Treat children <2 yrs old. If >2 yrs old, afebrile, no ear pain, neg./questionable exam—consider analgesic treatment without antimicrobials. Favorable results in mostly afebrile pts with waiting 48hrs before deciding on antibiotic use (JAMA 296:1235, 1290, 2006)	Overall detection in middle ear fluid: No pathogen 4% Virus 70% Bact. + virus 66% Bacteria 92% Bacterial pathogens from middle ear: S. pneumo 49%, H. influenzae 29%, M. catarrhalis 28%. Ref.: CID 43:1417, & 1423, 2006 Children 6 mo-3 yrs, 2 episodes AOM/yrs, & 63% are virus positive. (CID 46:815 & 824, 2008).	If **NO antibiotics in prior month:** Amox po HD[3] For dosage, see footnote[4]. **All doses are pediatric Duration of rx:** <2 yrs x 10 days; 22 yrs x 5–7 days. Appropriate duration unclear. 5 days may be inadequate for severe disease (NEJM 347:1169, 2002) For adult dosages, see Sinusitis, page 50, and Table 10A	Received antibiotics in prior month: Amox HD[3] or AM-CL extra-strength[3] or cefdinir or cefpodoxime or cefprozil or cefuroxime axetil	**If allergic to β-lactam drugs?** If history unclear or rash, effective oral ceph OK; avoid ceph if IgE-mediated allergy, e.g., anaphylaxis. High failure rate with TMP-SMX. S. pneumo etiology is DRSP or (if H. influenzae, azithro x 5 days or clarithro x 10 days (both have ↓ activity vs. DRSP). Up to 50% S. pneumo resistant to macrolides. Rationale & data for single dose azithro, 30 mg per kg: PIDJ 23:S102 & S108, 2004. Spontaneous resolution occurred in: 90% pts infected with M. catarrhalis, 50% with H. influenzae, 10% with S. pneumoniae, overall 80% resolve within 2–14 days (Ln 363:465, 2004). Risk of DRSP if age <2 yrs, antibiotics last 3 mos, &/or daycare attendance. Selection of drug based on (1) effectiveness against β-lactamase producing H. influenzae & M. catarrhalis & (2) effectiveness against S. pneumo, inc. DRSP. **Cefaclor, loracarbef, & ceftibuten less active vs. resistant S. pneumo.** than other agents listed.
Treatment for clinical failure after 3 days	Drug-resistant S. pneumoniae main concern	**NO antibiotics in month prior to last 3 days:** AM-CL high dose or cefdinir or cefpodoxime or cefprozil or cefuroxime axetil or IM ceftriaxone x 3 days. For dosage, see footnote[4] **All doses are pediatric**	Antibiotics in month prior to last 3 days: (IM ceftriaxone) or (clindamycin) and/or (tympanocentesis) See Clindamycin Comments	**Clindamycin** not active vs. H. influenzae or M. catarrhalis. S. pneumo resistant to macrolides are usually also resistant to clindamycin. Definition of failure: no change in ear pain, fever, bulging TM or otorrhea after 3 days of therapy. Tympanocentesis will allow culture. Newer FQs active vs. drug-resistant S. pneumo (DRSP), but not approved for children (PIDJ 23:390, 2004). **Vanco is active vs. DRSP.** Ceftriaxone IM x 3 days superior to 1-day treatment vs. DRSP (PIDJ 19:1040, 2000). AM-CL HD reported successful for pen-resistant S. pneumo AOM (PIDJ 20:829, 2001).
After >48hrs of nasotracheal intubation	Pseudomonas sp., Klebsiella, enterobacter	**Ceftazidime or CFP or IMP or MER or (PIP-TZ) or TC-CL or CIP** (For dosages, see Ear, Malignant otitis externa, page 10)		With nasotracheal intubation >48 hrs, about ½ pts will have otitis media with effusion.
Prophylaxis: acute otitis media PIDJ 22:10, 2003	Pneumococci, H. influenzae, Staph. aureus, Group A strep (see Comments)	**Sulfisoxazole** 50 mg/kg po at bedtime or **amoxicillin** 20 mg/kg po q24h	Use of antibiotics to prevent otitis media is a major contributor to emergence of antibiotic-resistant S. pneumo! Pneumococcal protein conjugate vaccine decreases freq. AOM due to vaccine serotypes. Adenoidectomy at time of tympanostomy tubes ↓ need for future hospitalization for AOM (NEJM 344:1188, 2001).

[3] **Amoxicillin UD or HD** = amoxicillin usual dose or high dose; **AM-CL HD** = amoxicillin-clavulanate high dose. **Dosages in footnote[4]**. Data supporting amoxicillin HD: PIDJ 22:405, 2003

[4] **Drugs & peds dosage** (all po unless specified) for acute otitis media: **Amoxicillin UD** = 40–45 mg/kg per day div q12h or q8h; **Amoxicillin HD** = 90 mg/kg per day div q12h; **AM-CL HD** = 90 mg/kg per day of amox component. **Extra-strength AM-CL oral suspension** (Augmentin ES-600) available as 600 mg AM & 42.9 mg CL per 5 mL; dose is 90 mg/kg per day bid. **Cefuroxime axetil** 30 mg/kg per day div q12h. **Ceftriaxone** 50 mg/kg IM x 3 days. **Clindamycin** 20–30 mg/kg per day div q8; may be effective vs. DRSP but no activity vs. H. influenzae. Other drugs suitable for drug (e.g., penicillin)-sensitive S. pneumo: **TMP-SMX**, 4 mg/kg of TMP q12h. **Erythro-sulfisoxazole** 50 mg/kg per day of erythro div q6-8h. **Clarithro** 15 mg/kg per day div q12h; **azithro** 10 mg/kg per day x 1, & then 5 mg/kg per day q24h on days 2–5. Other FDA-approved regimen: 10 mg/kg q24h x 3 days & 30 mg/kg x 1. **Cefprozil** 15 mg/kg q12h or **cefpodoxime proxetil** 10 mg/kg per day as single dose; **cefaclor** 40 mg/kg per day div q8h; **loracarbef** 15 mg/kg per day div q12h or 14 mg/kg q24h. **Cefdinir** 7 mg/kg q12h or 14 mg/kg q24h.

Abbreviations on page 2. NOTE: All dosage recommendations are for adults (unless otherwise indicated) and assume normal renal function.

TABLE 1 (9)

ANATOMIC SITE/DIAGNOSIS/ MODIFYING CIRCUMSTANCES	ETIOLOGIES (usual)	SUGGESTED REGIMENS* PRIMARY	SUGGESTED REGIMENS* ALTERNATIVE[$]	ADJUNCT DIAGNOSTIC OR THERAPEUTIC MEASURES AND COMMENTS
EAR (continued)				
Mastoiditis				
Acute				
Outpatient	Strep. pneumoniae 22%, S. pyogenes 16%, **Staph. aureus** 7%, H. influenzae 4%, others <1%	Empirically, same as Acute otitis media, above: need **vanco** for **nafcillin/oxacillin** if culture + for S. aureus.		Has become a rare entity, presumably as result of the aggressive treatment of acute otitis media. Small ↑ in incidence in Netherlands where use of antibiotics limited to children with complicated course or high risk (PIDJ 20:140, 2001). ↑ incidence reported from US also (Arch Otolaryngol Head Neck Surg 135: 638, 2009).
Hospitalized		**Cefotaxime** 1-2 gm IV q4-6h (depends on severity) or **ceftriaxone** 1 gm IV q24h)		Unusual causes of acute mastoiditis: nocardia (AIDS Reader 17: 402, 2007), TB, actinomyces (Ear Nose Throat Journal 79: 884, 2000).
Chronic	Often polymicrobic: anaerobes, Enterobacteriaceae, P. aeruginosa	Treatment for acute exacerbations or perioperatively. No treatment until surgical cultures obtained. Empiric regimens: **IMP** 0.5 gm IV q6h, **TC-CL** 3.1 gm IV q4-6h, **PIP-TZ** 3.375 gm q6h over 4.5 gm, or 4 hr infusion of 3.375 gm q8h. **MER** 1 gm IV q8h. If MRSA, add **vanco** to any of the listed agents.		May or may not be associated with chronic otitis media with drainage via ruptured tympanic membrane. Antimicrobials given in association with surgery. Mastoidectomy indications: chronic drainage and evidence of osteomyelitis by MRI or CT, evidence of spread to CNS (epidural abscess, suppurative phlebitis, brain abscess).
EYE				
Eyelid: Little reported experience with CA-MRSA (See Cochrane Database Syst Rev 5:CD005556, 2012)				
Blepharitis	Etiol. unclear. Factors include Staph. aureus & Staph. epidermidis, seborrhea, rosacea, & dry eye	Lid margin care with baby shampoo & warm compresses q24h. Artificial tears if assoc. dry eye (see Comment).		Usually topical ointments of no benefit. If associated rosacea, add doxy 100 mg po bid for 2 wks and then q24h.
Hordeolum (Stye)				
External (eyelash follicle)	Staph. aureus	Hot packs only. Will drain spontaneously.		Infection of superficial sebaceous gland.
Internal (Meibomian glands); Can be acute, subacute or chronic.	Staph. aureus, MSSA Staph. aureus, MRSA-CA Staph. aureus, MRSA-HA	Oral **dicloxacillin** ± hot packs **TMP-SMX-DS**, tabs ii q12h **Linezolid** 600 mg po bid possible therapy if multi-drug resistant.		Also called acute meibomianitis. Rarely drain spontaneously. I&D and culture. Role of fluoroquinolone eye drops is unclear. MRSA often resistant to lower conc.; may be susceptible to higher concentration of FQ in ophthalmologic solutions of gati, levo or moxi.
Conjunctiva: NEJM 343:345, 2000				
Conjunctivitis of the newborn (**ophthalmia neonatorum**): by day of onset post-delivery—all dose pediatric				
Onset 1st day	Chemical due to silver nitrate prophylaxis	None		Usual prophylaxis is erythro ointment; hence, silver nitrate irritation rare.
Onset 2–4 days	N. gonorrhoeae	**Ceftriaxone** 25–50 mg/kg IV x 1 dose (see Comment), not to exceed 125 mg		Treat mother and her sexual partners. Hyperpurulent. Topical rx inadequate. **Treat neonate for concomitant Chlamydia trachomatis.**
Onset 3–10 days	Chlamydia trachomatis	**Erythro** base or ethylsuccinate syrup 12.5 mg/kg q6h x 14 days. No topical rx needed.		Diagnosis by antigen detection. Alternative: **Azithro suspension** 20 mg/kg po q24h x 3 days. Treat mother & sexual partner.
Onset 2–16 days	Herpes simplex types 1, 2	Topical anti-viral rx under direction of ophthalmologist.		Also give Acyclovir 60 mg/kg/day IV div 3 doses (Red Book online, accessed Jan 2011).
Ophthalmia neonatorum prophylaxis: **erythro** 0.5% ointment x 1 or **tetra** 1% ointment[AUS] x 1 application				
Pink eye (viral conjunctivitis) Usually unilateral	Adenovirus (types 3 & 7 in children, 8, 11 & 19 in adults)	No treatment. If symptomatic, cold artificial tears may help.		Highly contagious. Onset of ocular pain and photophobia in an adult suggests associated keratitis–rare.

Abbreviations on page 2. NOTE: All dosage recommendations are for adults (unless otherwise indicated) and assume normal renal function.

TABLE 1 (10)

ANATOMIC SITE/DIAGNOSIS/ MODIFYING CIRCUMSTANCES	ETIOLOGIES (usual)	SUGGESTED REGIMENS* PRIMARY	SUGGESTED REGIMENS* ALTERNATIVE[1]	ADJUNCT DIAGNOSTIC OR THERAPEUTIC MEASURES AND COMMENTS
EYE/Conjunctiva (continued)				
Inclusion conjunctivitis (adult) Usually unilateral	Chlamydia trachomatis	**Azithro** 1 gm once or twice weekly (for 24,985, 2010 and Am J Ophthal 135:447, 2003)	**Erythro** 250 mg po qid × 1-3 wks	Oculogenital disease. Diagnosis by culture or antigen detection or PCR—availability varies by region and institution. Treat sexual partner. May need to repeat dose of azithro.
Trachoma —a chronic bacterial keratoconjunctivitis linked to poverty	Chlamydia trachomatis	**Azithro** 20 mg/kg po single dose—78% effective in children; Adults: 1 gm po	**Doxy** 100 mg po bid × minimum of 21 days or **tetracycline** 250 mg po qid × 14 days.	Starts in childhood and can persist for years with subsequent damage to cornea. Topical therapy of marginal benefit. Avoid doxy/tetracycline in young children. Mass treatment works (NEJM 358:1777 & 1870, 2008; JAMA 299:778, 2008).
Suppurative conjunctivitis: Children and Adults				
Non-gonococcal; non-chlamydial Med Lett 50:11, 2008	Staph. aureus, S. pneumoniae, H. influenzae, et al.	Ophthalmic solution: **Gati** 0.3%; **Levo** 0.5% or **Moxi** 0.5%. All 1-2 gtts q2h while awake 1st 2 days, then 1 gtt qid up to 7 days.	Polymyxin B + trimethoprim solution 1-2 gtts q3-6h × 7-10 days. **Azithro** 1%, 1 gtt bid × 2 days, then 1 gtt daily × 5 days.	**FQs** best spectrum for empiric therapy but expensive: $40-50 for 5 mL. High concentrations ↑ likelihood of activity vs S. aureus—even MRSA. **TMP** spectrum may include MRSA. Polymyxin B spectrum only Gm-neg. bacilli but no ophthal. prep of only **TMP**. Most S. pneumo resistant to **gent** & **tobra**. **Azithro** active vs. common gm+ pathogens.
Gonococcal (peds/adults)	N. gonorrhoeae	**Ceftriaxone** 25-50 mg/kg IV/IM (not to exceed 125 mg) as one dose in children; 1 gm IM/IV as one dose in adults		
Cornea (keratitis): Usually serious and often sight-threatening. Prompt ophthalmologic consultation essential for diagnosis, antimicrobial and adjunctive therapy! Herpes simplex most common etiology in developed countries; bacterial and fungal infections more common in underdeveloped countries.				
Viral				
H. simplex	H. simplex, types 1 & 2	**Trifluridine** ophthalmic soln, one drop q-2h until re-epithelialized, then one drop q4h up to 5x/day, for total not to exceed 21 days.	**Ganciclovir** 0.15% ophthalmic gel: Indicated for acute herpetic keratitis. One drop 5 times per day while awake until corneal ulcer heals, then one drop three times per day for 7 days. **Vidarabine** ointment—useful in children. Use 5x/day for up to 21 days (currently listed as discontinued in U.S.).	Approx. 30% recurrence rate within one year; consider prophylaxis with acyclovir 400 mg bid for 12 months to prevent recurrences (Arch Ophthal 130:108, 2012)
Varicella-zoster ophthalmicus	Varicella-zoster virus	**Famciclovir** 500 mg po tid or **valacyclovir** 1 gm po tid × 10 days	**Acyclovir** 800 mg po 5x/day × 7 days	Clinical diagnosis most common: dendritic figures with fluorescein staining in patient with varicella-zoster of ophthalmic branch of trigeminal nerve.
Bacterial				
Acute: No comorbidity	S. aureus, S. pneumo., S. pyogenes, Haemophilus sp.	**Moxi**: ophthalmic 0.5% 1 drop q1h for the first 48h taper according to response	All treatment listed for bacterial, fungal, protozoan is topical unless otherwise indicated **Gati**: ophthalmic 0.3%: 1 drop q1h for the first 48h then taper according to response	Moxi may be preferable because of enhanced lipophilicity and penetration into aqueous (Survey of Ophthal 50 (Suppl 1): 1, Nov 2005). Regimens vary, some start q 1h by applying drops every 5-30 min for several hours; some extend interval to q2h during sleep. In a clinical trial, drops were applied q1h for 48-72h, then q2h through day 6; then q2h during waking hours on days 7-9; then q6h until healing (Cornea 29:751, 2010). **Note**: despite high concentrations, may fail vs. MRSA.

NOTE: All dosage recommendations are for adults (unless otherwise indicated) and assume normal renal function.

TABLE 1 (11)

ANATOMIC SITE/DIAGNOSIS/ MODIFYING CIRCUMSTANCES	ETIOLOGIES (usual)	SUGGESTED REGIMENS* PRIMARY	ALTERNATIVE[1]	ADJUNCT DIAGNOSTIC OR THERAPEUTIC MEASURES AND COMMENTS
EYE/Cornea (keratitis) *(continued)*				
Contact lens users	P. aeruginosa	**Tobra or Gentamicin** (14 mg/mL) + **[Piperacillin or Ticarcillin** eye drops (6-12 mg/mL)] q15-60 min around the clock for 24-72h, then slowly reduce frequency depending upon response.	**CIP** ophthalmic 0.3% or **Levo** ophthalmic 0.5%: 1 drop q15-60 min around the clock for 24-72h, then slowly taper based on response	Recommend alginate swab culture and susceptibility testing.
Dry cornea, diabetes, immunosuppression	Staph. aureus, S. epidermidis, S. pneumoniae, S. pyogenes, Enterobacteriaceae, listeria	**Cefazolin** (50 mg/mL) + **Gent or Tobra** (14 mg/mL) q15-60 min around the clock for 24-72h, then slowly reduce frequency depending upon response.	**Vanco** (50 mg/mL) + **Ceftaz** (50 mg/mL) q15-60 min around the clock for 24-72h, then slowly reduce frequency depending upon response. See Comment.	Specific therapy guided by results of alginate swab culture.
Fungal	Aspergillus, fusarium, candida and others.	**Natamycin** (5%): 1 drop every 1-2 h for several days; then q3-4h for several days; can reduce frequency depending upon response.	**Amphotericin B** (0.15%): 1 drop every 1-2 hours for several days; can reduce frequency depending upon response.	Obtain specimens for fungal wet mount and cultures. Numerous other treatment options (1% topical fira for 6 wks, oral fira 100 mg bid x 3 wks, topical voriconazole 1% 1x/h for 5 wks, topical miconazole 1% 3x a day, topical silver sulphadiazine 0.5-1% 5x a day, all appear to have similar efficacy (Cochrane Database Syst Rev 2/04/241, 2012)
Mycobacteria. Post-refractive eye surgery	Mycobacterium cheloniae	**Gati or Moxi** eye drops: 1 gtt qid, probably in conjunction with other active antimicrobials		Used in conjunction with other topical and/or systemic anti-mycobacterial agents (J Cataract Refract Surg 33:1978, 2007; Ophthalmology 113:950, 2006)
Protozoan: Soft contact lens use. Ref: CID 35:434, 2002.	Acanthamoeba, sp.	Optimal regimen uncertain. Suggested regimen: [(**Chlorhexidine** 0.02% or Polyhexamethylene biguanide 0.02%) + (Propamidine isethionate 0.1% or Hexamidine 0.1%)] drops. Apply one drop every hour for 48h, then one drop every two hours while awake for 3-4 weeks, then reducing frequency based on response (Her Am J Ophthalmol 148:487, 2009; Curr Op Infect Dis 23:590, 2010).		Uncommon. Trauma and soft contact lenses are risk factors. To obtain suggested drops: Leiter's Park Ave Pharmacy (800-292-6773; www.leiterrx.com). Cleaning solution outbreak: MMWR 56: 532, 2007.
Lacrimal apparatus				
Canaliculitis	Actinomyces most common. Rarely, Arachnia, fusobacterium, nocardia, candida	Remove granules & irrigate with **pen G** (100,000 mcg/mL). **Child: AM-CL** or **cefprozil** or **cefuroxime** (See dose on Table 16)	If fungi, irrigate with **nystatin** approx. 5 mcg/mL; 1 gtt tid	Digital pressure produces exudate at punctum; Gram stain confirms diagnosis. Hot packs to punctal area qid. M. cheloniae reported after use of intracanalic plugs (Ophth Plast Reconstr Surg 24: 241, 2008).
Dacryocystitis (lacrimal sac)	S. pneumo, S. aureus, H. influenzae, S. pyogenes, P. aeruginosa	Often consequence of obstruction of lacrimal duct. Empiric systemic antimicrobial therapy based on Gram stain of aspirate—see Comment.		Need ophthalmologic consultation. Surgery may be required. Can be acute or chronic. Culture to detect MRSA.

NOTE: All dosage recommendations are for adults (unless otherwise indicated) and assume normal renal function.

Abbreviations on page 2.

TABLE 1 (12)

ANATOMIC SITE/DIAGNOSIS/ MODIFYING CIRCUMSTANCES	ETIOLOGIES (usual)	SUGGESTED REGIMENS* PRIMARY	SUGGESTED REGIMENS* ALTERNATIVE[1]	ADJUNCT DIAGNOSTIC OR THERAPEUTIC MEASURES AND COMMENTS
EYE/Cornea (keratitis) (continued)				
Endophthalmitis: Endogenous (secondary to bacteremia or fungemia) and exogenous (post-injection, post-operative) types				
Bacterial: Haziness of vitreous key to diagnosis. Needle aspirate of both vitreous and aqueous humor for culture prior to therapy. Intravitreal administration of antimicrobials essential.				
Postocular surgery (cataracts) Early, acute onset (incidence 0.05%)	S. epidermidis 60%, Staph. aureus, streptococci, & enterococci each 5–10%, Gm-neg. bacilli 6%		**Immediate ophthal. consult.** If only light perception or worse, immediate vitrectomy + intravitreal vanco 1 mg & intravitreal ceftazidime 2.25 mg. No clear data on intravitreal steroid. May need to repeat intravitreal antibiotics in 2–3 days. Can usually leave lens in. Adjunctive systemic antibiotics (e.g., Vancomycin, Ceftazidime, Moxifloxacin or Gatifloxacin[NUS]) not of proven value, but recommended in endogenous infection.	
Low grade, chronic	Propionibacterium acnes, S. epidermidis, S. aureus (rare)		Intraocular **vanco**. Usually requires vitrectomy, lens removal.	
Post filtering blebs for glaucoma	Strep. species (viridans & others), H. influenzae		Intravitreal agent (e.g., **Vanco** 1 mg + **Ceftaz** 2.25 mg) and a topical agent. Consider a systemic agent such as **Amp-Sulb** or **Cefuroxime** or **Ceftaz** (add **Vanco** if MRSA is suspected)	
Post-penetrating trauma	Bacillus sp., S. epiderm. S. pneumoniae.		Intravitreal agent as above + systemic **clinda** or **vanco**. Use topical antibiotics post-surgery (tobra & cefazolin drops).	
None, suspect hematogenous	N. meningitidis, Staph. aureus, Grp B Strep, K. pneumo		(**cefotaxime** 2 gm IV q4h or **ceftriaxone** 2 gm IV q24h) + **vanco** 30-60 mg/kg/day in 2-3 div doses to achieve target trough serum concentration of 15-20 mcg/mL. Intravitreal antibiotics as cultures pending. Intravitreal antibiotics as early post-operative.	
IV heroin abuse	Bacillus cereus, Candida sp.		Intravitreal agent + systemic agent based on etiology and antimicrobial susceptibility.	
Mycotic (fungal): Broad-spectrum antibiotics, often corticosteroids, indwelling venous catheters	Candida sp. Aspergillus sp.		Intravitreal **ampho B** 0.005–0.01 mg in 0.1 mL. Also see Table 11A, page 116 for concomitant systemic therapy. See Comment.	Patients with Candida spp. chorioretinitis usually respond to systemically administered antifungals (Clin Infect Dis 53:262, 2011). Intravitreal amphotericin and/or vitrectomy may be necessary for those with vitritis or endophthalmitis (Br J Ophthalmol 92:466, 2008; Pharmacotherapy 27:1711, 2007).
Retinitis				
Acute retinal necrosis	Varicella zoster, Herpes simplex, Cytomegalovirus	IV **acyclovir** 10–12 mg/kg IV q8h × 5–7 days, then 800 mg po 5x/day × 6 wks See Table 14, page 158		Strong association of VZ virus with atypical necrotizing herpetic retinopathy.
HIV+/AIDS[1] CD4 usually <100/mm[3]				Occurs in 5–10% of AIDS patients
Progressive outer retinal necrosis	VZV, H. simplex, CMV (rare)	**Acyclovir** 10–12 mg/kg IV q8h for 1–2 weeks, then (**valacyclovir** 1000 mg po tid, or **famciclovir** 500 mg po tid, or **acyclovir** 800 mg po tid). Ophthalmology consultation imperative: approaches have also included intra-vitreal injection of anti-virals (foscarnet, ganciclovir implant). In rare cases due to CMV use **ganciclovir/valganciclovir** (see CMV retinitis, Table 14A)		Most patients are highly immunocompromised (HIV with low CD4 or transplantation). In contrast to Acute Retinal Necrosis, lack of intraocular inflammation or arteritis. May be able to stop oral antivirals when CD4 recovers with ART (Ocul Immunol Inflammation 15:425, 2007).
Orbital cellulitis (see page 54 for erysipelas, facial)	S. pneumoniae, H. influenzae, M. catarrhalis, S. aureus, anaerobes, group A strep, occ. Gm-neg. bacilli post-trauma	**Nafcillin** 2 gm IV q4h (or for **MRSA**-**vanco** 30-60 mg/kg/day in 2-3 div doses to target trough serum concentration of 15–20 mcg/mL) + **ceftriaxone** 2 gm IV q24h + **metro** 1 gm IV q12h		**If penicillin/ceph allergy: Vanco** + **levo** 750 mg IV once daily + **metro** IV. Problem is frequent inability to make microbiologic diagnosis. Image orbit (CT or MRI). Risk of cavernous sinus thrombosis. If vanco intolerant, another option for S. aureus is dapto 6 mg/kg IV q24h.

NOTE: All dosage recommendations are for adults (unless otherwise indicated), and assume normal renal function.

Abbreviations on page 2.

15

TABLE 1 (13)

ANATOMIC SITE/DIAGNOSIS/ MODIFYING CIRCUMSTANCES	ETIOLOGIES (usual)	SUGGESTED REGIMENS* PRIMARY	SUGGESTED REGIMENS* ALTERNATIVE$	ADJUNCT DIAGNOSTIC OR THERAPEUTIC MEASURES AND COMMENTS
FOOT				
"**Diabetic**"—Two thirds of patients have friad of neuropathy, deformity and pressure-induced trauma. IDSA Guidelines *CID* 54:e132, 2012.				
Ulcer without inflammation	Colonizing skin flora	No antibacterial therapy.		**General:** 1. Glucose control, eliminate pressure on ulcer 2. **Assess for peripheral vascular disease** 3. Caution in use of TMP-SMX in patients with diabetes, as many have risk factors for hyperkalemia (e.g., advanced age, reduced renal function, concomitant medications) (*Arch Intern Med* 170:1045, 2010).
Mild infection	S. aureus (assume MRSA), S. agalactiae (gp B), S. pyogenes predominate	**Oral therapy:** Doxy or cephalexin or AM-CL (not MRSA) Doxy or TMP-SMX-DS (MRSA, may not cover strep) CLINDA (covers MSSA, MRSA, strep) *Dosages in footnote*[5]		**Principles of empiric antibacterial therapy:** 1. Obtain culture/ cover for MRSA in moderate, more severe infections pending culture data, local epidemiology. 2. Severe limb and/or life-threatening infections require initial parenteral therapy with predictable activity vs. Gm-positive cocci, coliforms & other aerobic Gm-neg. rods, & anaerobic Gm-neg. bacilli 3. **NOTE:** The regimens listed are suggestions consistent with above principles. Other alternatives exist & may be appropriate for individual patients. 4. Is there an associated osteomyelitis? Risk increased if ulcer area >2 cm², positive probe to bone, ESR >70 and abnormal plain x-ray. Negative MRI reduces likelihood of osteomyelitis (*JAMA* 299:806, 2008). MRI is best imaging modality (*CID* 47:519 & 528, 2008).
Moderate infection. **Osteomyelitis** See Comment.	As above, plus coliforms possible	**Oral:** As above **Parenteral therapy:** [based on prevailing susceptibilities: AM-SB or TC-CL or **PIP-TZ** or **ERTA** or other carbapenem) plus (**vanco** (or alternative anti-MRSA drug as below) until MRSA excluded] *Dosages in footnotes*[6,7]		
Extensive local inflammation plus systemic toxicity.	As above, plus anaerobic bacteria. Role of enterococci unclear.	**Parenteral therapy: (Vanco** plus (β-lactam/β-lactamase inhibitor) or (**vanco** plus (**Dori** or **IMP** or **MER**)). Other alternatives: 1. **Dapto** or **linezolid** for vanco 2. **CIP** or **Levo** or **Moxi** or **aztreonam** plus **metronidazole** for β-lactam/β-lactamase inhibitor *Dosages in footnote*[7] **Assess for arterial insufficiency**		
Onychomycosis: See Table 11, page 120. *fungal infections*				
Puncture wound: Nail/Toothpick	P. aeruginosa	Cleanse. Tetanus booster. Observe.		See page 4. 1–2% evolve to osteomyelitis. After toothpick injury (*PIDJ* 23:80, 2004). S. aureus, Strep sp. and mixed flora.

[5] **TMP-SMX-DS** 1-2 tabs bid, **minocycline** 100 mg po bid, **Pen VK** 500 mg po qid, (O Ceph 2, 3: **cefprozil** 500 mg po q12h; **cefuroxime axetil** 500 mg po q12h; **cefdinir** 300 mg po q12h or 600 mg po q24h, **cefpodoxime** 200 mg po q12h), **CIP** 750 mg po bid, **Diclox** 500 mg qid, **Cephalexin** 500 mg qid, **AM-CL** 875/125 bid, **Doxy** 100 mg bid, **CLINDA** 300-450 mg tid

[6] **AM-CL-ER** 2000/125 mg po bid, **TMP-SMX-DS** 1-2 tabs po bid, **CIP** 750 mg po bid or 400 mg IV q12h, **Levo** 750 mg po/IV q24h, **Moxi** 400 mg po/IV q24h, **linezolid** 600 mg IV or po q12h.

[7] Vanco 1 gm IV q12h, nafcillin/oxacillin 2 gm IV q4h, β-lactam/β-lactamase inhibitors: AM-SB 3 gm IV q6h, PIP-TZ 3.375 gm IV q6h or 4 hr infusion 3.375 gm q8h; TC-CL 3.1 gm IV q6h; carbapenems: Doripenem 500 mg (1-hr infusion) q8h, ERTA 1 gm IV q24h, IMP 0.5 gm IV q6h, MER 1 gm IV q8h, daptomycin 6 mg per kg IV q24h, linezolid 600 mg IV q12h, aztreonam 2 gm IV q8h. CIP 400 mg IV q12h, Levo 750 mg IV q24h, metro 1 gm IV loading dose & then 0.5 gm IV q6h or 1 gm IV q12h.

Abbreviations on page 2. NOTE: All dosage recommendations are for adults (unless otherwise indicated) and assume normal renal function.

TABLE 1 (14)

ANATOMIC SITE/DIAGNOSIS/ MODIFYING CIRCUMSTANCES	ETIOLOGIES (usual)	SUGGESTED REGIMENS* PRIMARY	SUGGESTED REGIMENS* ALTERNATIVE[1]	ADJUNCT DIAGNOSTIC OR THERAPEUTIC MEASURES AND COMMENTS
GALLBLADDER				
Cholecystitis, cholangitis, biliary sepsis, or common duct obstruction (partial; 2° to tumor, stones, stricture). Cholecystitis Ref: NEJM 358:2804, 2008	Enterobacteriaceae 68%, enterococci 14%, bacteroides 10%, Clostridium sp. 7%, rarely candida	PIP-TZ or AM-SB or TC-CL or ERTA. If life-threatening: IMP or MER or Dori	P Ceph 3 or Aztreonam* + metro or CIP* + metro or Moxi	In severely ill pts, antibiotic therapy complements adequate biliary drainage. 15-30% pts will require decompression: surgical, percutaneous or ERCP-placed stent.

Dosages in footnote on page 16.
*Add vanco to these regimens to cover gram-positives.

GASTROINTESTINAL

Gastroenteritis—Empiric Therapy (laboratory studies not performed or culture, microscopy, toxin results NOT AVAILABLE) (Ref.: *NEJM 350:38, 2004*)

Premature infant with necrotizing enterocolitis	Associated with intestinal flora	Antibiotic treatment should cover broad range of intestinal organisms, using regimens appropriate to age and local susceptibility patterns, rationale as in diverticulitis/peritonitis, page 22. See Table 16, page 203 for pediatric dosages.		Pneumatosis intestinalis, if present on x-ray confirms diagnosis. Bacteremia-peritonitis in 30-50%. If Staph. epidermidis isolated, add vanco (IV). For review and general management, see *NEJM 364:255, 2011*.
Mild diarrhea (≤3 unformed stools/day, minimal associated symptomatology)	Bacteria (see Severe, below), viral (norovirus), parasitic. Viral usually causes mild to moderate disease. For traveler's diarrhea, see page 20	Fluids only + lactose-free diet, avoid caffeine		**Rehydration: For po fluid replacement**, see *Cholera, page 19*. **Antimotility:** (Do not use if fever, bloody stools, or suspicion of HUS): Loperamide (Imodium) 4 mg po, then 2 mg after each loose stool to max. of 16 mg per day. Bismuth subsalicylate (Pepto-Bismol) 2 tablets (262 mg) po qid
Moderate diarrhea (≥4 unformed stools/day &/or systemic symptoms)		Antimotility agents (see Comments) + fluids		**Hemolytic uremic syndrome (HUS):** Risk in children infected with E. coli 0157:H7 is 8-10%. Early treatment with TMP-SMX or FQs ↑ risk of HUS (*NEJM 342:1930 & 1990, 2000*). Controversial meta-analysis: *JAMA 288:996 & 3110, 2002*.
Severe diarrhea (≥6 unformed stools/day, &/or temp ≥101°F, tenesmus, blood, or fecal leukocytes). NOTE: Severe afebrile bloody diarrhea should ↑ suspicion of Shiga toxin E. coli 0157:H7 & others (*MMWR 58 (RR-12):1, 2009*)	Shigella, salmonella, C. jejuni, Yersinia, E. coli, toxin-positive C. difficile, E. histolytica oxytoca, E. histolytica. For typhoid fever, see page 61	FQ (CIP 500 mg po q12h or Levo 500 mg q24h) times 3-5 days	TMP-SMX-DS bid times 3-5 days. Campylobacter resistance to TMP-SMX common in tropics.	**Norovirus:** Etiology of over 90% of non-bacterial diarrhea (± nausea/vomiting). Lasts 12-60 hrs. Hydrate. No effective antiviral. **Other potential etiologies:** Cryptosporidia—no treatment in immunocompetent host (see Table 13A & *JID 170:272, 1994*). Cyclospora—usually chronic diarrhea, responds to TMP-SMX (see *Table 13A, page 141 & AIM 123:409, 1995*). Klebsiella oxytoca identified as cause of antibiotic-associated hemorrhagic colitis (cytotoxin positive): *NEJM 355:2418, 2006*.
	If recent antibiotic therapy (C. difficile toxin colitis possible) add:	Metro 500 mg po qid times 10-14 days	Vanco 125 mg po qid times 10-14 days	

Gastroenteritis—Specific Therapy (results of culture, microscopy, toxin assay AVAILABLE) (Ref.: *NEJM 361:1560, 2009*)

If culture negative, probably Norovirus (Norwalk) other virus (*EID 17:1381, 2011*)—see Norovirus, page 165		CIP 750 mg po x3 days	Azithro 500 mg po once daily x3 days.	Although no absolute proof, increasing evidence for Plesiomonas as cause of diarrheal illness (*NEJM 361:1560, 2009*)
Aeromonas/Plesiomonas				
Amebiasis (Entamoeba histolytica, Cyclospora, Cryptosporidia and Giardia), see Table 13A				
Campylobacter jejuni	History of fever in 53-83%. Self-limited diarrhea in normal host.	Azithro 500 mg po x 3 days.	Erythro stearate 500 mg po qid x 5 days or CIP 500 mg po bid (CIP resistance increasing).	**Post-Campylobacter Guillain-Barré:** assoc: 15% of cases (*Ln 366:1653, 2005*). Assoc. with small bowel lymphoproliferative disease; may respond to antimicrobials (*NEJM 350:239, 2004*). **Reactive arthritis** another potential sequelae. See Traveler's diarrhea, page 20.
Campylobacter fetus	Campylobacter uncommon. More systemic disease in debilitated hosts	Gentamicin (See Table 10D)	AMP 100 mg/kg/day IV q6h or IMP 500 mg IV q6h	Draw blood cultures: 32% of C. fetus resistant to FQs (*CID 47:790, 2008*). Meropenem inhibits C. fetus at low concentrations in vitro.

Abbreviations on page 2. NOTE: *All dosage recommendations are for adults (unless otherwise indicated) and assume normal renal function.*

TABLE 1 (15)

GASTROINTESTINAL/Gastroenteritis—Specific Therapy (continued)

ANATOMIC SITE/DIAGNOSIS/ MODIFYING CIRCUMSTANCES	ETIOLOGIES (usual)	SUGGESTED REGIMENS* PRIMARY	SUGGESTED REGIMENS* ALTERNATIVE[1]	ADJUNCT DIAGNOSTIC OR THERAPEUTIC MEASURES AND COMMENTS
Differential diagnosis of toxin-producing diarrhea: • C. difficile • Klebsiella oxytoca • S. aureus • Shiga toxin producing E. coli (STEC) • Enterotoxigenic B. fragilis (CID 47:797, 2008)	C. difficile toxin positive antibiotic-associated colitis. po meds okay. WBC <15,000, <50% increase in serum creatinine.	**Metro** 500 mg po tid or 250 mg qid x 10-14 days	**Vanco** 125 mg po qid x 10-14 days **Teicoplanin**[NUS] 400 mg po bid x 10 days	D/C antibiotic if possible: avoid **antimotility agents, hydration, enteric isolation.** Recent review suggests antimotility agents can be used cautiously in certain pts with mild disease who are receiving rx (CID 48: 598, 2009), but others believe there is insufficient data re safety of this approach. **Nitazoxanide** 500 mg po bid for 7–10 days equivalent to **Metro** in phase 3 study (CID 43:421, 2006). Probiotics (lactobacillus or saccharomyces) inconsistent in prevention of C. difficile (NEJM 359:1932, 2008)
More on C. difficile: Treatment review: CID 51:1306, 2010. SHEA/IDSA treatment guidelines: ICHE 31:431, 2010; ESCMID guidelines: Clin Microbiol Infect 15:1067, 2009; AnIM 155:839, 2011.	Sicker; WBC >15,000; ≥ 50% increase in baseline creatinine	**Vanco** 125 mg po qid x 10-14 days. To use IV vanco po, see Table 10A, page 97	**Fidaxomicin** 200 mg po bid x 10 days	Vanco superior to metro in sicker pts. Relapse in 10-20% (not due to resistance: JAC 56:988, 2005). Fidaxomicin had lower rate of recurrence than Vanco for diarrhea with non-NAP1 strains (N Engl J Med 364:422, 2011).
	Post-treatment relapse	**1st relapse** **Metro** 500 mg po tid x 10 days	**2nd relapse** **Vanco** 125 mg po qid x 10-14 days, then immediately start taper (See Comments)	**Vanco** taper (all doses 125 mg po): week 1 – bid, week 2 – q24h; week 3 – qod; then every 3rd day for 5 doses (NEJM 359: 1932, 2006). Other options: 1) After vanco, **rifaximin**[NUS] 400-800 mg po daily divided bid or tid x 2 wks (CID 44:846, 2007. Rifaximin-resistant C. diff reported); 2) **nitazoxanide**[NUS] 500 mg bid x 10d (JAC 59:705, 2007). **Last resort: stool transplant** (CID 53:994, 2011).
	Post-op ileus: severe disease with toxic megacolon (NEJM 359:1932, 2008).	**Metro** 500 mg IV q6h + **vanco** 500 mg q6h via nasogastric tube (or naso-small bowel tube) ± retrograde catheter in cecum. See comment for dosage.		For vanco instillation into bowel, add 500 mg vanco to 1 liter of saline and perfuse at 1-3 mL/min to nasogastric and 2 gm in 24 hrs (CID 690, 2002). **Note:** **IV vanco not effective. IVIG:** Reports of benefit of 400 mg/kg x 1-3 doses (JAC 53:882, 2004) and lack of benefit (Am J Inf Cont 35:131, 2007). Indications for colectomy, see ICHE 31:431, 2010. Reported successful use of IV to treat severe C. diff refractory to standard rx (CID 48:1732, 2009).
	E. coli O157:H7 History of bloody stools 63% shiga toxin producing E. coli (STEC)	**NO TREATMENT** with antimicrobials or anti-motility drugs; may enhance toxin release and ↑ risk of hemolytic uremic syndrome (HUS) (Ln 365:1073, 2005).		5–10% of pts develop HUS (approx. 10% with HUS die or have permanent renal failure. 50% HUS pts have some degree of renal impairment). In US, no O157:H7 STEC emerging; for lab diagnosis, see MMWR 58 (RR-12), 2009. In the US, infection with non-O157 Shiga-toxin producing E. coli was associated with international outbreak (CID 53:269, 2011). In 2011, large outbreak centered in Germany of HUS from E. coli O104 H4, an E. coli enteroaggregative strain acquired Shiga toxin-mediating Shiga toxin 2 (NEJM 365:709, 2011; NEJM 365:1763, 2011). Suggested that stopping NSAIDs helps. Ref: NEJM 355:2418, 2006.
	Klebsiella oxytoca-antibiotic-associated diarrhea	Responds to stopping antibiotic		
	Listeria monocytogenes	Usually self-limited. Value of oral antibiotics (e.g., ampicillin or TMP-SMX) unknown, but their use might be reasonable in populations at risk for serious listeria infections (CID 40:1327, 2005; Wien Klin Wochenschr 121:149, 2009). Those meningitis may require parenteral therapy; see pages 9 & 60.		Recognized as a cause of food-associated febrile gastroenteritis. Not detected in standard stool cultures (NEJM 336:100 & 130, 1997). Percentage with complicating bacteremia/meningitis unknown. Among 292 children hospitalized during an outbreak, none developed sepsis (NEJM 342:1236, 2000). Pregnant women, debilitated older persons, those on corticosteroids, neonates, the elderly, and immunocompromised hosts (MMWR 57:1097, 2008).

(Continued on next page)

NOTE: All dosage recommendations are for adults (unless otherwise indicated) and assume normal renal function.

Abbreviations on page 2.

TABLE 1 (16)

GASTROINTESTINAL/Gastroenteritis—Specific Therapy (continued)

ANATOMIC SITE/DIAGNOSIS/ MODIFYING CIRCUMSTANCES	ETIOLOGIES (usual)	SUGGESTED REGIMENS* PRIMARY	SUGGESTED REGIMENS* ALTERNATIVE[1]	ADJUNCT DIAGNOSTIC OR THERAPEUTIC MEASURES AND COMMENTS
(Continued from previous page)	**Salmonella, non-typhi**—For typhoid (enteric) fever, see page 21. Fever in 71-91%, history of bloody stools in 34%	If pt asymptomatic or illness mild, antimicrobial therapy not indicated. **Treat if** < 1 yr old or >50 yrs old, if immunocompromised, if vascular grafts or prosthetic joints, bacteremic, hemoglobinopathy, or hospitalized with fever and severe diarrhea (see typhoid fever, page 61). **CIP 500 mg bid** or **Levo 500 mg qd x 7-10 days (14 days if immunocompromised).**	**Azithro 500 mg po once daily x 7 days (14 days if immunocompromised).**	If resistance to TMP-SMX and chloro. Ceftriaxone usually active if IV therapy required (see footnote, page 25, for dose). Ceftriaxone & FQ resistance in Asia (AAC 53:2696, 2009). **Primary treatment of enteritis is fluid and electrolyte replacement.**
	Shigella Fever in 58%, history of bloody stools 51%	**CIP 750 mg bid x 3 days**	**Azithro 500 mg po once daily x 3 days** See Comment for peds rx per dose	Recent expert review recommended adult CIP dose of 750 mg once daily for 3 days (NEJM 361:1560, 2009). Infection due to S. flexneri resistant to CIP, ceftriaxone and cefotaxime has been reported (MMWR 59:1619, 2010). **Peds doses: Azithro** 10 mg/kg/day once daily x 3 days. For severe disease, ceftriaxone 50-75 mg/kg/day x 2-5 days. CIP suspension 10 mg/kg bid x 5 days. CIP superior to ceftriaxone in children (LnID 3:537, 2003). **Immunocompromised children & adults: Treat for 7-10 days.** Azithro superior to cefixime in trial in children (PIDJ 22:374, 2003).
	Spirochetosis (Brachyspira pilosicoli)	Benefit of treatment unclear. Susceptible to **metro, ceftriaxone, and Moxi** (AAC 47:2354, 2003).		Anaerobic intestinal spirochete that colonizes colon of domestic & wild animals plus humans. Case reports of diarrhea with large numbers of the organism present (JCM 39:347, 2001; Am J Clin Path 120:828, 2003). Rarely, B. pilosicoli has been isolated from blood culture (Arch Int Med 162:1717, 2002).
	Vibrio cholerae Treatment decreases duration of disease, volume losses, & duration of excretion (CID 37:272, 2003; Ln 363:223, 2004)	**Primary therapy is rehydration.** Select antibiotics based on susceptibility of locally prevailing isolates. Options include: **Doxycycline** 300 mg po single dose **OR Azithromycin** 1 gm po single dose **OR Erythromycin** 500 mg po qid x 3 days **OR Tetracycline** 500 mg po qid x 3 days (these options are based on CDC recommendations for 2010 Haiti epidemic)	**For pregnant women: Azithromycin** 1 gm po single dose **OR Erythromycin** 500 mg po qid x 3 days. **For children: Azithromycin** 20 mg/kg po as single dose; for other age-specific alternatives, see CDC website http://www.cdc.gov/haiticholera/hcp_goingtohaiti.htm	Antimicrobial therapy shortens duration of illness, but rehydration is paramount. When IV hydration is needed, use Ringer's lactate. Switch to PO repletion with Oral Rehydration Salts (ORS) as soon as able to take oral fluids. ORS are commercially available for reconstitution in potable water. If not available, WHO suggests a substitute can be made by dissolving ½ teaspoon salt and 6 level teaspoons of sugar per liter of potable water (http://www.who.int/cholera/technical/en/). For additional practical considerations, see Lancet 363:223, 2004. CDC recommendations for other aspects of management developed for Haiti outbreak can be found at http://www.cdc.gov/haiticholera/hcp_goingtohaiti.htm Isolates from this outbreak demonstrate reduced susceptibility to ciprofloxacin and resistance to sulfisoxazole, nalidixic acid and furazolidone.

Abbreviations on page 2.   NOTE: All dosage recommendations are for adults (unless otherwise indicated) and assume normal renal function.

19

TABLE 1 (17)

ANATOMIC SITE/DIAGNOSIS/ MODIFYING CIRCUMSTANCES	ETIOLOGIES (usual)	SUGGESTED REGIMENS* PRIMARY	SUGGESTED REGIMENS* ALTERNATIVE[1]	ADJUNCT DIAGNOSTIC OR THERAPEUTIC MEASURES AND COMMENTS
GASTROINTESTINAL/Gastroenteritis—Specific Therapy *(continued)*				
	Vibrio parahaemolyticus	Antimicrobial rx does not shorten course. Hydration.		Shellfish exposure common. Treat severe disease: **FQ, doxy, P Ceph 3**
	Vibrio vulnificus	Usual presentation is skin lesions & bacteremia; life-threatening; treat early. **ceftaz** ± **doxy**—see page 54; levo (*AAC 46:3580, 2002*).
	Yersinia enterocolitica Fever in 68%, bloody stools in 26%	No treatment unless severe. If severe, combine **doxy** 100 mg IV bid + **(tobra** or **gent** 5 mg/kg per day once q24h). **TMP-SMX** or **FQs** are alternatives.		Mesenteric adenitis pain can mimic acute appendicitis. Lab diagnosis difficult; requires "cold" enrichment and/or yersinia selective agar. Desferrioxamine therapy increases severity, discontinue if pt on it. Iron overload states predispose to yersinia (*CID 27:1362 & 1367, 1998*).
Gastroenteritis—Specific Risk Groups—Empiric Therapy				
Anoreceptive intercourse Proctitis (distal 15 cm only)	Herpes viruses, gonococci, chlamydia, syphilis. See *Genital Tract, page 23*			
Colitis	*Shigella, salmonella, campylobacter, E. histolytica* (see Table 13A)			See specific GI pathogens, *Gastroenteritis, above*.
HIV-1 infected (AIDS): >10 days diarrhea	*G. lamblia*			
Acid-fast organisms:	*Cryptosporidium parvum, Cyclospora cayetanensis*			See Table 13A
Other:	*Isospora belli, microsporidia (Enterocytozoon bieneusi, Septata intestinalis)*			
Neutropenic enterocolitis or "typhlitis" (*CID 27:695 & 700, 1998*)	Most often caused by *Clostridium septicum*. Occasionally caused by *C. sordellii* or *P. aeruginosa*	As for peritoneal abscess, diverticulitis, pg 22. Ensure empiric regimen includes drug active vs Clostridia species. Empiric regimen should have predictive activity vs. P. aeruginosa also.		Tender right lower quadrant may be clue, but tenderness may be diffuse or absent in immunocompromised host. Need surgical consult. Surgical resection controversial but may be necessary. **NOTE**: Resistance of clostridia to clindamycin reported. Broad-spectrum agents such as PIP-TZ, IMP, MER, DORI should cover most pathogens
Traveler's diarrhea self-medication. Patient usually afebrile (*CID 44:338 & 347, 2007*)	Acute 60% due to diarrheagenic E. coli; shigella, salmonella, or campylobacter, C. difficile, amebiasis (see Table 13A). If chronic: cyclospora, cryptosporidia, giardia, isospora	**CIP** 500 mg po bid for 1-3 days **OR** **Levo** 500 mg po q24h for 1-3 days **OR** **Oflox** 300 mg po bid for 3 days **OR** **Rifaximin** 200 mg po tid for 3 days **OR** **Azithro** 1000 mg po once or 500 mg po q24h for 3 days		**For pediatrics:** Azithro 10 mg/kg/day as a single dose for 3 days or Ceftriaxone 50 mg/kg/day as single dose for 3 days. Avoid FQs. **For pregnancy:** Use Azithro. Avoid FQs. **Antimotility agent:** For non-pregnant adults with no fever or blood in stool, add loperamide 4 mg po x 1, then 2 mg po after each loose stool to a maximum of 16 mg per day. **Comments:** Rifaximin approved only for ages 12 and older. Works only for diarrhea due to non-invasive E. coli; do not use if fever or bloody stool. **References:** *NEJM 361:1560, 2009; BMJ 337: a1746, 2008;* http://wwwnc.cdc.gov/travel/yellowbook/2012/chapter-2-the-pre-travel-consultation/travelers-diarrhea.htm
Prevention of Traveler's diarrhea		Not routinely indicated. Current recommendation is to take **FQ** + **Imodium** with 1st loose stool.	Alternative during 1st – 3 wks & only if activities are essential: **Rifaximin** 200 mg po bid[ad] (*AnIM 142:805 & 861, 2005*).	

Abbreviations on page 2.   NOTE: All dosage recommendations are for adults (unless otherwise indicated) and assume normal renal function.

TABLE 1 (18)

ANATOMIC SITE/DIAGNOSIS/ MODIFYING CIRCUMSTANCES	ETIOLOGIES (usual)	SUGGESTED REGIMENS* PRIMARY	SUGGESTED REGIMENS* ALTERNATIVE[§]	ADJUNCT DIAGNOSTIC OR THERAPEUTIC MEASURES AND COMMENTS
GASTROINTESTINAL (continued)				
Gastrointestinal Infections by Anatomic Site: Esophagus to Rectum				
Esophagitis	Candida albicans, HSV, CMV	See SANFORD GUIDE TO HIV/AIDS THERAPY and Table 11A.		
Duodenal/Gastric ulcer; gastric cancer, MALT lymphomas (not 2° NSAIDs)	**Helicobacter pylori** See Comment Prevalence of pre-treatment resistance increasing	**Sequential therapy**: (**Rabeprazole** 20 mg + **amox** 1 gm) bid x 5 days, then (**rabeprazole** 20 mg + **clarithro** 500 mg + **tinidazole** 500 mg) bid for another 5 days. See footnote[§]	**Quadruple therapy (10-14 days)**: **Bismuth subsalicylate** 2 tabs qid + **metro** 500 mg tid + **omeprazole** 20 mg bid.	**Comment**: In many locations, failure rates with previously recommended triple regimens (**PPI + Amox + Clarithro**) are no longer acceptable (20%). With 10 days of quadruple therapy (**omeprazole** 20 mg twice daily) + (3 capsules po four times per day, each containing **Bismuth subcitrate potassium** 140 mg + **Metro** 125 mg + **Tetracycline** 125 mg), eradication rates were 93% in a per protocol analysis and 80% in an intention-to-treat population, both significantly better than with 7-day triple therapy regimen (PPI + Amox + Clarithro) (*Lancet* 377:905, 2011). Exercise caution regarding potential interactions with other drugs, contraindications in pregnancy and warnings for other special populations. For general review, see *NEJM* 362:1597, 2010. **Dx**: **Stool antigen**—Monoclonal EIA—96% sens. & 92% specific (*Amer. J. Gastro.* 101:921, 2006) Other tests: if endoscoped, rapid urease &/or histology &/or culture; urea breath test, but some office-based tests underperform (*CID* 48:1385, 2009). **Test of cure**: Repeat stool antigen and/or urea breath test >8 wks post-treatment. **Treatment outcome**: Failure rate of triple therapy 20% due to clarithro resistance. Cure rate with sequential therapy 90%.
Small intestine: Whipple's disease (*NEJM* 356:55, 2007; *LnID* 8:179, 2008) See *Infective endocarditis, culture-negative*, page 30.	Tropheryma whipplei	**Initial 10-14 days**: **Ceftriaxone** 2 gm IV q24h or **Pen G** 2 million units IV q4h **Then, for approx. 1 year**: **TMP-SMX-DS** 1 tab po bid	If sulfa-allergic: **Doxy** 100 mg po bid + hydroxychloroquine 200 mg po tid.	Therapy based on empiricism and retrospective analyses. Randomized trial reported that initial therapy with Meropenem 1 gm q8h was comparable to Ceftriaxone 2 gm q24h, each administered for 14 days and then followed by TMP-SMX for 12 months, in maintaining remission of Whipple's disease for at least 3 years (*Gastroenterology* 138:478, 2010; editorial *ibid* 138:422, 2010). TMP-SMX: CNS relapses during therapy have been reported. Late relapses with resistance to TMP-SMX have been described (*ibid* 141:1553, 2006). Another (4th) patient with CSF involvement with intestinal disease and no neurological findings. For review of Whipple's pathogenesis, see *Lancet Infect Dis* 8:179, 2008.

* Can substitute other proton pump inhibitors for omeprazole or rabeprazole—all bid: **esomeprazole** 20 mg (FDA-approved), **lanzoprazole** 30 mg (FDA-approved), **pantoprazole** 40 mg (not FDA-approved for this indication).

Bismuth preparations: (1) In U.S., **bismuth subsalicylate (Pepto-Bismol)** 262 mg tabs; adult dose for helicobacter is 2 tabs (524 mg) qid. (2) Outside U.S., colloidal bismuth subcitrate (De-Nol) 120 mg chewable tablets; dose is 1 tablet qid. In the U.S., bismuth subcitrate is available in combination cap only (Pylera: each cap contains bismuth subcitrate 140 mg + Metro 125 mg + Tetracycline 125 mg), given as 3 caps po 4x daily for 10 days **together with** a twice daily PPI.

Abbreviations on page 2. NOTE: All dosage recommendations are for adults (unless otherwise indicated) and assume normal renal function.

TABLE 1 (19)

ANATOMIC SITE/DIAGNOSIS/ MODIFYING CIRCUMSTANCES	ETIOLOGIES (usual)	SUGGESTED REGIMENS* PRIMARY	SUGGESTED REGIMENS* ALTERNATIVE[1]	ADJUNCT DIAGNOSTIC OR THERAPEUTIC MEASURES AND COMMENTS
GASTROINTESTINAL/Gastrointestinal Infections by Anatomic Site: Esophagus to Rectum *(continued)*				
Diverticulitis, perirectal abscess, peritonitis. *Also see Peritonitis, page 47*	Enterobacteriaceae, occasionally P. aeruginosa, Bacteroides sp., enterococci	**Outpatient rx—mild diverticulitis, drained perirectal abscess:** [(**TMP-SMX-DS** bid) or (**CIP** 500 mg bid or **Levo** 750 mg q24h)] + **metro** 500 mg q6h. All po x 7–10 days. **Mild-moderate disease—Inpatient—Parenteral Rx:** (e.g. focal periappendiceal peritonitis, peridiverticular abscess, endomyometritis) **PIP-TZ** 3.375 gm IV q6h or 4.5 gm IV q8h or **AM-SB** 3 gm IV q6h or **TC-CL** 3.1 gm IV q6h or **ERTA** 1 gm IV q24h or **MOXI** 400 mg IV q24h **Severe life-threatening disease, ICU patient:** IMP 500 mg IV q6h or MER 1 gm IV q8h or Dori 500 mg q8h (1-hr infusion).	**AM-CL-ER** 1000/62.5 mg 2 tabs po bid x 7–10 days **OR Moxi** 400 mg po q24h x 7–10 days [(**CIP** 400 mg IV q12h) or **Levo** 750 mg IV q24h)] + (**metro** 500 mg IV q6h or 1 gm IV q12h) **OR tigecycline** 100 mg IV 1st dose & then 50 mg IV q12h **OR Moxi** 400 mg IV q24h **AMP** + **metro** + (**CIP** 400 mg IV q12h or **Levo** 750 mg IV q24h) **OR AMP** 2 gm IV q6h + **metro** 500 mg IV q6h + **aminoglycoside**[10] (see Table 10D, page 109)	Must "cover" both Gm-neg. aerobic & Gm-neg. anaerobic bacteria. **Drugs active only vs. aerobic Gm-neg. bacilli:** APAG[10], FQs. **Drugs active only vs. anaerobic Gm-neg. bacilli:** metro, clinda, tinido. **Drugs active vs. both aerobic/anaerobic Gm-neg. bacteria:** cefoxitin, cefotetan, TC-CL, PIP-TZ, AM-SB, ERTA, Dori, IMP, MER, Moxi, & tigecycline. Increasing resistance of **Bacteroides species** (AAC 51:1649, 2007): Cefoxitin Cefotetan Clindamycin % Resistant: 5–30 17–87 19–35 **Resistance:** Resistance to metro, PIP-TZ rare. Resistance to FQ increased in enteric bacteria, particularly if any FQ used recently. Ertapenem poorly active vs. P. aeruginosa/Acinetobacter sp. **Concomitant surgical management important**, esp. with moderate-severe disease. Role of enterococci remains debatable. Probably pathogenic in infections of biliary tract. Probably need drugs active vs. enterococci in pts with valvular heart disease. Severe penicillin/cephalosporin allergy: **aztreonam** 2 gm IV q6h to q8h) + [**metro** (500 mg IV q6h) or (1 gm IV q12h)] **OR** [(**CIP** 400 mg IV q12h) or (**Levo** 750 mg IV q24h) + **metro**].

[10] **Aminoglycoside** = **antipseudomonal aminoglycosidic aminoglycoside**, e.g., **amikacin, gentamicin, tobramycin**

NOTE: All dosage recommendations are for adults (unless otherwise indicated) and assume normal renal function.

Abbreviations on page 2.

TABLE 1 (20)

ANATOMIC SITE/DIAGNOSIS/ MODIFYING CIRCUMSTANCES	ETIOLOGIES (usual)	SUGGESTED REGIMENS* PRIMARY	ALTERNATIVE[1]	ADJUNCT DIAGNOSTIC OR THERAPEUTIC MEASURES AND COMMENTS
GENITAL TRACT: Mixture of empiric & specific treatment. Divided by sex of the patient. For sexual assault (rape), see Table 15A, page 192 & MMWR 59 (RR-12), 2010. See Guidelines for Dx of Sexually Transmitted Diseases, MMWR 59 (RR-12), 2010.				
Both Women & Men: Chancroid	H. ducreyi	Ceftriaxone 250 mg IM single dose OR **azithro** 1 gm po single dose	CIP 500 mg bid po x 3 days OR erythro base 500 mg qid po x 7 days.	In HIV+ pts, failures reported with single dose azithro (CID 21:409, 1995). Evaluate after 7 days, ulcer should objectively improve. Symptoms improve in 7 days. All patients treated for chancroid should be tested for HIV and syphilis. All sex partners of pts who had sex with index pt within the last 10 days have evidence of disease or have had sex with index pt within the last 10 days (AJM 102:914, 2000). Test all urethritis/cervicitis pts for HIV & syphilis. For additional erythromycin regimens, see MMWR (RR-11), 2006.
Chlamydia, et al. non-gono-coccal or post-gonococcal urethritis, cervicitis UTR cervicitis, concomitant N. gonorrhoeae Chlamydia conjunctivitis, see page 12.	Chlamydia 50%, Mycoplasma hominis. Other known etiologies (10%) include her-pes simplex virus, Mycoplasma genitalium. Ref: JID 193:333, 336, 2006.	(**Doxy** 100 mg po x 7 days) or (**azithro** 1 gm po as single dose). Evaluate & treat sex partners. In pregnancy: **Azithromycin** 1 gm po single dose OR amox 500 mg po tid x 7 days.	(**Erythro base** 500 mg po x 7 days) or (**Ofiox** 300 mg po bid x 7 days) or (**Levo** 500 mg po qd x 7 days) in pregnancy: Erythro base 500 mg po qd for 7 days. Doxy & FQs contraindicated	Evaluate & treat sex partners. Re-test for cure in pregnancy. Azithromycin 1 gm was superior to doxycycline for M. genitalium male urethritis (CID 48:1649, 2009), but may select resistance leading to ↑ failure of multi-dose azithromycin retreatment regimens (CID 48:1655, 2009). In men with NGU, 20% infected with trichomonas (JID 188:465, 2003). See above re M. genitalium.
Recurrent/persistent urethritis	Occult trichomonas, tetra-resistant U. urealyticum	Metro 2 gm po x 1	Tinidazole 2 gm po x 1 + azithromycin 1 gm po x 1 (if not used for initial episode)	
Gonorrhea (MMWR 59 (RR-12) :49, 2010). **FQs no longer recommended for treatment of gonococcal infections** (MMWR 59 (RR-12):49, 2010). **Cephalosporin resistance**: JAMA 309:163 & 185, 2013.				
Conjunctivitis (adult)	N. gonorrhoeae	Ceftriaxone 1 gm IM or IV single dose		Consider one-time saline lavage of eye.
Disseminated gonococcal infection (DGI, dermatitis-arthritis syndrome)	N. gonorrhoeae	Ceftriaxone 1 gm IV q24h—see Comment	(**Cefotaxime** 1 gm q8h IV) or (**ceftizoxime** 1 gm q8h IV). Most pts respond in 24-48 hr after rx; change to cefixime 400 mg po bid. If meningitis/endocarditis. Treat presumptively for concomitant C. trachomatis.	Continue IM or IV regimen for 24hr after symptoms ↓; reliable pts may be discharged 24hr after sx resolve to complete 7 days rx with **cefixime** 400 mg po bid. If meningitis/endocarditis. Treat presumptively for concomitant C. trachomatis.
Endocarditis	N. gonorrhoeae	Ceftriaxone 1-2 gm IV q24h x 4 wks	Due to resistance concerns, do not use FQs.	Ref. JID 157:1281, 1988.
Pharyngitis	N. gonorrhoeae	Ceftriaxone 250 mg IM x 1 PLUS (**Azithro** 1 gm po x 1) or **doxy** 100 mg bid x 7 days.		Pharyngeal GC more difficult to eradicate. Some suggest test of cure culture after 1 wk. **Spectinomycin, cefixime, cefpodoxime & ceftixime not effective**
Urethritis, cervicitis, proctitis (uncomplicated) For prostatitis, see page 27. **Diagnosis**: Nucleic acid amplification test (NAAT) on urine or urethral swab—see AnIM 142:914, 2005. MMWR 59 (RR-12):49, 2010. **NO FQs**.	N. gonorrhoeae, cervicitis in pts with urethritis, cervicitis have concomitant C. trachomatis—**treat for both unless NAAT indicates single pathogen**).	(**Ceftriaxone** 250 mg IM x 1) **PLUS** - [(**doxy** 100 mg po bid x 7 days) or (**azithro** 1 gm po x 1)]. Severe pen/ceph allergy? Maybe **azithro**—see comment. Increasing risk of FQ-resistance, could try FQ therapy with close follow-up.		Screen for syphilis. Other alternatives for **GC** (Test of Cure recommended one week after Rx for ALL of these approaches listed below): • **Cefixime** 400 mg po x 1 OR Cefpodoxime 400 mg po x 1 (Note: not effective for pharyngeal disease); oral cephalosporin use is no longer recommended as primary therapy owing to emergence of resistance, MMWR 61:590, 2012. • Other single-dose cephalosporins: ceftizoxime 500 mg IM, cefotaxime 500 mg IM, cefoxitin 2 gm IM + probenecid 1 gm po. • **Azithro** 1 gm po x 1 effective for chlamydia but need 2 gm for GC; not recommended for GC due to GI side-effects, expense & rapid emergence of resistance.

[**] Cefixime oral preparations now available as oral suspension, 200 mg/5 mL, and 400 mg tablets (Lupine Pharmaceuticals, (+1) 866-587-4617). (MMWR 57:435, 2008).

Abbreviations on page 2. NOTE: All dosage recommendations are for adults (unless otherwise indicated) and assume normal renal function.

TABLE 1 (21)

GENITAL TRACT/Both Women & Men (continued)

ANATOMIC SITE/DIAGNOSIS/ MODIFYING CIRCUMSTANCES	ETIOLOGIES (usual)	SUGGESTED REGIMENS* PRIMARY	SUGGESTED REGIMENS* ALTERNATIVE[1]	ADJUNCT DIAGNOSTIC OR THERAPEUTIC MEASURES AND COMMENTS
Granuloma inguinale (Donovanosis)	Klebsiella (formerly Calymmatobacterium) granulomatis	**Doxy** 100 mg po bid x 3–4 wks	**TMP-SMX** one DS tablet bid x 3 wks **OR Erythro** 500 mg po qid x 3 wks **OR CIP** 750 mg po bid x 3 wks **OR azithro** 1 gm po q wk x 3 wks	Clinical response usually seen in 1 wk. **Rx until all lesions healed**, may take 4 wks. Relapse seen with failures & recurrence with TMP-SMX. Report of efficacy with FQ and chloro. Ref: *CID* 25:24, 1997. Relapse can occur 6-18 months after apparently effective Rx. If improvement not evidence in first few days, some experts add gentamicin 1 mg/kg IV q8h.
Herpes simplex virus Human papilloma virus (HPV)	See Table 14A, page 160 See Table 14A, page 166			
Lymphogranuloma venereum	Chlamydia trachomatis, serovars, L1, L2, L3	**Doxy** 100 mg po bid x 21 days	**Erythro** 0.5 gm po qid x 21 days **or Azithro** 1 gm po qwk X 3 weeks (clinical data lacking) See Table 13A, page 151	Dx based on serology; biopsy contraindicated because sinus tracts develop. Nucleic acid ampli tests for *C. trachomatis* will be positive. In MSM, presents as fever, rectal ulcer, anal discharge (*CID* 39:996, 2004; *Dis Colon Rectum* 52:507, 2009).
Phthirus pubis ("public lice, "crabs") & scabies	Phthirus pubis & Sarcoptes scabiei			
Syphilis (*JAMA* 290:1510, 2003): Early, primary, secondary, or latent <1 yr. Screen with treponemal Ab; if positive, test with RPR/VDRL, see *JCM* 50:2 & 148, 2012.	T. pallidum NOTE: Test all pts with syphilis for HIV, test all HIV patients for latent syphilis.	**Benzathine pen G (Bicillin L-A)** 2.4 million units IM x 1 or **Azithro** 2 gm po x 1 dose (See Comment)	**Doxy** 100 mg po bid x 14 days **or tetracycline** 500 mg po qid x 14 days) **or (ceftriaxone** 2 tubes i.d at 12 mo. With 1°, 50% will be RPR seronegative at 12 mos., 24% neg. FTA/ABS at 2-3 yrs (*AnIM* 114:1005, 1991). If titers fail to fall, examine CSF; if CSF (+), treat as neurosyphilis; if CSF is negative, retreat with benzathine Pen G 2.4 mu IM weekly x 3 wks. **Azithro** 2 gm po x 1 dose is alternative to benzathine Pen 2.4 M x 1 dose in early syphilis (*N Infect Dis* 201:1729, 2010). **Azithro-resistant syphilis** documented in California, Ireland, & elsewhere (*CID* 44:S130, 2007; *AAC* 54:583, 2010). NOTE: Use of **benzathine procaine penicillin** is inappropriate!!	If early or congenital syphilis, quantitative VDRL at 0, 3, 6, 12 & 24 mos after rx. If 1° or 2° syphilis, VDRL should ↓ 2 tubes at 6 mos, 3 tubes 12 mos, & 4 tubes 24 mos. Update on congenital syphilis (*MMWR* 59:413, 2010).
More than 1 yr's duration (latent of indeterminate duration, cardiovascular, late benign gumma)	For penicillin desensitization method, see Table 7, page 80 and *MMWR* 59 (RR-12): 26, 2010.	**Benzathine pen G (Bicillin L-A)** 2.4 million units IM q week x 3 = 7.2 million units total	**Doxy** 100 mg po bid x 28 days **or tetracycline** 500 mg po qid x 28 days; **Ceftriaxone** 1 gm IV or IM daily x 10–14 days as an alternative (No clinical data; consult ID specialist)	No published data on efficacy of alternatives. **Indications for LP (CDC): neurologic symptoms, treatment failure, any eye or ear involvement, other evidence of active syphilis (aortitis, gumma, iritis).**
Neurosyphilis—Very difficult to treat. Includes ocular (retrobulbar neuritis) syphilis **All need CSF exam.** HIV infection (AIDS) *CID* 44:S130, 2007.		**Pen G** 18–24 million units per day either as continuous infusion or as 3–4 million units IV q4h x 10–14 days. Treatment same as HIV uninfected with closer follow-up. Treat as neurosyphilis: for 10-14 days regardless of CD4 count, *MMWR* 59:S25, 2007.	**Procaine pen G** 2.4 million units IM q24h **+ probenecid** 0.5 gm po qid; both x 10–14 days—See Comment	**Ceftriaxone** 2 gm (IV or IM) q24h x 14 days. 23% failure rate reported (*AJM* 93:481, 1992). For penicillin allergy; desensitize to penicillin or obtain infectious diseases consultation. **Serologic criteria for response to rx: 4-fold or greater ↓ in VDRL titer over 6–12 mos.** (*CID* 28 *Suppl. 1*:S21, 1999). See Syphilis discussion in *MMWR* 59 (RR-12), 2010.

Abbreviations on page 2.   NOTE: All dosage recommendations are for adults (unless otherwise indicated) and assume normal renal function.

TABLE 1 (22)

ANATOMIC SITE/DIAGNOSIS/ MODIFYING CIRCUMSTANCES	ETIOLOGIES (usual)	SUGGESTED REGIMENS* PRIMARY	SUGGESTED REGIMENS* ALTERNATIVE[†]	ADJUNCT DIAGNOSTIC OR THERAPEUTIC MEASURES AND COMMENTS
GENITAL TRACT/Both Women & Men (continued)				
Pregnancy and syphilis		Same as for non-pregnant, some recommend 2nd dose of benzathine pen G 1 wk after initial dose esp. in 3rd trimester or with 2° syphilis	Skin test for penicillin allergy. Desensitize if necessary, as parenteral pen G is only therapy with documented efficacy!	Monthly quantitative VDRL or equivalent. If 4-fold ↑, re-treat. Doxy, tetracycline contraindicated. Erythro not recommended because of high risk of failure to cure fetus.
"Congenital syphilis" (Update on Congenital Syphilis: MMWR 59 (RR-12): 36, 2010)	T. pallidum	Aqueous crystalline pen G 50,000 units/kg per dose IV q12h x 7 days, then q8h for 10 day total.	Procaine pen G 50,000 units/kg IM q24h for 10 days	Another alternative: Ceftriaxone ≤30 days old, 75 mg/kg IV/IM q24h (use with caution in infants with jaundice); or >30 days old 100 mg/kg IV/IM q24h. Treat 10–14 days. If symptomatic, ophthalmologic exam indicated. If more than 1 day of rx missed, restart entire course. **Need serologic follow-up!**
Warts, anogenital	See Table 14A, page 166			
Women:				
Amnionitis, septic abortion	Bacteroides, esp. Prevotella bivius; Group B, A streptococci; Enterobacteriaceae; C. trachomatis	[(Cefoxitin or TC-CL or Dori[NAI] or IMP or MER or ERTA or PIP-TZ) + doxy] OR [Clinda + (aminoglycoside or ceftriaxone)[12]] Dosage: see footnote[12]		D&C of uterus. **In septic abortion,** Clostridium perfringens may cause fulminant intravascular hemolysis. **In postpartum patients with enigmatic fever and/or pulmonary emboli, consider septic pelvic vein thrombophlebitis** (see *Vascular, septic pelvic vein thrombosis,* page 66). After discharge: doxy or clinda for C. trachomatis.
Cervicitis, mucopurulent Treatment based on results of nucleic acid amplification test	N. gonorrhoeae Chlamydia trachomatis	Treat for Gonorrhea, page 23 Treat for non-gonococcal urethritis, page 23 **Note:** in US and Europe, 1/3 of Grp B Strep resistant to clindamycin.		Criteria for diagnosis: 1) (muco) purulent endocervical exudate and/or 2) sustained endocervical bleeding after passage of cotton swab; >10 WBC/hpf of vaginal fluid is suggestive, intracellular gram-neg diplococci are specific but insensitive. If not available, send swab or urine for culture, EIA or nucleic acid amplification test and treat for both.
Endomyometritis/septic pelvic phlebitis Early postpartum (1st 48 hrs) (usually after C-section)	Bacteroides, esp. Prevotella bivius; Group B, A streptococci; Enterobacteriaceae; C. trachomatis	[(Cefoxitin or TC-CL or ERTA or PIP-TZ) + doxy] or [Clinda + (aminoglycoside or ceftriaxone)[12]] Dosage: see footnote[12]		See Comments under Amnionitis, septic abortion, above
Late postpartum (48 hrs to 6 wks) (usually after vaginal delivery)	Chlamydia trachomatis, M. hominis	Doxy 100 mg IV or po q12h times 14 days		Tetracyclines not recommended in nursing mothers; discontinue nursing. M. hominis sensitive to tetra, clinda, not erythro.
Fitzhugh-Curtis syndrome	C. trachomatis, N. gonorrhoeae	Treat as for pelvic inflammatory disease immediately below.		Perihepatitis (violin-string adhesions).
Pelvic actinomycosis; usually tubo-ovarian abscess	A. Israelii most common	AMP 50 mg/kg/day IV div 3–4 doses x 4–6 wks, then Pen VK 2–4 gm/day po x 3–6 mos.	Doxy or ceftriaxone or clinda or erythro	Complication of intrauterine device (IUD). Remove IUD. Can use **Pen G** 10-20 million units/day IV instead of **AMP** x 4–6 wks.

[12] **P Ceph 2** (cefoxitin 2 gm IV q6-8h; cefotetan 2 gm IV q12h; ceturoxime 750 mg IV q8h); **TC-CL** 3.1 gm IV q6h; **PIP-TZ** 3.375 gm q6h or for nosocomial pneumonia: 4.5 gm IV q6h or 4-hr infusion of 3.375 gm IV q8h; **doxy** 100 mg IV/po q12h; **clinda** 450-900 mg IV q8h; **aminoglycoside** (**gentamicin,** see Table 10D, page 109); **P Ceph 3** (**cefotaxime** 2 gm IV q8h; **ceftriaxone** 2 gm IV q24h); **doripenem** 500 mg IV q8h (1-hr infusion); **ertapenem** 1 gm IV q24h; **IMP** 0.5 gm IV q6h; **MER** 1 gm IV q8h; **azithro** 500 mg IV q/po q12h; **vanco** 1 gm IV q12h

Abbreviations on page 2. NOTE: All dosage recommendations are for adults (unless otherwise indicated) and assume normal renal function.

TABLE 1 (23)

ANATOMIC SITE/DIAGNOSIS/ MODIFYING CIRCUMSTANCES	ETIOLOGIES (usual)	SUGGESTED REGIMENS* PRIMARY	SUGGESTED REGIMENS* ALTERNATIVE[1]	ADJUNCT DIAGNOSTIC OR THERAPEUTIC MEASURES AND COMMENTS
GENITAL TRACT/Women (continued)				
Pelvic Inflammatory Disease (PID), salpingitis, tubo-ovarian abscess Outpatient rx: limit to pts with <38°C, WBC <11,000 per mm³, minimal evidence of peritonitis, active bowel sounds & able to tolerate oral nourishment *CID 44:953 & 961, 2007; MMWR 59 (RR-12):63, 2010 & www.cdc.gov/std/treatment*	N. gonorrhoeae, chlamydia, Bacteroides, Enterobacteriaceae, streptococci, especially S. agalactiae. Less commonly: G. vaginalis, Haemophilus influenzae, cytomegalovirus (CMV), U. urealyticum, and M. genitalium.	**Outpatient rx:** (ceftriaxone 250 mg IM or IV x 1) **+ metro** 500 mg po bid x 14 days) + **doxy** 100 mg po bid x 14 days). **OR cefoxitin** 2 gm IM with **probenecid** 1 gm po both as single dose plus **doxy** 100 mg po bid x 14 days with **metro** 500 mg bid — both times 14 days	**Inpatient rx:** [(**Cefotetan** 2 gm IV q12h or **cefoxitin** 2 gm IV q6h) + **doxy** 100 mg IV/po q12h)] **Clinda** 900 mg IV q8h) + **gentamicin** 2 mg/kg loading dose, then 1.5 mg/kg q8h or 4.5 mg/kg once per day), then **doxy** 100 mg bid x 14 days	Another alternative parenteral regimen: **AM-SB** 3 gm IV q6h + **doxy** 100 mg IV/po q12h. Remember: Evaluate and treat sex partner. FQs not recommended due to increasing resistance (*MMWR 59 (RR-12), 2010 & www.cdc.gov/std/treatment*). Suggest initial inpatient evaluation/therapy for pts with tubo-ovarian abscess. For inpatient regimens, continue treatment until satisfactory response for ≥24-hr before switching to outpatient regimen.
Vaginitis—*MMWR 59 (RR-12):63, 2010 or CID 36 (Suppl 2):S135, 2002* **Candidiasis** Pruritus, thick cheesy discharge, pH <4.5 See Table 11A, page 116	Candida albicans 80-90%. C. glabrata, C. tropicalis may be increasing—they are less susceptible to azoles	**Oral azoles: Fluconazole** 150 mg po x 1; **itraconazole** 200 mg po bid x 1 day. For milder cases, Topical Therapy with one of the over the counter preparations usually is successful (e.g. clotrimazole, butoconazole, miconazole, or tioconazole) as creams or vaginal suppositories.	**Intravaginal azoles:** variety of strengths—from 1 dose to 7-14 days. Drugs available (all end in -azole): butocon, clotrim, micon, ticon, tercon doses: *Table 11A*)	Nystatin vag. tabs times 14 days less effective. Other rx for azole-resistant strains: gentian violet, boric acid. If recurrent candidiasis (4 or more episodes per yr): 6 mos. suppression with: fluconazole 150 mg po q week or itraconazole 100 mg po q24h or clotrimazole vag. suppositories 500 mg a week.
Trichomoniasis Copious foamy discharge, pH >4.5 Treat sexual partners—see Comment	Trichomonas vaginalis	**Metro** 2 gm as single dose or 500 mg po bid x 7 days OR **Tinidazole** 2 gm po single dose **Pregnancy:** See Comment	**For rx failure:** Re-treat with metro 500 mg po bid x 7 days; if 2nd failure: metro 2 gm po q24h x 3-5 days. If still failure, suggest ID consultation and/or contact CDC: 770-488-4115 or www.cdc.gov/std	Treat **male sexual partners (2 gm metronidazole as single dose).** Nearly 20% men with NGU are infected with trichomonas (*JID 188:465, 2003*). For alternative option in refractory cases, see *CID 33:1341, 2007*. **Pregnancy:** No data indicating metro teratogenic or mutagenic (*MMWR 51(RR-6), 2002*). For discussion of treating trichomonas, including issues in pregnancy, see *MMWR 59 (RR-12), 2010; CID 44:S123, 2007*.
Bacterial vaginosis Malodorous vaginal discharge, pH >4.5 Data on recurrence & review: *JID 193:1475, 2006*	Etiology unclear: associated with Gardnerella vaginalis, mobiluncus, Mycoplasma hominis, Prevotella sp., & Atopobium vaginae et al.	**Metro** 0.5 gm po bid x 7 days OR **metro vaginal gel** 5 gm (1 applicator intravaginally) 1x/day x 5 days OR **Tinidazole** (2 gm po once daily x 3 days or 1 gm po once daily x 5 days) 2% **clinda vaginal cream** 5 gm intravaginally at bedtime x 7 days	**Clinda** 0.3 gm po x 7 days OR **clinda ovules** 100 mg intravaginally at bedtime x 3 days.	Reported 50% 1 yr cure rate if abstain from sex or use condoms: *CID 44:213 & 220, 2007*. Treatment of male sex partner **not** indicated unless balanitis present. Metro extended release tabs 750 mg po q24h x 7 days available; no published data. **Pregnancy:** Oral **metro** or oral **clinda**; 7-day regimens (see Canadian OB/GYN practice guidelines in *J.ObstetGynCan 30:702, 2008*). Atopobium resistant to metro in vitro, susceptible to clinda (*BMC Inf Dis 6:51, 2005*); importance unclear.

[13] 1 applicator contains 5 gm of gel with 37.5 mg metronidazole

NOTE: All dosage recommendations are for adults (unless otherwise indicated) and assume normal renal function.

TABLE 1 (24)

ANATOMIC SITE/DIAGNOSIS/ MODIFYING CIRCUMSTANCES	ETIOLOGIES (usual)	SUGGESTED REGIMENS* PRIMARY	SUGGESTED REGIMENS* ALTERNATIVE[†]	ADJUNCT DIAGNOSTIC OR THERAPEUTIC MEASURES AND COMMENTS
GENITAL TRACT (continued)				
Men:				
Balanitis	Candida 40%, Group B strep, gardnerella	**Metro** 2 gm po as a single dose OR **Fluc** 150 mg po x 1 OR **Itra** 200 mg po bid x 1 day.		Occurs in 1/4 of male sex partners of women infected with candida. Exclude circinate balanitis (Reiter's syndrome). Plasma cell balanitis (non-infectious) responds to hydrocortisone cream.
Epididymo-orchitis *Reviews in Brit J Urol Int 87:747, 2001; Andrologia 40:76, 2008.*				
Age <35 years	N. gonorrhoeae, Chlamydia trachomatis	**Ceftriaxone** 250 mg IM x 1 + **doxy** 100 mg po bid x 10 days		Also: bed rest, scrotal elevation, and analgesics. Enterobacteriaceae occasionally encountered. All patients treated for epididymo-orchitis <35 yrs of age should be tested for HIV and syphilis.
Age >35 years or homosexual men (insertive partners in anal intercourse)	Enterobacteriaceae (coliforms)	**Levo** 500-750 mg IV/po once daily) OR (**cipro** 500 mg po bid) or (400 mg IV twice daily) for 10-14 days.	**AM-SB, P Ceph 3, TC-CL, PIP-TZ** *(Dosage: see footnote page 25)*	Also: bed rest, scrotal elevation, and analgesics. Midstream pyuria and scrotal pain and edema. NOTE: Do urine NAAT (nucleic acid amplification test) to ensure absence of N. gonorrhoeae with concomitant risk of FQ-resistant gonorrhoeae or of chlamydia if using agents without reliable activity. Other causes include: mumps, brucella, TB, intravesical BCG, B. pseudomallei, coccidioides, Behçet's *(see Brit J Urol Int 87:747, 2001).*
Non-gonococcal urethritis	*See Chlamydia et al, Non-gonococcal urethritis, Table 1(20), page 23*			
Prostatitis—Review CiD 50:1641, 2010.				
Acute				
Uncomplicated (with risk of STD; age < 35 yrs)	N. gonorrhoeae, C. trachomatis	(**ceftriaxone** 250 mg IM x 1 OR **cefixime** 400 mg po x 1) then **doxy** 100 mg bid x 10 days.		FQs no longer recommended for gonococcal infections. Test for HIV. In AIDS pts, prostate may be focus of Cryptococcus neoformans.
Uncomplicated with low risk of STD	Enterobacteriaceae (coliforms)	**FQ** *(Dosage: see Epididymo-orchitis, >35 yrs, above)* or **TMP-SMX** 1 DS tablet (160 mg TMP) po bid x 10-14 days (minimum). Some authorities recommend 4 weeks of therapy.		Treat as acute urinary infection, 14 days (not single dose regimen). Some authorities recommend 3-4 wks therapy. If uncertain, do urine test for C. trachomatis and of N. gonorrhoeae. If resistant enterobacteriaceae, use ERTA 1 gm IV q24h. If resistant pseudomonas, use IMP or MER (500 mg IV q6 or q8 respectively).
Chronic bacterial	Enterobacteriaceae 80%, enterococci 15%, P. aeruginosa	**FQ** (**CIP** 500 mg po bid x 4-6 wks, **Levo** 750 mg po q24h x 4 wks—see Comment)	**TMP-SMX-DS** 1 tab po bid x 1-3 mos	With treatment failures consider infected prostatic calculi. FDA approved dose of levo is 500 mg; editors prefer higher dose.
Chronic prostatitis/chronic pain syndrome (New NIH classification, *JAMA 282:236, 1999*)	The most common prostatitis syndrome. Etiology is unknown; molecular probe data suggest infectious etiology (*Clin Micro Rev 11: 604, 1998*).	α-adrenergic blocking agents are controversial (*AnIM 133:367, 2000*).		Pt has 3x of prostatitis but negative cultures and no cells in prostatic secretions. Rev. *JAC 46:157, 2000*. In randomized double-blind study, CIP and an alpha-blocker of no benefit (*AnIM 141:581 & 639, 2004*).

Abbreviations on page 2.   NOTE: All dosage recommendations are for adults (unless otherwise indicated) and assume normal renal function.

TABLE 1 (25)

ANATOMIC SITE/DIAGNOSIS/ MODIFYING CIRCUMSTANCES	ETIOLOGIES (usual)	SUGGESTED REGIMENS* PRIMARY	SUGGESTED REGIMENS* ALTERNATIVE[†]	ADJUNCT DIAGNOSTIC OR THERAPEUTIC MEASURES AND COMMENTS
HAND (Bites: See Skin)				
Paronychia Nail biting, manicuring	Staph. aureus (maybe MRSA)	Incision & drainage; do culture	TMP-SMX-DS 1-2 tabs po bid while waiting for culture result.	See Table 6 for alternatives. Occasionally—candida, gram-negative rods.
Contact with oral mucosa—dentists, anesthesiologists, wrestlers	Herpes simplex (Whitlow)	Acyclovir 400 mg tid po x 10 days	Famciclovir or valacyclovir should work, see Comment	Gram stain and routine culture negative. Famciclovir/valacyclovir doses used for primary genital herpes should work; see Table 14A, page 160.
Dishwasher (prolonged water immersion)	Candida sp.	Clotrimazole (topical)		Avoid immersion of hands in water as much as possible.
HEART				
Infective endocarditis—Native valve—empirical rx awaiting cultures—No IV illicit drugs Valvular or congenital heart disease but no modifying circumstances See Table 15C, page 197 for prophylaxis	**NOTE:** Diagnostic criteria include evidence of continuous bacteremia (multiple positive blood cultures), new murmur (worsening of old murmur) of valvular insufficiency, definite emboli, and echocardiographic (transthoracic or transesophageal) evidence of valvular vegetations. Refs.: *Circulation* 111:3167, 2005; *Eur Heart J* 30:2369, 2009. For antimicrobial prophylaxis, see Table 15C, page 197. Viridans strep 30-40%, "other" strep 15-25%, enterococci 5-18%, staphylococci 20-35% (including coag-neg staph)/nococci-CID 46:232, 2008)	[(Pen G 20 million units IV q24h, continuous or div. q4h) or **AMP** 12 gm IV q24h, continuous or div q4h) + (**nafcillin** or **oxacillin** 2 gm IV q4h)] + **gentamicin** 1 mg/kg IM or IV q8h (see Comment)	Vanco 30-60 mg/kg/d in 2-3 divided doses to achieve trough of 15-20 mg/mL + **gentamicin** 1 mg/kg IV q8h) **OR** **dapto** 6 mg/kg IV q24h	If patient not acutely ill and not in heart failure, wait for blood culture results. If initial 3 blood cultures neg. after 24-48 hrs, obtain 2-3 more blood cultures before empiric therapy started. **Nafcillin/oxacillin + gentamicin** may not cover enterococci, hence addition of penicillin or ampicillin pending cultures. When blood cultures +, modify regimen to appropriate therapy for organism. **Gentamicin** used for synergy; peak levels need not exceed 4 mcg per mL. **Surgery indications:** See *Ann Thoracic Surg* 91:2012, 2011.
Infective endocarditis—Native valve—IV illicit drug use ± evidence rt-sided endocarditis—empiric therapy	S. aureus (MSSA & MRSA). All others rare	**Vanco** 30-60 mg/kg per day in 2-3 divided doses to achieve target trough concentrations of 15-20 mg/mL; recommended for serious infections.	**Dapto** 6 mg/kg IV q24h Approved for right-sided endocarditis.	
Infective endocarditis—Native valve—culture positive Viridans strep, S. bovis (S. gallolyticus subsp. gallolyticus) MIC ≤0.12 mcg/mL	Viridans strep, S. bovis (S. gallolyticus subsp. gallolyticus)	[(**Pen G** 12-18 million units/day IV, divided - q4h **x 2 wks**) PLUS (**gentamicin** IV 1 mg/kg IV **x 2 wks**)] **OR** (**Pen G** 12-18 million units/day IV, divided - q4h **x 4 wks**) **OR** (**ceftriaxone** 2 gm IV q24h **x 4 wks**)	(**Ceftriaxone** 2 gm IV q24h + **gentamicin** 1 mg per kg IV q8h both **x 2 wks**). If allergy to pen G or ceftriax, use **vanco** 15 mg/kg IV q12h to 2 gm/day max unless serum levels measured **x 4 wks**	• Target **gent levels:** peak 3 mcg/mL, trough <1 mcg/mL. If very obese pt, recommend consultation for dosage adjustment. • Infuse vanco over ≥1 hr to avoid "red man" syndrome. • **S. bovis suggests occult bowel pathology (new name: S. gallolyticus).** • Since relapse rate may be greater in pts ill for > 3 mos. prior to start of rx, the penicillin-gentamicin synergism theoretically may be advantageous in this group.

Abbreviations on page 2. NOTE: All dosage recommendations are for adults (unless otherwise indicated) and assume normal renal function.

TABLE 1 (26)

ANATOMIC SITE/DIAGNOSIS/ MODIFYING CIRCUMSTANCES	ETIOLOGIES (usual)	SUGGESTED REGIMENS* PRIMARY	ALTERNATIVE[†]	ADJUNCT DIAGNOSTIC OR THERAPEUTIC MEASURES AND COMMENTS
HEART/Infective endocarditis—Native valve—culture positive (continued)				
Viridans strep, S. bovis (S. gallolyticus) with **penicillin G MIC >0.12 to ≤0.5 mcg/mL**	Viridans strep, S. bovis, nutritionally variant streptococci, (e.g., S. abiotrophila) tolerant strep[14].	Pen G 18 million units/day IV (divided q4h) x **4 wks PLUS Gent** 1 mg/kg IV q8h 2 wks **NOTE: Low dose of Gent**	Vanco 15 mg/kg IV q12h to max. 2 gm/day unless serum levels documented x **4 wks**	Can use cefazolin for pen G in pt with allergy that is not IgE-mediated (e.g., anaphylaxis). Alternatively, can use vanco. (See Comment above **NOTE: If necessary to remove infected valve & valve culture neg., 2 weeks antibiotic treatment post-op sufficient** (CID 41:187, 2005). 4 wks of rx if symptoms <3 mos.; 6 wks of rx if symptoms >3 mos. Vanco for pen-allergic pts: do not use cephalosporins
For viridans strep or S. bovis with **pen G MIC >0.5** and enterococci susceptible to AMP/pen G, vanco, gentamicin **NOTE:** Inf. Dis. consultation suggested	"Susceptible" enterococci, viridans strep, S. bovis, nutritionally variant streptococci (new names are: Abiotrophia sp. & Granulicatella sp.)	(Pen G 18-30 million units per 24h IV, divided q4h x **6 wks) PLUS gentamicin** 1-1.5 mg/kg q8h IV x 4-6 wks) **OR (AMP** 12 gm/day IV, divided q4h + **gent** as above x 4-6 wks)	Vanco 15 mg/kg IV q12h to max of 2 gm/day unless serum levels measured **PLUS gentamicin** 1-1.5 mg/kg q8h IV x 4-6 wks **NOTE: Low dose of gent**	Do **not** give gent alone for enterococcal endocarditis. Target gent levels: peak 3 mcg/mL, trough <1 mcg/mL. Vanco target serum levels: peak 20-50 mcg/mL, trough 5-12 mcg/mL. **NOTE:** Because of frequency of resistance (see below), all enterococci causing endocarditis should be tested in vitro for susceptibility to penicillin, gentamicin and vancomycin plus β-lactamase production. 10-25% E. faecalis and 45-50% E. faecium resistant to high gent levels. May be sensitive to streptomycin, check MIC. AMP + Dapto may be another option (Eur J Micro Infect Dis 30:807, 2011).
Enterococci, high-level aminoglycoside resistance		Pen G or AMP IV as above x 8-12 wks (approx. 50% cure)	If prolonged pen G or AMP fails, consider surgical removal of infected valve. See Comment	Case report of success with combination of AMP, IMP, and vanco (Scand J Infect Dis 29:628, 1997). **Cure rate of 67% with IV AMP 2 gm/4h plus ceftriaxone 2 gm/q12h x 6 wks** (AnIM 146:574, 2007). Based on sequential blocking of PBPs 4&5 (Amp) and 2&3 (ceftriaxone).
Enterococci, intrinsic pen G/AMP resistance	Enterococci: pen G MIC >16 mcg/mL; no gentamicin resistance	No reliable effective rx. Can try quinupristin-dalfopristin (Synercid) or linezolid—see Comment, and Table 5A	Teicoplanin active against a subset of vanco-resistant enterococci. Teicoplanin is not available in U.S. Dapto is an option.	Desired vanco serum levels: trough 5-12 mcg/mL. **Gentamicin** used for synergy; peak levels need not exceed 4 mcg/mL. **Synercid** activity limited to E. faecium and is usually bacteriostatic, therefore expect high relapse rate. Dose: 7.5 mg per kg IV (via central line) q8h. **Linezolid** active most enterococci, but bacteriostatic. Dose: 600 mg IV or po q12h. Linezolid failed in pt with E. faecalis endocarditis (CID 37:e29, 2003). **Dapto** bactericidal in vitro, clinical experience in CID 41:1134, 2005. Avoid under dosing (consider 8-10 mg/kg) as resistance may emerge on therapy (CID 52:228, 2011; see also, JAC 65:1126, 2010).
Enterococci: Pen/AMP resistant + high-level gent/strep resistant, usually VRE resistant **Consultation suggested**				
Staphylococcal endocarditis Aortic &/or mitral valve infection—MSSA Surgery indications: see Comment page 28.	Staph. aureus, methicillin-sensitive **Note: Low dose of gentamicin for only 3-5 days.**	Nafcillin (oxacillin) 2 gm IV q4h x 4-6 wks	(Cefazolin 2 gm IV q8h **OR Vanco** 30-60 mg/kg/d in 2-3 divided doses to achieve trough of 15-20 mcg/mL) x 4-6 wks	If IgE-mediated penicillin allergy, 10% cross-reactivity to cephalosporins (AnIM 141:16, 2004). Gentamicin optional. The benefit of low dose gentamicin in improving outcome is unproven and even low-dose gentamicin for only a few days is nephrotoxic (CID 48:713, 2009). If used at all it should be administered for <3-5 days. Cefazolin better tolerated (AAC 55:5122, 2011); in clinical trial (AAC 50:2398, 2006), high failure rate with both vanco and dapto in small numbers of pts. For other alternatives, see Table 6, pg 78. Daptomycin references: JAC 65:1126, 2010; Eur J Clin Micro Infect Dis 30:807, 2011. Case reports of success with Telavancin (JAC 65:1315, 2010; AAC 54:5376, 2010; JAC (Jun 8), 2011) and ceftaroline (JAC 67:1267, 2012; J Infect Chemo online 7/14/12).
Aortic and/or mitral valve—MRSA	Staph. aureus, methicillin-resistant	Vanco 30-60 mg/kg/d IV in 2-3 divided doses to achieve target trough concentrations of 15-20 mcg/mL recommended for serious infections.	Dapto 6 mg/kg IV q24h (NOT FDA approved for this indication or dose)	

[14] Tolerant streptococci = MBC 32-fold greater than MIC NOTE: All dosage recommendations are for adults (unless otherwise indicated) and assume normal renal function.

Abbreviations on page 2.

TABLE 1 (27)

ANATOMIC SITE/DIAGNOSIS/ MODIFYING CIRCUMSTANCES	ETIOLOGIES (usual)	SUGGESTED REGIMENS* PRIMARY	SUGGESTED REGIMENS* ALTERNATIVE[1]	ADJUNCT DIAGNOSTIC OR THERAPEUTIC MEASURES AND COMMENTS
HEART/Infective endocarditis—Native valve—culture positive (continued)				
Tricuspid valve infection (usually IVDUs): MSSA	Staph. aureus, methicillin-sensitive	**Nafcillin (oxacillin)** 2 gm IV q4h **PLUS gentamicin** 1 mg/kg IV q8h x 2 wks. **NOTE: low dose of gent**	If penicillin allergy: **Vanco** 30-60 mg/kg/d in 2-3 divided doses to achieve trough of 15-20 mcg/mL x 4 wks **OR Dapto** 6 mg/kg IV q24h (avoid if concomitant left-sided endocarditis); 8-12 mg/kg IV q24h used in some cases, but not FDA approved	**2-week regimen not long** enough if metastatic infection (e.g. osteo) or left-sided endocarditis. If **Dapto** is used treat for at least 4 weeks. **Dapto** resistance can occur de novo, after or during vanco, or after/during dapto therapy. **Dapto** resistant MRSA killed by combination of **dapto** + **TMP/SMX** or nafcillin (AAC 54:5187, 2010, AAC 56:6192, 2012; worked in 7 pts (CID 53:158, 2011).
Tricuspid valve—MRSA	Staph. aureus, methicillin-resistant	**Vanco** 30-60 mg/kg IV q24h in 2-3 divided doses to achieve target trough concentrations of 15-20 mcg/mL recommended for serious infections	**Dapto** 6 mg/kg IV q24h 4-6 wks equiv to **vanco** for rt-sided endocarditis; both vanco & dapto did poorly if lt-sided endocarditis (NEJM 355: 653, 2006). (See Comments & table 6, page 78)	**Linezolid:** Limited experience (see JAC 58:273, 2006) in patients with few treatment options; 64% cure rate; clear failure in 21%; thrombocytopenia in 31%. **Dapto** dose of 8-12 mg/kg may help in selected cases, but not FDA-approved
Slow-growing fastidious Gm-neg. bacilli–any valve	HACEK group (see Comments)	**Ceftriaxone** 2 gm IV q24h x 4 wks (Bartonella resistant – see below).	**AMP** 2 gm q4h IV (continuous or div. q4h) x 4 wks + **gentamicin** 1 mg/kg IV/IM q8h x 4 wks.	**HACEK** (acronym for **H**aemophilus parainfluenzae, **H. aphrophilus**) **A**ggregatibacter, **A**ctinobacillus, **B**artonella, **C**ardiobacterium, **E**ikenella, **K**ingella). H. aphrophilus resistant to vanco, clinda and methicillin. Penicillinase-positive HACEK organisms should be susceptible to AM-SB + gentamicin.
Bartonella species—any valve	B. henselae, B. quintana	**Ceftriaxone** 2 gm IV q24h x 6 wks + **gentamicin** 1 mg/kg IV q8h x 14 days) 100 mg IV/po bid x 6 wks. If Gent toxicity precludes its use, substitute **Rifampin** 300 mg IV/po bid.		Do immunofluorescent antibody titer ≥1:800; blood cultures only occ. positive, or PCR of tissue from surgery. **Surgery:** Over ½ pts require valve surgery; relation to cure unclear. B. quintana transmitted by body lice among homeless
Infective endocarditis—"culture negative"				
Fever, valvular disease, and ECHO vegetations ± emboli and neg. cultures.		Etiology in 348 cases studied by serology, culture, histopath, & molecular detection: C. burnetti 48%, Bartonella sp. 28%, and rarely (Abiotrophia elegans (nutritionally variant strep), Mycoplasma hominis, Legionella pneumophila, Tropheryma whipplei—together 1%), & test without etiology identified (most on antibiotic). See CID 51:131, 2010 for approach to work-up.		
Infective endocarditis—Prosthetic valve—empiric therapy (cultures pending)	S. aureus now most common etiology (JAMA 297:1354, 2007)			
Early (<2 mos post-op)	S. epidermidis, S. aureus, Rarely, Enterobacteriaceae, diphtheroids, fungi	**Vanco** 15 mg/kg IV q12h + **gentamicin** 1 mg/kg IV q8h + **RIF** 600 mg po q24h		Early surgical consultation advised especially if etiology is S. aureus, evidence of heart failure, new conduction abnormalities, presence of diabetes and/or renal failure, or concern for valve ring abscess (JAMA 297:1354, 2007; CID 44:364, 2007).
Late (>2 mos post-op)	S. epidermidis, viridans strep, enterococci, S. aureus			

Abbreviations on page 2. NOTE: All dosage recommendations are for adults (unless otherwise indicated) and assume normal renal function.

TABLE 1 (28)

ANATOMIC SITE/DIAGNOSIS/ MODIFYING CIRCUMSTANCES	ETIOLOGIES (usual)	SUGGESTED REGIMENS* PRIMARY	ALTERNATIVE[1]	ADJUNCT DIAGNOSTIC OR THERAPEUTIC MEASURES AND COMMENTS
HEART (continued)				
Infective endocarditis—Prosthetic valve—positive blood cultures Treat for 6 weeks even if suspect Viridans Strep. **Surgical consultation advised:** Indications for surgery; severe heart failure, S. aureus infection, prosthetic dehiscence, resistant organism, emboli due to large vegetation (JACC 48 e1, 2006). See also, Eur J Clin Micro Infect. Dis 38:528, 2010.	Staph. epidermidis	(**Vanco** 15 mg IV q12h + **RIF** 300 mg po q8h) **× 6 wks** + **gentamicin** 1 mg/kg IV q8h **× 14 days**		If S. epidermidis is susceptible to nafcillin/oxacillin in vitro (not common), then substitute nafcillin (or oxacillin) for vanco.
	Staph. aureus	Methicillin sensitive: (**Nafcillin** 2 gm IV q4h + **RIF** 300 mg po q8h) **times 6 wks** + **gentamicin** 1 mg per kg IV q8h **times 14 days.** Methicillin resistant: (**Vanco** 1 gm IV q12h + **RIF** 300 mg po q8h) **times 6 wks** + **gentamicin** 1 mg per kg IV q8h **times 14 days.**		
	Viridans strep, enterococci	See infective endocarditis, native valve, culture positive, page 28. Treat for 6 weeks.		
	Enterobacteriaceae or P. aeruginosa.	**Aminoglycoside** (**tobra** if P. aeruginosa) + (**AP Pen** or **P Ceph 3 AP** or **P Ceph 4**)		In theory, could substitute CIP for aminoglycoside, but no clinical data.
	Candida, aspergillus	Table 11, page 113		High mortality. Valve replacement plus antifungal therapy standard therapy but some success with antifungal therapy alone.
Infective endocarditis—Q fever LnID 10:527, 2010; NEJM 356:715, 2007.	Coxiella burnetii	**Doxy** 100 mg po bid + **hydroxychloroquine** 600 mg/day for at least 18 mos (Mayo Clin Proc 83:574, 2008). Pregnancy: Need long term **TMP-SMX** (see CID 45:548, 2007).		**Dx:** Phase 1 IgG titer >800 plus clinical evidence of endocarditis. Treatment duration: 18 mos for native valve, 24 mos for prosthetic valve. Monitor serologically for 5 yrs.
Pacemaker/defibrillator infections	S. aureus (40%), S. epidermidis (40%), Gram-negative bacilli (5%), fungi (5%)	**Device removal** + **vanco** 1 gm IV q12h + **RIF** 300 mg po bid	**Device removal** + **dapto** 6 mg per kg IV q24h[NAI] + **RIF** (no data) 300 mg po bid	**Duration of rx after device removal:** For "pocket" or subcutaneous infection, 10–14 days; if lead-assoc. endocarditis, 4–6 wks depending on organism. Device removal and absence of valve vegetation assoc. with significantly higher survival at 1 yr (JAMA 307:1727, 2012).
Pericarditis, purulent— empiric therapy Ref: Medicine 88: 52, 2009.	Staph. aureus, Strep. pneumoniae, Group A strep, Enterobacteriaceae	**Vanco** + **CIP** (Dosage, see footnote[5])	**Vanco** + **CFP** (see footnote[5])	Drainage required if signs of tamponade. Forced to use empiric vanco due to high prevalence of MRSA.
Rheumatic fever with carditis Ref: Ln 366:155, 2005	Post-infectious sequelae of Group A strep infection (usually pharyngitis)	ASA, and usually prednisone 2 mg/kg q24h for symptomatic treatment of fever, arthritis, arthralgia. May not influence carditis.		Clinical features: Carditis, polyarthritis, chorea, subcutaneous nodules, erythema marginatum. Prophylaxis: see page 61
Ventricular assist device-related infection Ref: LnID 6:426, 2006	S. aureus, S. epidermidis, aerobic gm-neg bacilli, Candida sp	After culture of blood, wounds, drive line, device pocket and maybe pump: **Vanco** 15-20 mg/kg IV q8-12h + (**Cip** 400 mg IV q12h or **levo** 750 mg IV q24h).		Can substitute **daptomycin** 10 mg/kg/d[NAI] for **vanco, cefepime** 2 gm IV q12h for FQ, and (**vori, caspo, micafungin or anidulafungin**) for **fluconazole**. Modify regimen based on results of culture and susceptibility tests. Higher than FDA-approved Dapto dose because of potential emergence of resistance.
JOINT—Also see Lyme Disease, page 58				
Reiter's syndrome (See Comment for definition)		Only treatment is non-steroidal anti-inflammatory drugs		Definition: Urethritis, conjunctivitis, arthritis, and sometimes uveitis and rash. Arthritis: asymmetrical oligoarthritis of ankles, knees, feet, sacroiliitis. Rash: keratoderma blennorrhagica, keratotic lesions, circinate balanitis of glans penis. HLA-B27 positive predisposes to Reiter s.
Reactive arthritis	Occurs wks after infection with C. trachomatis, Campylobacter jejuni, Yersinia enterocolitica, Shigella/Salmonella sp.			

Aminoglycosides (see Table 10D, page 109), **IMP** 0.5 gm IV q6h, **MER** 1 gm IV q8h, **nafcillin** or **oxacillin** 2 gm IV q4h, **TC-CL** 3.1 gm IV q6h or 4.5 gm IV q8h, **AM-SB** 3 gm IV q6h, **P Ceph** 1 (cephapirin 2 gm IV q4h or ceftazidim 2 gm IV q8h), **CIP** 750 mg po bid or 400 mg IV q12h, **vanco** 1 gm IV q12h, **aztreonam** 2 gm IV q8h, **CFP** 2 gm IV q12h

Abbreviations on page 2.   NOTE: All dosage recommendations are for adults (unless otherwise indicated) and assume normal renal function.

TABLE 1 (29)

ANATOMIC SITE/DIAGNOSIS/ MODIFYING CIRCUMSTANCES	ETIOLOGIES (usual)	SUGGESTED REGIMENS* PRIMARY	SUGGESTED REGIMENS* ALTERNATIVE[$\dagger$]	ADJUNCT DIAGNOSTIC OR THERAPEUTIC MEASURES AND COMMENTS
JOINT/Reactive arthritis (continued)				
Poststreptococcal reactive arthritis (See Rheumatic fever, above)	Immunologic reaction after strep pharyngitis; (1) arthritis onset in <10 days, (2) lasts months; (3) unresponsive to ASA	Treat strep pharyngitis and then NSAIDs (prednisone needed in some pts)		A reactive arthritis after a β-hemolytic strep infection in absence of sufficient Jones criteria for acute rheumatic fever. Ref.: Mayo Clin Proc 75:144, 2000.
Septic arthritis: Treatment requires both adequate drainage of purulent joint fluid and appropriate antimicrobial therapy. **There is no need to inject antimicrobials into joints.** Empiric therapy after collection of blood and joint fluid for culture; review Gram stain of joint fluid.				
Infants <3 mos (neonate)	Staph. aureus, Enterobacteriaceae, Group B strep	If MRSA not a concern: (Nafcillin or oxacillin) + P Ceph 3	If MRSA a concern: (Cefotaxime, ceftizoxime or ceftriaxone)	Blood cultures frequently positive. Adjacent bone involved in 2/3 pts. Group B strep and gonococci most common community-acquired etiologies.
Children (3 mos-14 yrs)	Staph. aureus 27%, S. pyogenes & S. pneumo 14%, H. influenzae 3%, Gm-neg. bacilli 6%, other (GC, N. meningitidis) 14%, unknown 36%.	Vanco + (Dosage, see Table 16, page 203) until culture results available See Table 16 for dosage Steroids—see Comment		Marked ↓ in H. influenzae since use of conjugate vaccine. NOTE: Septic arthritis due to salmonella has no association with sickle cell disease, unlike salmonella osteomyelitis. 10 days of therapy as effective as a 30-day treatment course if there is a good clinical response and CRP levels normalize quickly (CID 48:1201, 2009).
Adults (review Gram stain): See page 58 for Lyme Disease and page 58 for gonococcal arthritis				
Acute monoarticular At risk for sexually-transmitted disease	N. gonorrhoeae (see page 23), S. aureus, streptococci, rarely aerobic Gm-neg. bacilli	Gram stain negative: Ceftriaxone 1 gm IV q24h or cefotaxime 1 gm IV q8h or ceftizoxime 1 gm IV q8h	If Gram stain shows Gm+ cocci in clusters: vanco 1 gm IV q12h; if >100 kg, 1.5 gm IV q12h.	For treatment comments, see Disseminated GC, page 23
Not at risk for sexually-transmitted disease	S. aureus, streptococci, Gm-neg. bacilli	All empiric choices guided by Gram stain Vanco + P Ceph 3	Vanco + (CIP or Levo) For dosage, see footnote page 70 For treatment duration, see Table 3, page 34 See Table 2 & Table 12	Differential includes gout and chondrocalcinosis (pseudogout). **Look for crystals in joint fluid.** NOTE: See Table 6 for MRSA treatment.
Chronic monoarticular	Brucella, nocardia, mycobacteria, fungi			
Polyarticular, usually acute	Gonococci, B. burgdorferi, acute rheumatic fever, viruses, (e.g. hepatitis B, rubella vaccine, parvo B19	Gram stain usually negative for GC. If sexually active, culture urethra, cervix, anal canal, throat, blood, joint fluid, and then: ceftriaxone 1 gm IV q24h		If GC, usually associated petechiae and/or pustular skin lesions and tenosynovitis. Consider Lyme disease if exposure areas known to harbor infected ticks. See page 58. Expanded differential includes gout, pseudogout, reactive arthritis (HLA-B27 pos.).
Septic arthritis, post intra-articular injection	MSSE/MRSE 40%, MSSA/MRSA 20%, P. aeruginosa, Propionibacteria, mycobacteria	NO empiric therapy. Arthroscopy for culture/sensitivity, crystals, washout		Treat based on culture results × 14 days (assumes no foreign body present).

Abbreviations on page 2.   NOTE: All dosage recommendations are for adults (unless otherwise indicated) and assume normal renal function.

TABLE 1 (30)

ANATOMIC SITE/DIAGNOSIS/ MODIFYING CIRCUMSTANCES	ETIOLOGIES (usual)	SUGGESTED REGIMENS* PRIMARY	ALTERNATIVE[†]	ADJUNCT DIAGNOSTIC OR THERAPEUTIC MEASURES AND COMMENTS
JOINT (continued)				
Infected prosthetic joint (PJI) • Suspect if: new sinus tract or wound drainage; acutely painful prosthesis; chronically painful prosthesis; or high ESR/CRP assoc. w/painful prosthesis. • **Empiric therapy is NOT recommended.** Treat based on culture and sensitivity results. • **3 surgical options:** 1) debridement and prosthesis retention (if sx < 3 wks or implantation < 30 days); 2) 1 stage, direct exchange; 3) 2 stage: debridement, removal, reimplantation. • **IDSA Guidelines:** *CID 56:e1, 2013.*	MSSA/MSSE	**Debridement/Retention:** [(Nafcillin 2 gm IV q4h or Oxacillin 2 gm IV q4h IV) + Rifampin 300 mg po bid] OR (Cefazolin 2 gm IV q8h + Rifampin 300 mg po bid) x 2-6 wks-followed by [(Ciprofloxacin 750 mg po bid or Levofloxacin 750 mg po q24h) + Rifampin 300 mg po bid] for 3-6 months (shorter duration for total hip arthroplasty) **1-stage exchange:** IV/PO regimen as above for 3 mos **2-stage exchange:** regimen as above for 4-6 wks	**Debridement/Retention:** (Vancomycin 15-20 mg/kg IV q8-12h + Rifampin 300 mg po bid) x 2-6 weeks followed by [(Ciprofloxacin 750 mg po bid OR Levofloxacin 750 mg po q24h) + Rifampin 300 mg po bid] for 3-6 months (shorter duration for total hip arthroplasty) **1-stage exchange:** IV/PO regimen as above for 3 mos **2-stage exchange:** regimen as above for 4-6 wks	**Confirm isolate susceptibility to fluoroquinolone and rifampin:** consider using other active highly bioavailable agent, e.g., TMP-SMX, Doxy, Minocycline, Amoxicillin-Clavulanate, Clindamycin, or Cefadroxil. Enterococcal infection: addition of aminoglycoside optional. *P. aeruginosa* infection: consider adding aminoglycoside if isolate is susceptible (but if this improves outcome unclear). Prosthesis retention most important risk factor for treatment failure *(Clin Microbiol Infect 16:1789, 2010).*
	MRSA/MRSE	**Debridement/Retention:** (Vancomycin 15-20 mg/kg IV q8-12h + Rifampin 300 mg po bid) x 2-6 weeks followed by [(Ciprofloxacin 750 mg po bid OR Levofloxacin 750 mg po q24h) + Rifampin 300 mg po bid] for 3-6 months (shorter duration for total hip arthroplasty) **1-stage exchange:** IV/PO regimen as above for 3 mos **2-stage exchange:** regimen as above for 4-6 wks	(Daptomycin 6-8 mg/kg IV q24h OR Linezolid 600 mg po/IV bid) ± Rifampin 300 mg po bid	(Linezolid 600 mg + Rifampin 300 mg) may be effective as salvage therapy if device removal not possible *(Antimicrob Agents Chemother 55:4308, 2011).* If prosthesis is retained, consider long-term, suppressive therapy, particularly for staphylococcal infections, depending on in vitro susceptibility options include TMP-SMX, Doxycycline, Minocycline, Amoxicillin, Ciprofloxacin, Cephalexin. Culture yield may be increased by sonication of prosthesis *(N Engl J Med 357:654, 2007).*
	Streptococci (Grps A, B, C, D, viridans, other)	**Debridement/Retention: Pen-susceptible:** Penicillin G 20 million units IV continuous infusion q24h or in 6 divided doses OR Ceftriaxone 2 gm IV q24h x 4-6 weeks	Vancomycin 15 mg/kg IV q12h	Other treatment consideration: Rifampin is bactericidal vs. biofilm-producing bacteria. Never use Rifampin alone due to rapid development of resistance. Rifampin 300 mg po bid + Fusidic acid[NUS] 500 mg IV bid is another option *(Clin Micro Inf 12(S3):93, 2006).*
	Enterococci	**Debridement/Retention: Pen-susceptible:** Ampicillin 12 gm IV OR Penicillin G 20 million units IV continuous infusion q24h or in 6 divided doses x 4-6 weeks **Pen-resistant:** Vancomycin 15 mg/kg IV q12h x 4-6 weeks **1 or 2 stage exchange:** regimen as above for 4-6 wks	Daptomycin 6-8 mg/kg IV q24h OR Linezolid 600 mg po/IV bid	
	Propionibacterium acnes	**Debridement/Retention:** Ertapenem 1 gm IV q24h OR continuous infusion or in 4 divided doses OR Ceftriaxone 2 gm IV q24h x 4-6 weeks **1 or 2 stage exchange:** regimen as above for 4-6 wks	Vancomycin 15 mg/kg IV q12h OR Clindamycin 300-450 mg po qid	Watch for toxicity of Linezolid if used for more than 2 weeks of therapy.
	Gm-neg enteric bacilli	**Debridement/Retention:** Cefepime 1 gm IV q8h or other beta-lactam (e.g., Ceftazidime 2 gm IV q24h OR Cefepime 2 gm IV q12h, based on susceptibility) x 4-6 weeks **1 or 2 stage exchange:** regimen as above for 4-6 wks	Ciprofloxacin 750 mg po bid	
	P. aeruginosa	**Debridement/Retention:** Meropenem 1 gm IV q8h + Tobramycin 5.1 mg/kg once daily IV **1 or 2 stage exchange:** regimen as above for 4-6 wks	Ciprofloxacin 750 mg po bid or 400 mg IV q8h	
Rheumatoid arthritis	TNF inhibitors (adalimumab, certolizumab, etanercept, golimumab, infliximab) ↑ risk of TBc, fungal infection, listeria, and malignancy. (LnID 8:601, 2008; Med Lett 51:55, 2009) treat latent TBc first. Tocilizumab (IL-6 receptor inhibitor) and James kinase inhibitor (tofacitinib) also increase infection risk (Cell Microbiol 12:301, 2010; Expert Rev Clin Immunol 7:229, 2011).				Immunosuppression, not duration of therapy, is a risk factor for recurrence; 7 days of therapy may be sufficient for immunocompetent patients undergoing one-stage bursectomy. (JAC 65:1008, 2010).
Septic bursitis; Olecranon bursitis; prepatellar bursitis	Staph. aureus >80%, M. tuberculosis (rare), M. marinum (rare)	**Nafcillin or oxacillin** 2 gm IV q4h or **dicloxacillin** 500 mg po qid if **MSSA**	(**Vanco** 15-20 mg/kg IV q8-12h or **linezolid** 600 mg po bid) if **MRSA**	

Other doses, see footnote page 34

Abbreviations on page 2.   NOTE: All dosage recommendations are for adults (unless otherwise indicated) and assume normal renal function.

TABLE 1 (31)

ANATOMIC SITE/DIAGNOSIS/ MODIFYING CIRCUMSTANCES	ETIOLOGIES (usual)	SUGGESTED REGIMENS* PRIMARY	SUGGESTED REGIMENS* ALTERNATIVE[1]	ADJUNCT DIAGNOSTIC OR THERAPEUTIC MEASURES AND COMMENTS
KIDNEY, BLADDER AND PROSTATE				
Acute uncomplicated urinary tract infection (cystitis-urethritis) in females				
NOTE: Resistance of E. coli to TMP-SMX approx. 15–20% & correlates with microbiological clinical failure. **Recent reports of resistance to FQs as well.** 5-day **nitrofurantoin** IDSA Treatment Guidelines, CID 52:e103, 2011.	Enterobacteriaceae (E. coli), Staph. saprophyticus, enterococci	**<20% of Local E. coli resistant to TMP-SMX & no sulfa allergy: TMP-SMX-DS** bid x 3 days. If sulfa allergy, **Nitrofurantoin** 100 mg po bid x 5 days or **fosfomycin** 3 gm po x one dose. All plus **Pyridium**	**>20% Local E. coli resistant to TMP-SMX or sulfa allergy:** then 3 days of **CIP** 250 mg bid, **CIP-ER** 500 mg q24h, **Levo** 250 mg q24h, **OR Moxi** 400 mg q24h **OR Nitrofurantoin** 100 mg q24h or **fosfomycin** 3 gm po x one dose. All plus **Pyridium**	7-day rx recommended **in pregnancy** (discontinue or do not use sulfonamides (TMP-SMX) near term (2 weeks before EDC) because of potential f in kernicterus). If failure on 3-day course, culture and rx 2 weeks. **Fosfomycin** 3 gm po times 1 less effective vs. E. coli than multi-dose rx, but OK for Enterococci & 15–20% more active vs E. faecalis, and other coliforms. **Moxifloxacin:** Not approved for UTIs. Moxi equivalent to comparator drugs in unpublished clinical trials (on file with Bayer). Therapy of **ESBL producing E. coli and Klebsiella spp.** problematic because of multiple drug resistances; ESBL producers susceptible to fosfomycin, ertapenem, and combo of amox-clav + cefdinir in vitro (AAC 53:1278, 2009). Amox-Clav or an oral cephalosporin are options, but generally less efficacious. **Phenazopyridine (Pyridium)**—non-prescription— may relieve dysuria: 200 mg po tid times 2 days. Hemolysis if G6PD deficient. Pelvic exam for vaginitis & herpes simplex, urine LCR/PCR for GC and C. trachomatis.
Risk factors for STD. Dipstick-positive leukocyte esterase or hemoglobin, neg. Gram stain. **Recurrent** (3 or more episodes/year) in young women	C. trachomatis	Azithro 1 gm po single dose	Doxy 100 mg po bid 7 days	
	Any of the above bacteria	Eradicate infection, then **TMP-SMX** 1 single-strength tab po q24h long term		A cost-effective alternative to continuous prophylaxis is self-administered single dose rx (TMP-SMX DS 2 tabs, 320/1600 mg) at symptom onset. Another alternative: 1 DS tablet TMP-SMX post-coitus.
Child: ≤5 yrs old & grade 3–4 reflux	Coliforms	**TMP-SMX** 8-12 mg/kg/day (based on TMP comp) div q12h (or **nitrofurantoin** 2 mg per kg po q24h)	**CIP** approved as alternative drug ages 1–17 yrs.	
Recurrent UTI in postmenopausal women	E. coli & other Enterobacteriaceae, enterococcus, S. saprophyticus	Treat as for uncomplicated UTI. Evaluate for potentially correctable urologic factors—see Comment. **Nitrofurantoin** more effective than vaginal cream in decreasing frequency, but Editors worry about pulmonary fibrosis with long-term NF use.		Definition: ≥3 culture + symptomatic UTIs in 6 months. Urologic factors: (1) cystocele, (2) incontinence, (3) ↑ residual urine volume
Acute uncomplicated pyelonephritis (usually women 18–40 yrs., temperature >102°F., definite costovertebral tenderness) [NOTE: Culture of urine and blood indicated prior to therapy.] **If male, look for obstructive uropathy or other complicating pathology.**				
Moderately ill (outpatient) **NOTE:** May need one IV dose due to nausea. Resistance of E. coli to TMP/SMX, 30% in a collaborative ER study (CID 47:1150, 2008).	Enterobacteriaceae (most likely E. coli, enterococci (Gm stain of uncentrifuged urine may allow identification of Gm-neg. bacilli vs. Gm+ cocci)	**FQ** po times 5–7 days: **CIP** 500 mg bid or **CIP-ER** 1000 mg q24h, **Levo** 750 mg q24h, **Oflox** 400 mg bid, **Moxi**[NA] 400 mg q24h possibly ok—see comment.	**AM-CL, O Ceph, or TMP-SMX-DS po.** Treat for 14 days. **Beta-lactams** not as effective as FQs: JAMA 293:949, 2005	7 day course of **Cipro** 500 mg bid as effective as 14 day course in women (Lancet 380:484, 2012) Since **CIP** worked with 7-day rx, suspect other FOs effective with 7 days of therapy; **Levo** 750 mg FDA-approved for 5 days. Ref: NEJM 366:1028, 2012.

[16] **AM-CL** 875/125 mg po q12h or 500/125 mg po tid or 2000/125 mg po bid or Antipseudomonal penicillins: **AM-SB**, 3 gm IV q4-6h; **PIP** 3 gm IV q4-6h; **PIP-TZ** 3.375 gm IV q6h (4.5 gm IV q8h for pseudomonas; **TC-CL** 3.1 gm IV q6h. Antipseudomonal cephalosporins: **ceftaz** 2 gm IV q8h, **cefepime** 2 gm IV q8h; Carbapenems: **DORI** 500 mg IV q8h (1 hr infusion); **ERTA** 1 gm IV q24h; **IMP** 0.5 gm IV q12h (max 4 gm/day); **MER** 1 gm IV q8h; Parenteral cephalosporins: **cefotaxime** 1 gm IV q8h (2 gm IV q4h for severe infection); **cefoxitin** 1-2 gm IV q6h; **ceftriaxone** 1-2 gm IV q24h; Oral cephalosporins— see Table 10A page 96; **dicloxacillin** 500 mg po q6h; **FQs:** Oral **Cipro** 500-750 mg po q12h; **Levo** 750 mg IV q24h; **gentamicin**— see Table 10D, page 109; **linezolid** 600 mg IV/po q12h; **metro** 500 mg po q6h or 15 mg/kg IV q12h (max 4 gm/day); **nafcillin/oxacillin** 2 gm IV q4h; **TMP-SMX** 2 mg/kg (TMP component) IV q6h; **vanco** 1 gm IV q12h (if over 100 kg, 1.5 gm IV q12h).

Abbreviations on page 2.   NOTE: All dosage recommendations are for adults (unless otherwise indicated) and assume normal renal function.

TABLE 1 (32)

KIDNEY, BLADDER AND PROSTATE/Acute uncomplicated pyelonephritis (continued)

ANATOMIC SITE/DIAGNOSIS/ MODIFYING CIRCUMSTANCES	ETIOLOGIES (usual)	SUGGESTED REGIMENS* PRIMARY	SUGGESTED REGIMENS* ALTERNATIVE[1]	ADJUNCT DIAGNOSTIC OR THERAPEUTIC MEASURES AND COMMENTS
Acute pyelonephritis—Hospitalized	E. coli most common, enterococci 2nd in frequency	FQ (IV) or (AMP + gentamicin) or ceftriaxone or PIP-TZ. Treat for 14 days. Dosages in footnote[16] on page 34. Do not use cephalosporins or ampicillin for suspect or proven enterococcal infection	TC-CL or AM-SB or PIP-TZ or ERTA or DORI: 500 mg q8h. Treat for 14 days.	Treat IV until pt afebrile 24–48 hrs, then complete 2-wks course with oral drugs (as Moderate); ill, above). DORI approved for 10 day treatment. If pt hypotensive, prompt imaging (Ultrasound or CT) is recommended to ensure absence of obstructive uropathy. NOTE: Cephalosporins and ertapenem not active vs. enterococci.
Complicated UTI/catheters—obstruction, reflux, azotemia, transplant, Foley catheter-related, R/O obstruction; multi-drug resistant gram-neg bacilli. For IDSA Guidelines: CID 50:625, 2010.	Enterobacteriaceae, P. aeruginosa, enterococci, rarely S. aureus	(AMP + gent) or PIP-TZ, TC-CL, or DORI or IMP or MER for up to 2-3 wks Switch to po FQ or TMP-SMX when possible. For dosages, see footnote[16] on page 34.	Ceftaz or CFP for 2–3 wks	Not all listed drugs predictably active vs. enterococci or P. aeruginosa. CIP approved for children (1-17 yrs) as alternative. Not 1st choice secondary to increased incidence joint adverse effects. Peds dose: 6-10 mg/kg (400 mg max) IV q8h or 10-20 mg/kg (750 mg max) po q12h. Treat for 7 days for catheter-associated UTI if prompt resolution of symptoms and 10-14 days if delayed response; a 3-day course of therapy may be consider for women < 65 years of age (CID 50:625, 2010)
Asymptomatic bacteriuria. IDSA Guidelines; CID 40:643, 2005; U.S. Preventive Services Task Force AnIM 149:43, 2008. Base regimen on C&S, not empirical				
Preschool children				Diagnosis requires ≥10⁵ CFU per mL urine of same bacterial species in 2 specimens obtained 3-7 days apart.
Pregnancy	Aerobic Gm-neg. bacilli & Staph. hemolyticus	Screen 1st trimester. If positive, rx 3-7 days with amox. nitrofurantoin, O Ceph. TMP-SMX or TMP alone		Screen monthly for recurrence. Some authorities treat continuously until delivery (stop TMP-SMX 2 wks before EDC); ↑ resistance of E. coli to TMP-SMX.
Before and after invasive urologic intervention, or Foley catheter	Aerobic Gm-neg. bacilli	Obtain urine culture and then rx 3 days with TMP-SMX DS, bid. For prevention of UTI: Consider removal after 72 hrs (CID 46:243 & 251, 2008).		Clinical benefit of antimicrobial-coated Foley catheters is uncertain (AnIM 144:116, 2006). (CID 60:625, 2010).
Neurogenic bladder – see "spinal cord injury" below		No therapy if asymptomatic patient; intermittent catheterization if possible		Ref.: AJM 113(1A):67S, 2002 - Bacteriuria in spinal cord injured patient
Asymptomatic, advanced age, male or female. Ref: CID 40:643, 2005		No therapy indicated unless in conjunction with surgery to correct obstructive uropathy; measure residual urine vol. in females; prostate exam/PSA in males. No screening recommended in men and non-pregnant women (AnIM 149:43, 2008)		
Malacoplakia	E. coli	Bethanechol chloride + (CIP or TMP-SMX)		Chronic pyelo with abnormal inflammatory response.
Perinephric abscess Associated with staphylococcal bacteremia	Staph. aureus	If MSSA: Nafcillin/oxacillin or cefazolin (Dosage, see footnote[6], page 34)	If MRSA: Vanco 1 gm IV q12h OR dapto 6 mg/kg IV q24h	Drainage, surgical or image-guided aspiration
Associated with pyelonephritis	Enterobacteriaceae	See pyelonephritis, complicated UTI, above		Drainage, surgical or image-guided aspiration
Post Renal Transplant Obstructive Uropathy (CID 46:825, 2008)	Corynebacterium urealyticum	Vanco or Teicoplanin[NUS]		Organism can synthesize struvite stones. Requires 48-72 hr incubation to detect in culture
Prostatitis		See prostatitis, page 27		
Spinal cord injury pts with UTI	E. coli, Klebsiella sp, enterococci	CIP 250 mg po bid x 14 days		If fever, suspect assoc. pyelonephritis. Microbiologic cure greater after 14 vs. 3 days of CIP (CID 39:658 & 665, 2004); for asymptomatic bacteriuria see AJM 113(1A):67S, 2002.

Abbreviations on page 2. NOTE: All dosage recommendations are for adults (unless otherwise indicated) and assume normal renal function.

TABLE 1 (33)

ANATOMIC SITE/DIAGNOSIS/ MODIFYING CIRCUMSTANCES	ETIOLOGIES (usual)	SUGGESTED REGIMENS* PRIMARY	SUGGESTED REGIMENS* ALTERNATIVE[1]	ADJUNCT DIAGNOSTIC OR THERAPEUTIC MEASURES AND COMMENTS
LIVER (for spontaneous bacterial peritonitis, see page 47)				
Cholangitis		See Gallbladder, page 17		
Cirrhosis & variceal bleeding	Esophageal flora	(Norfloxacin 400 mg po bid or CIP 400 mg IV q12h) x max. of 7 days	Ceftriaxone 1 gm IV once daily for max. of 7 days	Short term prophylactic antibiotics in cirrhotics with G-I hemorr., with or without ascites, decreases rate of bacterial infection & ↑ survival (Hepatology 46:922, 2007).
Hepatic abscess Klebsiella liver abscess ref.: Ln 12:881, 2012	Enterobacteriaceae (esp. Klebsiella sp.), bacteroides, enterococci, Entamoeba histolytica, with anaerobes without. For cat-scratch disease (CSD), see pages 45 & 57	Metro + (ceftriaxone or cefoxitin or TC-CL or PIP-TZ or AM-SB or CIP or levo) (Dosage, see footnote[15] on page 34)	Metro (for amoeba) + either IMP, MER or Dori (Dosage, see footnote on page 34)	Serological tests for amebiasis should be done on all patients; if neg., surgical drainage or percutaneous aspiration. In pyogenic abscess, ½ have identifiable GI source or underlying biliary tract disease. If amoeba serology positive, treat with metro alone without surgery. Empiric metro included for both E. histolytica & bacteroides. Hemochromatosis associated with Yersinia enterocolitica liver abscess; regimens listed are effective for yersinia. Klebsiella pneumonia genotype K1 associated ocular & CNS Klebsiella infections (CID 45:284, 2007).
Hepatic encephalopathy	Urease-producing gut bacteria	Rifaximin 550 mg po bid (take with lactulose)		Refs: NEJM 362:1071, 2010; Med Lett 52:87, 2010.
Leptospirosis	Leptospirosis, see page 60	See page 57		
Peliosis hepatis in AIDS pts	Bartonella henselae and B			
Post-transplant infected "bilioma"	Enterococci (incl. VRE), candida, Gm-neg. bacilli (P. aeruginosa 8%), anaerobes 5%	Linezolid 600 mg IV bid + CIP 400 mg IV q12h + fluconazole 400 IV q24h	Dapto 6 mg/kg per day + Levo 750 mg IV q24h + fluconazole 400 IV q24h	Suspect if fever & abdominal pain post-transplant. Exclude hepatic artery thrombosis. Presence of candida and/or VRE bad prognosticators.
Viral hepatitis	Hepatitis A, B, C, D, E, G	See Table 14F and Table 14G		
LUNG/Bronchi				
Bronchiolitis/wheezy bronchitis (expiratory wheezing) Infants/children (≤ age 5) See RSV, Table 14A, page 167 Ref: Ln 368:312, 2006	Respiratory syncytial virus (RSV) 50%, parainfluenza 25%, human metapneumovirus	Antibiotics not useful, mainstay of therapy is oxygen. Ribavirin for severe disease: 6 gm vial (20 mg/mL) in sterile H₂O by SPAG-2 generator over 18-20 hrs daily times 3-5 days.		RSV most important. Rapid diagnosis with antigen detection methods. For prevention a humanized monoclonal antibody, **palivizumab** See Table 14A, page 167. RSV immune globulin is no longer available. Review: Red Book of Peds 2006, 27ᵗʰ Ed.
Bronchitis				
Infants/children (≤ age 5)	< Age 2: Adenovirus; age 2-5: parainfluenza 3 virus, human metapneumovirus	Antibiotics not indicated.		
Adolescents and adults with acute tracheobronchitis (Acute bronchitis) Ref.: NEJM 355:2125, 2006	Usually viral. M. pneumoniae 5%, C. pneumoniae 5%. See Persistent cough, below	Antitussive ± inhaled bronchodilators		Antibiotics indicated only with associated sinusitis for S. pneumo., Group A strep, H. influenzae or no improvement in 1 week. Otherwise rx is symptomatic. Purulent sputum alone not an indication for antibiotic therapy. Expect cough to last 2 weeks. If fever/rigors, get chest x-ray. If mycoplasma documented, prefer doxy over macrolides.

Abbreviations on page 2. NOTE: All dosage recommendations are for adults (unless otherwise indicated) and assume normal renal function.

TABLE 1 (34)

LUNG/Bronchi/Bronchus (continued)

ANATOMIC SITE/DIAGNOSIS/ MODIFYING CIRCUMSTANCES	ETIOLOGIES (usual)	SUGGESTED REGIMENS* PRIMARY	SUGGESTED REGIMENS* ALTERNATIVE[1]	ADJUNCT DIAGNOSTIC OR THERAPEUTIC MEASURES AND COMMENTS
Persistent cough (>14 days), afebrile during community outbreak: Pertussis (whooping cough) >14 days have pertussis (MMWR 54:(RR-14), 2005). Review: *Chest* 130:547, 2006	Bordetella pertussis & occ. Bordetella parapertussis. Also consider asthma, gastroesophageal reflux, post-nasal drip	**Peds doses: Azithro / clarithro** OR **erythro estolate**[17] OR **erythro base**[17] OR **TMP-SMX** (doses in footnote[17])	**Adult doses: Azithro** po 500 mg day 1, then 250 mg q24h days 2-5 OR **erythro estolate** 500 mg po qid times 14 days OR **TMP-SMX DS** 1 tab po bid times 14 days OR **clarithro** 500 mg po bid or 1 gm ER q24h times 7 days)	**3 stages of illness:** catarrhal (1-2 wks), paroxysmal coughing (2-4 wks), and convalescence (1-2 wks). Treatment may abort or eliminate pertussis in catarrhal stage, but does not shorten paroxysmal stage. **Diagnosis:** PCR for nasal aspirates, or nasopharyngeal washings, or culture of NP swab. **Rx aimed at eradication of NP carriage.** In non-outbreak setting, likelihood of pertussis increased if post-tussive emesis or inspiratory whoop present (*JAMA* 304:890, 2010).
Pertussis: Prophylaxis of household contacts	Drugs and doses as per treatment immediately above			Recommended by Am. Acad. Ped. Red Book 2006 for all household or close contacts; community-wide prophylaxis not recommended
Acute bacterial exacerbation of chronic bronchitis (ABECB) adults (almost always smokers with COPD) Ref: *NEJM* 359:2355, 2008.	Viruses 20–50%, C. pneumoniae 5%, M. pneumoniae <1%; role of S. pneumo, H. influenzae & M. catarrhalis controversial. Tobacco use, air pollution contribute. Non-pathogenic H. haemolyticus may be mistaken for H. influenza (*IJID* 195:81, 2007).	**Severe ABECB** = ↑ dyspnea, ↑ sputum viscosity/purulence; ↑ sputum volume. For severe ABECB: (1) consider chest x-ray, esp. if febrile &/or low O₂ sat, (2) inhaled anticholinergic bronchodilator; (3) oral corticosteroid; taper over 2 wks (*Cochrane Library* 3, 2006); (4) D/C tobacco use; (5) non-invasive positive pressure ventilation. **Role of antimicrobial therapy debated even for severe disease, no antimicrobial treatment** or may be AM-CL, azithro/clarithro, or O Ceph or FQs with enhanced activity vs. drug-resistant S. pneumo (Gemi, Levo, or Moxi). **For severe disease,** AM-CL, azithro/clarithro, or O Ceph or FQs with enhanced activity vs. drug-resistant S. pneumo (Gemi, Levo, or Moxi). **Drugs & doses in footnote. Duration** varies with drug; range 3–10 days. Limit Gemi to 5 days to decrease risk of rash. Azithro 250 mg daily x 1 yr modestly reduced frequency of acute exacerbations in pts with milder disease (*NEJM* 365:689, 2011).		
Fever, cough, myalgia during Influenza season, 2009 regarding novel H1N1 Influenza A)	Influenza A & B	See *Influenza,* Table 14A, page 164.		**Complications: Influenza pneumonia, secondary bacterial pneumonia** Community MRSA and MSSA, S. pneumoniae, H. influenzae.
Bronchiectasis. Ref: *Chest* 134:815, 2008 Acute exacerbation	H. influ., P. aeruginosa, and rarely S. pneumo.	**Gemi, levo, or moxi** bid x 7-10 days. *Dosage in footnote*.	One option: **Erythro** 500 mg po bid or **azithro** 250 mg q24h x 8 wks.	Many potential etiologies: obstruction, ↓ immune globulins, cystic fibrosis, dyskinetic cilia, tobacco, prior severe or recurrent necrotizing bronchitis e.g. pertussis.
Prevention of exacerbation	Not applicable			
Specific organisms	Aspergillus (see *Table 11*) MAI (*Table 12*) and P. aeruginosa (*Table 5A*).			

[17] **ADULT DOSAGE: AM-CL:** 875/125 mg po bid or 500/125 mg po bid or 2000/125 mg po bid; **azithro** 500 mg po x 1 dose, then 250 mg q24h x 3 days; *Oral cephalosporins:* **cefaclor** 500 mg po q8h or 500 mg extended release q12h; **cefdinir** 300 mg po q12h or 600 mg po q24h; **cefditoren** 200-400 mg q24h; **cefixime** 400 mg po q24h; **cefpodoxime proxetil** 200 mg q12h; **cefprozil** 500 mg po q12h; **ceftibuten** 400 mg po q24h; **cefuroxime axetil** 250 or 500 mg po q12h; **clarithro** extended release 1000 mg po q24h; **doxy** 100 mg po bid; **erythro base** 40 mg/kg/day po div q6h; **erythro estolate** 40 mg/kg/day po div qid; FQs: **CIP** 750 mg po q12h; **gemi** 320 mg po q24h; **levo** 500 mg po q24h; **moxi** 400 mg po q24h; **TMP-SMX** 1 DS tab po bid.
PEDS DOSAGE: azithro 10 mg/kg/day po div q24h x 4 days; **clarithro** 7.5 mg/kg po q24h x 4 days; **erythro base** 40 mg/kg/day div q8-12h; **erythro estolate** 40 mg/kg/day div q6h (>6 mos. of age) 8 mg/kg/day (TMP component) div bid.
TMP-SMX (>6 mos. of age) 8 mg/kg/day (TMP component) div bid.

Abbreviations on page 2.   NOTE: *All dosage recommendations are for adults (unless otherwise indicated) and assume normal renal function.*

TABLE 1 (35)

ANATOMIC SITE/DIAGNOSIS/ MODIFYING CIRCUMSTANCES	ETIOLOGIES (usual)	SUGGESTED REGIMENS* PRIMARY	ALTERNATIVE[1]	ADJUNCT DIAGNOSTIC OR THERAPEUTIC MEASURES AND COMMENTS
LUNG/Bronchi (continued)				
Pneumonia: CONSIDER TUBERCULOSIS IN ALL PATIENTS; ISOLATE ALL SUSPECT PATIENTS				
Neonatal: Birth to 1 month	Viruses: CMV, rubella, H. simplex. Bacteria: Group B strep, listeria, coliforms, S. aureus, P. aeruginosa. Other: Chlamydia trachomatis, syphilis	AMP + gentamicin ± cefotaxime. Add vanco if MRSA a concern. For chlamydia therapy, erythro 12.5 mg per kg po or IV qid times 14 days.		Blood cultures indicated. Consider C. trachomatis if afebrile pneumonia, staccato cough, IgM >1:8; therapy with erythro or sulfisoxazole. If MRSA documented, vanco. TMP-SMX & linezolid alternatives. Linezolid dosage from birth to age 11 yrs is **10 mg per kg q8h.**
Age 1–3 months Pneumonitis syndrome. Usually afebrile	C. trachomatis, RSV, parainfluenza virus 3, human metapneumovirus, Bordetella, S. pneumoniae, S. aureus (rare)	**Outpatient: po** erythro 12.5 mg/kg q6h x 14 days or po azithro 10 mg/kg x dose, then 5 mg/kg x 4 days.	**Inpatient: If afebrile erythro** 10 mg/kg IV q6h or azithro 2.5 mg/kg IV q12h (see Comment). **If febrile,** add cefotaxime 200 mg/kg per day div q8h.	Pneumonitis syndrome: Cough, tachypnea, dyspnea, diffuse infiltrates, afebrile. Usually requires hospital care. Reports of hypertrophic pyloric stenosis after erythro under age 6 wks; not sure about azithro, bid azithro dosing theoretically might ↑ risk of hypertrophic pyloric stenosis. If lobar pneumonia, give AMP 200–300 mg per kg per day for S. pneumoniae. No empiric coverage for S. aureus, as it is rare etiology.
		For RSV, see Bronchiolitis, page 36		
Infants and Children, age > 3 months to 18 yrs (IDSA Treatment Guidelines: CID 53:617, 2011).				
Outpatient	RSV, human metapneumovirus, rhinovirus, influenza virus, adenovirus, parainfluenza virus, Mycoplasma, H. influenzae, S. pneumoniae, S. aureus (rare)	**Amox** 90 mg/kg in 2 divided doses x 5 days	**Azithro** 10 mg/kg x 1 dose (max 500 mg), then 5 mg/kg (max 250 mg). x 4 days OR **Amox-Clav** 90 mg/kg (Amox) in 2 divided doses x 5 days	Antimicrobial therapy not routinely required for preschool-aged children with CAP as most infections are viral etiologies.
Inpatient	As above	Fully immunized **AMP** 50 mg/kg IV q6h Not fully immunized: **Cefotaxime** 150 mg/kg IV divided q8h	Fully immunized: **Cefotaxime** 150 mg/kg IV divided q8h	If atypical infection suspected, add **Azithro** 10 mg/kg x 1 dose (max 500 mg), then 5 mg/kg (max 250 mg) x 4 days. If community MRSA suspected, add **Vanco** 40-60 mg/kg/day divided q6-8h OR **Clinda** 40 mg/kg/day divided q6-8h. Depending on clinical response, may switch to oral agents as early as 2-3 days. Duration of therapy: 10-14 days.

(Continued on next page)

Abbreviations on page 2.   NOTE: All dosage recommendations are for adults (unless otherwise indicated) and assume normal renal function.

TABLE 1 (36)

LUNG/Bronchi/Pneumonia (continued)

ANATOMIC SITE/DIAGNOSIS/ MODIFYING CIRCUMSTANCES	ETIOLOGIES (usual)	SUGGESTED REGIMENS* PRIMARY	ALTERNATIVE[1]	ADJUNCT DIAGNOSTIC OR THERAPEUTIC MEASURES AND COMMENTS
Adults (over age 18) — IDSA/ATS Guideline for CAP in adults: *CID* 44 (Suppl 2): S27-S72, 2007. **Community-acquired, not hospitalized** **Prognosis prediction: CURB-65** (*AnIM* 118:384, 2005): C: confusion = 1 pt U: BUN >19 mg/dL = 1 pt R: RR >30 = 1 pt B: BP <90/60 = 1 pt Age ≥65 = 1 pt **If score = 1, ok for outpatient therapy; if >1, hospitalize.** The higher the score, the higher the mortality. Lab diagnosis of invasive pneumococcal disease: *CID* 46:926, 2008.	Varies with clinical setting. **No co-morbidity:** Atypicals—M. pneumoniae, et al; S. pneumo, viral **Co-morbidity:** Alcoholism: S. pneumo, anaerobes, coliforms Bronchiectasis: see Cystic fibrosis, page 43 COPD [1] S. pneumo, H. influenzae, M. catarrhalis, S. pneumo IVDU: Hematogenous S. aureus Post-CVA aspiration: Oral flora, incl. S. pneumo Post-obstruction of bronchi: S. pneumo, anaerobes Post-influenza: S. pneumo, and S. aureus	**No co-morbidity:** Azithro 0.5 gm po times 1, then 0.25 gm per day **OR** clarithro-ER 1 gm po q24h **OR** clarithro 500 mg po bid **OR** clarithro-ER 1 gm po q24h **OR** doxy 100 mg po bid **OR** If prior antibiotic within 3 months: (azithro or clarithro) + (amox 1 gm po tid or high dose AM-CL-ER) **Respiratory FQ** **Duration of rx:** S. pneumo—Not bacteremic: until afebrile 3 days C. pneumoniae—Unclear. Some reports suggest 21 days. Some bronchitis pts required 5–6 wks of clarithro (*J Med Micro* 52:265, 2003) Legionella—10-21 days M. pneumoniae 2° to coliforms, S. aureus, anaerobes: 2-2 weeks **Cautions:** 1. If local macrolide resistance to *S. pneumoniae* >25%, use alternative empiric therapy. 2. Esp. during influenza season, look for *S. aureus*.	**Co-morbidity present: Respiratory FQ** (see footnote[19]) **OR** (azithro or clarithro) + (high dose amox, high dose AM-CL, cefdinir, cefpodoxime, cefprozil[20]) Doses in footnote[20]	**Azithro/clarithro:** Pro: appropriate spectrum of activity; more in vitro resistance than clinical failure would predict; usually better tolerated than erythro. Con: If pen G resist., S. pneumo resistance in vitro 20-30% and may be increasing. If pen G resist., up to 50%+ resistance to azithro/clarithro. Increased risk of macrolide resistance with prior use. **Amoxicillin:** Pro: Active vs. 80-95% S. pneumo at 3-4 gm per day. Con: No activity atypicals or β-lactamase positive organisms. **AM-CL:** Pro: Spectrum of activity includes β-lactamase producing organisms. Con: No activity atypicals. **Cephalosporins—po:** Cefditoren, cefpodoxime, cefprozil, cefuroxime & others—see footnote[20]. Pro: Active 75-85% S. pneumo & H. influenzae. Cefuroxime least active & higher mortality rate when S. pneumo resistant. Con: Inactive vs. atypical pathogens. **FQs—Respiratory FQs:** Moxi, levo & gemi Pro: In vitro & clinically effective vs. pen-sensitive & pen-resistant S. pneumo. **NOTE: dose of Levo is 750 mg q24h dosing.** Gemi only available po. Con: Geographic pockets of resistance with clinical failure. Important drug-drug interactions (see Table 22A, page 217). Reversible rash in young females given Gemi for >7 days.
Community-acquired, hospitalized—NOT in the ICU Empiric therapy Treat for minimum of 5 days, afebrile for 48-72 hrs, with stable BP, adequate oral intake, and room air O₂ saturation of >90% (*COID* 20:177, 2007).	Etiology by % co-morbidity & risk factors as above. Culture sputum & blood. S. pneumo urine antigen reported helpful (*CID* 40:1608, 2005). Legionella urine antigen—sensitivity is only ca. 75% but specificity high, & it can pick up the pt. In general, blood culture is the more valuable culture data. Look for S. aureus.	**Ceftriaxone** 1 gm IV q24h + **azithro** 500 mg IV q24h **OR** **Ertapenem** 1 gm IV q24h plus **azithro** 500 mg IV q24h	**Levo** 750 mg IV q24h or **Moxi** 400 mg IV q24h (gati 400 mg IV q24h (gati no longer marketed in US due to hypo- and hyperglycemic reactions) If diagnosis of pneumonia vague, OK for admitting MD to hold antibiotics until diagnosis of "uncertain." (*Chest* 130:16, 2006)	**Ceftriaxone:** Pro: Drug of choice for pen-sens. S. pneumo, active H. influenzae, M. catarrhalis, & MSSA. Con: Not active atypicals or pneumonia due to bioterrorism pathogens. Add macrolide for atypicals and perhaps their anti-inflammatory activity. Administration of antibiotic in pneumonia with associated sepsis improved survival in pneumonia and pts with CAP. (*Eur Respir J* 39:156, 2012); in ER, first dose in ER. **Ceftaroline:** FDA approved at a dose of 600 mg q12h IV for 5-7 days for hospitalized patients with CAP. Pro: Clinical response rates at day 4 and clinical cure rates at days 8-15 post-treatment were similar for ceftaroline and ceftriaxone (see ceftaroline package insert). Con: More expensive; no data for MRSA yet.

[19] Atypical pathogens: Chlamydophila pneumoniae, C. psittaci, Legionella sp., M. pneumoniae, C. burnetii (Q fever). (Ref.: *LnID* 3:709, 2003)
Respiratory FQs with enhanced activity vs. S. pneumo with high-level resistance to penicillin: **Gati**[NUS] 400 mg IV/po q24h (no longer marketed in US due to hypo- and hyperglycemic reactions), **Gemi** 320 mg po q24h; **Levo** 750 mg po/IV q24h; **Moxi** 400 mg IV/po q24h. Ketolide: **telithro** 800 mg po q24h (physicians warned about rare instances of hepatotoxicity).
[20] **O Ceph** dosage: **Cefdinir** 300 mg po q12h, **cefditoren pivoxil** 200 mg, 2 tabs po bid, **cefpodoxime proxetil** 200 mg po q12h, **cefprozil** 500 mg po q12h, **high dose amox** 1 gm po tid, **high dose AM-CL** = use AM-CL-ER 1000/62.5 mg, 2 tabs po bid.

Abbreviations on page 2. NOTE: All dosage recommendations are for adults (unless otherwise indicated) and assume normal renal function.

TABLE 1 (37) (continued)

ANATOMIC SITE/DIAGNOSIS/ MODIFYING CIRCUMSTANCES	ETIOLOGIES (usual)	SUGGESTED REGIMENS* PRIMARY	ALTERNATIVE[1]	ADJUNCT DIAGNOSTIC OR THERAPEUTIC MEASURES AND COMMENTS
LUNG/Bronchi/Pneumonia/Adults (over age 18)				
Community-acquired, hospitalized—NOT in ICU Empiric therapy NOTE: Not all ICU admissions meet IDSA/ATS/or Guideline criteria for severe CAP. Some believe that all ICU pneumonia patients need 2 drugs with activity vs. gram-negative bacilli. Hence, 4 example clinical settings are outlined: **severe COPD; post-influenza, suspect gm-neg bacilli; risk of pen-resistant S. pneumo**	Severe COPD pt with pneumonia. S. pneumoniae, H. influenzae, Moraxella sp. Legionella sp. Rarely S. aureus. Culture sputum, blood and maybe pleural fluid. Look for respiratory viruses. Urine antigen for both Legionella and S. pneumoniae. Sputum PCR for Legionella.	**Levo** 750 mg IV q24h or **Moxi** 400 mg IV q24h Gati not available in US due to hypo- and hyperglycemic reactions	**Ceftriaxone** 1 gm IV q24h + **azithro** 500 mg IV q24h or **ERTA** 1 gm q24h IV + **azithro** 500 mg IV q24h (see Comment)	**Various studies** indicate improved outcome when azithro added to a β-lactam (CID 36:389 & 1239, 2003; AnM 164:1837, 2001 & 159:2562, 1999). Similar results in prospective study of critically ill pts with pneumococcal bacteremia (AJRCCM 170:440, 2004). **Ertapenem** could substitute for ceftriaxone; need azithro for atypical coverage. Not active vs. P. aeruginosa. **Legionella**: Not all Legionella species detected by urine antigen; if suspicious culture or PCR on airway secretions. Value of specific diagnosis: CID 46:1356 & 1385, 2008. In patients with normal sinus rhythm and not receiving beta-blockers, relative bradycardia suggests Legionella, psittacosis, Q-fever, or typhoid fever.
	Addition of a macrolide to beta-lactam empiric regimens lowers mortality for patients with bacteremic pneumococcal pneumonia (CID 36:389, 2003). Benefit NOT found with use of FQ or tetracycline for "atypicals" (Chest 131:466, 2007). Combination therapy benefitted patients with concomitant "shock." (CCM 35:1493 & 1617, 2007.)			
Community-acquired, hospitalized—IN ICU Empiric therapy	If concomitant with or post-influenza, S. aureus and S. pneumoniae possible.	**Vanco** 1 gm IV q12h + (**Levo** 750 mg IV q24h or **moxi** 400 mg IV q24h)	**Linezolid** 600 mg IV bid + (**levo** or **moxi**)	Sputum gram stain may help. S. aureus post-influenza ref: EID 12:894, 2006 Empiric therapy vs. MRSA decreases risk of mortality (CCM 34:2069, 2006)
Community-acquired, hospitalized—IN ICU Empiric therapy	Suspect aerobic gm-neg bacilli: e.g., P. aeruginosa and/or life-threatening infection (see comment). Hypoxic and/or hypotensive "Cover" S. pneumo & Legionella	Anti-pseudomonal beta-lactam[1] + (respiratory FQ or aminoglycoside) + azithro if no FQ	If severe (g)-mediated beta-lactam allergy, aztreonam + aminoglycoside + azithro Drugs and doses in footnote[1]	At risk for gm-neg rod pneumonia due to: alcoholism with necrotizing pneumonia, underlying chronic bronchiectasis (e.g. cystic fibrosis), chronic tracheostomy and/or mechanical ventilation, febrile neutropenia and pulmonary infiltrates, septic shock, underlying malignancy, or organ failure.
	Risk of Pen G-resistant S. pneumoniae 2° antibiotic use in last 3 months.	High dose IV amp (or Pen G) + azithro + respiratory FQ	Beta-lactam allergy: vanco + respiratory FQ	If Pen G MIC>4 mg/mL, vanco. Very rare event.
Health care-associated pneumonia (HCAP) Ref: CID 46 (Suppl 4): S296, 2008.	HCAP used to designate large diverse population of pts with many co-morbidities who reside in nursing homes, other long-term care facilities, require home IV therapy or are dialysis pts. Pneumonia in these pts frequently resembles hospital-acquired pneumonia (see next section).			

[1] Antipseudomonal beta-lactams: **Aztreonam** 2 gm IV q6h; **piperacillin** 3 gm IV q4h; **piperacillin/tazobactam** 3.375 gm IV q4h or 4.5 gm IV q8h (high dose for Pseudomonas); **cefepime** 2 gm IV q12h; **ceftazidime** 2 gm IV q8h; **doripenem** (do NOT use to treat pneumonia); **imipenem/cilastatin** 500 mg IV q6h; **meropenem** 1 gm IV q8h; **gentamicin or tobramycin** (see Table 10D, page 98); **P. aeruginosa dose** 2 mg/kg load, then 1.7 mg/kg q8h or **levo** 750 mg IV once daily. **Respiratory FQs: levofloxacin** 750 mg IV q24h or **moxifloxacin** 400 mg IV q24h; **high-dose ampicillin** 2 gm IV q6h; **azithromycin** 500 mg IV q24h; **vanco** 1 gm IV q12h.

Abbreviations on page 2.   NOTE: All dosage recommendations are for adults (unless otherwise indicated) and assume normal renal function.

TABLE 1 (38)

LUNG/Bronchi/Pneumonia/Adults (over age 18) (continued)

ANATOMIC SITE/DIAGNOSIS/ MODIFYING CIRCUMSTANCES	ETIOLOGIES (usual)	SUGGESTED REGIMENS* PRIMARY	ALTERNATIVE[1]	ADJUNCT DIAGNOSTIC OR THERAPEUTIC MEASURES AND COMMENTS
Hospital-acquired—usually with mechanical ventilation (VAP) (empiric therapy) Refs: U.S. Guidelines: AJRCCM 171:388, 2005; U.S. Review: JAMA 297:1583, 2007; Canadian Guidelines: JAC 62:5, 2008	Highly variable depending on clinical setting: S. pneumo, S. aureus, Legionella, coliforms, P. aeruginosa, stenotrophomonas, acinetobacter, anaerobes all possible	**IMP** 0.5 gm IV q6h or **MER** 1 gm IV q8h[22] plus, if suspect legionella or bioterrorism, respiratory FQ (Levo or Moxi) See Comment regarding diagnosis Dosages: See footnote[24] on page 40. Duration of therapy, see footnote[24]	If suspect P. aeruginosa, empirically start 2 anti-P. are drugs to increase likelihood that at least one will be active, e.g., **IMP** or **CFP** or **PIP-TZ**[23] plus tobra. Ref.: CCM 35:1888, 2007 NOTE: Regimen not active vs. **MRSA**: see specific rx below	**Dx of ventilator-associated pneumonia**: Fever & lung infiltrates often **not** pneumonia. Quantitative cultures helpful: bronchoalveolar lavage (>10⁴ per mL pos.) or protect. spec. brush (>10³ per mL pos). Ref.: AJRCCM 165:867, 2002; AnIM 132:621, 2000. **Microbiology**: No empiric regimen covers all possibilities. Regimens active vs. majority of S. pneumo, legionella, & most coliforms. Regimens **not active vs. MRSA, Stenotrophomonas & others**; see below. Specific therapy when culture known. **Ventilator-associated pneumonia—Prevention**: Keep head of bed elevated 30° or more. Remove N-G, endotracheal tubes as soon as possible. If available, continuous subglottic suctioning. Chlorhexidine oral care. Chest 130:251, 2006; AJRCCM 173:1297, 1348, 2006. **Misc**: clarithro. accelerated resolution of VAP (CID 46:1157, 2008). Silver-coated endotracheal tubes reported to reduce incidence of VAP (JAMA 300:805 & 842, 2008). See consensus document on management of febrile neutropenic pt: CID 34:730, 2002.
Hospital- or community-acquired, neutropenic pt (<500 neutrophils per mm³)	Any of organisms listed under community- and hospital-acquired + fungi (aspergillus). See Table 11.	See Hospital-acquired, immediately above. Vanco not included in initial therapy unless high suspicion of infected IV access or drug-resistant S. pneumo. Ampho not used unless still febrile after 3 days or high clinical likelihood. See Comment		

Adults—Selected therapy after culture results (sputum, blood, pleural fluid, etc.) available. Also see Table 2, page 67

Acinetobacter baumannii (See also Table 5A); Ref.: NEJM 358:1271, 2008	Patients with VAP	Use **IMP** or **MER** if susceptible	If IMP resistant: **colistin** + (IMP or MER). Colistin Dose: Table 10A, page 101	Sulbactam portion of AM-SB often active; dose: 3 gm IV q6h. For second-line agents: see Pharmacother 30:1279, 2010; J Inten Care Med 25:343, 2010
Burkholderia (Pseudomonas) pseudomallei (etiology of melioidosis) Can cause primary or secondary skin infection See Curr Opin Infect Dis 23:554, 2010	Gram-negative	Initial parenteral rx: **Ceftazidime** 30-50 mg per kg IV q8h or **IMP** 20 mg per kg IV q8h. Rx minimum 10 days & improving, then po therapy → See Alternative column	**Post-parenteral po rx**: **TMP-SMX** (See Comment for children) **TMP-SMX** 5 mg/kg (TMP component) bid + **Doxy** 2 mg/kg bid x 3 mos.	**Children ≤8 yrs old & pregnancy**: For oral regimen, use **AM-CL-ER** Dosage: 20 wks to term 2 tabs bid or 3 tabs tid. Even with compliance, relapse rate is 10%. Max. daily ceftazidime dose: 6 gm. Tigecycline: No clinical data but active in vitro (AAC 50:1555, 2006)
Haemophilus influenzae	β-lactamase negative β-lactamase positive	**AMP** IV, **amox** po, **TMP-SMX**, **azithro/clarithro**, **doxy** **AM-CL**, **O Ceph 2/3**, **P Ceph 3**, **FQ** Dosage: Table 10A		25–35% strains β-lactamase positive. ↑ resistance to both TMP-SMX (CID 41:758, page 111 for dosage). High % of otitis media H. influenza isolated as H. influenza (JID 195:81, 2007). ESBL[25] inactivates all cephalosporins, β-lactam/β-lactamase inhibitor drug activity, not predictable; co-resistance to all FQs & often aminoglycosides.
Kiebsiella sp.—ESBL pos. & other coliforms[25]	β-lactamase positive	**IMP** or **MER**; if resistant, **Colistin** + (IMP or MER) Usually several weeks of therapy.		

[22] If Acinetobacter sp., **susceptibility to IMP & MER** may be discordant (CID 41:758, 2005).
[23] **PIP-TZ** for P. aeruginosa pneumonia: 3.375 gm IV over 4 hrs & repeat q8h (CID 44:357, 2007) plus **tobra**.
[24] Dogma on duration of therapy not consistent with data on so many variables: i.e. certainty of diagnosis, infecting organism, severity of infection and number/severity of co-morbidities. Agree with efforts to de-escalate & shorten course: Treat at least 7-8 days. Need clinical evidence of response: fever resolution, improved oxygenation, falling WBC. Refs: AJRCCM 171:388, 2005; CID 43:S75, 2006; COID 19:185, 2006.
[25] **ESBL** = Extended spectrum beta-lactamase

Abbreviations on page 2. NOTE: *All dosage recommendations are for adults (unless otherwise indicated) and assume normal renal function.*

TABLE 1 (39)

ANATOMIC SITE/DIAGNOSIS/ MODIFYING CIRCUMSTANCES	ETIOLOGIES (usual)	SUGGESTED REGIMENS* PRIMARY	ALTERNATIVE[1]	ADJUNCT DIAGNOSTIC OR THERAPEUTIC MEASURES AND COMMENTS
LUNG/Pneumonia/Adults—Selected specific therapy after culture results (sputum, blood, pleural fluid, etc.) available (continued)				
Legionella species Relative bradycardia common feature	Hospitalized/ immunocompromised	**Azithro** 500 mg IV or **Levo** 750 mg IV or **Moxi** 400 mg IV. See Table 10A, pages 98 & 100 for dosages. Treat for 7-14 days (CID 39:1734, 2004)		Legionella website: www.legionella.org. Two studies support superiority of **Levo** over macrolides (CID 40:794 & 800, 2005), although not FDA-approved.
Moraxella catarrhalis	93% β-lactamase positive	**AM-CL**, **O Ceph 2/3**, **P Ceph 2/3**, **macrolide**[26], **FQ**, **TMP-SMX**, **Doxy** another option. See Table 10A, page 93 for dosages		
Pseudomonas aeruginosa	Often ventilator-associated	**PIP-TZ** 3.375 gm IV q4h or prefer 4-hr infusion of 3.375 gm q8h) + **tobra** 5 mg/kg IV once q24h (see Table 10D, page 109). Could substitute anti-pseudomonal **cephalosporin** or **carbapenem** (**IMP**, **MER**) for **PIP-TZ** if P. strain is susceptible.		NOTE: **PIP-TZ** for P. aeruginosa (CID 44:357, 2007); other options: **CFP** 2 gm IV q 12h; **CIP** 400 mg IV q8h + **PIP-TZ**; **IMP** 500 mg IV q6h + **CIP** 400 mg IV q12h. If multi-drug resistant, **Colistin** IV + (**IMP** or **MER**) + **Colistin** by inhalation 80 mg bid.
Staphylococcus aureus Duration of treatment: 2-3 wks if just pneumonia; 4-6 wks if concomitant endocarditis and/or osteomyelitis. IDSA Guidelines, CID 52 (Feb 1):1, 2011.	Nafcillin/oxacillin susceptible	**Nafcillin/oxacillin** 2 gm IV q4h	**Vanco** 30-60 mg/kg/d IV in 2-3 divided doses or **linezolid** 600 mg IV q12h.	Adjust dose of vancomycin to achieve target concentrations of 15-20 mcg/mL. Some authorities recommend 25-30 mg/kg loading dose (actual body weight in severely ill patients (CID 49:325, 2009). A prospective trial comparing Linezolid to Vanco for MRSA pneumonia showed higher cure rate (p=0.042) for Linezolid (95/165, 57.6%) than for Vancomycin (81/174, 46.6%) but no difference in mortality (15.7% for Linezolid vs. 17% for Vanco) (CID 54:621, 2012).
	MRSA	**Vanco** 30-60 mg/kg/d IV in 2-3 divided doses or **Linezolid** 600 mg IV q12h.	**Dapto** probably not an option; pneumonia developed during dapto rx (CID 49:1286, 2009).	
Stenotrophomonas maltophilia		**TMP-SMX** up to 20 mg/kg/day div q8h	**TC-CL** 3.1 gm IV q4h	Potential synergy: **TMP-SMX** + **TC-CL** (JAC 62:889, 2008).
Streptococcus pneumoniae	Penicillin-susceptible	**AMP** 2 gm IV q6h, **amox** 1 gm po tid, **macrolide**[26], **pen G**[27], **doxy**. **O Ceph 2**, **P Ceph 2/3**. See Table 10A, page 111 for other dosages. Treat until afebrile, 3-5 days (min. of 5 days).		
	Penicillin-resistant, high level	**FQs** with enhanced activity: **Gemi**, **Levo**, **Moxi**. **vanco** IV—see Table 5A, page 77 for more data. If all options not possible (IV, allergy), linezolid active: 600 mg IV or q12h. Dosages Table 10A. Treat until afebrile, 3-5 days (min. of 5 days). Ceftaroline 600 mg IV q12h superior to Ceftriaxone (CID 51:641, 2010).		
Yersinia pestis (Plague) CID 49:736, 2009	Aerosol Y. pestis.	**Gentamicin** 5 mg/kg IV q24h	**Doxy** 200 mg IV times 1, then 100 mg IV bid	TMP-SMX used as prophylaxis for bubonic pneumonia (CID 40:1166, 2005). Chloro effective but potentially toxic. Cephalosporins and FQs effective in animal models.
LUNG—Other Specific Infections				
Actinomycosis	A. Israelii and rarely others	**AMP** 50 mg/kg/day IV div in 3-4 doses x 4-6 wks, then **Pen VK** 2-4 gm/day po x 3-6 wks	**Doxy** or **ceftriaxone** or **clinda** or **erythro**	Can use **Pen G** instead of AMP. 10-20 million units/day IV x 4-6 wks.

[26] Macrolide = azithromycin, clarithromycin and erythromycin.
[27] IV Pen G dosage: no meningitis, 2 million units IV q4h. If concomitant meningitis, 4 million units IV q4h.

Abbreviations on page 2.   NOTE: All dosage recommendations are for adults (unless otherwise indicated) and assume normal renal function.

TABLE 1 (40)

ANATOMIC SITE/DIAGNOSIS/ MODIFYING CIRCUMSTANCES	ETIOLOGIES (usual)	SUGGESTED REGIMENS* PRIMARY	SUGGESTED REGIMENS* ALTERNATIVE†	ADJUNCT DIAGNOSTIC OR THERAPEUTIC MEASURES AND COMMENTS
LUNG—Other Specific Infections *(continued)*				
Anthrax Inhalation (applies to oropharyngeal & gastrointestinal forms): **Treatment** (Cutaneous: See page 51) Ref: www.bt.cdc.gov	Bacillus anthracis **To report possible bioterrorism event: 770-488-7100** Plague, tularemia: See page A. Chest x-ray, mediastinal widening & pleural effusion	**Adults (including pregnancy): CIP** 400 mg IV q12h) or **doxy** 100 mg IV q12h) **plus clindamycin** 900 mg IV q8h &/or **RIF** 300 mg IV q12h). Switch to po when able & lower dose to 500 mg po bid: clinda to 450 mg po q8h; & RIF 300 mg po bid. Treat times 60 days.	**Children:** CIP 10 mg/kg IV q12h or 15 mg/kg IV q12h) or (**doxy** >8 y/o & >45 kg: 100 mg IV q12h; >8 y/o & ≤45 kg: 2.2 mg/kg IV q12h; ≤8 y/o: 2.2 mg/kg IV q12h) **plus clindamycin** 7.5 mg/kg IV q6h **and/or RIF** 20 mg/kg IV q12h (max. 600 mg) IV q24h. Treat times 60 days. See Table 16, page 203 for oral dosage.	1. Clinda may block toxin production 2. Rifampin penetrates CSF & intracellular sites. 3. If isolate shown penicillin-susceptible: a. **Adults: Pen G** 4 million units IV q4h b. **Children: Pen G** <12 y/o: 50,000 units per kg IV q6h; >12 y/o: 4 million units every 4 hours. c. Pregnancy, induced β-lactamases—do not use pen or amp alone. 4. Do not use cephalosporins or TMP-SMX. 5. Erythro, azithro activity borderline; clarithro active. 6. No person-to-person spread. 7. Monoclonal antitoxin activity approved: **raxibacumab** single 2 hr IV infusion. 8. Moxi should work, but no clinical data 9. Case report of survival with use of anthrax immunoglobulin (*CID 54:968, 2007; CID 54:1848, 2012*).
Anthrax, prophylaxis	Info: www.bt.cdc.gov	**Adults (including pregnancy) or children >50 kg: Levo** 500 mg po bid or **CIP** 500 mg po bid x 60 days. **Children <50 kg:** CIP 20-30 mg/kg/day div q12h x 60 days; or **levo** 8 mg/kg q12h x 60 days	**Adults (including pregnancy): Doxy** 100 mg po bid x 60 days. **Children (See Comment): Doxy** >8 y/o & >45 kg: 100 mg po bid; >8 y/o & ≤45 kg: 2.2 mg/kg po bid; ≤8 y/o: 2.2 mg/kg po bid. All for 60 days.	1. Once organism shows suscept. to penicillin, switch to amoxicillin 80 mg per kg per day div q8h (max. 500 mg q8h); pregnant pt to amoxicillin 500 mg po tid. 2. Do **not** use cephalosporins or TMP-SMX. 3. Other FQs (Gati, Moxi) & clarithro should work but no clinical experience.
Aspiration pneumonia/anaerobic lung infection/lung abscess	Transthoracic culture in 90 pts—% of total isolates: anaerobes 34%, Gm-pos. cocci 26%, S. milleri 16%, Klebsiella pneumoniae 25%, nocardia 3%	Clindamycin 300-450 mg po tid OR Ampicillin-sulbactam 3 g IV q6h OR a carbapenem (e.g., ertapenem 1 g IV q24h)	Ceftriaxone 1 gm IV q24h plus metro 500 mg IV q6h or 1 gm IV q12h	Typically an aerobic infection of the lung including aspiration pneumonitis, necrotizing pneumonia, lung abscess and empyema (REF: Anaerobe 18:235, 2012) Other treatment options: PIP-TZ 3.325 g IV q6h (for mixed infections with resistant Gram-negative aerobes) or Moxi 400 mg IV q24h (*CID 42:1264, 2005*).
Chronic pneumonia with fever, night sweats and weight loss	M. tuberculosis, coccidioidomycosis, histoplasmosis	See Table 11, Table 12. For risk associated with TNF inhibitors, see *CID 41(Suppl 3):S187, 2005.*		HIV+, foreign-born, alcoholism, contact with TB, travel into developing countries
Cystic fibrosis **Acute exacerbation of pulmonary symptoms** Ref: *AJRCCM 180:802, 2009* *(Continued on next page)*	S. aureus or H. influenzae early in disease; P. aeruginosa later in disease	**For P. aeruginosa:** (Peds doses) **Tobra** 3.3 mg/kg div q8h or 12 mg/kg IV q24h (*Ref 16*). Combine tobra with **(PIP** or **ticarcillin** 100 mg/kg q6h or **ceftaz** 50 mg/kg IV q8h to max of 6 gm per day. **CIP**, if resistant to above, CIP, Levo if used if P. aeruginosa susceptible. See footnote²⁸ & Comment.	**For S. aureus: (1) MSSA oxacillin/nafcillin** 2 gm IV q4h (*see Table 6*); (2) **MRSA—vanco** 1 gm q12h & check serum levels. See Comment	Cystic Fibrosis Foundation Guidelines: 1. Combination therapy for P. aeruginosa infection. 2. Once-daily dosing for aminoglycosides. 3. Need more data on continuous infusion beta-lactam therapy. 4. Routine use of steroid not recommended. For chronic suppression of P. aeruginosa, **inhaled phenol-free tobra** 300 mg bid x 28 days, then no rx x 28 days, then repeat cycle. (*AJRCCM 167:841, 2003*); **Aztreonam** (Cayston) 75 mg inhaled tid; pre-dose bronchodilator. (*Chest 135:1223, 2009*)

²⁸ Other options: (Tobra + aztreonam 50 mg per kg IV q8h); (IMP 15-25 mg per kg IV q8h + tobra); **CIP commonly used in children.**

* NOTE: All dosage recommendations are for adults (unless otherwise indicated) and assume normal renal function.
† Abbreviations on page 2.

43

TABLE 1 (41)

ANATOMIC SITE/DIAGNOSIS/ MODIFYING CIRCUMSTANCES	ETIOLOGIES (usual)	SUGGESTED REGIMENS* PRIMARY	ALTERNATIVE[1]	ADJUNCT DIAGNOSTIC OR THERAPEUTIC MEASURES AND COMMENTS
LUNG—Other Specific Infections *(continued)*				
(Continued from previous page)	Burkholderia (Pseudomonas) cepacia	TMP-SMX 5 mg per kg (TMP) IV q6h	Chloro 15–20 mg per kg IV q6h	B. cepacia has become a major pathogen. Patients develop progressive respiratory failure, 62% mortality at 1 yr. **Fail to respond to aminoglycosides,** piperacillin, & ceftazidime. Patients with B. cepacia should be isolated from other CF patients.
Empyema. Refs.: Pleural effusion review: *CID 45:1480, 2007*; IDSA Treatment Guidelines for Children, *CID 53:617, 2011*.			For other alternatives, see Table 2	
Neonatal	Staph. aureus, Strep. pneumoniae, E. coli	See Pneumonia, neonatal, page 38		Drainage indicated.
Infants/children (1 month–5 yrs)	Staph. aureus, Strep. pneumoniae, H. influenzae	See Pneumonia, age 1 month–5 years, page 38		Drainage indicated.
Child >5 yrs to ADULT—Diagnostic thoracentesis; chest tube for empyema Acute, usually parapneumonic Strep. pneumoniae Group A strep For dosage, see Table 10B or footnote page 25 Microbiologic diagnosis: Check for MRSA		Cefotaxime or ceftriaxone (Dosage, see footnote[12] page 25)	Vanco	Tissue Plasminogen Activator (10 mg) + DNase (5 mg) bid x 3 days via chest tube improves outcome (*NEJM 365:518, 2011*).
	Staph. aureus: Check for MRSA	Nafcillin or oxacillin if MSSA	Vanco or linezolid if MRSA.	Usually complication of S. aureus pneumonia &/or bacteremia.
	H. influenzae	Ceftriaxone		Pleomorphic Gm-neg. bacilli, ↑ resistance to TMP-SMX.
Subacute/chronic	Anaerobic strep, Strep. milleri, Bacteroides sp., Enterobacteriaceae, M. tuberculosis	Clinda 450–900 mg IV q8h + ceftriaxone	Cefoxitin or IMP or TC-CL or PIP-TZ or AM-SB (Dosage, see footnote[12] page 25)	If organisms not seen, treat as subacute. Drainage. R/O tuberculosis or tumor. Pleural biopsy with culture for mycobacteria and histology if TBc suspected.
Human immunodeficiency virus infection (HIV+): See SANFORD GUIDE TO HIV/AIDS THERAPY				
CD4 T-lymphocytes <200 per mm³ or clinical AIDS Dry cough, progressive dyspnea, & diffuse infiltrate **Prednisone first if suspect pneumocystis** (see Comment)	Pneumocystis carinii most likely; also M. TBc, fungi, Kaposi's sarcoma, & lymphoma. NOTE: AIDS pts may develop pneumonia due to DRSP or other pathogens—see next box below	Rx listed here is for **severe** pneumocystis; see Table 13A, page 145 for regimens for mild disease. **Prednisone 1**° (see Comment) TMP-SMX [IV: 15 mg per kg per day div q8h (TMP component) or po: 2 DS tabs q8h], total of 21 days	(Clinda 600 mg IV q8h + primaquine 30 mg po q24h) or (pentamidine 4 mg per kg per day IV times 21 days—See Comment)	**Diagnosis (induced sputum or bronchial wash) for:** histology or monoclonal antibody strains or PCR. Serum beta-glucan (Fungitell) levels under study (*CID 46:1928 & 1930, 2008*). **Prednisone 40 mg bid po times 5 days then 40 mg q24h po times 5 days then 20 mg q24h po times 11 days is indicated with PCP rx (pO₂ <70 mmHg), should be given at initiation of anti-PCP rx; don't wait until pt's condition deteriorates.** If PCP studies negative, consider bacterial pneumonia, TBc, cocci, histo, crypto, Kaposi's sarcoma or lymphoma. **Pentamidine** not active vs. bacterial pathogens. **NOTE: Pneumocystis resistant to TMP-SMX, albeit rare, does exist.**
CD4 T-lymphocytes normal Acute onset, purulent sputum & pulmonary infiltrates ± pleuritic pain. **Isolate pt until TBc excluded: Adults**	Strep. pneumoniae, H. influenzae, aerobic Gm-neg. bacilli (including P. aeruginosa), Legionella rare, M. TBc	Ceftriaxone 1 gm IV q24h (over age 65 1 gm IV q24h) + azithro. Could use Levo, Moxi IV as alternative (see Comment)		Gram stain of sputum shows Gm-neg. bacilli, options include **P Ceph 3** AP PCN, PIP-TZ, AP Carb; all ± aminoglycoside. Gati not available in US due to hypo- & hyperglycemic reactions. FQs: Levo 750 mg po/IV q24h. Moxi 400 mg po/IV q24h. Gati not available in US due to hypo- & hyperglycemic reactions.
As above: Children	Same as above with HIV+ lymphoid interstitial pneumonia (LIP)	As for HIV+ adults with pneumonia. If diagnosis is LIP, rx with steroids.		In children with AIDS, LIP responsible for 1/3 of pulmonary complications, usually >1 yr of age vs. PCP, which is seen at <1 yr of age. Clinically: clubbing, hepatosplenomegaly, salivary glands enlarged (take up gallium), lymphocytosis.

NOTE: All dosage recommendations are for adults (unless otherwise indicated) and assume normal renal function.

TABLE 1 (42)

ANATOMIC SITE/DIAGNOSIS/ MODIFYING CIRCUMSTANCES	ETIOLOGIES (usual)	SUGGESTED REGIMENS* PRIMARY	SUGGESTED REGIMENS* ALTERNATIVE[1]	ADJUNCT DIAGNOSTIC OR THERAPEUTIC MEASURES AND COMMENTS
LUNG—Other Specific Infections *(continued)*				
Nocardia pneumonia Expert Help: Wallace Lab (+1) 903-877-7680; CDC (+1) 404-639-3158 Ref: *Medicine* 88:250, 2009.	N. asteroides, N. brasiliensis	TMP-SMX 15 mg/kg/day IV/po in 2-4 divided doses + Imipenem 500 mg IV q6h for first 3-4 weeks then TMP-SMX 10 mg/kg/day in 2-4 divided doses x 3-6 mos.	IMP 500 mg IV q6h + amikacin 7.5 mg/kg IV q12h x 3-4 wks & then po TMP-SMX	**Duration:** 3 mos. if immunocompetent; 6 mos. if immunocompromised. **Measure peak sulfonamide levels:** Target is 100-150 mcg/mL, 2 hrs post po dose. Linezolid active in vitro (*Ann Pharmacother* 41:1694, 2007). In vitro resistance to TMP-SMX may be increasing (*Clin Infect Dis* 51:1445, 2010), but whether this is associated with worse outcomes is not known.
Tularemia Inhalational tularemia Treatment Ref: *JAMA* 285:2763, 2001 & www.bt.cdc.gov	Francisella tularemia	(Streptomycin 15 mg per kg IV bid) or (gentamicin 5 mg per kg IV q8h) times 10 days	Doxy 100 mg IV or po bid times 14-21 days or CIP 100 mg IV (or 750 mg po) bid times 14-21 days.	For pediatric doses, see *Table 16, page 203*. Pregnancy: as for non-pregnant adults. **Tobramycin** should work.
Post-exposure prophylaxis		Doxy 100 mg po bid times 14 days	CIP 500 mg po bid times 14 days	For pediatric doses, see *Table 16, page 203*. Pregnancy: As for non-pregnant adults
Viral (interstitial) pneumonia suspected See *Influenza, Table 14A, page 164*. Ref: *Chest* 133:1221, 2008	Consider: **Influenza**, adenovirus, coronavirus (SARS), hantavirus, metapneumovirus, parainfluenza virus, respiratory syncytial virus	Oseltamivir 75 mg po bid for 5 days or zanamivir two 5 mg inhalations twice a day for 5 days.		No known efficacious drugs for adenovirus, coronavirus (SARS), hantavirus, metapneumovirus, parainfluenza or RSV. Need travel (SARS) & exposure (Hanta) history. RSV and human metapneumovirus as serious as influenza in the elderly (*NEJM* 352:1749 & 1810, 2005; *CID* 44:1152 & 1159, 2007).
LYMPH NODES (approaches below apply to lymphadenitis without an obvious primary source)				
Lymphadenitis, acute Generalized	Etiologies: EBV, early HIV infection, syphilis, toxoplasma, tularemia, Lyme disease, sarcoid, lymphoma, systemic lupus erythematosus, and Kikuchi-Fujimoto disease. Complete history and physical examination followed by appropriate serological tests. Treat specific agent(s).			
Regional Cervical—see cat-scratch disease (CSD), below				History & physical exam directs evaluation. If nodes fluctuant, aspirate and base rx on Gram & acid-fast stains. **Kikuchi-Fujimoto** disease causes fever and benign self-limited adenopathy; the etiology is unknown (*CID* 39:138, 2004).
Inguinal	HSV, chancroid, syphilis, LGV			
Sexually transmitted				
Not sexually transmitted	GAS, SA, tularemia, CSD, Y. pestis (plague)			Consider bubonic plague & glandular tularemia
Axillary	GAS, SA, CSD, tularemia, Y. pestis			Consider bubonic plague & glandular tularemia.
Extremity, with associated nodular lymphangitis	Sporotrichosis, leishmania, Nocardia brasiliensis, Mycobacterium marinum, Mycobacterium chelonae, tularemia			Assess distal site for primary lesion. Lymphangitis is characterized by subcutaneous swellings along draining lymphatic channels. Primary site of skin invasion usually present; regional adenopathy variable.
Nocardia lymphadenitis & skin abscesses	N. asteroides, N. brasiliensis	TMP-SMX 5-10 mg/kg/day based on TMP IV/po in 2-4 doses	Sulfisoxazole 2 gm po qid or minocycline 100-200 mg po bid.	**Duration:** 3 mos. if immunocompetent; 6 mos. if immunocompromised. **Linezolid:** 600 mg po bid reported effective (*Ann Pharmacother* 41:1694, 2007).
Cat-scratch disease—immunocompetent patient Typically right supraclavicular nodes 46%, neck 26%, inguinal 17%. Ref: *Amer Fam Physician* 83:152, 2011.	Bartonella henselae	**Azithro dosage—Adults** (>45.5 kg): 500 mg po x 1, then 250 mg po x 4 days. **Children** (<45.5 kg): liquid azithro 10 mg/kg x 1, then 5 mg/kg per day x 4 days. Rx is controversial	No therapy; resolves in 2-6 mos. Needle aspiration relieves pain in suppurative nodes. Avoid I&D.	**Clinical:** Approx. 10% nodes suppurate. Atypical presentation in <5% pts, i.e., lung nodules, liver/spleen lesions, Parinaud's oculoglandular syndrome, CNS manifestations in 2% of pts (encephalitis, peripheral neuropathy, retinitis), FUO. **Dx:** Cat exposure. Positive IFA serology. Rarely need biopsy.

Abbreviations on page 2.   NOTE: *All dosage recommendations are for adults (unless otherwise indicated) and assume normal renal function.*

45

TABLE 1 (43)

ANATOMIC SITE/DIAGNOSIS/ MODIFYING CIRCUMSTANCES	ETIOLOGIES (usual)	SUGGESTED REGIMENS* PRIMARY	ALLERNATIVE[$\dagger$]	ADJUNCT DIAGNOSTIC OR THERAPEUTIC MEASURES AND COMMENTS
MOUTH				
Aphthous stomatitis, recurrent	Etiology unknown	Topical steroids (Kenalog in Orabase) may ↓ pain and swelling; If AIDS, see SANFORD GUIDE TO HIV/AIDS THERAPY.		
Buccal cellulitis Children <5 yrs	H. influenzae	Cefuroxime or ceftriaxone	AM-CL or TMP-SMX	With Hib immunization, invasive H. influenzae infections have ↓ by 95%. Now occurring in infants prior to immunization.
		Dosage: see Table 16, page 203		
Candida Stomatitis ("Thrush")	C. albicans	Fluconazole	Echinocandin	See Table 11, page 113.
Herpetic stomatitis	Herpes simplex virus 1 & 2	See Table 14		
Submandibular space infection, bilateral (Ludwig's angina)	Oral anaerobes, facultative streptococci, S. aureus (rare)	(PIP-TZ or TC-CL) or Pen G IV + Metro IV)	Clinda 600 mg IV q6-8h (for Pen-allergic pt)	Ensure adequate airway and early surgical debridement. Add Vanco IV if gram-positive cocci on gram stain.
Ulcerative gingivitis (Vincent's angina or Trench mouth)	Oral anaerobes + vitamin deficiency	Pen G po/IV + Metro po/IV	Clinda	Replete vitamins (A-D). Can mimic scurvy. Severe form is NOMA (Cancrum oris) (Ln 368:147, 2006)
MUSCLE				
"Gas gangrene": Contaminated traumatic wound. Can be spontaneous without trauma.	Cl. perfringens, other histotoxic Clostridium sp.	**Clinda** 900 mg IV q8h) + (**pen G** 24 million units/day div. q4-6h IV	**Ceftriaxone** 2 gm IV q12h or **erythro** 1 gm IV q6h IV (not by bolus)	Surgical debridement primary therapy. **Hyperbaric oxygen** adjunctive efficacy debated, consider if debridement not complete or possible. Clinda given to decrease toxin production.
Pyomyositis	Staph aureus, Group A strep, (rarely Gm-neg, bacilli), variety of anaerobic organisms	(**Nafcillin** or **oxacillin** 2 gm IV q4h) or [**P Ceph 1** **ceftriaxone** 2 gm IV q8h)] if **MSSA**	**Vanco** 1 gm IV q12h if **MRSA**	Common in tropics; rare, but occurs, in temperate zones. Follows exercise or muscle injury. Necrotizing fasciitis. Now seen in HIV/AIDS. Add **metro** if anaerobes suspected or proven.
PANCREAS: Review: NEJM 354:2142, 2006.				
Acute alcoholic (without necrosis) or (idiopathic) pancreatitis	Not bacterial	None No necrosis on CT		1-9% become infected but prospective studies show no advantage of prophylactic antimicrobials. Observe for pancreatic abscesses or necrosis which require therapy.
Post-necrotizing pancreatitis; infected pseudocyst; pancreatic abscess	Enterobacteriaceae, enterococci, S. aureus, S. epidermidis, anaerobes, candida	Need culture of abscess/infected pseudocyst to direct therapy; **PIP-TZ** is reasonable empiric therapy		Can often get specimen by fine-needle aspiration. **Moxi**, **MER**, **IMP**, **ERTA** are all options (AAC 56:6434, 2012).
Antimicrobic prophylaxis, necrotizing pancreatitis	As above	If > 30% pancreatic necrosis on CT scan (with contrast), initiate antibiotic therapy: **IMP** 0.5-1 gm IV q6h or **MER** 1 gm IV q8h. No need for empiric Fluconazole. If patient worsens CT guided aspiration for culture & sensitivity. Controversial: Cochrane Database Sys Rev 2003: CD 002941; Gastroenterol 126:977, 2004; Ann Surg 245:674, 2007.		
PAROTID GLAND				
"Hot" tender parotid swelling	S. aureus, S. pyogenes, oral flora, & aerobic Gm-neg. bacilli (rare), mumps, rarely enteroviruses/ influenza	**Nafcillin** or **oxacillin** 2 gm IV q4h if MSSA, **vanco** if MRSA		Predisposing factors: stone(s) in Stensen's duct, dehydration. Therapy depends on ID of specific etiologic organism.
"Cold" non-tender parotid swelling	Granulomatous disease (e.g., mycobacteria, fungi, sarcoidosis, Sjögren's syndrome), drugs (iodides, et al.), diabetes, cirrhosis, tumors			History/lab results may narrow differential; may need biopsy for diagnosis

Abbreviations on page 2.   NOTE: All dosage recommendations are for adults (unless otherwise indicated) and assume normal renal function.

TABLE 1 (44)

ANATOMIC SITE/DIAGNOSIS/ MODIFYING CIRCUMSTANCES	ETIOLOGIES (usual)	SUGGESTED REGIMENS* PRIMARY	ALTERNATIVE†	ADJUNCT DIAGNOSTIC OR THERAPEUTIC MEASURES AND COMMENTS
PERITONEUM/PERITONITIS: Reference: CID 50:133, 2010				
Primary (spontaneous bacterial peritonitis), SBP Hepatology 49:2087, 2009; Dx: Pos. culture & ≥ 250 neutrophils/µL of ascitic fluid	Enterobacteriaceae 63%, *S. pneumoniae* 15%, enterococci 6–10%, anaerobes <1%. Extended β-lactamase (ESBL) positive Klebsiella species	**Cefotaxime** 2 gm IV q8h (if life-threatening, q4h)) or **TC-CL** or **PIP-TZ** (Doses, Table 10D) or **ERTA** 1 gm IV q24h)	**ceftriaxone** 2 gm IV q24h) or (**FQ: CIP, Levo, Moxi**) If resistant E. coli/Klebsiella species (ESBL+), then: (**DORI, ERTA, IMP** or **MER**) or (**FQ: CIP, Levo, Moxi**) (Dosage in footnote²⁰). Check in vitro susceptibility.	One-yr **risk of SBP** in pts with ascites about as high as 29% (Am J Gastro 104:133, 1994). If clinical diagnosis of SBP, 30–40% of pts have neg. cultures (blood and ascitic fluid). To ↑ yield, inject 10 ml of pt's ascitic fluid into blood culture bottles (JAMA 299:1166, 2008). **Duration of rx unclear.** Treat for at least 5 days, perhaps longer if pt bacteremic (Pharm & Therapeutics 34:204, 2009). **IV albumin** (1.5 gm/kg at dx & 1 gm/kg on day 3) may ↓ frequency of renal impairment (p 0.02) & ↓ hospital mortality (p 0.01) (NEJM 341:403, 1999).
Prevention of SBP [Amer J Gastro 104:993, 2009] Cirrhosis & ascites For prevention after UGI bleeding, see Liver, page 36		**TMP-SMX-DS** 1 tab po 5 days/wk or **CIP** 750 mg po q wk	**TMP-SMX**, peritonitis or mortality. Ref. for CIP: Hepatology 22:1171, 1995	
Secondary (bowel perforation, ruptured appendix, ruptured diverticulus). Ref: CID 50:133, 2010 (IDSA Guidelines) Antifungal rx? No need if successful uncomplicated 1st surgery for viscus perforation. Treat for candida if: repeat surg. perforation(s), anastomotic leaks, necrotizing pancreatitis, liver or pancreas transplant, pure peritoneal culture, candidemia (Ln 2:1437, 1989; Am Surg 76:197, 2010).	Enterobacteriaceae, Bacteroides sp., enterococci. *P. aeruginosa* (3-15%), *C. albicans* (may contribute with recurrent perforation/multiple surgeries) If VRE documented, daptomycin may work. (Int J Antimicrob Agents 32:369, 2008)	**Mild-moderate disease—Inpatient—parenteral rx:** (e.g. focal periappendiceal peritonitis, peridiverticular abscess). Usually need surgery for source control. **PIP-TZ** 3.375 gm IV q6h or 4.5 gm IV q8h (4-hr infusion) of 3.375 gm, **TC-CL** 3.1 gm IV q6h **OR ERTA** 1 gm IV q24h **OR MOXI** 400 mg IV q24h	(**CIP** 400 mg IV q12h or **Levo** 750 mg IV q24h) + **metro** 1 gm IV q12h) + **metro**) or (**CFP** 2 gm q12h + **metro**) or **tigecycline** 100 mg IV times 1 dose, then 50 mg q12h	Must "cover" both Gm-neg. aerobic & Gm-neg. anaerobic bacteria. Empiric coverage of MRSA, enterococci and candida not necessary unless culture indicates infection. Cover enterococci if valvular heart disease. **Drugs active only vs. anaerobic Gm-neg. bacilli:** metro. **Drugs active vs. aerobic Gm-neg. bacilli:** aminoglycosides, P Cφh 2/3/4, aztreonam, AP Pen, CIP, Levo. **Drugs active vs. both aerobic/anaerobic Gm-neg. bacteria:** cefoxitin, TC-CL, PIP-TZ, Dori, IMP, MER, Moxi. Increasing resistance (R) of Bacteroides species (AAC 51:1649, 2007; AAC 56:1247, 2012): % R Cefotetan Cefoxitin Clindamycin Essentially no resistance of Bacteroides to **metro**. **PIP-TZ**. Case reports of metro resistance to: (CID 40:e67, 2005; JCM 42:4127, 2004. **Ertapenem** not active vs. P. aeruginosa/Acinetobacter species. If absence of ongoing fecal contamination, **aerobic/anaerobic culture** of peritoneal exudate/abscess may be of help in guiding specific therapy. Less need for aminoglycosides. **With severe pen allergy,** can "cover" Gm-neg. aerobes with **CIP** or **aztreonam**. Remember **DORI/IMP/MER are β-lactams.** If VRE documented, daptomycin may work (Int J Antimicrobial Agents 32:369, 2008).
		Severe life-threatening disease—ICU patient: Surgery for source control - **IMP** 500 mg IV q6h or **MER** 1 gm IV q8h or **DORI** 500 mg IV q8h (1-hr infusion). See Comments.	(**AMP + metro + (CIP** 400 mg IV q12h or **Levo** 750 mg IV q24h) **OR (AMP** 1 gm IV q6h + **metro** 500 mg q6h) + **aminoglycoside** (see Table 10D, page 109)	IMP dose increased to 1 gm q6h if suspect P. aeruginosa and pt. is critically ill.
		Concomitant surgical management important.		
Abdominal actinomycosis	*A. Israelii* and rarely others	**AMP** 50 mg/kg/day IV div in 3–4 doses x 4–6 wks, then **Pen VK** 2–4 gm/day po x 3–6 mos.	**Doxy** or **ceftriaxone** or **clinda**	Presents as mass +/– fistula tract after abdominal surgery, e.g., for ruptured appendix. Can use IV Pen G instead of AMP: 10–20 million units/day IV x 4–6 wks.

²⁰ Parenteral IV therapy for peritonitis: **TC-CL** 3.1 gm q6h, **PIP-TZ** 3.375 gm q6h or 4.5 gm q8h (4-hr infusion of 3.375 gm q8h (See Table 10), **Dori** 500 mg IV q8h (1-hr infusion), **IMP** 0.5-1 gm q6h, **MER** 1 gm q8h, **FQ: CIP** 400 mg q12h, **Ofloxa** 400 mg q12h, **Levo** 750 mg q24h, **Moxi** 400 mg q24h, **AMP** 1 gm q6h, **aminoglycoside** (see Table 10D, page 109), **cefotetan** 2 gm q12h, **cefoxitin** 2 gm q6h, **cefotaxime** 2 gm q4–8h, **ceftriaxone** 1–2 gm q24h, **ceftizoxime** 2 gm q12h, **cefepime** 2 gm q12h, **clinda** 600–900 mg q8h, **metronidazole** 1 gm (15 mg/kg) loading dose IV, then 1 gm IV q12h (Some data supports once-daily dosing, see Table 10A, page 102), **AP Pen** (ticarcillin 4 gm q6h, **PIP** 4 gm q8h), **aztreonam** 2 gm q8h).

NOTE: All dosage recommendations are for adults (unless otherwise indicated) and assume normal renal function.

Abbreviations on page 2.

TABLE 1 (45)

ANATOMIC SITE/DIAGNOSIS/ MODIFYING CIRCUMSTANCES	ETIOLOGIES (usual)	SUGGESTED REGIMENS* PRIMARY	SUGGESTED REGIMENS* ALTERNATIVE[†]	ADJUNCT DIAGNOSTIC OR THERAPEUTIC MEASURES AND COMMENTS
PERITONEUM/PERITONITIS *(continued)*				
Associated with chronic ambulatory peritoneal dialysis (Abdominal pain, cloudy dialysate, dialysate WBC >100 cells/µL with >50% neutrophils, normal = <8 cells/µL. Ref: *Perit Dial Int* 30:393, 2010).	Gm-: 45%; Gm+: 15%; Multiple 11%; Fungi 2%; No Etiol. 20% (*Perit Dial Int* 24-424, 2004).	**Empiric therapy:** Need activity vs. MRSA (Vanco) & aerobic gram-negative bacilli (**Ceftaz, CFP, Carbapenem, Grp 2 Aztreonam if gram stain not evident).** Add **Fluconazole** if gram stain shows yeast. Use intraperitoneal dosing, unless bacteremia (rare). For bacteremia, IV dosing. For dosing detail, see Table 19, page 213.		**For diagnosis:** concentrate several hundred mL of removed dialysis fluid by centrifugation. Gram stain concentrate and then inject into aerobic/anaerobic blood culture bottles. A positive Gram stain will guide initial therapy. If culture shows Staph. epidermidis and no S. aureus, good chance of "saving" dialysis catheter. **If multiple Gm-neg. bacilli cultured, consider catheter-induced bowel perforation and need for catheter removal.** See *Perit Dialysis Int* 29:5, 2009. Other indications for catheter removal: relapsing/refractory peritonitis, fungal peritonitis, catheter tunnel infection.
PHARYNX				
Pharyngitis/Tonsillitis				
Exudative or Diffuse Erythema Associated cough, rhinorrhea, hoarseness and/or oral ulcers suggest viral etiology. IDSA Guidelines on Group A Strep: *CID* 55:1279, 2012.	Group A, C, G Strep; Fusobacterium (in research studies); Infectious Mono.; Primary HIV, N. gonorrhoeae; Respiratory viruses	**For Strep pharyngitis: (Pen)** V po x 10 days or **Benzathine Pen** 1.2 million units IM x 1 dose) OR (**Cefdinir** or **Cefpodoxime**) x 5 days. **Cephalosporin doses in footnote**[30] (adult and peds). (Durations are FDA-approved).	**For Strep, pharyngitis: Pen allergic: Clinda** 300-450 mg po q8h x 10 days. **Azithro, Clarithro** are alternatives, but resistance has been reported (*JAC* 63:42, 2009). *S. pyogenes* resistance to Sulfonamides and FQ's not recommended due to questionable efficacy.	Dx: Rapid Strep test. No need for post-treatment test of cure rapid strep test or culture. Complications of Strep pharyngitis: 1) Acute rheumatic fever 48 - follows Grp A S. pyogenes infection, rare after Grp C/G infection. See footnote[31]. For prevention, start treatment within 9 days of onset of symptoms. 2) Children age < 7yrs at risk for post-streptococcal glomerulonephritis. 3) Possibly, acute neuropsychiatric disorder associated with Grp A (PANDAS) infection.
	Gonococcal pharyngitis	**Ceftriaxone** 250 mg IM x 1 dose + **Azithro** 1 gm po x 1 dose) or **Doxy** 100 mg po bid x 7 days		4) Peritonsillar abscess, Suppurative phlebitis see complications. Not effective for pharyngeal GC: spectinomycin, cefixime, cefpodoxime and cefuroxime. Ref: *MMWR* 61:590, 2012.
	Proven S. pyogenes recurrence Grp A >3 x in 6 mo or 4 in 2 consecutive yrs	**Cefdinir** or **Cefpodoxime** Tonsillectomy not recommended to decrease Strep infections	**AM-CL** or **Clinda**.	Hard to distinguish true Grp A Strep infection from chronic Grp A Strep carriage and/or repeat viral infections.
Peritonsillar abscess – Serious complication of exudative pharyngitis	F. necrophorum (44%) Grp A Strep (33%) Grp C/G Strep (9%) (*CID* 49:1467, 2009)	Surgical drainage plus **PIP-TZ** or **TC-CL** or (**Metro** + **Ceftriaxone**)	Pen allergic: **Clinda** IV	**Avoid macrolides**. Fusobacterium is resistant. Reports of beta-lactamase production by oral anaerobes (*Anaerobe* 9:105, 2003). See jugular vein suppurative phlebitis, page 49.
Other complications		See parapharyngeal space infection and jugular vein suppurative phlebitis (below)		

[30] **Treatment of Group A, C & G strep; Treatment durations are from approved package inserts. Subsequent studies indicate efficacy of shorter treatment courses.** All po unless otherwise indicated. **PEDIATRIC DOSAGE: Benzathine penicillin** 25,000 units per kg IM to max. 1.2 million units; **Pen V** 25-50 mg per kg per day div. q6h x 10 days; **amox** 1000 mg once daily x 10 days; **AM-CL** 45 mg per kg per day div. q12h x 10 days; **cephalexin** 25-50 mg/kg/dose bid (max 500 mg/dose) bid x 10 days; **cefuroxime axetil** 20 mg per kg per day div. bid x 10 days; **cefpodoxime proxetil** 10 mg per kg per day bid x 5 days; **cefdinir** 7 mg per kg per day q12h x 5-10 days or 14 mg per kg q24h x 10 days; **cefprozil** 15 mg per kg per day div. bid x 10 days; **cefadroxil** 30 mg/kg once daily (max 1 gm/day) x 10 days; **clarithro** 15 mg per kg per day div. bid x 10 days; **azithro** 12 mg per kg once daily x 5 days; clinda 20–30 mg per kg per day div. q8h x 10 days. **ADULT DOSAGE: Benzathine penicillin** 1.2 million units IM x 1; **Pen V** 500 mg bid or 250 mg qid x 10 days; **cefditoren** 200 mg bid x 10 days; **cefpodoxime axetil** 100 mg bid x 5-10 days or 200 mg bid x 4-6 days of strep. pharyngitis; 5 days; **cefdinir** 300 mg q12h x 5-10 days or 600 mg q24h x 10 days; **cefprozil** 500 mg q24h x 10 days or 250 mg bid x 10 days; **cefuroxime axetil** 250 mg bid x 10 days; increasing number of studies show efficacy of 4-6 day courses; **clarithro** 250 mg bid x 10 days, **clarithro ext release** 1 gm q24h x 4 days; **azithro** 500 mg q24h x 3 days.

[31] Primary rationale for therapy is eradication of Group A strep (GAS) and prevention of acute rheumatic fever (ARF). Benzathine penicillin G has been shown in clinical trials to ↓ rate of ARF from 2.8 to 0.2%. This was associated with clearance of GAS on pharyngeal cultures (*CID* 19:1110, 1994). Subsequent studies have been based on cultures, not actual prevention of ARF. Treatment decreases duration of symptoms.

Abbreviations on page 2. NOTE: All dosage recommendations are for adults (unless otherwise indicated) and assume normal renal function.

TABLE 1 (46)

ANATOMIC SITE/DIAGNOSIS/ MODIFYING CIRCUMSTANCES	ETIOLOGIES* (usual)	SUGGESTED REGIMENS* PRIMARY	ALTERNATIVE[†]	ADJUNCT DIAGNOSTIC OR THERAPEUTIC MEASURES AND COMMENTS
PHARYNX/Pharyngitis/Tonsillitis: Exudative or Diffuse Erythema *(continued)*				
Membranous pharyngitis due to Diphtheria. Respiratory isolation, nasal & pharyngeal cultures, obtain antitoxin.	*C. diphtheriae* (human to human), *C. ulcerans* and *C. pseudotuberculosis* (animal to human) (rare)	**Treatment: antibiotics + antitoxin. Antibiotic therapy:** Erythro 500 mg IV qid OR Pen G 50,000 units/kg (max. 1.2 million units) IV q12h. Can switch to Pen VK 250 mg po qid when able. Treat for 14 days.	**Diphtheria antitoxin:** Horse serum. Obtain from CDC: +1 404-639-2889. Do scratch test before IV therapy. Dose depends on stage of illness: < 48hrs: 20,000-40,000 units; If NP membranes: 40,000-60,000 units; > 3 days & bull neck: 80,000-120,000 units	Ensure adequate airway. EKG & cardiac enzymes. F/U cultures post-treatment to document cure. Then, diphtheria toxoid immunization. Culture contacts, treat contacts with either single dose of **Pen G** IM 600,000 units if age < 6 yrs, 1.2 million units if age ≥ 6 yrs. If Pen-allergic, **Erythro** 500 mg po qid x 7-10 days.
Vesicular, ulcerative pharyngitis (viral)	Coxsackie A9, B1-5, ECHO (multiple types), Enterovirus 71, Herpes simplex 1,2	Antibacterial agents not indicated. For HSV-1,2: **acyclovir** 400 mg tid po x 10 days.		Small vesicles posterior pharynx suggests enterovirus. Viruses are most common etiology of acute pharyngitis. Suspect viral if concurrent conjunctivitis, coryza, cough, skin rash, hoarseness.
Epiglottitis (Supraglottis) Children	H. influenzae (rare), S. pyogenes, S. pneumoniae, S. aureus (includes MRSA)	**Peds dosage: Cefotaxime** 50 mg per kg IV q8h **or ceftriaxone** 50 mg per kg IV q24h) ± **Vanco**	**Peds dosage: Levo** 10 mg/kg IV q24h + **Clinda** 7.5 mg/kg IV q8h	Have tracheostomy set "at bedside." **Levo** use in children is justified as emergency empiric therapy in pts with severe beta-lactam allergy. *Ref: Ped Clin No Amer 53:215, 2006.*
Adults	Group A strep, H. influenzae (rare) & many others	Same regimens as for children. Adult dosage: See footnote[3]		
Parapharyngeal space infection; peritonsillar abscess [Spaces include: sublingual, submandibular (Ludwig's angina), lateral pharyngeal, retropharyngeal, pretracheal] Poor dental hygiene, dental extractions, foreign bodies (e.g., toothpicks, fish bones) Ref: CID 49:1467, 2009	Polymicrobic: Strep sp. anaerobes, Eikenella corrodens. Anaerobes outnumber aerobes 10:1.	[(**Clinda** 600-900 mg IV q8h) or (**pen G** 24 million units/day by cont. infusion of div. q4-6h IV) + **metro** 1 gm IV load and then 0.5 gm IV q6h]	**Cefoxitin** 2 gm IV q8h or **clinda** 600-900 mg IV q8h or **TC-CL** or **PIP-TZ** (Dosage, see footnote[3])	Close observation of airway. 1/3 require intubation. MRI or CT to identify abscess; **surgical drainage**. **Metro** may be given 1 gm IV q12h. Complications: infection of carotid (rupture possible) & jugular vein phlebitis.
Jugular vein suppurative phlebitis (Lemierre's syndrome) *LnID 12:808, 2012.*	Fusobacterium necrophorum in vast majority	**PIP-TZ** 4.5 gm IV q8h or **IMP** 500 mg IV q6h or (**Metro** 500 mg po/IV q8h + **ceftriaxone** 2 gm IV once daily)	**Clinda** 600-900 mg IV q8h. Avoid macrolides: Fusobacterium are resistant	Emboli: pulmonary and systemic common. Erosion into carotid artery can occur. Lemierre described F. necrophorum in 1936; other anaerobes & Gm-positive cocci are less common etiologies of suppurative phlebitis post-pharyngitis.
Laryngitis (hoarseness)	Viral (90%)	Not indicated		

[3] Parapharyngeal space infection: **Ceftriaxone** 2 gm IV q24h; **cefotaxime** 2 gm IV q4-8h; **PIP-TZ** 3.375 gm IV q6h or 4-hr infusion of 3.375 gm IV q8h; **TC-CL** 3.1 gm IV q4-6h; **TMP-SMX** 8-10 mg per kg per day (based on TMP component); div q6h, q8h, or q12h. **Clinda** 600-900 mg IV q6-8h; **Levo** 750 mg IV q24h.

Abbreviations on page 2. NOTE: All dosage recommendations are for adults (unless otherwise indicated) and assume normal renal function.

TABLE 1 (47)

ANATOMIC SITE/DIAGNOSIS/ MODIFYING CIRCUMSTANCES	ETIOLOGIES (usual)	SUGGESTED REGIMENS* PRIMARY	SUGGESTED REGIMENS* ALTERNATIVE[†]	ADJUNCT DIAGNOSTIC OR THERAPEUTIC MEASURES AND COMMENTS
SINUSES, PARANASAL				
Sinusitis, acute: current terminology: acute rhinosinusitis Obstruction of sinus ostia, viral infection, allergens Refs: Otolaryn-Head & Neck Surg. 137:1 2007; JAMA 301:1798, 2009; JAMA 307:685, 2012. For rhinovirus infections (common cold), see Table 14A, page 167	**acute rhinosinusitis:** S. pneumoniae 33%, H. influenzae 32%, M. catarrhalis 9%, anaerobes 6%, viruses 15% **By CT scans, sinus mucosa inflamed in 87% of viral URIs; only 2% develop bacterial rhinosinusitis**	Reserve antibiotic therapy for pts given decongestants, analgesics for 10 days who have (1) maxillary/facial pain & (2) purulent nasal discharge. If severe illness (pain, fever), treat sooner—usually requires hospitalization. Viral infections which resolve within 10 days. For mild/mod. disease: Ask if recent antibiotic use (recent = in last month).		**Rx goals:** (1) Resolve infection, (2) prevent bacterial complications, e.g., subdural empyema, epidural abscess, brain abscess, meningitis and cavernous sinus thrombosis (LnID 7:62, 2007), (3) avoid chronic sinus disease, (4) avoid unnecessary antibiotic rx. 40-60% rate of spontaneous resolution. **For pts with pen/cephalosporin allergy, esp. severe IgE-mediated allergy, e.g., hives, anaphylaxis, treatment options: clarithro, azithro, TMP-SMX, doxy or FQs. Avoid FQs if under age 18. Do not use Clinda**—no activity vs. Haemophilus or Moraxella sp. Dosages in footnote[33], page 50. If allergy just skin rash, po cephalosporin OK.
Meta-analysis of 9 double-blind trials found no clinical signs/symptoms that justify treatment—even after 7-10 days of symptoms (Ln 371:908, 2008).	S. pneumoniae 33%, H. influenzae 32%, M. catarrhalis 9%, Group A strep 2%, anaerobes 6%, viruses 15%, Staph. aureus 10%. CID 45:e121, 2007.	**No Recent Antibiotic Use:** **Amox-HD** or **AM-CL-ES** or **cefdinir** or **cefpodoxime** or **cefprozil**	**Recent Antibiotic Use:** **AM-CL-ER** (adults) or resp. **FQ** (adults). For pen. allergy, see Comments; previous page. Use AM-CL suspension in peds.	Usual rx 10 days; but same efficacy with 3-7 days vs. 6-10 days (LnID 8:543, 2008) (meta-analysis). **S. aureus is not considered an etiology of acute uncomplicated sinusitis.** Isolation of S. aureus in pts same incidence as in healthy controls. Hence, empiric therapy is not aimed at S. aureus. NOTE: Levo 750 mg q24h x 5 days vs. Levo 500 mg q24h x 10 days has equivalent microbiologic and clinical efficacy (Otolaryngol Head Neck Surg 134:10, 2006).
Clinical failure after 3 days	As above; consider diagnostic tap/aspirate	In general, treat 10 days (see Comment; Adult and pediatric doses, footnote[33,34] and footnote1, page 11 (Otitis). **Mild/Mod. Disease: AM-CL-ER** OR (**cefpodoxime, cefprozil**, or **cefdinir**) Treat 5-10 days. Adult doses in footnote[34] & Comment	**Severe Disease:** **Gati[NUS], Gemi, Levo, Moxi** Adjunctive rx in footnote[34]	**Complications:** From acute viral rhinosinusitis—transient hyposmia. From acute bacterial rhinosinusitis—orbital infections, meningitis, epidural abscess, brain abscess & cavernous sinus thrombosis. Adjunctive therapy for cavernous sinus thrombosis: topical decongestant (oxymetazoline) for < 3 d; nasal steroids of possible benefit; antihistamines (minor role), saline irrigation may help.
		See Table 11, pages 117 & 122.		
Hospitalized + nasotracheal or nasogastric intubation	Gm-neg. bacilli 47% (pseudomonas, klebsiella, enterobacter, E. coli common), Gm+ (S. aureus) 35%, yeasts 18% Polymicrobial in 60%	Remove nasotracheal tube if fever persists and ENT available; recommend sinus aspiration for C/S prior to empiric therapy **IMP** 0.5 gm IV q6h or **MER** 1 gm IV q8h. **AM-CL-ER** 2000/125 mg bid, **amox high-dose (HD)** 1 gm po q6h; add **clarithro** 500 mg po or **vanco** 1 gm IV for MRSA if Gram stain suggestive.	(**Ceftaz** 2 gm IV q8h + **vanco**) or (**CFP** 2 gm IV q12h + **vanco**)	After 7 days of nasotracheal or nasogastric tubes, 95% have x-ray "sinusitis" (fluid in sinuses), but on transnasal puncture only 38% culture + (AJRCCM 150:776, 1994). For pts requiring mechanical ventilation with nasotracheal tube for ≥1 wk, bacterial sinusitis occurs in <10% (CID 27:851, 1998). May need fluconazole if yeast on Gram stain of sinus aspirate.

[33] **Pediatric doses for sinusitis (all oral): Amox HD** high dose 90 mg per kg per day div. q8h or q12h; **AM-CL-ES** (extra strength) pediatric susp.: 90 mg **amox** component per kg per day, div. q12h; **azithro** 10 mg per kg times 1, then 5 mg per kg per day times 4 days; **cefdinir** 7 mg per kg per day div. q24h or divided bid; **cefpodoxime** 10 mg per kg per day div. q12h; **cefuroxime axetil** 30 mg per kg per day div. q12h; **clarithro** 7.5 mg per kg per day div. q12h; **cefprozil** 15 mg/kg/day divided bid (max 1 gm/day); **TMP-SMX** 8-12 mg TMP/40-60 mg SMX per kg per day div. q12h.

[34] **Adjunctive therapy for sinusitis (all oral): AM-CL-ER** 2000/125 **mg** bid, **amox high-dose (HD)** 1 gm po q6h; **clarithro** 500 mg po or **clarithro ext. release** 1 gm po q24h; **doxy** 100 mg bid, **respiratory FQs** (**Gati** 400 mg q24h[NUS] due to hypo/hyperglycemia. **Gemi** 320 mg q24h (not FDA indication but should work), **Levo** 750 mg q24h x 5 days. **Moxi** 400 mg q24h); **O Ceph** (**cefdinir** 300 mg q12h or 600 mg q24h, **cefpodoxime** 200 mg bid, **cefuroxime** 250-500 mg bid). **TMP-SMX** 1 double-strength (TMP 160 mg) bid (results after 3- and 10-day rx similar).

Abbreviations on page 2. *NOTE: All dosage recommendations are for adults (unless otherwise indicated) and assume normal renal function.*

TABLE 1 (48)

ANATOMIC SITE/DIAGNOSIS/ MODIFYING CIRCUMSTANCES	ETIOLOGIES (usual)	SUGGESTED REGIMENS* PRIMARY	SUGGESTED REGIMENS* ALTERNATIVE[$]	ADJUNCT DIAGNOSTIC OR THERAPEUTIC MEASURES AND COMMENTS
SINUSES, PARANASAL *(continued)*				
Sinusitis, chronic Adults	Prevotella, anaerobic strep, & fusobacterium—most common anaerobes. Strep sp., haemophilus, P. aeruginosa, S. aureus, & moraxella—aerobes. *(CID 35:428, 2002)*	Antibiotics usually not effective	Otolaryngology consultation. If acute exacerbation, treat as acute sinusitis.	Pathogenesis unclear and may be polyfactorial: damage to ostiomeatal complex, underlying acute bacterial disease, allergy ± polyps, occult immunodeficiency, and/or odontogenic disease (periodontitis in maxillary teeth).
SKIN				
Acne vulgaris *(Med Lett Treatment Guidelines 11 (Issue 125): 1, 2013).* Comedonal acne, "blackheads," whiteheads, earliest form, no inflammation.	Excessive sebum production & gland obstruction. No Propionibacterium acnes	All once-q24h: Topical **tretinoin** (cream 0.025% or 0.05%) or (gel 0.01 or 0.025%)	Topical **adapalene** 0.1% gel OR **azelaic acid** 20% cream or **tazarotene** 0.1% cream	Goal is prevention. ↓ number of new comedones and create an environment unfavorable to P. acnes. Adapalene causes less irritation than tretinoin. Azelaic acid less potent but less irritating than retinoids. **Tazarotene: Do not use in pregnancy.**
Mild inflammatory acne: small papules or pustules	Proliferation of P. acnes + abnormal desquamation of follicular cells	Topical **erythro** 3% + **benzoyl peroxide** 5%, bid	Can substitute **clinda** 1% gel for erythro	In random. controlled trial, topical benzoyl peroxide + erythro of equal efficacy to oral minocycline & tetracycline and not affected by antibiotic resistance of propionibacteria (*Ln 364:2188, 2004*).
Inflammatory acne: comedones, papules & pustules. Less common: deep nodules (cysts)	Progression of above events. Also, drug induced, e.g., glucocorticoids, phenytoin, lithium, INH & others.	(Topical **erythro** 3% + **benzoyl peroxide** 5% bid) + oral antibiotic. See *Comment* for mild acne	Oral drugs: (**doxy** 50 mg bid) or (**minocycline** 50 mg bid). Others: **tetracycline**, **erythro**, **TMP-SMX**, **clinda**. Extended release **minocycline** (Solodyn) 1 mg/kg/d	Systemic **isotretinoin** reserved for pts with severe widespread nodular cystic lesions that fail oral antibiotic rx: 4-5 mos. course of 0.1–1 mg per kg per day. Aggressive/violent behavior reported. **Tetracyclines** stain developing teeth. **Doxy** can cause photosensitivity. **Minocycline** side-effects: urticaria, vertigo, pigment deposition in skin or oral mucosa. Rare induced autoimmunity in children: fever, polyarthralgia, positive ANCA (*J Peds* 153:314, 2008).
Acne rosacea Ref: *NEJM 352:793, 2005.*	Skin mite: Demadex folliculorum	**Azelaic acid** gel bid, topical or **Metro** topical cream once daily or q24h	**Doxy** 50 mg po once daily.	Avoid activities that provoke flushing, e.g. alcohol, spicy food, sunlight. Ref: *Med Lett 49:5, 2007.*
Anthrax, cutaneous. Inhalation. To report bioterrorism event: 770-488-7100. For info: www.bt.cdc.gov See *JAMA* 281:1735, 1999; *MMWR* 50:909, 2001. Treat as inhalation if systemic illness.	B. anthracis Spores are introduced subcutaneous into the skin by contact with infected animals/animal products. See **Lung**, page 43.	**Adults (including pregnancy) and children >50 kg: CIP** 500 mg po bid or **Levo** 500 mg IV/po q24h x 60 days. **Children: CIP** 30 mg/kg/day div q12h po (to max. 1 gm per day) or **levo** 8 mg/kg po q24h x 60 days	**Adults (including pregnancy): Doxy** 100 mg po bid x 60 days. **Children:** Doxy: >8 y/o & >45 kg: 100 mg po bid; ≤8 y/o & ≤45 kg: 2.2 mg/kg po bid. All for 60 days.	1. If penicillin susceptible, then: **Adults: Amox** 500 mg po q8h times 60 days. **Children: Amox** 80 mg per kg per day, q8h (max. 500 mg, q8h). 2. Usual treatment of cutaneous anthrax is 7–10 days; 60 days in setting of bioterrorism with presumed aerosol exposure. 3. Other **FQs** (Levo, Moxi) should work based on in vitro susceptibility data. 4. Intestinal anthrax can also occur (*NEJM 363:766, 2010*). 5. Anthrax vaccine absorbed recommended at 0, 2, 4 wks postexposure for postexposure prophylaxis.
Bacillary angiomatosis: For other Bartonella infections, see **Cat-scratch disease** lymphadenitis, page 45, and **Bartonella** systemic infections, page 57	Bartonella henselae and quintana	**Clarithro** 500 mg po qid or ext. release 1 gm po q24h or **azithro** 250 mg po q24h (see *Comment*)	**Clarithro** 500 mg po qid or (**Doxy** 100 mg po bid + **RIF** 300 mg po bid)	For AIDS pts, continue suppressive therapy until HIV treated and CD > 200 cells/μL for 6 mos.

Abbreviations on page 2.   NOTE: All dosage recommendations are for adults (unless otherwise indicated) and assume normal renal function.

TABLE 1 (49)

ANATOMIC SITE/DIAGNOSIS/ MODIFYING CIRCUMSTANCES	ETIOLOGIES (usual)	SUGGESTED REGIMENS* PRIMARY	SUGGESTED REGIMENS* ALTERNATIVE†	ADJUNCT DIAGNOSTIC OR THERAPEUTIC MEASURES AND COMMENTS
SKIN (continued)				
Bite: Remember tetanus prophylaxis— See Table 20B, page 215 for rabies prophylaxis.				For extensive review of microbiology of animal bite caused infections, see CMR 24:231, 2011.
Bat, raccoon, skunk	Strep & staph from skin; rabies	AM-CL 875/125 mg po bid	Doxy 100 mg po bid	In Americas, **anti-rabies rx indicated**: rabies immune globulin + vaccine. (See Table 20B, page 215)
Camel	S. aureus, P. aeruginosa, Pasteurella sp.	PIP-TZ 3.375-4.5 gm IV q6h + CIP 750 mg po bid	Cephalexin 500 mg po qid + CIP 750 mg po bid	See EJCMID 18:918, 1999
Cat: 80% get infected; culture & treat empirically.	Pasteurella multocida, Streptococci, Staph. aureus, Nesseria, Moraxella	AM-CL 875/125 mg po bid or 500/125 mg po bid	Cefuroxime axetil 0.5 gm q12h or doxy 100 mg po bid	P. multocida resistant to dicloxacillin, cephalexin, clinda; many strains resistant to erythro (most sensitive to azithro but no clinical data). P. multocida infection develops within 24 hrs. Observe for osteomyelitis. If culture + for only P. multocida, can switch to pen G IV or pen VK po. See Dog Bite
Cat-scratch disease, page 45				
Catfish sting	Toxins	See Comments		Presents as immediate pain, erythema and edema. Resembles strep cellulitis.
Dog: Only 5% get infected; treat only if bite severe or bad co-morbidity (e.g. diabetes).	Pasteurella canis, S. aureus, Streptococci, Fusobacterium sp. Capnocytophaga canimorsus	AM-CL 875/125 mg po bid or 500/125 mg po bid	Clinda 300 mg po qid (adults) + (either FQ or TMP-SMX) (children)	May become secondarily infected. AM-CL is reasonable choice for prophylaxis. Consider anti-rabies prophylaxis: rabies immune globulin + vaccine (see Table 20B). Capnocytophaga in splenectomized pts may cause local eschar, sepsis with DIC. **P. canis resistant to diclox, cephalexin, clinda and erythro;** sensitive to ceftriaxone, cefuroxime, cefpodoxime and FQs. **Do not use cephalexin.** Sens. to FQs in vitro.
Human: For bacteriology, see CID 37:1481, 2003	Viridans strep 100%, Staph epidermidis 53%, corynebacterium 41%, **Staph. aureus 29%, eikenella 15%,** bacteroides 82%, peptostrep 26%	Early (not yet infected): AM-CL 875/125 mg po bid times 5 days; Later: Signs of infection (usually in 3-24 hrs): (AM-SB 1.5 gm IV q6h or cefoxitin 2 gm IV q8h) or (TC-CL 3.1 gm IV q4h or PIP-TZ 3.375 gm IV q6h or 4.5 gm q8h or 4-hr infusion of 3.375 gm q8h) Pen allergy: **Clinda** 1 tab + (either **CIP** or **TMP-SMX**)	TMP-SMX DS 1 tab po bid	**Cleaning, irrigation and debridement most important.** Bites inflicted by hospitalized pts, consider aerobic Gm-neg. bacilli. **Eikenella resistant to clinda, nafcillin/oxacillin, metro, P Ceph 1, and erythro; susceptible to FQs and TMP-SMX.**
Leech (Medicinal)	Aeromonas hydrophila	**CIP** (400 mg IV or 750 mg po) bid		Aeromonas found in 5 tract of leeches. Some use prophylactic antibiotics when leeches used medically, but not universally accepted or necessary (IDCP 10:211, 2001). Avoid Amp or 1st gen Cephalosporins (CID 35:e1, 2002). Information limited but infection is common and serious (Ln 348:888, 1996).
Pig (swine)	Polymicrobic: Gm+ cocci, Gm-neg. bacilli, anaerobes, Pasteurella sp.	AM-CL 875/125 mg po bid	P. Ceph 3 or TC-CL or AM-SB IV or IMP	CID 20:421, 1995
Prairie dog	Monkeypox	See Table 14A, page 165. No rx recommended		
Primate, non-human	Herpesvirus simiae	Acyclovir: See Table 14B, page 168		Anti-rabies rx not indicated. Tetanus prophylaxis. Penicillin generally used but would not be effective vs. organisms monilliformis). Pen G or doxy, alternatively erythro or clinda.
Rat	Spirillum minus & Streptobacillus moniliformis	AM-CL 875/125 mg po bid	Doxy	Can take weeks to appear after bite (Ln 364:448, 2004)
Seal	Marine mycoplasma	Tetracycline times 4 wks		
Snake: pit viper (Ref: NEJM 347:347, 2002)	Pseudomonas sp. Enterobacteriaceae, Staph. epidermidis, Clostridium sp.	Primary therapy is antivenom		**Primary therapy is antivenom**. Ceftriaxone should be more effective vs. organisms isolated. Ceftriaxone should be more effective vs. organisms isolated. Ref: CID 43:1309, 2006; cutaneous anthrax (Ln 364:549, 2004) or **MRSA infection** (spider bite painful; anthrax not painful).
Spider bite: Most necrotic ulcers attributed to spiders are probably due to another cause, e.g., cutaneous anthrax				
Widow (Latrodectus)	Not infectious	None		May be confused with "acute abdomen." Diazepam or calcium gluconate helpful to control pain, muscle spasm. Tetanus prophylaxis.
Brown recluse (Loxosceles) NEJM 352:700, 2005	Not infectious. "Overdiagnosed." Spider distribution limited to Central & desert SW of US	Bite usually self-limited & self-healing. No therapy of proven efficacy.	Dapsone 50 mg q24h	Dapsone causes hemolysis (check for G6PD deficiency). "Can cause hepatitis; baseline & weekly liver panels suggested.

NOTE: All dosage recommendations are for adults (unless otherwise indicated) and assume normal renal function.

Abbreviations on page 2.

TABLE 1 (50)

ANATOMIC SITE/DIAGNOSIS/ MODIFYING CIRCUMSTANCES	ETIOLOGIES (usual)	SUGGESTED REGIMENS* PRIMARY	ALTERNATIVE†	ADJUNCT DIAGNOSTIC OR THERAPEUTIC MEASURES AND COMMENTS
SKIN (continued)				
Boils—Furunculosis—Subcutaneous abscesses in drug addicts ("skin poppers"). Carbuncles = multiple connecting furuncles; Emergency Dept Perspective (IDC No Amer 22:89, 2008).				
Active lesions See Table, page 78 Community-associated MRSA widespread. I&D mainstay of therapy. Ref. CID 46:1032, 2008. No difference between TMP-SMX and placebo in peds pts–most with abscesses <5 cm (An Emer Med (ePub, Apr 29), 2009	Staph. aureus, both MRSA & MSSA. Concern for community-associated MRSA (See Comments) IDSA Guidelines: CID 52 (Feb 1):1, 2011.	If afebrile & abscess <5 cm in diameter: I&D, culture, hot packs. No drugs. If ≥5 cm in diameter: TMP-SMX-DS 1 tab po bid times 5–10 days. Alternatives (Adult dosage) clinda 300–600 mg po q6-8h or doxy or minocycline 100 mg po q12h	Febrile, large &/or multiple abscesses, outpatient care: I&D, culture abscess & maybe blood, hot packs. TMP-SMX-DS 1 tab po bid ± RIF 300 mg bid) times 10 days. If no response after 2–3 days, look for complications and consider IV therapy.	One TMP-SMX-DS tab bid as effective as 2 tabs bid in prospective case control study (AAC 55:5430, 2011). TMP-SMX activity vs streptococci uncertain. Usually clear clinical separation of strep "cellulitis" (erysipelas) from S. aureus abscess. If unclear or strep, use clinda or TMP-SMP plus beta-lactam. Few data to support TMP-SMP alone first. Other options: (1) Linezolid 600 mg po bid x 10 days; (2) Fusidic acid[NUS] 250-500 mg po q8-12h ± RIF (CID 42:394, 2006); (3) FQs only if in vitro susceptibility known.
		Incision and Drainage mainstay of therapy!		
To lessen number of furuncle recurrences—decolonization For surgical prophylaxis, see Table 15B, page 193.	MSSA & MRSA. IDSA Guidelines, CID 52 (Feb 1):1, 2011; AAC 56:1084, 2012.	7-day therapy: Chlorhexidine (2%) washes daily, 2% mupirocin ointment in anterior nares bid x 7 days + doxy 100 mg bid)	Mupirocin ointment in anterior nares bid x 7 days + chlorhexidine (2%) washes daily + TMP-SMX DS 1 tab po bid ± RIF 300 mg po bid) x 7 days	Optimal regimen uncertain. In randomized prospective study of combined topical & systemic therapy, negative MRSA cultures at 3 mos. in 74% of treated vs. 32% of not treated (CID 44:178, 2007). Mupirocin trials: CID 48:922, 2009; AAC 54:4415, 2009. No benefit from decolonizing household contacts (CID 54:743, 2012). Can substitute bleach baths for chlorhexidine (Inf Control Hosp Epidemiol 32:872, 2011). Bacitracin oint. inferior to Mupirocin (ICHE 43:351, 1999).
Hidradenitis suppurativa Not infectious disease, but bacterial superinfection occurs	Lesions secondarily infected: S. aureus, Enterobacter, anaerobes, Pseudomonas anaerobes	Clinda 1% topical cream Adalimumab 40 mg once weekly beneficial (AnIM 157:846, 2012)	Tetracycline 500 mg po bid x 3 months	Caused by keratinous plugging of apocrine glands of axillary, inguinal, perianal, perineal, infra-mammary areas. Other therapy: antiperspirants, loose clothing and anti-androgens. Dermatol Clin 28:779, 2010.
Burns. For overall management: NEJM 360:810, 2004—step-by-step procedure outlined.				
Initial burn wound care (CID 37:543, 2003& BMJ 332:649, 2006) Topical therapy options: NEJM 359:1037, 2008.	Not infected Prophylactic measures.	Early excision & wound closure; Variety of skin grafts and skin substitutes: see JAMA 283:717, 2000 & Adv Skin Wound Care 18:323, 2005; shower hydrotherapy. Role of topical antimicrobials unclear.	Silver sulfadiazine cream, 1%, apply 1–2 times per day or 0.5% silver nitrate solution or mafenide acetate cream. Apply bid.	Marrow-induced neutropenia can occur during 1st wk of sulfadiazine but resolves even if use is continued. Silver nitrate leaches electrolytes from wounds & stains everything. Mafenide inhibits carbonic anhydrase and can cause metabolic acidosis.
Burn wound sepsis	Strep. pyogenes, Enterobacter sp., S. aureus, S. epidermidis, E. faecalis, E. coli, P. aeruginosa Fungi rare. Herpesvirus rare.	Vanco 1 gm IV q12h) + (amikacin 10 mg per kg loading dose then 7.5 mg per kg IV q12h) + (PIP 4 gm IV q4h every ½ q24h dose of piperacillin into subeschar tissues with surgical eschar removal within 12 hours]) Can use PIP-TZ if PIP not available.		Monitor serum levels of Vanco and AMK as T½ of most antibiotics ↓. Staph. aureus tend to remain localized to burn wound; if toxic, consider toxic shock syndrome. Candida sp. colonize but seldom invade. Pneumonia is the major non-infectious complication, often staph. Complications include septic thrombophlebitis at IV sites. Dapto (6-8 mg per kg IV q24h) alternative for vanco.

Abbreviations on page 2. NOTE: All dosage recommendations are for adults (unless otherwise indicated) and assume normal renal function.

53

TABLE 1 (51)

ANATOMIC SITE/DIAGNOSIS/ MODIFYING CIRCUMSTANCES	ETIOLOGIES (usual)	SUGGESTED REGIMENS* PRIMARY	ALTERNATIVE[$]	ADJUNCT DIAGNOSTIC OR THERAPEUTIC MEASURES AND COMMENTS
SKIN (continued)				
Cellulitis, erysipelas: Be wary of macrolide (erythro-resistant) Streptococcus sp. Review: NEJM 350:904, 2004. **NOTE:** Consider diseases that masquerade as cellulitis (AVIM 142:47, 2005)				
Extremities, non-diabetic For diabetes, see below. Practice guidelines: CID 41:1373, 2005.	Strep. sp. (Gp A, B, C & G); Staph. aureus, including MRSA (but rare).	**Pen G** 1-2 million units IV q6h or **cefazolin** 1 gm IV q8h. If Pen-allergic: **Vanco** 15 mg/kg IV q12h. When afebrile: Pen VK 500 mg po q6h & hs. Total therapy: 10 days.	**Pen VK** 500 mg po qid & hs x 10 days. If Pen-allergic: Azithro 500 mg po x 1 dose, then 250 mg once daily x 4 days (total 5 days). Rarely, might need Linezolid 600 mg po bid. (expensive).	Look for tinea pedis as portal of entry. Treat if present. If S. aureus suspected (esp. for fluctuance or positive gram stain: MSSA: Diclox 500 mg po qid or Nafcillin/Oxacillin 2 gm IV q4h; MRSA: Doxy 100 mg po bid or TMP-SMX-DS 1 tab po bid or Vanco 1 gm IV q12h (inpatient). If S. aureus confirmed, usually need I&D. S. pyogenes: S. pyogenes may fail in vivo even if active in vitro (Eur J Clin Micro 3:424, 1984).
Facial, adult (erysipelas)	Strep. sp. (Gp A, B, C & G); Staph. aureus to include MRSA, S. pneumo	**Vanco** 1 gm IV q12h. If over 100 kg, 1.5 gm IV q12h	**Dapto** 4 mg/kg IV q24h or **Linezolid** 600 mg IV q12h	**Choice of empiric therapy must have activity vs. S. aureus**. S. aureus erysipelas of face can mimic streptococcal erysipelas of an extremity. Forced to treat empirically for MRSA until in vitro susceptibilities available.
Diabetes mellitus and erysipelas (See Foot, "Diabetic", page 16)	Strep. sp. (Grp A, B, C & G). Staph. aureus, Enterobacteriaceae, Anaerobes	**Early mild: TMP-SMX-DS** 1-2 tabs po bid + **cephalexin** 500 mg po qid or **cefazolin** 500 mg po qid or for severe disease: **IMP, MER, ERTA** or **Dori IV** + (**linezolid** 600 mg IV/po bid or **vanco** IV or **dapto** 4 mg/kg IV q24h). Dosage, see page 16.		Prompt surgical debridement indicated to rule out necrotizing fasciitis and to obtain cultures. If septic, consider x-ray of extremity to demonstrate gas. **Prognosis dependent on blood supply: assess arteries.** See diabetic foot, page 16. For severe disease, use regimen that targets both aerobic gram-neg bacilli & MRSA.
Erysipelas 2° to lymphedema (congenital = Milroy's disease); post-breast surgery with lymph node dissection	Streptococcus sp. Groups A, C, G	**Benzathine pen G** 1.2 million units IM q4 wks		Indicated if pt. is having > 2 episodes of cellulitis. Pen V 250 mg po bid should be effective. If not aware of clinical trials. In pen-allergic pts: erythro 500 mg po q24h, azithro 250 mg po q24h, or clarithro 500 mg po q24h.
Dandruff (seborrheic dermatitis)	Malassezia species	Ketoconazole shampoo 2% or selenium sulfide 2.5% (see page 10, chronic external otitis)		
Erythema multiforme	H. simplex, type 1, mycoplasma, Strep. pyogenes, drugs (sulfonamides, phenytoin, penicillin)			**Rx: Acyclovir** if due to H. simplex (Dermatology 207:349, 2003).
Erythema nodosum	Sarcoidosis, inflammatory bowel disease, M. TBc, coccidioidomycosis, yersinia, sulfonamides, Whipple's disease.			**Rx: NSAIDs; glucocorticoids** if refractory. Identify and treat precipitant disease if possible.
Erythrasma	Corynebacterium minutissimum	Localized infection: **Topical Clinda** 2-3 x daily x 7-14 days	Widespread infection: **Clarithro** 500 mg po bid or **Erythro** 250 mg po bid x 14 days	Dx: Coral red fluorescence with Wood's lamp. If infection recurs, prophylactic bathing with anti-bacterial soap or wash with benzyl peroxide.
Folliculitis	S. aureus, candida, P. aeruginosa common	Usually self-limited, no Rx needed. Could use topical mupirocin for Staph and topical antifungal for Candida.		
Furunculosis	Staph. aureus	See Boils, page 53		
Hemorrhagic bullous lesions Hx of sea water-contaminated abrasion or eating raw seafood in cirrhotic pt.	Vibrio vulnificus (CID 52:788, 2011)	**Ceftazidime** 2 gm IV q8h + **doxy** 100 mg IV/po bid	Either **cefotaxime** 2 gm IV or **CIP** 750 mg po bid or 400 mg IV bid)	Wound infection in healthy hosts, but bacteremia mostly in cirrhotics. Pathogenesis: Open wound exposure to contaminated seawater. Can cause necrotizing fasciitis (JAC 67:488, 2012).
Herpes zoster (shingles) See Table 14				

NOTE: All dosage recommendations are for adults (unless otherwise indicated) and assume normal renal function.

TABLE 1 (52)

ANATOMIC SITE/DIAGNOSIS/ MODIFYING CIRCUMSTANCES	ETIOLOGIES (usual)	SUGGESTED REGIMENS* PRIMARY	SUGGESTED REGIMENS* ALTERNATIVE[1]	ADJUNCT DIAGNOSTIC OR THERAPEUTIC MEASURES AND COMMENTS
SKIN (continued)				
Impetigo—children, military "Honey-crust" lesions Non-bullous Ecthyma is closely related. Causes "punched out" skin lesions.	Group A strep impetigo (rarely C or G); crusted lesions can be Group A (or C or G); crusted lesions can be Staph. aureus. Staph. aureus may be secondary colonizer.	Mupirocin ointment 2% tid or retapamulin cream 1%, times 7-12 days or retapamulin 1% bid times 5 days *For dosages, see Table 10A and Table 16, page 203 for children*	Should be no need for oral antibiotics.	In meta-analysis that combined strep & staph impetigo, mupirocin had higher cure rates than placebo. Mupirocin superior to oral erythro. Penicillin. Few placebo-controlled trials. Ref.: *Cochrane Database Systemic Reviews, 2004 (2): CD003261*. 46% of USA-300 CA-MRSA isolates carry gene encoding resistance to Mupirocin (*Ln 367:731, 2006*). **Note:** While resistance to Mupirocin continues to evolve, over-the-counter triple antibiotic ointment (Neomycin, polymyxin B, Bacitracin) remains active in vitro (*CMID 54:63, 2006*). **Ecthyma:** Infection deeper into epidermis than impetigo. May need parenteral penicillin. Military outbreaks reported: *CID 48: 1213 & 1220, 2009 (good images)*.
Bullous (if ruptured, thin "varnish-like" crust)	Staph. aureus. MSSA & MRSA. strains that produce exfoliative toxin A.	For MSSA: po therapy with dicloxacillin, oxacillin, cephalexin, AM-CL, azithro, clarithro, or mupirocin ointment or retapamulin ointment	For MRSA: Mupirocin ointment or po therapy with TMP-SMX-DS, minocycline, doxy, clinda. *For dosages, see Table 10A*	
Infected wound, extremity *(for bites, see page 52; for post-operative, see page 52)*— Gram stain negative				
Mild to moderate, uncomplicated. Debride wound, if necessary.	Polymicrobic: S. aureus (MSSA & MRSA), aerobic & anaerobic strep.	TMP-SMX-DS 1-2 tabs po bid or clinda 300-450 mg po tid (see Comment)	Mino-cycline 100 mg po bid or linezolid 600 mg po bid (see Comment)	**Culture & sensitivity, check Gram stain. Tetanus toxoid if indicated. Mild infection:** Suggested drugs focus on S. aureus & Strep species. If suspect Gm-neg. bacilli, add **AM-CL-ER** 1000/62.5 two tabs po bid. If MRSA is erythro-resistant, use **linezolid** 600 mg IV/po q12h.
Febrile with sepsis—hospitalized. Debride wound, if necessary.	Enterobacteriaceae, C. perfringens, Cl. tetani; if water exposure, Pseudomonas sp., Ae(o) bacillus sp. Acinetobacter in soldiers in Iraq (see *CID 47:444, 2008*).	TC-CL, PIP-TZ, DORI[NA] or IMP or MER or ERTA *(Dosage, page 25)* + vanco 1 gm IV q12h (1.5 gm if > 100 kg).	Mino-cycline 1 gm IV q12h + dapto 6 mg per kg IV q24h or ceftaroline 600 mg IV q12h or telavancin 10 mg/kg IV q24h + (CIP or Levo IV—dose in Comment)	**Fever—sepsis:** Another alternative is **linezolid** 600 mg IV/po q12h (q8h if P. aeruginosa) or **Levo** 750 mg IV q24h. Why 1-2 **TMP-SMX-DS?** See discussion in footnote 1 of Table 6 (*MRSA*) **TMP-SMX** not predictably active vs. strep species.
Infected wound, post-operative—Gram stain negative; for Gram stain positive cocci - see below				
Surgery not involving GI or female genital tract Without sepsis (mild, afebrile) With sepsis (severe, febrile)	Staph. aureus, Group A, B, C or G strep sp.	**TMP-SMX-DS** 1 tab po bid **Vanco** 1 gm IV q12h, if >100 kg., 1.5 gm q12h.	**Clinda** 300-450 mg po tid **Dapto** 6 mg per kg IV q24h or **televancin** 10 mg/kg IV q24h	Check Gram stain of exudate. If Gm-neg. bacilli **add** β-lactam/β-lactamase inhibitor: **AM-CL-ER** po or (**ERTA** or **PIP-TZ**, or **TC-CL**) IV. *Dosage on page 25.* Why 1-2 **TMP-SMX-DS?** See discussion in footnote 1 of Table 6 (*MRSA*). **TMP-SMX** not predictably active vs. strep species.
Surgery involving GI tract (includes oropharynx, esophagus) or female genital tract—fever, neutrophilia	MSSA/MRSA, coliforms, bacteroides & other anaerobes	(**PIP-TZ** or **P Ceph 3** + metro) or **DORI** or **ERTA** or **IMP** or **MER**) + (vanco 1 gm IV q12h). If severely ill: **TMP-SMX-DS** 1-2 tabs po bid if Gm+ cocci on Gram stain. *Dosages Table 10A & footnote 36, page 62.*	Mild infection: **AM-CL-ER** 1000/62.5, 1-2 tabs po bid	For all treatment options, see *Peritonitis, page 47.* Most important: Drain wound & get cultures. Can sub **linezolid** for vanco. Can sub **CIP** or **Levo** for β-lactams. Why 2 **TMP-SMX-DS?** See discussion in footnote 1 of Table 6 (*MRSA*)
Meleney's synergistic gangrene	See *Necrotizing fasciitis, page 56*			

Abbreviations on page 2.   NOTE: All dosage recommendations are for adults (unless otherwise indicated) and assume normal renal function.

TABLE 1 (53)

ANATOMIC SITE/DIAGNOSIS/ MODIFYING CIRCUMSTANCES	ETIOLOGIES (usual)	SUGGESTED REGIMENS* PRIMARY	SUGGESTED REGIMENS* ALTERNATIVE[†]	ADJUNCT DIAGNOSTIC OR THERAPEUTIC MEASURES AND COMMENTS
SKIN/Infected wound, post-operative—Gram stain negative (continued)				
Infected wound, post-op, febrile patient— Positive gram stain: Gram-positive cocci in clusters	S. aureus, possibly MRSA	**Do culture & sensitivity: open & drain wound** Oral: **TMP-SMX-DS** 1-2 tabs po bid or **clinda** 300-450 mg po tid (see Comment)	IV: **Vanco** 1 gm IV q12h or **dapto** 4-6 mg/kg IV q24h or **linezolid** 600 mg po q12h (expensive) or **telavancin** 10 mg/kg IV q24h	Need culture & sensitivity to verify MRSA. Other po options for CA-MRSA include minocycline 100 mg po q12h or **Doxy** 100 mg po bid (inexpensive) & linezolid 600 mg po q12h (expensive). If MRSA clinda-sensitive but erythro-resistant, watch out for inducible clinda resistance.
Necrotizing fasciitis ("flesh-eating bacteria") Post-surgery, trauma, or strepto-coccal skin infections See **Gas gangrene, page 46**, & **Toxic shock, page 64**. Refs. CID 44:705, 2007; NEJM 360:281, 2009	5 types: (1) Strep sp. Grp A, C, G; (2) Clostridia sp.; (3) polymicrobic: aerobic + anaerobic strep = Meleney's synergistic gangrene); (4) Community-associated MRSA; (5) K. pneumoniae (CID 55:930 & 946, 2012)	For treatment of clostridia, see **Muscle, gas gangrene, page 46**. The terminology of **polymicrobic** wound infections is not precise. Meleney's synergistic gangrene, Fournier's gangrene, necrotizing fasciitis have common pathophysiology. **All require prompt surgical debridement + antibiotics.** Dx of necrotizing fasciitis req incision & probing. If no resistance to blunt probing with facial plane involvement, (fascial plane), diagnosis = necrotizing fasciitis → polymicrobial, or S. aureus. **Need Gram stain/culture** to determine etiology is strep, clostridia, polymicrobial, or S. aureus. **Treatment: Pen G** if strep or clostridia: **DORI**™ **IMP** or **MER** if polymicrobial; add vanco OR dapto if MRSA suspected. **NOTE:** If strep necrotizing fasciitis, reasonable to treat with penicillin & clinda.; if clostridia is gas gangrene, add clinda to penicillin (see **page 46**). MRSA ref: NEJM 352:1445, 2005. **See toxic shock syndrome, streptococcal, page 64**.		
Puncture wound—nail, toothpick	Through nails shoe: P. aeruginosa	Local debridement to remove foreign body & tetanus prophylaxis, no antibiotic therapy.		Osteomyelitis evolves in only 1–2% of plantar puncture wounds. Consider x-ray if chance of radio-opaque foreign body.
Staphylococcal scalded skin syndrome Ref: PIDJ 19:819, 2000	Toxin-producing S. aureus	**Nafcillin** or **oxacillin** 2 gm IV q4h (children: 150 mg/kg/ div q6h) x 5-7 days for MSSA, **vanco** 1 gm IV q12h (children 40-60 mg/kg/day div. q6h) for MRSA		Toxin causes **intraepidermal split** and positive Nikolsky sign. Biopsy differentiates: drugs cause epidermal/dermal split, **called toxic epidermal necrolysis—more serious**.
Ulcerated skin lesions: Differential Dx	Consider: anthrax, tularemia, P. aeruginosa (ecthyma gangrenosum), plague, blastomycosis, mycobacteria, leishmania, spider (rarely), mucormycosis, YAWS, arterial insufficiency, venous stasis, and others.			
Ulcerated skin: venous/arterial insufficiency; pressure with secondary infection (infected decubiti)	Polymicrobic: Streptococcus sp. (Groups A, C, G), S. aureus & anaerobic strep., Enterobacteriaceae, Pseudomonas sp., Bacteroides sp., Staph. aureus	Severe local or possible bacteremia: **IMP** or **MER** or **DORI** or **TC-CL** or **PIP-TZ** or **ERTA** If Gm-pos cocci on gram stain, add **Vanco**	(**CIP** or **Levo**) + **Metro**) or (**CFP** or **Ceftaz**) + **Metro**) If Gm-pos cocci on gram stain, add **Vanco**	If ulcer clinically inflamed, treat IV with no topical rx. If not clinically inflamed, consider debridement, removal of foreign body, lessening direct pressure on weight-bearing limbs, & leg elevation (if no arterial insufficiency). Topical rx to reduce bacterial counts: silver sulfadiazine 1% or combination antibiotic ointment. **Chlorhexidine & povidone iodine may harm "granulation tissue"—Avoid.**
Whirlpool: (Hot Tub) folliculitis	Pseudomonas aeruginosa	Usually self-limited; treatment not indicated	Dosages, see footnotes 6, 6, 7, 12, 15, 36	
Whirlpool: Nail Salon, soft tissue infection	Mycobacterium (fortuitum or chelonae)	Minocycline, doxy or CIP		Decontaminate hot tub; drain and chlorinate. Also associated with exfoliative beauty aids (loofah sponges). Ref: CID 38:38, 2004.
SPLEEN. For post-splenectomy prophylaxis, see Table 15B, page 193; for Septic Shock Post-Splenectomy, see Table 1, pg 63.				
Splenic abscess Endocarditis, bacteremia Contiguous from intra-abdominal site Immunocompromised	Staph. aureus, streptococci Polymicrobic Candida sp.	**Nafcillin** or **oxacillin** 2 gm IV q4h if MSSA **Amphotericin B** (Dosage, see Table 11, page 113)	**Vanco** 1 gm IV q12h if MRSA, see **page 47** **Fluconazole, caspofungin**	Burkholderia (Pseudomonas) pseudomallei is common cause of splenic abscess in SE Asia.

Abbreviations on page 2. NOTE: All dosage recommendations are for adults (unless otherwise indicated) and assume normal renal function.

TABLE 1 (54)

ANATOMIC SITE/DIAGNOSIS/ MODIFYING CIRCUMSTANCES	ETIOLOGIES (usual)	SUGGESTED REGIMENS* PRIMARY	SUGGESTED REGIMENS* ALTERNATIVE[1]	ADJUNCT DIAGNOSTIC OR THERAPEUTIC MEASURES AND COMMENTS
SYSTEMIC SYNDROMES (FEBRILE/NON-FEBRILE) Spread by infected TICK, FLEA, or LICE. Epidemiologic history crucial. **Babesiosis, Lyme disease, & Anaplasma (Ehrlichiosis)** have same reservoir & tick vector.				
Babesiosis: see NEJM 366:2397, 2012; Etiol.: B. microti et al. Vector: Usually Ixodes ticks Babesiosis can be fatal if asymptomatic, young, has spleen, and immunocompromised.	Etiol.: B. microti et al. Vector: Usually Ixodes ticks Hosts: white-footed mouse & others	[(**Atovaquone** 750 mg po q12h) + (**azithro** 600 mg po day 1, then 500-1000 mg per day) times 7-10 days]. Duration of infection: Not clear but 7-10 days for mild, times 7 days + **quinine** 650 mg po tid times 7 days. **Ped. dosage: Clinda** 20-40 mg per kg per day and **quinine** 25 mg per kg per day). **Exchange transfusion--See Comment**		**Seven diseases where pathogen visible in peripheral blood smear:** African/American trypanosomiasis; babesia; bartonellosis; filariasis; malaria; plague; relapsing fever. **Dx: Giemsa-stained blood smear;** antibody test available. PCR if available. **Rx: Exchange transfusions successful adjunct if used early, in severe disease. May need treatment for 6 or more wks if immunocompromised. Look for Lyme and/or Anaplasma co-infection.**
Bartonella infections: Review E/D 12:389, 2006 Bacteremia, asymptomatic	B. quintana, B. henselae	**Doxy** 100 mg po/IV times 15 days		Can lead to endocarditis &/or trench fever; found in homeless, alcoholics, esp. if lice/leg pain. Often missed since asymptomatic.
Cat-scratch disease	B. henselae	**Azithro** 500 mg po x 1 dose, then 250 mg/day po x 4 days.		Or symptomatic only--see Lymphadenitis, page 45; usually lymphadenitis, hepatitis, splenitis, FUO, neuroretinitis, osteomyelitis, oculoglandular syndrome
Bacillary angiomatosis; Peliosis hepatis--pts with AIDS MMWR 58(RR-4):39, 2009; AAC 48:1921, 2004.	B. henselae, B. quintana	**Erythro** 500 mg po qid or **Doxy** 100 mg po bid x 3 months or longer. If CNS involvement: **Doxy** 100 mg IV/po bid + **RIF** 300 mg po bid	**Azithro** 250 mg po once daily x 3 months or longer	**Do not use:** TMP-SMX, CIP, Pen, Ceph. **Manifestations of Bartonella infections: HIV/AIDS Patient:** Bacteremia/endocarditis/FUO encephalitis Bacillary angiomatosis Bacteremia/endocarditis/FUO **Immunocompetent Patient:** Bacteremia/endocarditis/FUO/ encephalitis Cat scratch disease Vertebral osteo Trench fever Parinaud's oculoglandular syndrome
Endocarditis (see page 29) (Circ 111:3167, 2005); AAC 48:1921, 2004)	B. henselae, B. quintana	Regardless of CD4 count, DC therapy after 3-4 mos. & observe. If no relapse, no suppressive rx. If relapse, single **azithro** or **erythro** x 3 mos. Stop when CD4 ≥200, x 6 mos. Surgical removal of infected valve	If suspect endocarditis: **Doxy** 100 mg IV/po bid x 6 wks + **Gent** 1 mg/kg IV q8h x 11 days	**Gentamicin toxicity:** If Gent toxicity, substitute **Rifampin** 300 mg IV/po bid x 14 days. Role of valve removal surgery to cure unclear. Presents as SBE. Diagnosis: ECHO, serology & PCR of resected heart valve.
Oroya fever (acute) & Verruga peruana (chronic) (AAC 48:1921, 2004)	B. bacilliformis	If suspect endocarditis: **Ceftriaxone** 2 gm IV once daily x 6 weeks + **Gent** 1 mg/kg IV q8h x 14 days + **Doxy** 100 mg IV/po bid x 6 wks Oroya fever: **CIP** 500 mg po bid or **Doxy** 100 mg po bid) x 14 d. Alternative: **Chloro** 500 mg IV/po q6h x 10 days, or **Azithro** 500 mg po q24h x 7 days.	**Verruga peruana:** RIF 10 mg/kg/day po bid x 14 d or **Streptomycin** 15-20 mg/kg IM once daily x 10 days	Oroya fever transmitted by sand-fly bite in Andes Mtns. Related Bartonella (B. rochalimae) caused bacteremia, fever and splenomegaly (NEJM 356:2346 & 2381, 2007). CIP and Chloro preferred due to prevention of secondary Salmonella infections.
Trench fever (FUO) (AAC 48:1921, 2004)	B. quintana	No endocarditis: **Doxy** 100 mg po bid x 4 wks; If endocarditis: **Doxy** + **Gentamicin** 3 mg/kg once daily for 1st 2 wks of therapy (AAC 48:1921, 2004)		Vector is body louse. Do not use: TMP-SMX, FQs, cefazolin or Pen

NOTE: All dosage recommendations are for adults (unless otherwise indicated) and assume normal renal function.

Abbreviations on page 2.

57

TABLE 1 (55)

ANATOMIC SITE/DIAGNOSIS/ MODIFYING CIRCUMSTANCES	ETIOLOGIES (usual)	SUGGESTED REGIMENS* PRIMARY	SUGGESTED REGIMENS* ALTERNATIVE[§]	ADJUNCT DIAGNOSTIC OR THERAPEUTIC MEASURES AND COMMENTS
SYSTEMIC SYNDROMES (FEBRILE/NON-FEBRILE/Spread by infected TICK, FLEA, or LICE (continued)				
Ehrlichiosis[36]. CDC def. is one of: (1) 4x↑ IFA antibody, (2) detection of Ehrlichia DNA in blood or SF by PCR, (3) visible morulae in WBC and IFA ≥1:64. New species in WI, MN (NEJM 365:422, 2011). **Human monocytic ehrlichiosis (HME)** Chaffeensis (Lone Star tick is vector) MMWR 55(RR-4), 2006; CID 43:1089, 2006	E. chaffeensis (Lone Star tick is vector)	**Doxy** 100 mg po/IV bid times 7-14 days	**Tetracycline** 500 mg po qid x 7-14d. No current rec. for children or pregnancy	30 states; mostly SE of line from NJ to IL to Missouri to Oklahoma to Texas. History of outdoor activity and tick exposure. April-Sept. Fever, rash (36%), leukopenia and thrombocytopenia. Blood smears no help. PCR for early dx.
Human Anaplasmosis (formerly known as Human granulocytic ehrlichiosis)	Anaplasma (Ehrlichia) phagocytophilum (Ixodes sp. ticks are vector. Dog variant is Ehrlichia ewingii) NEJM 341:148 & 195, 1999	**Doxy** 100 mg bid po or IV times 7-14 days	**Tetracycline** 500 mg po qid times 7-14 days. Not in children or pregnancy. See Comment	Upper Midwest, NE, West Coast & Europe. H/O tick exposure. April-Sept. Febrile flu-like illness after outdoor activity. Doxy: Up to 80% have ↑ Leukopenia, thrombocytopenia less common. Dx: PCR on blood, serology, buffy coat smear test for confirmation (all difficult in pregnancy (CID 27:213, 1998) but worry about resistance developing. Based on in vitro studies, no clear alternative rx—Levo activity marginal (AAC 47:413, 2003).
Lyme Disease NOTE: Think about concomitant tick-borne disease—e.g., babesiosis and ehrlichiosis. **Guidelines:** CID 43:1089, 2006; CID 51:1, 2010 Bite by ixodes-infected tick in an endemic area— Post-exposure prophylaxis	Borrelia burgdorferi **IDSA guidelines:** CID 43:1089, 2006; CID 51:1, 2010	**If endemic area,** if nymphal partially engorged deer tick: **doxy** 200 mg po times 1 dose with food	**If not endemic area,** not engorged, not deer tick: No treatment	Prophylaxis study in endemic area: erythema migrans developed in 3% of the control group and 0.4% doxy group (NEJM 345:79 & 133, 2001).
Early (erythema migrans)	Western blot diagnostic criteria: **IgM**—Need 2 of 3 positive of 3 kilocatons (kD): 23, 39, 41 **IgG**—Need 5 of 10 positive of KD: 18, 21, 28, 30, 39, 41, 45, 58, 66, 93	**Doxy** 100 mg po bid, or **amoxicillin** 500 mg po tid or **cefuroxime axetil** 500 mg po bid. All regimens for 14-21 days (10 days as good as 20). See Comment for peds doses	**Tetracycline** 500 mg po qid times 14-21 days	High rate of clinical failure with azithro & erythro (Drugs 57:157, 1999). **Peds** (all po for 14-21 days): **Amox** 50 mg per kg per day in 3 div. doses or **cefuroxime axetil** 30 mg per kg per day in 2 div. doses or **erythro** 30 mg per kg per day in 4 div. doses. Lesions usually homogeneous—not target-like (AnIM 136:423, 2002).
Carditis See Comment		**(Ceftriaxone** 2 gm IV q24h) or **(cefotaxime** 2 gm IV q4h) or **(Pen G** 3 million units IV q4h) times 14-21 days	**Doxy** 100 mg po bid times 14-21 days or **amoxicillin** 500 mg po tid times 14-21 days	First degree AV block. Oral regimen. Generally self-limited. High degree AV block (PR >0.3 sec.): IV therapy—permanent pacemaker not necessary.
Facial nerve paralysis (isolated finding, early)		**Doxy** 100 mg po bid) or **amoxicillin** 500 mg po tid) times 14-21 days	**Ceftriaxone** 2 gm IV q24h times 14-21 days	LP suggested excluding central neurologic disease. If LP neg, oral regimen OK. If abnormal or not done, suggest parenteral Ceftriaxone.
Meningitis, encephalitis For encephalopathy, see Comment		**Ceftriaxone** 2 gm IV q24h times 14-28 days	**(Pen G** 20 million units IV q24h in div. doses) or **(cefotaxime** 2 gm IV q8h) times 14-28 days	Encephalopathy: memory difficulty, depression, somnolence, or headache. CSF abnormalities. 89% had objective CSF abnormalities. 18/18 pts improved with ceftriaxone 2 gm per day times 30 days (JID 180:377, 1999). No compelling evidence that prolonged treatment has any benefit in post-Lyme syndrome (Neurology 69:91, 2007).
Arthritis	For chronic lyme disease discussion see CID 51:1, 2010	**Doxy** 100 mg po bid, or **amoxicillin** 500 mg po tid), both times 30-60 days. Choice should **not** include doxy. **amoxicillin** 500 mg po tid times 21 days	**(Ceftriaxone** 2 gm IV q24h) or **(cefotaxime** 2 gm IV q24h) or **Pen G** 20-24 million units per day IV times 14-28 days **If pen. allergic: azithro** 500 mg po q24h times 7-10 days) or **erythro** 500 mg po qid times 14-21 days	Start with 1 mo of therapy; if only partial response, treat for a second mo.
Pregnant women		None indicated		
Post-Lyme Disease Syndromes				No benefit from treatment (CID 51:1, 2010; NEJM 345:85, 2001).

[36] In endemic area (New York), high % of both adult ticks and nymphs were jointly infected with Anaplasma (HGE) and B. burgdorferi.

[§] NOTE: All dosage recommendations are for adults (unless otherwise indicated) and assume normal renal function.

Abbreviations on page 2.

TABLE 1 (56)

ANATOMIC SITE/DIAGNOSIS/ MODIFYING CIRCUMSTANCES	ETIOLOGIES (usual)	SUGGESTED REGIMENS* PRIMARY	SUGGESTED REGIMENS* ALTERNATIVE[†]	ADJUNCT DIAGNOSTIC OR THERAPEUTIC MEASURES AND COMMENTS
SYSTEMIC SYNDROMES (FEBRILE/NON-FEBRILE)/Spread by infected TICK, FLEA, or LICE *(continued)*				
Relapsing fever Louse-borne (LBRF)	*Borrelia recurrentis* Reservoir: human Vector: Louse pediculus humanus	**Tetracycline** 500 mg IV/po x 1 dose	**Erythro** 500 mg IV/po x 1 dose	Jarisch-Herxheimer (fever, ↑ pulse, ↑ resp., ↓ blood pressure) in most patients (occurs in ~2 hrs). Not prevented by prior steroids. **Dx: Examine peripheral blood smear during fever for spirochetes.** Can relapse up to 10 times. Postexposure **doxy** pre-emptive therapy highly effective (*NEJM* 355:148, 2006) *B. miyamoto* ref: *EID* 17:816, 2011.
Tick-borne (TBRF)	No Amer: *B. hermsii, B. turicata;* Africa: *B. hispanica, B. crocidurae, B. duttonii;* Russia: *B. miyamoto*	**Doxy** 100 mg po bid x 7-10 days	**Erythro** 500 mg po qid x 7-10 days	
Rickettsial diseases. Review—Disease in travelers (*CID* 39:1493, 2004)				
Spotted fevers (NOTE: Rickettsial pox not included) Rocky Mountain spotted fever (**RMSF**) (*LnID* 8:143, 2008 and *MMWR* 55 (RR-4), 2007)	*R. rickettsii* (Dermacentor tick vector)	**Doxy** 100 mg IV/po bid times 7 days or for 2 days after temp. normal. Do not use in pregnancy. Some suggest single 200 mg loading dose.	**Chloro** 50 mg/kg/day in 4 div doses. Use in pregnancy.	Fever, rash (88%), petechiae 40–50%. **Rash spreads from distal extremities to trunk.** Rash in <50% pts in 1st 72 hr. Dx: Immunohistology on skin biopsy; confirmation with antibody titers. Highest incidence in SE and South Central states; also seen in Oklahoma, S. Dakota, Montana. Cases reported from 42 U.S. states. **NOTE: Only 3–18% of pts present with fever, rash, and hx of tick exposure; many early deaths in children & empiric doxy reasonable** (*MMWR* 49:885, 2000).
NOTE: Can mimic ehrlichiosis. Pattern of rash important—see Comment				
Other spotted fevers, e.g., Rickettsial pox, African tick bite fever	At least 8 species on 6 continents (*CID* 45 (Suppl 1): S39, 2007)	**Doxy** 100 mg po bid times 7 days	**Chloro** 500 mg po/IV qid times 7 days Children <8 y.o.: **azithro** or **clarithro** (if mild disease)	Clinical diagnosis supported by: 1) fever, intense myalgia, headache; 2) exposure to mites or ticks; 3) localized eschar (tache noire) or rash. Definitive Dx: PCR of blood, skin biopsy or sequential antibody tests.
Typhus group—Consider in returning travelers with fever				
Louse-borne: epidemic typhus Ref: *LnID* 8:417, 2008.	*R. prowazekii* (vector is body or head louse)	**Doxy** 100 mg IV/po bid times 7 days; single 200 mg dose 95% effective.	**Chloro** 500 mg IV/po qid times 5 days	**Brill-Zinsser disease** (*Ln* 357:1198, 2007) is a relapse of typhus acquired during WWII. Truncal rash (64%) spreads centrifugally—opposite of RMSF. Louse borne typhus is a winter disease. Diagnosis by serology. *R. prowazekii* found in flying squirrels in SE US. Delouse clothing of infected pt.
Murine typhus (cat flea typhus) (*Eid* 14:1019, 2008)	*R. typhi* (rat reservoir and flea vector); *CID* 46:913, 2008	**Doxy** 100 mg IV/po bid times 7 days	**Chloro** 500 mg IV/po qid times 5 days	Rash in 20–54%, not diagnostic. Despite clothing of infected pt. 2 wks. Faster recovery with treatment. Dx based on suspicion; confirmed serologically.
Scrub typhus	*O. tsutsugamushi* (rodent reservoir; vector is larval stage of mites (chiggers)	**Doxy** 100 mg po/IV bid x 7 days. In pregnancy: **Azithro** 500 mg po x one dose	**Chloro** 500 mg po/IV qid x 7 days	Asian/W Pacific. Suspect Dx in endemic area. Confirm with serology. If Doxy resistance suspected, alternatives are **Doxy** + **RIF** 900 or 600 mg once daily (*Ln* 356:1057, 2000) or **Azithro**.
Tularemia, typhoidal type Ref: **bioterrorism**; see *JAMA* 285:2763, 2001; *ID Clin No Amer* 22:489, 2008; *MMWR* 58:744, 2009.	*Francisella tularensis* (Vector depends on geography: ticks, biting flies, mosquitoes identified)	Moderate/severe: (**Gentamicin** or **tobra** 5 mg per kg per day q8h IV) or (**Streptomycin** 1 gm IM/IV q12h) x 10 days.	Mild: (**CIP** 400 mg IV or 750 mg po) bid or **Doxy** 100 mg IV/po bid) x 14-21 days	Diagnosis: Culture on cysteine-enriched media & serology. Dangerous in the lab. Hematogenous meningitis is a complication; treatment is **Streptomycin** + **Chloro** 50-100 mg/kg/day IV in 4 divided doses (*Arch Neurol* 66:523, 2009).

NOTE: All dosage recommendations are for adults (unless otherwise indicated) and assume normal renal function.

Abbreviations on page 2.

TABLE 1 (57)

SYSTEMIC SYNDROMES (FEBRILE/NON-FEBRILE)

Other Zoonotic Systemic Bacterial Febrile Illnesses: Obtain careful epidemiologic history

ANATOMIC SITE/DIAGNOSIS/ MODIFYING CIRCUMSTANCES	ETIOLOGIES (usual)	SUGGESTED REGIMENS* PRIMARY	SUGGESTED REGIMENS* ALTERNATIVE[1]	ADJUNCT DIAGNOSTIC OR THERAPEUTIC MEASURES AND COMMENTS
Brucellosis Refs: NEJM 352:2325, 2005; CID 62:126, 2008; MMWR 57:603, 2008; BMJ 336:701, 2008; PLoS One 7:e32090, 2012.	B. abortus–cattle B. suis–swine B. melitensis–goats B. canis–dogs	**Non focal disease:** [**Doxy** 100 mg po bid x 6 wks + **Gent** 5 mg/kg once daily for 1st 7 days] **Spondylitis, Sacroiliitis:** [**Doxy** + **Gent** (as above) + **RIF**] x min 3 mos **Neurobrucellosis:** [**Doxy** + **RIF** (as above) + **ceftriaxone** 2 gm IV q12h until CSF returned to normal (AAC 56:1523, 2012)] **Endocarditis:** Surgery + [(**RIF** + **Doxy** + **Gent**) for 2-4 wks] **Pregnancy:** Not much data. **RIF** 900 mg po once daily x 6 wks	[**Doxy** 100 mg po bid x 6 wks + **RIF** 600-900 mg po once daily] x 6 wks [(**CIP** 750 mg po bid + **RIF** 600-900 mg po once daily) x min 3 mos] **Pregnancy:** **RIF** 900 mg po once daily + **TMP-SMX** 5 mg/kg (TMP comp) po bid x 4 wks	CIP active in vitro but clinical response not good. Clinical response to ceftriaxone is variable. Bone involvement, esp. sacroiliitis in 20-30%. **Neurobrucellosis:** Usually meningitis; 1% of all pts with brucellosis. Role of corticosteroids unclear; not recommended. **Endocarditis:** Rare but most common cause of death. Need surgery + antimicrobials. **Pregnancy:** TMP-SMX may cause kernicterus if given during last week of pregnancy.
Leptospirosis CID 36:1507 & 1514, 2003; LnID 3:757, 2003	Leptospira—in urine of domestic livestock, dogs, small rodents	Severe illness: **Pen G** 1.5 million units IV q6h or **ceftriaxone** 1 gm q24h. Duration: 7 days	Mild illness: **Doxy** 100 mg IV/po q12h or **AMP** 0.5–1 gm IV q6h x 7 days	**Severity varies.** Two-stage mild anicteric disease to severe icteric disease (Weil's disease) with renal failure and myocarditis. **Rx:** Azithro 1 gm once, then 500 mg daily x 2 days; non-inferior to, and fewer side effects than, doxy in standard dose (AAC 51:3259, 2007). Jarisch-Herxheimer reaction can occur post-Pen therapy.
Salmonella bacteremia other than S. typhi (non-typhoidal)	Salmonella enteritidis— a variety of serotypes from animal sources	If NOT acquired in Asia: **CIP** 400 mg IV q12h or **Levo** 750 mg po once daily x 14 days (See Comment)	If acquired in Asia: **Ceftriaxone** 2 gm IV q24h or **Azithro** 1 gm po once daily x 5-7 days or 500 mg IV once daily until susceptibility determined. Do NOT use FQs until susceptibility determined. (See Comment)	In vitro resistance to nalidixic acid indicates relative resistance to FQs. Bacteremia can infect any organ/tissue: look for infection of atherosclerotic aorta, osteomyelitis in sickle cell pts. Duration range 14 days (immunocompetent) to ≥6 wks if mycotic aneurism or endocarditis. Alternative, if susceptible: **TMP-SMX** 8-10 mg/kg/day (TMP comp) divided q8h.

Abbreviations on page 2.   NOTE: All dosage recommendations are for adults (unless otherwise indicated) and assume normal renal function.

TABLE 1 (58)

SYSTEMIC SYNDROMES (FEBRILE/NON-FEBRILE)

Miscellaneous Systemic Febrile Syndromes

ANATOMIC SITE/DIAGNOSIS/ MODIFYING CIRCUMSTANCES	ETIOLOGIES (usual)	SUGGESTED REGIMENS* PRIMARY	ALTERNATIVE[§]	ADJUNCT DIAGNOSTIC OR THERAPEUTIC MEASURES AND COMMENTS
Fever in Returning Travelers (NEJM 354:119, 2006; COID 20:449, 2007)	Dengue		Supportive care: see Table 14A, page 156	Average incubation period 4 days; serodiagnosis.
	Malaria		Diagnosis: peripheral blood smear	See table 13A, page 143
	Typhoid fever		See Table 1, page 60.	Average incubation 7-14 days; diarrhea in 45%.
Kawasaki syndrome 6 weeks to 12 yrs of age, peak at 1 yr of age; 85% below age 5. Ref: Pediatrics 124:1, 2009.	Acute self-limited vasculitis of skin, rash, conjunctivitis, stomatitis, cervical adenitis, red hands/feet & coronary artery aneurysms (25% if untreated)	IVIG 2 gm per kg over 8-12 hrs x 1 + **ASA** 20-25 mg per kg qid THEN **ASA** 3-5 mg per kg per day po q24h times 6-8 wks	If still febrile after 1st dose of IVIG, some give 2nd dose. In Japan: **IVIG** + prednisolone 2 mg/kg/day. Continue steroid until 4-d normal for 15 days (Lancet 379:1571, 2012).	IV gamma globulin (2 gm per kg over 10 hrs) in pts rx before 10th day of illness ↓ coronary artery lesions (Ln 347:1128, 1996). See Table 14A, page 11 for IVIG adverse effects; Pulsed steroids of NO value: NEJM 356:659 & 663, 2007.
Rheumatic Fever, acute Ref: Ln 366:155, 2005 Prophylaxis Primary prophylaxis: Treat S. pyogenes pharyngitis	Post-Group A strep pharyngitis (not Group B, C, or G) (see Pharyngitis, p. 48)	(1) Symptom relief: **ASA** 80-100 mg per kg per day in children; 4-8 gm per day in adults. (2) Eradicate Group A strep: **Pen times** (see below)		
		Benzathine pen G 1.2 million units IM	Penicillin for 10 days prevents rheumatic fever when started 7-9 days after onset of illness (see page 48). Alternative: **Penicillin V** 250 mg po bid or **sulfadiazine (sulfisoxazole)** 1 gm po q24h or **erythro** 250 mg po bid.	
Secondary prophylaxis (previous documented rheumatic fever)		**Benzathine pen G** 1.2 million units IM q3-4 wks	**Duration?** No carditis: 5 yrs or until age 21, whichever is longer; carditis without residual valvular disease: 10 yrs since last episode or until age 40 whichever is longer (PEDS 96:758, 1995).	
Typhoidal syndrome (typhoid fever, enteric fever) BMJ 333:78, 2006; LnID 5:623, 2005. Global susceptibility results: C/D 50:241, 2010.	Salmonella typhi, S. paratyphi. NOTE: FQ resistance to nalidixic acid predicts clinical failure of CIP (FQs); Do not use empiric FQs if Asia-acquired infection. Need susceptibility results: AAC 54:5201, 2010; BMJ 333:78, 2006.	If NOT acquired in Asia: **CIP** 400 mg IV q12h or **Levo** 750 mg po/IV q24h) x 7-10 d (See Comment)	If acquired in Asia: **Ceftriaxone** 2 gm IV daily x 1 dose, then 500 mg po daily x 5-7 d; or **Chloro** 500 mg po/IV q6h x 14 d) In children, CIP superior to ceftriaxone (LnID 3:537, 2003)	**Dexamethasone:** Chloro + dex vs. Chloro alone (NEJM 310:82, 1984). No data on dex + FQs or ceftriaxone. **Use in severely ill pts: 1st dose just prior to antibiotic, 3 mg/kg IV, then 1 mg/kg q6h x 8 doses.** Complications: perforation of terminal ileum &/or cecum, osteo, septic arthritis, **mycotic aneurysm** (approx. 10% over age 50, AJM 110:60, 2001), meningitis.

Sepsis: Following suggested **empiric** therapy, all regimens pt is bacteremic, mimicked by BMI, rickettsial infections and pancreatitis (Intensive Care Medicine 34:17, 2008; IDC No Amer 22:1, 2008)

| **Neonatal**—early onset <1 week old | Group B strep, E. coli, klebsiella, enterobacter, Staph aureus (uncommon), listeria (rare in U.S.) | (**AMP** 25 mg per kg IV q8h + **cefotaxime** 50 mg per kg q8h) or (**AMP** 25 mg per kg IV q8h) + **ceftriaxone** 75 mg per kg IV q24h) | (**AMP** 25 mg per kg IV q8h + **gent** 2.5 mg per kg IV/IM q12h) or (**AMP** + **ceftriaxone** 50 mg per kg IV/IM q24h) | Blood cultures any day, but only 5-10% if blood culture after 72 hrs if cultures and x-ray do not support diagnosis. In Spain, listeria predominates; in S. America, salmonella. If Grp B Strep infection + severe beta-lactam allergy, alternatives include: erythro & clinda; report of clinda resistance at 38% & erythro resistance at 51% (AAC 56:739, 2012). |
| **Neonatal**—late onset 1-4 weeks old | As above + H. influenzae & S. epidermidis | | **AMP** + **gent** 2.5 mg per kg q8h IV or IM | If MSSA/MRSA a concern, add **vanco**. |

Abbreviations on page 2. NOTE: All dosage recommendations are for adults (unless otherwise indicated) and assume normal renal function.

61

TABLE 1 (59)

ANATOMIC SITE/DIAGNOSIS/ MODIFYING CIRCUMSTANCES	ETIOLOGIES (usual)	SUGGESTED REGIMENS* PRIMARY	SUGGESTED REGIMENS* ALTERNATIVE[$\dagger$]	ADJUNCT DIAGNOSTIC OR THERAPEUTIC MEASURES AND COMMENTS
SYSTEMIC SYNDROMES (FEBRILE/NON-FEBRILE)/Sepsis (continued)				
Child: not neutropenic	Strep. pneumoniae, meningococci, Staph. aureus (MSSA & MRSA), H. influenzae now rare	(Cefotaxime 50 mg per kg IV q6h, or ceftriaxone 100 mg per kg IV q24h) + vanco 15 mg per kg IV q6h	Aztreonam 7.5 mg per kg IV q6h + linezolid (see Table 16, page 203 for dose)	Major concerns are S. pneumoniae & community-associated MRSA. Coverage for Gm-neg. bacilli indicated but H. influenzae infection now rare. Meningococcemia mortality remains high (Ln 356:961, 2000).
Adult: not neutropenic; NO HYPOTENSION but LIFE-THREATENING — For Septic shock, see page 63				Systemic inflammatory response syndrome (**SIRS**): 2 or more of the following:
Source unclear—consider primary bacteremia, intra-abdominal or skin source. May be bacteremic. Survival greater with quicker, effective empiric antibiotic Rx (CCM 38:1045 & 1211, 2010).	Aerobic Gm-neg. bacilli; Staph. aureus; streptococci; others	ERTA or IMP or MER) + vanco	(Dapto 6 mg per kg IV q24h) + (cefepime or PIP-TZ or TC-CL)[$\dagger$] Could substitute linezolid for vanco or dapto; however, linezolid bacteriostatic vs. S. aureus. Dosages in footnote[36]	1. Temperature >38°C or <36°C 2. Heart rate >90 beats per min. 3. Respiratory rate >20 breaths per min. 4. WBC >12,000 per mcL or >10% bands **Sepsis**: SIRS + a documented infection (+ culture) **Severe sepsis**: Sepsis + organ dysfunction: hypotension or hypoperfusion abnormalities (lactic acidosis, oliguria, mental status) **Septic shock**: Sepsis-induced hypotension (systolic BP <90 mmHg) not responsive to 500 mL IV fluid challenge + peripheral hypoperfusion.
if suspect biliary source (see p.12)	Enterococci + aerobic Gm-neg. bacilli	PIP-TZ or TC-CL	Ceftriaxone + metro. (CIP or Levo) + metro.	
if community-acquired pneumonia (see page 39 and following pages)	S. pneumoniae; MRSA; Legionella, Gm-neg. bacillus	Levo (or moxi) + (PIP-TZ) + Vanco	Aztreonam + (Levo or moxi) + linezolid Dosages—footnote[36]	Many categories of CAP, see material beginning at page 39. Suggestions based on most severe CAP, e.g., MRSA after influenza or Klebsiella pneumonia in an alcoholic.
if illicit use IV drugs	S. aureus			Vanco if high prevalence of MRSA. Do NOT use empiric vanco + oxacillin pending organism ID. In vitro nafcillin increased production of toxins by CA-MRSA (JID 195:202, 2007). Dosages—footnote[36], page 62
If suspect intra-abdominal source	Mixture aerobic & anaerobic Gm-neg. bacilli			See secondary peritonitis, page 47.
If petechial rash	Meningococcemia	Ceftriaxone 2 gm IV q12h (until sure no meningitis), consider Rocky Mountain spotted fever—see page 59		
if suspect urinary source, e.g. pyelonephritis	Aerobic Gm-neg. bacilli & enterococci	See pyelonephritis, page 34		
Neutropenia: Child or Adult (absolute PMN count <500 per mm3) in cancer and transplant patients. Guideline: CID 52:427, 2011				
Prophylaxis (IJAD 9:97, 9.07)		Meta-analysis demonstrates substantive reduction in mortality with **CIP** 500 mg po bid (AnIM 142:979, 2005). Similar results in observational study using **Levo** 500 mg po q24h (CID 40:1087 & 1094, 2005). Also NEJM 353:977, 988 & 1052, 2005		
Post-chemotherapy—impending neutropenia				
Post-chemotherapy in AIDS patient	↑ risk pneumocystis, aerobic Gm-neg bacilli	**TMP-SMX-DS** 1 tab po once daily—adults; 10 mg per kg IV day bid po—children	**TMP-SMX DS** has prophylactic efficacy vs. PCP and E. coli.	
Post-marrow ablation, bone marrow transplant	↑ risk aerobic Gm-neg. bacilli, ↑ risk viruses, Candida, herpes viruses	**TMP-SMX** as above + [either **acyclovir** or **ganciclovir**] + **fluconazole**		Combined regimen justified by combined effect of neutropenia and immunosuppression.

[36] P Ceph 3 (**cefotaxime** 2 gm IV q8h, use q4h if life-threatening; **ceftazidime** 2 gm IV q8h; **ceftriaxone** 2 gm IV q24h); **Levo** 750 mg IV q24h; **ticarcillin** 3 gm IV q4h; **TC-CL** 3.1 gm IV q4h; **PIP-TZ** 3.375 gm IV q6h (or 4-hr infusion of 3.375 gm q8h, see Table 10D, page 109). **AP Pen** (**piperacillin** 3 gm IV q4h; **ticarcillin** 3 gm IV q4h; **TC-CL** 3.1 gm IV q4h; **ERTA** 1 gm IV q24h; **DORI** 500 mg IV q8h (1-hr infusion). **Naf/cillin** or **oxacillin** 2 gm IV q4h; **aztreonam** 2 gm IV q8h; **metro** 1 gm loading dose then 0.5 gm q6h or 1 gm IV q12h; **vanco** 1 gm IV q12h; **ceftazidime** 2 gm IV q12h (q8h if neutropenic), **cefepime** 2 gm IV q12h (q8h if neutropenic); **CIP** 400 mg IV q12h; **linezolid** 600 mg IV q12h.

Abbreviations on page 2. NOTE: All dosage recommendations are for adults (unless otherwise indicated) and assume normal renal function.

TABLE 1 (60)

ANATOMIC SITE/DIAGNOSIS/ MODIFYING CIRCUMSTANCES	ETIOLOGIES (usual)	SUGGESTED REGIMENS*		ADJUNCT DIAGNOSTIC OR THERAPEUTIC MEASURES AND COMMENTS
		PRIMARY	ALTERNATIVE[†]	
SYSTEMIC SYNDROMES (FEBRILE/NON-FEBRILE)/Neutropenia (continued)				
Empiric therapy—febrile neutropenia (<38.3°C for > 1 hr or sustained >38°C and absolute neutrophil count <500 cells/µL) (Practice Guidelines: CID 52:427, 2022).				
Low-risk adults Anticipate < 7 days neutropenia, no co-morb, can take po meds	Aerobic Gm-neg. bacilli; Viridans strep	CIP 750 mg po bid + AM-CL 875 /125 mg po bid. Treat until absolute neutrophil count >1000 cells/µL	Treat as outpatients with 24/7 access to inpatient care if: no focal findings, no hypotension, no COPD, no fungal infection, no dehydration, age range 16-60 yrs; motivated and compliant pts & family.	Increasing resistance of viridans streptococci to penicillins, cephalosporins & FQs (IDSA Guidelines: CID 52:e56, 2011). **What if severe IgE-mediated β-lactam allergy?** No formal trials, but (aminoglycoside (or CIP) + aztreonam] ± vanco should work.
High-risk adults (Anticipate > 7 days profound neutropenia, active co-morbidities)	Aerobic Gm-neg. bacilli; to include P. aeruginosa; cephalosporin-resistant viridans strep; MRSA	**Monotherapy:** cefta or (cefepime) or (tobra) + (TC-CL or Gent or tobra) + (TC-CL or PIP-TZ) or MER or DORI or CFP or PIP-TZ	**Combination therapy:** (Gent or tobra) + (TC-CL or PIP-TZ)	IMP: 0.5 gm q6h achieved MIC90 coverage in only 53%. If GFR OK, dose of 500 mg q4h or 750 mg (over 2 hrs) may be better (AAC 53:785, 2009). If cultures remain neg, but pt afebrile, treat until absolute neutrophil count ≥ 500 cells/µL.
		Dosages: Footnote* and Table 10B		
		Include empiric vanco if: suspect IV access infected; colonized with drug-resistant S. pneumo or MRSA; blood culture pos. for Gm-pos. cocci; pt hypotensive		
Persistent fever and neutropenia after 5 days of empiric antibacterial therapy—see CID 52:427, 2011				
	Candida species, aspergillus, VRE, resistant GNB	Add either **(caspofungin** 70 mg IV day 1, then 50 mg IV q24h or **Micafungin** 100 mg IV q24h) or **Anidulafungin** 200 mg IV x 1 dose, then 100 mg IV q24h) **OR voriconazole** 6 mg per kg IV q12h times 2 doses, then 3 mg per kg IV q12h		Conventional **ampho B** causes more fever & nephrotoxicity & lower efficacy than lipid-based ampho B. both **caspofungin & voriconazole** better tolerated & perhaps more efficacious than lipid-based ampho B (NEJM 346:225, 2002 & 351:1391 & 1445, 2005).
Shock syndromes				
Septic shock: Fever & hypotension **Bacteremic shock, endotoxin shock** Antimicrobial therapy: Surviving Sepsis Campaign: CCM 36:296, 2008 & Intensive Care Med 34:17, 2008; JAMA 305:1469, 2011.	Bacteremia with aerobic Gm-neg. bacteria or Gm+ cocci	**Proven Therapies:** - Replete intravascular vol. with IV saline; goal is CVP >8 cm within 6 hr of admission - Attempt to correct source of bacteremia. - Blood cultures, then antibiotics appropriate for clinical syndrome. Time to effective rx crucial (Chest 136:1237, 2009; CCM 38:1045 & 1211, 2010). - If still hypotensive & lactate elevated either nor-epinephrine or dopamine (NEJM 362:779 & 841, 2010). ----------- Other management as per Septic shock, above -----------		- Low dose glucocorticoids: data controversial. Currently, consider use if pt still hypotensive & vasopressor dependent after 2+ days of fluids, antibiotics & success w/source control (JAMA 301:2362, 2009; CID 49:93, 2009). Hard to interp. ACTH stim. data. Review. Am J Respir Crit Care Med 185:133, 2012. - Insulin Rx. Current target is glucose levels of 140-180 mg/dL. Attempts at tight control (80-110 mg/dL) resulted in excessive hypoglycemia (NEJM 363:2540, 2010). - A polymyxin B fiber column reduced 28 day mortality in pts with intra-abdominal gram-negative infections (not available in U.S.); Ln 11:55, 2011.
Septic shock: post-splenectomy or functional asplenia	S. pneumoniae, N. meningitidis, H. influenzae, Capnocytophaga (DF-2)	Ceftriaxone 2 gm IV q24h (1 to 2 gm q12h if meningitis)	**Levo** 750 mg IV q24h or **Moxi** 400 mg) once IV q24h	Howell-Jolly bodies in peripheral blood smear confirm absence of functional spleen. Often results in **symmetrical peripheral gangrene of digits** due to severe DIC. For prophylaxis, see Table 15A, page 192.

NOTE: All dosage recommendations are for adults (unless otherwise indicated) and assume normal renal function.

TABLE 1 (61)

SYSTEMIC SYNDROMES (FEBRILE/NON-FEBRILE)/Neutropenia (continued)

ANATOMIC SITE/DIAGNOSIS/ MODIFYING CIRCUMSTANCES	ETIOLOGIES (usual)	SUGGESTED REGIMENS* PRIMARY	SUGGESTED REGIMENS* ALTERNATIVE[1]	ADJUNCT DIAGNOSTIC OR THERAPEUTIC MEASURES AND COMMENTS
Toxic shock syndrome, Clostridium sordellii Clinical picture: shock, capillary leak, hemoconcentration, leukemoid reaction, afebrile Ref. CID 43:1436 & 1447, 2006.	Clostridium sordellii —hemorrhagic & lethal toxins	Fluids, aq. **penicillin G** 18–20 million units per day div. q4–6h + **clindamycin** 900 mg IV q8h; **Surgical debridement is key**.		Occurs in variety of settings that produce anaerobic tissue, e.g., illicit drug use, post-partum. Several deaths reported after use of abortifacient regimen of mifepristone (RU486) & misoprostol. 2001-2006 standard medical abortion: po mifepristone & then vaginal misoprostol. Since 2006, switch to buccal; instead of vaginal misoprostol. Mortality nearly 100% if WBC > 50,000/μL. (NEJM 361:145, 2009).
Toxic shock syndrome, staphylococcal. Review: LnID 9:281 Colonization by toxin-producing Staph. aureus of: vagina (tampon-assoc.), surgical/traumatic wounds, endometrium, burns	Staph. aureus (toxic shock toxin-mediated)	1096 (**Nafcillin** or **oxacillin** 2 gm IV q4h (if MRSA: **vanco** 1 gm IV q12h) + **Clinda** 600–900 mg IV q8h + **IVIG** (Dose in Comment)	**Cefazolin** 1–2 gm IV q8h) or (if MRSA: **vanco** 1 gm IV q12h OR **dapto** 6 mg/kg IV q24h) Clinda 600–900 mg IV q8h + **IVIG** (Dose in Comment)	**IVIG reasonable** (see Streptococcal TSS) — dose 1 gm per kg on day 1, then 0.5 gm per kg days 2 & 3 — antitoxin antibodies present. If suspect TSS, "turn off" toxin production with clinda; report of success with **linezolid** (JID 195:202, 2007). Exposure of MRSA to nafcillin increased toxin production in vitro; JID 195:202, 2007.
Toxic shock syndrome, streptococcal. NOTE: For Necrotizing fasciitis without toxic shock, see page 56. Ref: LnID 9:281, 2009. Associated with invasive disease, i.e., erysipelas, necrotizing fasciitis, secondary strep infection of varicella. Recent NASS cases reported (NEJM 335:547 & 590, 1996; CID 27:150, 1998).	Group A, B, C, & G Strep. pyogenes, Group B strep ref. EID 15:223, 2009.	(**Pen G** 24 million units per day IV div. doses) + (**clinda** 900 mg IV q8h) IVIG associated with 1 in sepsis-related organ failure (CID 37:333 & 341, 2003). IVIG dose: 1 gm per kg day 1, then 0.5 gm per kg days 2 & 3. IVIG preps vary in neutralizing antibody content (CID 43:743, 2006). In multicenter retrospective study, no benefit from IVIG controversial (CID 9:69 & 1377, 2009).	**Ceftriaxone** 2 gm IV q24h + **clinda** 900 mg IV q8h	**Definition**: Isolation of Group A strep. hypotension and ≥2 of: renal impairment, coagulopathy, liver involvement, ARDS, generalized rash, soft tissue necrosis. Associated with massive tissue destruction, **usually requires surgical intervention**. Mortality 30–50%; mortality 80% even with early rx (CID 14:2, 1992). Clinda ↓ toxin production. Use of NSAID may predispose to TSS. For reasons pen G may fail in fulminant S. pyogenes infections (see JID 167:1401, 1993).

Toxin-Mediated Syndromes—no fever unless complicated

Botulism (CID 41:1167, 2005. As biologic weapon: JAMA 285:1059, 2001; www.bt.cdc.gov)	Clostridium botulinum		for all types: Follow vital capacity, other supportive care. If no ileus, purge GI tract	**Equine antitoxin**: Heptavalent currently only antitoxin available (U.S) for non-infant botulism: CDC (+1 404-639-2206 M-F OR +1 404-639-2888 evenings/weekends). For infants, use Baby BIG (human botulism immune globulin): California Infant Botulism Treat & Prevent Program.
Food-borne Dyspnea at presentation bad sign (CID 43:1247, 2006)		Human botulism immunoglobulin (BIG) IV, single dose. Call (+1) 510-540-2646. Do not use equine antitoxin.	Heptavalent—CDC (see Comment)	**Antimicrobials**: May make infant botulism worse. Untested in wound botulism. When used, pen G 10–20 million units per day usual dose. If complications (pneumonia, UTI) occur, avoid antimicrobials with assoc. neuromuscular blockade, i.e., aminoglycosides, tetracycline, polymyxin. **Differential dx**: Guillain-Barré, myasthenia gravis, tick paralysis, organophosphate toxicity, West Nile virus.
Infant (Adult intestinal botulism is rare variant: EIN 18:1, 2012)			**No antibiotics**: may lyse C. botulinum in gut and ↑ load of toxin	
Wound		Debridement & anaerobic cultures. No proven value of local antitoxin. Role of antibiotics untested.	Trivalent equine antitoxin (see Comment)	Wound botulism can result from spore contamination of tar heroin. Ref: CID 31:1018, 2000. Mouse bioassay failed to detect toxin in 1/3 of patients (CID 48:1669, 2009).

Abbreviations on page 2. NOTE: All dosage recommendations are for adults (unless otherwise indicated) and assume normal renal function.

TABLE 1 (62)

ANATOMIC SITE/DIAGNOSIS/ MODIFYING CIRCUMSTANCES	ETIOLOGIES (usual)	SUGGESTED REGIMENS* PRIMARY	SUGGESTED REGIMENS* ALTERNATIVE[1]	ADJUNCT DIAGNOSTIC OR THERAPEUTIC MEASURES AND COMMENTS
SYSTEMIC SYNDROMES/Neutropenia (continued)				
Tetanus: Trismus, generalized muscle rigidity, muscle spasm Ref. *Ann* 154:329, 2011.	C. tetani–production of tetanosporium toxin	**Six treatment steps:** 1—Urgent endotracheal intubation to protect the airway. Laryngeal spasm is common. Early tracheostomy. 2—Eliminate reflex spasms with diazepam, 20 mg/kg/day IV or midazolam. Reports of benefit combining diazepam with magnesium sulfate (*Ln* 368:1436, 2006). Worst cases: need neuromuscular blockade with vecuronium. 3—Neutralize toxin. Human hyperimmune globulin IM; start tetanus immunization, from clinical tetanus. 4—Surgically debride infected source tissue. Start antibiotic: (**Pen G** 3 million units IV q4h or **Doxy** 100 mg IV q12h or **Metro** 1000 mg IV q12h) x 7-10 days. 5—Avoid light as may precipitate muscle spasms. 6—Use beta blockers, e.g., short acting esmolol, to control sympathetic hyperactivity.		
VASCULAR				
IV line infection (See IDSA Guidelines *CID* 49:1, 2009). Heparin lock, midline catheter, **non-tunneled** central venous catheter (subclavian, internal jugular), peripherally inserted central catheter (PICC). 2008 study found ↑ infection risk/thrombosis if femoral vein used, esp. if BMI >28.4 (*JAMA* 299:2413, 2008). Recent meta-analysis did not confirm an increased risk (*CCM* 40: 2479 & 2528, 2012).	Staph. epidermidis, Staph. aureus (MSSA/MRSA). **Diagnosis:** Fever & either + blood cult from line & peripheral vein OR culture >15 colonies on tip of removed line OR culture from catheter positive 2 hrs earlier than peripheral vein culture.	**Vanco** 1 gm IV q12h. Other rx and duration: (1) If **S. aureus**, remove catheter. Can use TEE result to determine if 2 or 4 wks of therapy (*JAC* 57:1172, 2006). (2) If **S. epidermidis**, can try IV "save" catheter: 80% cure after 7-10 days of therapy. With only systemic antibiotics, high rate of recurrence (*CID* 49:1187, 2009).	Other alternatives—see Comment. If **leuconostoc** or **lactobacillus** are Vanco resistant: need **Pen G, Amp** or **Clinda.**	If no response to, or intolerant of, **vanco**: switch to **daptomycin** 6 mg per kg IV q24h. **Quinupristin-dalfopristin** an option: 7.5 mg per kg IV q8h via central line. Culture removed catheter. With "roll" method, >15 colonies (*NEJM* 312:1142, 1985) suggests infection. Lines do not require "routine" changing when not infected. When infected, do not insert new catheter over a wire. Antimicrobial-impregnated catheters may ↓ infection risk; the debate is lively (*CID* 37:65, 2003 & 38:1287, 2004 & 39:1829, 2004).
Tunnel type indwelling venous catheters and ports (Broviac, Hickman, Groshong, Quinton), dual lumen hemodialysis catheters (Permacath). For prevention, see below.	Staph. epidermidis, Staph. aureus, (Candida sp.). Rarely: leuconostoc or lactobacillus—both resistant to vanco (See Table 2, page 67) (Dx, see above)	(**Vanco** + (**Cefepime** or **Ceftaz**) or (**Vanco** + **Pip-Tazo**) or **IMP** or ((**Cefepime** or **Ceftaz**) + **Aminoglycoside**). (Dosage in footnotes[29,36]; pages 47 and 62).	If candida, **voriconazole** or an echinocandin (**anidulafungin, micafungin, caspofungin**) if clinically stable. Dosage: see *Table 11B, page 124*.	If subcutaneous tunnel infected, very low cure rates; need to remove catheter. Beware of silent infection in clotted hemodialysis catheters. Indium scans detect (*Am J Kid Dis* 40:832, 2002).
Impaired host (burn, neutropenic)	As above + Pseudomonas sp., Enterobacteriaceae, Corynebacterium jeikeium, aspergillus, rhizopus			Usually have associated septic thrombophlebitis: biopsy of vein to rule out fungi. If fungal, surgical excision + amphotericin B. Surgical drainage, ligation or removal often indicated.
Hyperalimentation	As with tunnel, Candida sp. resistant (Candida species) common (see *Table 11, page 124*).	**Vanco** 1 gm IV q12h **Fluconazole** 400 mg IV q24h		Remove venous catheter and discontinue antimicrobial agents if possible. Ophthalmologic consultation recommended. **Rx all patients with + blood cultures.** See *Table 11A, Candidiasis, page 113*
Intravenous lipid emulsion	Staph. epidermidis Malassezia furfur			Discontinue intralipid

Abbreviations on page 2.   NOTE: *All dosage recommendations are for adults (unless otherwise indicated) and assume normal renal function.*

TABLE 1 (63)

ANATOMIC SITE/DIAGNOSIS/ MODIFYING CIRCUMSTANCES	ETIOLOGIES (usual)	SUGGESTED REGIMENS* PRIMARY	SUGGESTED REGIMENS* ALTERNATIVE[1]	ADJUNCT DIAGNOSTIC OR THERAPEUTIC MEASURES AND COMMENTS
VASCULAR/IV line Infection (continued)				
Prevention of Infection of Long-Term IV Lines CID 52:1087, 2011	To minimize risk of infection. **Hand washing and** 1. Maximal sterile barrier precautions during catheter insertion 2. Use >0.5% chlorhexidine prep with alcohol for skin antisepsis 3. If infection rate high despite # 1 & 2, use either chlorhexidine/silver sulfadiazine or minocycline/rifampin-impregnated catheters or "lock" solutions (see Comment). 4. If possible, use subclavian vein, avoid femoral vessels. Lower infection risk in jugular vs. femoral vein if BMI >28.4 (JAMA 299:2413, 2008)			**IV line "lock" solutions under study. No FDA-approved product.** Reports of the combination of TMP, EDTA, & ethanol (AAC 55:4430, 2011). Trials to begin in Europe. Another report: lock soln of sodium citrate, methylene blue, methylparabens (CCM 39:613, 2011). Recent meeting abstracts support 70% ethanol.
Mycotic aneurysm	S. aureus, (28–71%), S. epidermidis, Salmonella sp. (15-24%), M.TBc, S pneumonia, many others	**Vanco** (dose sufficient to achieve trough level of 15-20 µg/mL) + **ceftriaxone** or **PIP-TZ** or **CIP**) **Treatment is combination of antibiotic + surgical resection with revascularization.**	**Dapto** could be substituted for Vanco. For GNB: **cefepime** or **carbapenems**. For MDR-GNB, **colistin** in combination therapy	No data for ceftaroline or telavancin. Best diagnostic imaging: CT angiogram. Blood cultures positive in 50-85%. **De-escalate to specific therapy when culture results known.** Treatment duration varies but usually 6 wks from date of definitive surgery.
Suppurative Phlebitis				
Pelvic thrombophlebitis (with or without septic pulmonary emboli) Postpartum or post abortion or post pelvic surgery	Streptococci, bacteroides, Enterobacteriaceae	(**Metro** 1 gm IV q12h +) **PIP-TZ** Dosages: Table 10A, page 93	**IMP** or **MER** or **ERTA** or (**clinda** + (**aztreonam** or **gent**)) q12h	Use heparin during antibiotic regimen. Duration unclear; one study shows benefit of anticoagulation (Am J Obstet Gyn 181:143, 1999). Decreasing activity of cefoxitin & cefotetan vs. Bacteroides sp.
Cavernous sinus thrombosis	Staph. aureus, Streptococcus sp. H. influenzae, aspergillus/mucor/rhizopus	**Vanco** 1 gm IV q12h + **ceftriaxone** 2 gm IV q12h	(**Dapto** 6 mg per kg IV q24h[NAI] or **linezolid** 600 mg IV q12h) + **ceftriaxone** 2 gm IV q12h	CT or MRI scan for diagnosis. **Heparin** usually used. If, fungal etiology, see specific organism in Table 11.
Other: Femoral, saphenous, internal jugular, subclavian	S. aureus, S. pyogenes, Strep sp. (Group B), Fusobacterium necrophorum (Lemierre's Syndrome)	**Vancomycin** 15 mg/kg IV q12h (normal weight) + **ceftriaxone** 1 gm IV q24h	**Daptomycin** 6 mg/kg IV q12h + **ceftriaxone** 1 gm IV q24h	Retrospective study: 2-3 weeks IV specific therapy + 2 weeks po therapy was efficacious (CID 49:741, 2008). If involved vein accessible, surgical I&D or excision may help, esp. if bacteremic pt.

Abbreviations on page 2. NOTE: All dosage recommendations are for adults (unless otherwise indicated) and assume normal renal function.

TABLE 2 – RECOMMENDED ANTIMICROBIAL AGENTS AGAINST SELECTED BACTERIA

BACTERIAL SPECIES	ANTIMICROBIAL AGENT (See page 2 for abbreviations)		
	RECOMMENDED	**ALTERNATIVE**	**ALSO EFFECTIVE[1] (COMMENTS)**
Achromobacter xylosoxidans spp xylosoxidans (formerly Alcaligenes)	IMP, MER, DORI (no DORI for pneumonia)	TMP-SMX. Some strains susc. to ceftaz, PIP-TZ	Resistant to aminoglycosides, most cephalosporins & FQs.
Acinetobacter calcoaceticus—baumannii complex	If suscept: IMP or MER or DORI. For MDR strains: Colistin + (IMP or MER) (no DORI for pneumonia)	AM-SB used for activity of sulbactam (CID 51:79, 2010). Perhaps Minocycline IV	Resistant to aminoglycosides, FQs. Minocycline, effective against many strains (CID 51:79, 2010) (See Table 5A, pg 77)
Actinomyces israelii	AMP or Pen G	Doxy, ceftriaxone	Clindamycin, erythro
Aeromonas hydrophila & other sp.	CIP or Levo	TMP-SMX or (P Ceph 3, 4)	See AAC 56:1110, 2012.
Arcanobacterium (C.) haemolyticum	Erythro; azithro	Benzathine Pen G, Clinda	Sensitive to most drugs, resistant to TMP-SMX (AAC 38:142, 1994)
Bacillus anthracis (anthrax): inhalation	See Table 1, page 43		
Bacillus cereus, B. subtilis	Vancomycin, clinda	FQ, IMP	
Bacteroides sp., B. fragilis & others	Metronidazole or PIP-TZ	Dori, ERTA, IMP, MER, AM-CL	Increasing resistance to: clinda, cefoxitin, cefotetan.
Bartonella henselae, quintana See Table 1, pages 30, 45, 51, 57	Varies with disease entity & immune status. Active: Azithro, clarithro, erythro, doxy & in combination: RIF, gent, ceftriaxone. Not active: CIP, TMP-SMX, Pen, most cephalosporins, aztreonam		
Bordetella pertussis	Azithro or clarithro	TMP-SMX	See PIDJ 31:78, 2012.
Borrelia burgdorferi, B. afzelii, B. garinii (Lyme & relapsing fever)	See specific disease entity		
Brucella sp.	Drugs & duration vary with localization or non-localization. See specific disease entities. PLoS One 7:e32090, 2012.		
Burkholderia (Pseudomonas) cepacia	TMP-SMX or MER or CIP	Minocycline or chloramphenicol	(Usually resist to aminoglycosides, polymyxins) (AAC 37: 123, 1993 & 43:213, 1999; Int Med 18:49, 2001) (Some resist to carbapenems) May need combo rx (AJRCCM 161:1206, 2000)
Burkholderia (Pseudomonas) pseudomallei Curr Opin Infect Dis 23:554, 2010; CID 41:1105, 2005	Initially, IV ceftaz or IMP or MER, then po (TMP-SMX + Doxy x 3 mos) ± Chloro (AAC 49:4010, 2005).		(Thai, 12-80% strains resist to TMP-SMX). FQ active in vitro. MER also effective (AAC 48: 1763, 2004)
Campylobacter jejuni	Azithro	Erythro or CIP	TMP-SMX, Pen & cephalosporins not active.
Campylobacter fetus	Gentamicin	IMP or ceftriaxone	AMP, chloramphenicol
Capnocytophaga ochracea (DF-1)	Dog bite: Clinda or AM-CL	Septic shock, post-splenectomy: PIP-TZ, Clinda, IMP, DORI, MER	FQ activity variable; aminoglycosides, TMP-SMX & Polymyxins have limited activity. LN ID 9:439, 2009.
Capnocytophaga canimorsus (DF-2)	Dog bite: AM-CL		
Chlamydophila pneumoniae	Doxy	Erythro, FQ	Azithro, clarithro
Chlamydia trachomatis	Doxy or azithro	Erythro	
Citrobacter diversus (koseri), C. freundii	Life threatening illness: IMP, MER, DORI	Non-life threatening illness: CIP or Gent	Emergence of resistance: AAC 52:995, 2007.
Clostridium difficile	Mild illness: Metronidazole (po)	Moderate/severe illness: Vancomycin (po) or Fidaxomicin (CID 51:1306, 2010).	Bacitracin (po); Nitazoxanide (CID 43:421, 2006; JAC 59:705, 2007). Rifaximin (CID 44:846, 2007). See also Table 1, page 18 re severity of disease.
Clostridium perfringens	Pen G ± clindamycin	Doxy	Erythro, chloramphenicol, cefazolin, cefoxitin, AP Pen, carbapenems
Clostridium tetani	Metronidazole or Pen G	Doxy	Role of antibiotics unclear.
Corynebacterium. diphtheriae	Erythro + antitoxin	Pen G + antitoxin	RIF reported effective (CID 27:845, 1998)
Corynebacterium jeikeium	Vancomycin + aminoglycoside	Pen G + aminoglycoside	Many strains resistant to Pen (EJCMID 25:349, 2006).
Corynebacterium minutissimum	Clinda 1% lotion	Clarithro or Erythro	Causes erythrasma
Coxiella burnetii (Q fever) acute disease (CID 52:1431, 2011)	Doxy, FQ (see Table 1, page 31)	Erythro, Azithro, Clarithro	Endocarditis: doxy + hydroxychloroquine (JID 188:1322, 2003; LnID 3:709, 2003; LnID 10:527, 2010).
chronic disease, e.g., endocarditis	Doxy + hydroxy chloroquine	TMP-SMX, Chloro	

67

TABLE 2 (2)

BACTERIAL SPECIES	ANTIMICROBIAL AGENT (See page 2 for abbreviations)		
	RECOMMENDED	**ALTERNATIVE**	**ALSO EFFECTIVE[1] (COMMENTS)**
Ehrlichia chaffeensis, Ehrlichia ewubguum Anaplasma (Ehrlichia) phagocytophillium	Doxy	RIF (CID 27:213, 1998), Levo (AAC 47:413, 2003).	CIP, ofloxacin, chloramphenicol also active in vitro. Resist to clinda, TMP-SMX, IMP, AMP, erythro, & azithro (AAC 41:76, 1997).
Eikenella corrodens	AM-CL, IV Pen G	TMP-SMX, FQ	Resistant to clinda, cephalexin, erythro, metro, diclox
Elizabethkingae meningosepticum (formerly Chryseobacterium)	Levo or TMP-SMX	CIP, Minocycline	Resistant to Pen, cephalosporins, carbapenems, aminoglycosides, vancomycin (JCM 44:1181, 2006)
Enterobacter species	Recommended agents vary with clinical setting and degree and mechanism of resistance.		
Enterococcus faecalis	Highly resistant. See Table 5A, page 77		
Enterococcus faecium	Highly resistant. See Table 5A, page 77		
Erysipelothrix rhusiopathiae	Penicillin G or amox	P Ceph 3, FQ	IMP, AP Pen (vancomycin, APAG, TMP-SMX resistant)
Escherichia coli	Highly resistant. Treatment varies with degree & mechanism of resistance, see TABLE 5B.		
Francisella tularensis (tularemia) See Table 1, page 45	Gentamicin, tobramycin, or streptomycin	Mild infection: Doxy or CIP	Chloramphenicol, RIF. Doxy/chloro bacteriostatic → relapses CID 53:e133, 2011.
Gardnerella vaginalis (bacterial vaginosis)	Metronidazole or Tinidazole	Clindamycin	See Table 1, pg 26 for dosage
Helicobacter pylori	See Table 1, pg 21		Drugs effective in vitro often fail in vivo.
Haemophilus aphrophilus (Aggregatibacter aphrophilus)	[(Penicillin or AMP) + gentamicin] or [AM- SB ± gentamicin]	(Ceftriaxone + Gent) or CIP or Levo	Resistant to vancomycin, clindamycin, methicillin
Haemophilus ducreyi (chancroid)	Azithro or ceftriaxone	Erythro, CIP	Most strains resistant to tetracycline, amox, TMP-SMX
Haemophilus influenzae Meningitis, epiglottitis & other life-threatening illness	Cefotaxime, ceftriaxone	AMP if susceptible and β-lactamase neg, FQs	Chloramphenicol (downgrade from 1st choice due to hematotoxicity).
non-life threatening illness	AM-CL, O Ceph 2/3		Azithro, clarithro, telithro
Klebsiella ozaenae/ rhinoscleromatis	CIP	Levo	Acta Otolaryngol 131:440, 2010.
Klebsiella species	Treatment varies with degree & mechanism of resistance, see TABLE 5B.		
Lactobacillus species	Pen G or AMP	Clindamycin	**May be resistant to vancomycin**
Legionella sp.	Levo or Moxi	Azithro	Telithro active in vitro.
Leptospira interrogans	Mild: Doxy or amox	Severe: Pen G or ceftriaxone	
Leuconostoc	Pen G or AMP	Clinda	**NOTE: Resistant to vancomycin**
Listeria monocytogenes	AMP + Gent for synergy	TMP-SMX	Erythro, penicillin G (high dose), APAG may be synergistic with β-lactams. Meropenem active in vitro. **Cephalosporin-resistant!**
Moraxella (Branhamella) catarrhalis	AM-CL or O Ceph 2/3, TMP-SMX	Azithro, clarithro, dirithromycin, telithro	Erythro, doxy, FQs
Mycoplasma pneumoniae	Doxy	Azithro	Clindamycin & B lactams NOT effective. Increasing macrolide resistance in Asia (>30% reported in Japan) (AAC 52:348, 2008).
Neisseria gonorrhoeae (gonococcus)	Ceftriaxone,	Azithro (high dose)	FQs and oral cephalosporins no longer recommended: high levels of resistance.
Neisseria meningitidis (meningococcus)	Ceftriaxone	Chloro, MER	Chloro-resist strains in SE Asia (NEJM 339:868, 1998) (Prophylaxis: pg 10)
Nocardia asteroides or **Nocardia brasiliensis**	TMP-SMX + IMP	Linezolid	Amikacin + (IMP or ceftriaxone or cefotaxime)
Pasteurella multocida	Pen G, AMP, amox, cefuroxime, cefpodoxime	Doxy, Levo, Moxi, TMP-SMX	Resistant to cephalothin, oxacillin, clindamycin, erythro, vanco.
Plesiomonas shigelloides	CIP	TMP-SMX	AM-CL, Ceftriaxone & Chloro active. Resistant to: Amp, Tetra, aminoglycosides
Propionibacterium acnes (not acne)	Penicillin, Ceftriaxone	Vanco, Dapto, Linezolid	May be resistant to Metro.
Proteus sp, **Providencia sp**, Morganella sp. (Need in vitro susceptibility)	CIP, PIP-TZ; avoid cephalosporins	May need carbapenem if critically ill	Note: Proteus sp. & Providencia sp. have intrinsic resistance to Polymyxins.
Pseudomonas aeruginosa (ID Clin No Amer 23:277, 2009). Combination therapy? See Clin Micro Rev 25:450, 2012.	No in vitro resistance: AP Pen, AP Ceph 3, Dori, IMP, MER, tobramycin, CIP, aztreonam. For serious inf., use AP β-lactam + (tobramycin or CIP)	For UTI, if no in vitro resistance, single drugs effective: AP Pen, AP Ceph 3, cefepime, IMP, MER, aminoglycoside, CIP, aztreonam	If resistant to all beta lactams, FQs, aminoglycosides: Colistin + MER or IMP. Do not use DORI for pneumonia.

TABLE 2 (3)

BACTERIAL SPECIES	ANTIMICROBIAL AGENT (See page 2 for abbreviations)		
	RECOMMENDED	**ALTERNATIVE**	**ALSO EFFECTIVE[1] (COMMENTS)**
Rhodococcus (C. equi)	Two drugs: Azithro, Levo or RIF	(Vanco or IMP) + (Azithro, Levo or RIF)	Vancomycin active in vitro; intracellular location may impair efficacy (CID 34:1379, 2002). Avoid Pen, cephalosporins, clinda, tetra, TMP-SMX.
Rickettsia species (includes spotted fevers)	Doxy	Chloramphenicol (in pregnancy), azithro (age < 8 yrs)	See specific infections (Table 1).
Salmonella typhi (CID 50:241, 2010; AAC 54:5201, 2010; BMC ID 51:37, 2005)	If FQ & nalidixic acid susceptible: CIP	Ceftriaxone, cefixime, azithro, chloro	Concomitant steroids in severely ill. Watch for relapse (1-6%) & ileal perforation. FQ resistance reported with treatment failures (AAC 52:1278, 2008).
Serratia marcescens	If no in vitro resistance: PIP-TZ, CIP, LEVO, Gent	If in vitro resistance: Carbapenem	Avoid extended spectrum Ceph if possible.
Shigella sp.	FQ or azithro		Ceftriaxone is alternative; TMP-SMX depends on susceptibility.
Staph. aureus, methicillin-susceptible	Oxacillin/nafcillin	P Ceph 1, vanco, teicoplanin[NUS], clinda ceftaroline	ERTA, IMP, MER, BL/BLI, FQ, erythro, clarithro, azithro, telithro, quinu-dalfo, linezolid, dapto, televancin.
Staph. aureus, methicillin-resistant (health-care associated) IDSA Guidelines: CID 52 (Feb 1):1, 2011.	Vancomycin	Teicoplanin[NUS], TMP-SMX (some strains resistant), quinu-dalfo, linezolid, daptomycin, telavancin, ceftaroline	Fusidic acid[NUS], >60% CIP-resistant in U.S. (Fosfomycin + RIF). Partially vancomycin-resistant strains (GISA, VISA) & highly resistant strains now described—see Table 6, pg 78.
Staph. aureus, methicillin-resistant [community-associated (CA-MRSA)]			
Mild-moderate infection	(TMP-SMX or doxy or mino)	Clinda (if D-test neg—see Table 5A & 6.	CA-MRSA usually not multiply-resistant. Oft resist. to erythro & variably to FQ. Vanco, teico[NUS], telavancin or daptomycin can be used in pts requiring hospitalization (see Table 6, pg 78). Also, ceftaroline.
Severe infection	Vanco or teico[NUS]	Linezolid or daptomycin	
Staph. epidermidis	Vancomycin ± RIF	RIF + (TMP-SMX or FQ), daptomycin (AAC 51:3420, 2007)	Cephalothin or nafcillin/oxacillin if sensitive to nafcillin/oxacillin but 75% are resistant. FQs. (See Table 5A).
Staph. haemolyticus	TMP-SMX, FQ, nitrofurantoin	Oral cephalosporin	Recommendations apply to UTI only.
Staph. lugdunensis	Oxacillin/nafcillin or penicillin G (if β-lactamase neg.)	P Ceph 1 or vancomycin or teico[NUS]	Approx. 75% are penicillin-susceptible.
Staph. saprophyticus (UTI)	Oral cephalosporin or AM-CL	FQ	Suscept to most agents used for UTI; occ. failure of sulfonamides, nitrofurantoin reported (JID 155:170, 1987). Resist to fosfomycin.
Stenotrophomonas (Xanthomonas, Pseudomonas) maltophilia	TMP-SMX	TC-CL	Minocycline, tigecycline, CIP, Ceftriaxone, moxifloxacin, ceftaz (LnID 9:312, 2009; JAC 62:889, 2008). [In vitro synergy (TC-CL + TMP-SMX) & (TC-CL + CIP), JAC 62:889, 2008].
Streptobacillus moniliformis	Penicillin G	Doxy	Maybe erythro, clinda, ceftriaxone
Streptococcus, anaerobic (Peptostreptococcus)	Penicillin G	Clindamycin	Doxy, vancomycin, linezolid, ERTA (AAC 51:2205, 2007).
Streptococcus anginosus group	Penicillin	Vanco or Ceftriaxone	Avoid FQs; macrolide resistance emerging
Streptococcus pneumoniae penicillin-susceptible	Penicillin G, Amox	Multiple agents effective, e.g., Ceph 2/3, Clinda	If meningitis, higher dose, see Table 1, page 9.
penicillin-resistant (MIC ≥2.0)	Vancomycin, Levo, ceftriaxone, Amox (HD), Linezolid		
Streptococcus pyogenes, Groups A, B, C, G: bacteremia	Penicillin G + Clinda	Pen (alone) or Clinda (alone)	JCM 49:439, 2011. Pockets of macrolide resistance
Vibrio cholerae	Doxy, FQ	Azithro, erythro	Maybe CIP or Levo; some resistance.
Vibrio parahaemolyticus	Doxy	Azithro, CIP	If bacteremic, treat as for V. vulnificus
Vibrio vulnificus, alginolyticus, damsela	Doxy + ceftriaxone	Levo	CID 52:788, 2011
Yersinia enterocolitica	CIP or ceftriaxone	TMP-SMX; CIP (if bacteremic)	CIP resistance (JAC 53:1068, 2004), also resistant to Pen, AMP, erythro.
Yersinia pestis (plague)	Streptomycin or Gent	Doxy or CIP	Maybe TMP-SMX (for bubonic, but sub-optimal).

[1] Agents are more variable in effectiveness than "Recommended" or "Alternative." Selection of "Alternative" or "Also Effective" based on in vitro susceptibility testing, pharmacokinetics, host factors such as auditory, renal, hepatic function, & cost.

TABLE 3 – SUGGESTED DURATION OF ANTIBIOTIC THERAPY IN IMMUNOCOMPETENT PATIENTS[1,2]

SITE	CLINICAL SITUATION / CLINICAL DIAGNOSIS	DURATION OF THERAPY (Days)
Bacteremia	Bacteremia with removable focus (no endocarditis)	10–14 (CID 14:75, 1992) (See Table 1)
Bone	Osteomyelitis, adult; acute	42
	adult; chronic	Until ESR normal (often > 3 months)
	child; acute; staph. and enterobacteriaceae[3]	21
	child; acute; strep, meningococci, haemophilus[3]	14
Ear	Otitis media with effusion	<2 yrs: 10 (or 1 dose ceftriaxone); ≥2 yrs: 5–7
	Recent meta-analysis suggests 3 days of azithro (JAC 52:469, 2003) or 5 days of "short-acting" antibiotics effective for uncomplicated otitis media (JAMA 279:1736, 1998), but may be inadequate for severe disease (NEJM 347:1169, 2002).	
Endo-cardium	Infective endocarditis, native valve	
	Viridans strep	14 or 28 (See Table 1, page 28)
	Enterococci	28 or 42 (See Table 1, page 29)
	Staph. aureus	14 (R-sided only) or 28 (See Table 1, page 29)
GI Also see Table 1	Bacillary dysentery (shigellosis)/traveler's diarrhea	3
	Typhoid fever (S. typhi): Azithro	5 (children/adolescents)
	Ceftriaxone	14 [Short course † effective (AAC 44:450, 2000)]
	FQ	5–7
	Chloramphenicol	14
	Helicobacter pylori	10–14. For triple-drug regimens, 7 days probably adequate (AJM 147:553, 2007).
	Pseudomembranous enterocolitis (C. difficile)	10
Genital	Non-gonococcal urethritis or mucopurulent cervicitis	7 days doxy or single dose azithro
	Pelvic inflammatory disease	14
Heart	Pericarditis (purulent)	28
Joint	Septic arthritis (non-gonococcal) Adult	14–28 (Ln 351:197, 1998)
	Infant/child	Rx as osteomyelitis above. Recent study suggests 10-14 days of therapy sufficient (CID 48:1201, 2009), but not complete agreement on this (CID 48:1211, 2009).
	Gonococcal arthritis/disseminated GC infection	7 (See Table 1, page 23)
Kidney	Cystitis (bladder bacteriuria)	3 (Single dose extended-release cipro also effective) (AAC 49:4137, 2005)
	Pyelonephritis	14 (7 days if CIP used; 5 days if levo 750 mg)
	Recurrent (failure after 14 days rx)	42
Lung	Pneumonia, pneumococcal	Until afebrile 3–5 days (minimum 5 days).
	Community-acquired pneumonia	Minimum 5 days and afebrile for 2-3 days (CID 44:S55, 2007; AJM 120:783, 2007).
	Pneumonia, enterobacteriaceae or pseudomonal	21, often up to 42
	Pneumonia, staphylococcal	21–28
	Pneumocystis carinii, in AIDS;	21
	other immunocompromised	14
	Legionella, mycoplasma, chlamydia	7–14
	Lung abscess	Usually 28–42[4]
Meninges[5] (CID 39:1267, 2004)	N. meningitidis	7
	H. influenzae	7
	S. pneumoniae	10–14
	Listeria meningoencephalitis, gp B strep, coliforms	21 (longer in immunocompromised)
Multiple systems	Brucellosis (See Table 1, page 60)	42 (add SM or gent for 1st 7–14 days) (JAC 65:1028, 2010)
	Tularemia (See Table 1, pages 45, 59)	7–14
Muscle	Gas gangrene (clostridial)	
Pharynx	Group A strep pharyngitis Also see Pharyngitis, Table 1, page 48	10 O Ceph 2/3, azithromycin effective at 5 days (JAC 45, Topic TI 23, 2000; JIC 14:213, 2008). 3 days less effective (Inf Med 18:515, 2001). Single dose extended rel Azithro (2 gm) as effective as 3 days of immediate rel Azithro (CMI 15:1103, 2009). See also 2009 Cochrane Review (www.thecochranelibrary.com).
	Diphtheria (membranous)	7–14
	Carrier	7
Prostate	Chronic prostatitis (TMP-SMX)	30–90
	(FQ)	28–42
Sinuses	Acute sinusitis	5–14[6]
Skin	Cellulitis	Until 3 days after acute inflamm disappears
Systemic	Lyme disease	See Table 1, page 58
	Rocky Mountain spotted fever (See Table 1, page 59)	Until afebrile 2 days

[1] Early change from IV to po regimens (about 72 hrs) is cost-effective with many infections, i.e., intra-abdominal (AJM 91:462, 1991). There is emerging evidence that serum **procalcitonin** level determination (a measure of bacterial or fungal infection) may allow early stopping of empiric therapy (JCM 48:2325, 2010).
[2] The recommended duration is a minimum or average time and should not be construed as absolute.
[3] These times are with proviso: sx & signs resolve within 7 days and ESR is normalized (J.D. Nelson, APID 6:59, 1991).
[4] In children relapses seldom occur until 3 days or more after termination of rx. For meningitis in children, see Table 1, page 8.
[5]
[6] Duration of therapy dependent upon agent used and severity of infection. Longer duration (10-14 days) optimal for beta-lactams and patients with severe disease. For sinusitis of mild-moderate severity shorter courses of therapy (5-7 days) effective with "respiratory FQs" (including gemifloxacin, levofloxacin 750 mg), azithromycin. Courses as short as 3 days reported effective for TMP-SMX and azithro and one study reports effectiveness of single dose extended-release azithro. Authors feel such "super-short" courses should be restricted to patients with mild-mod disease (JAMA 273:1015, 1995; AAC 47:2770, 2003; Otolaryngol-Head Neck Surg 133:194, 2005; Otolaryngol-Head Neck Surg 127:1, 2002; Otolaryngol-Head Neck Surg 134:10, 2006).

TABLE 4 – COMPARISON OF ANTIBACTERIAL SPECTRA

Editorial Note: Choice of antibacterial agent must be made in consideration of local/institutional patterns of organism susceptibility and drug resistance. Patterns vary considerably based on geography and temporal changes in patterns are continuous. These data are intended to convey a generalized image of susceptibility/resistance to provide a basis for making decisions concerning empiric as well as specific antibacterial therapy. These data reflect in vitro susceptibilities, drawn from package inserts and/or reports in the published literature. In vitro susceptibility is not a predictor of in vivo efficacy.

Organisms	Penicillin G	Penicillin V	Methicillin	Nafcillin/Oxacillin	Cloxacillin[NUS]/Diclox.	AMP/Amox	Amox/Clav	AMP-Sulb	Ticarcillin	Ticar-Clav	Pip-Tazo	Piperacillin	Doripenem	Ertapenem	Imipenem	Meropenem	Aztreonam	Ciprofloxacin	Ofloxacin	Pefloxacin[NUS]	Levofloxacin	Moxifloxacin	Gemifloxacin	Gatifloxacin
GRAM-POSITIVE:																								
Strep, Group A, B, C, G	+	+	+	+	+	+	+	+	+	+	+	+	+	+	+	+	0	+	±	0	+	+	+	+
Strep. pneumoniae	+	+	+	+	+	+	+	+	+	+	+	+	+	+	+	+	0	+	±	0	+	+	+	+
Viridans strep	+	+	±	±	±	±	±	±	±	±	±	±	±	±	±	±	0	±	±		±	±	±	±
Strep. milleri	+	+	+	+	+	+	+	+	+	+	+	+	+	+	+	+	0	+	+		+	+	+	+
Enterococcus faecalis	+	+	0	0	0	+	+	+	+	+	+	+	+	±	+	±	0	±	0	0	±	±	±	±
Enterococcus faecium	+	+	0	0	0	+	+	+	0	0	0	0	0	0	±	0	0	0	0	0	0	0	0	0
Staph. aureus (MSSA)	0	0	+	+	+	0	+	+	0	+	+	0	+	+	+	+	0	+	+	+	+	+	+	+
Staph. aureus (MRSA)	0	0	0	0	0	0	0	0	0	0	0	0	0	0	0	0	0	±	0	0	±	±	±	±
Staph. aureus (CA-MRSA)	0	0	0	0	0	0	0	0	0	0	0	0	+	±	+	+	0	+	±	+	+	+	+	+
Staph. epidermidis	0	0	0	0	0	0	0	0	0	0	0	0	+	+	+	+	0	±	±	0	±	±	±	±
C. jeikeium	0	0	0	0	0	0	0	0	0	0	0	0					0							
L. monocytogenes	+	+	0	0	0	+	+	+	+	+	+	+	+	±	+	+	0	+	+	0	+	+	+	+
GRAM-NEGATIVE:																								
N. gonorrhoeae	0	0	0	0	0	0	+	+	+	+	+	+	+	+	+	+	+	+	+	+	+	+	+	+
N. meningitidis	+	+	0	0	0	+	+	+	+	+	+	+	+	+	+	+	+	+	+	+	+	+	+	+
M. catarrhalis	0	0	0	0	0	0	+	+	0	+	+	±	+	+	+	+	+	+	+	+	+	+	+	+
H. influenzae	0	0	0	0	0	±	+	+	+	+	+	±	+	+	+	+	+	+	+	+	+	+	+	+
Klebsiella sp	0	0	0	0	0	0	+	+	0	+	+	+	+	+	+	+	+	+	+	+	+	+	+	+
E. coli/Klebs sp ESBL+	0	0	0	0	0	0	0	0	0	0	±	0	+	+	+	+	0	±	±	±	±	±	±	±
E. coli/Klebs sp KPC+	0	0	0	0	0	0	0	0	0	0	0	0	0	0	0	0	0	0	0	0	0	0	0	0
Enterobacter sp.	0	0	0	0	0	0	0	0	+	+	+	+	+	+	+	+	+	+	+	+	+	+	+	+

[1] Prevalence of quinolone-resistant GC varies worldwide from <1% in Europe and >30.9% in Taiwan. In US in 2006 it was 6.7% overall and as a result, CDC no longer recommends FQs for first line therapy of GC (MMWR 56:332, 2007; JAC 58:587, 2006; CID 40:188, 2005; AHM 147:81, 2007).

** Most strains ±, can be used in UTI, not in systemic infection

+ = **usually susceptible**;   ± = **variably susceptible/resistant**;   0 = **usually resistant**;   blank = **no data**

TABLE 4 (2)

Organisms	Penicillins		Antistaphylococcal Penicillins			Amino-Penicillins			Anti-Pseudomonal Penicillins				Carbapenems					Fluoroquinolones						
	Penicillin G	Penicillin V	Methicillin	Nafcillin/Oxacillin	Cloxacillin[NUS]/Diclox.	AMP/Amox	Amox/Clav	AMP-Sulb	Ticarcillin	Ticar-Clav	Pip-Tazo	Piperacillin	Doripenem	Ertapenem	Imipenem	Meropenem	Aztreonam	Ciprofloxacin	Ofloxacin	Pefloxacin[NUS]	Levofloxacin	Moxifloxacin	Gemifloxacin	Gatifloxacin
Serratia sp.	0	0	0	0	0	0	0	0	+	+	+	0	+	+	+	+	+	+	+	+	+	+		+
Salmonella sp.	0	0	0	0	0	±	±	+	+	+	+	+	+	+	+	+	+	+	+	+	+	+		+
Shigella sp.	0	0	0	0	0	±	+	+	+	+	+	+	+	+	+	+	+	+	+	+	+	+	+	+
Proteus mirabilis	+	0	0	0	0	+	+	+	+	+	+	+	+	+	+	+	+	+	+	+	+	+		+
Proteus vulgaris	0	0	0	0	0	0	+	+	+	+	+	+	+	+	+	+	+	+	+	+	+	+		+
Providencia sp.	0	0	0	0	0	0	0	+	+	+	+	+	+	+	+	+	+	+	+	+	+	+		+
Morganella sp.	0	0	0	0	0	0	0	0	+	+	+	+	+	+	+	+	+	+	+	+	+	+		+
Citrobacter sp.	0	0	0	0	0	0	0	+	+	+	+	+	+	+	+	+	+	+	+	+	+	+	±	+
Aeromonas sp.	0	0	0	0	0	0	+	+	+	+	+	+	+	+	+	+	0	+	+		+	+		+
Acinetobacter sp.	0	0	0	0	0	0	+	+	+	+	±	+	±	0	±	±	+	+	+	0	±	±		±
Ps. aeruginosa	0	0	0	0	0	0	0	0	+	+	+	+	+	0	+	+	0	0	0	0	±	0		0
B. (Ps.) cepacia	0	0	0	0	0	0	0	0	0	+	0	+	+	0	0	0	+	0	0	+	+	+		+
S. (X.) maltophilia	0	0	0	0	0	0	+	0	0	+	0	0	0	0	0	0	0	0	+	+	+	+		+
Y. enterocolitica	0	0	0	0	0	+	+	+	+	+	+	+	+	+	+	+	+	+	+	+	+	+		+
Legionella sp.	0	0	0	0	0	0	0	0	0	0	0	0	0	0	0	0	0	0	0	0	0	0		0
P. multocida	+	±	0	0	0	+	+	+	+	+	+	+	+	+	+	+	+	+	+		+	+		+
H. ducreyi	+	0	0	0	0	0	+	+	+	+	+	+	+	+	+	+	0	+	+		+	+		+
MISC.:																								
Chlamydophila sp	0	0	0	0	0	0	0	0	0	0	0	0	0	0	0	0	0	+	+	0	+	+	+	+
M. pneumoniae	0	0	0	0	0	0	0	0	0	0	0	0	0	0	0	0	0	+	±		+	+	+	±
ANAEROBES:																								
Bacteroides fragilis	0	0	0	0	0	0	+	+	0	+	+	0	+	+	+	+	0	0	±	0	0	+		+
P. melaninogenica	+	+	0	0	0	+	+	+[a]	+	+	+	+[a]	+	+	+	+	0	0	±		0	+		+
Clostridium difficile	+[a]	±	0	0	0	0	+	+	+	+	+	+	+	+	+	+	0	0			0	0		0
Clostridium (not difficile)	+	+	+	+	+	+	+	+	+	+	+	+	+	+	+	+	0	0	±		+	±		±
Fusobacterium necrophorum	+	±	+	+	+	+	+	+	+	+	+	+	+	+	+	+	0	0	±		+	+		0
Peptostreptococcus sp.	+	+	+	+	+	+	+	+	+	+	+	+	+	+	+	+	0	±	±		+	+		+

[a] No clinical evidence that penicillins or fluoroquinolones are effective for C. difficile enterocolitis (but they may cover this organism in mixed intra-abdominal and pelvic infections).

+ = **usually susceptible**; ± = **variably susceptible/resistant**; 0 = **usually resistant**; blank = **no data**
* A 1-carbacephem best classified as a cephalosporin

TABLE 4 (3)

CEPHALOSPORINS

Organisms	1st Generation	2nd Generation			3rd/4th Generation (including anti-MRSA)						Oral Agents						
											1st Generation		2nd Generation			3rd Generation	
	Cefazolin	Cefotetan	Cefoxitin	Cefuroxime	Cefotaxime	Ceftizoxime	Ceftriaxone	Ceftaroline	Ceftazidime	Cefepime	Cefadroxil	Cephalexin	Cefaclor/Loracarbef*	Cefprozil	Cefuroxime axetil	Cefixime	Ceftibuten	Cefpodox/Cefdinir/Cefditoren
GRAM-POSITIVE:																		
Strep. Group A, B, C, G	+	+	+	+	+	+	+	+	+³	+	+	+	+	+	+	+	+	+
Strep. pneumoniae³	+	+	+	+	+	+	+	+	±	+	+	+	+	+	+	+	±	+
Viridans strep	+	+	+	+	+	+	+	+	±	+	+	+	+	+	+	+	+	+
Enterococcus faecalis	0	0	0	0	0	0	0	+	0	0	0	0	0	0	0	0	0	0
Staph. aureus (MSSA)	+	+	+	+	+	+	+	+	+	+	+	+	+	+	+	0	0	0
Staph. aureus (MRSA)	0	0	0	0	0	0	0	+	0	0	0	0	0	0	0	0	0	0
Staph. aureus (CA-MRSA)	0	0	0	0	0	0	0	+	0	0	0	0	0	0	0	0	0	0
Staph. epidermidis	±	±	±	±	±	±	±	+	±	±	±	±	±	±	±	±	±	±
C. jelkeium	0	0	0	0	0	0	0	+	0	0	0	0	0	0	0	0	0	0
L. monocytogenes	0				0	0	0		0	0	0	0	0	0	0	0	0	0
GRAM-NEGATIVE																		
N. gonorrhoeae	+	±	±	+	+	+	+	+	+	+	0	0	±	±	±	+	+	+
N. meningitidis	0	±	±	+	+	+	+	+	+	+	0	0	±	±	±	±	±	±
M. catarrhalis	±	+	+	+	+	+	+	+	+	+	0	0	+	+	+	+	+	+
H. influenzae	±	+	+	+	+	+	+	+	+	+	0	0	+	+	+	+	+	+
E. coli	+	+	+	+	+	+	+	+	+	+	+	+	+	+	+	+	+	+
Klebsiella sp.	+	+	+	+	+	+	+	+	+	+	+	+	+	+	+	+	+	+
E. coli/Klebs sp. ESBL+	0	0	0	0	0	0	0	0	0	0	0	0	0	0	0	0	0	0
E. coli/Klebs sp. KPC+	0	0	0	0	0	0	0	0	0	0	0	0	0	0	0	0	0	0
Enterobacter sp.	0	0	0	0	+	+	+	+	+	+	0	0	0	0	0	0	0	0
Serratia sp.	0	±	0	0	+	+	+	+	+	+	0	0	0	0	0	0	0	0
Salmonella sp.					+	+	+		+	+						+	+	+
Shigella sp.					+	+	+		+	+						+	+	+
Proteus mirabilis	+	+	+	+	+	+	+	+	+	+	+	+	+	+	+	+	+	+
Proteus vulgaris	0	+	+	±	+	+	+	+	+	+	0	0	0	0	±	+	+	+
Providencia sp.	0	+	+	0	+	+	+	+	+	+	0	0	0	0	0	+	+	+
Morganella sp.	0	+	±	0	+	+	+	+	+	+	0	0	0	0	0	+	0	0

³ Ceftaz 8–16 times less active than cefotax/ceftriax, effective only vs Pen-sens. strains (AAC 39:2193, 1995). Oral cefuroxime, cefprozil, cefpodoxime most active in vitro vs resistant S. pneumo (PIDJ 14:1037, 1995).

* A 1-carbacephem best classified as a cephalosporin

+ = **usually susceptible**; ± = **variably susceptible/resistant;** 0 = **usually resistant;** blank = **no data**

TABLE 4 (4)

CEPHALOSPORINS

Organisms	1st Generation: Cefazolin	2nd Generation: Cefotetan	2nd Generation: Cefoxitin	2nd Generation: Cefuroxime	3rd/4th Generation (including anti-MRSA): Cefotaxime	Ceftizoxime	Ceftriaxone	Ceftaroline	Ceftazidime	Cefepime	Oral 1st Gen: Cefadroxil	Cephalexin	Oral 2nd Gen: Cefaclor/Loracarbef*	Cefprozil	Cefuroxime axetil	Oral 3rd Gen: Cefixime	Ceftibuten	Cefpodox/Cefdinir/Cefditoren
C. freundii	0	0	0	0	+	0	+		0	+	0	0	0	0	0	0		
C. diversus	0	+	+	+	+	+	+		+	+	0	0	0	0	±	+	+	+
Citrobacter sp.	0	+	+	+	+	+	+	+	+	+	0	0	±	0	±	+	+	0
Aeromonas sp.	0	+	±	±	+	+	+		+	+	0	0	0	0	0	0		
Acinetobacter sp.	0	0	0	0	0	0	0		±	±	0	0	0	0	0	0	0	0
Ps. aeruginosa	0	0	0	0	±	±	±	0	+	+	0	0	0	0	0	0	0	0
B. (Ps.) cepacia	0	0	0	0	+	+	+	0	+	±	0	0	0	0	0	0	+	0
S. (X.) maltophilia	0	0	0	0	0	0	0	0	±	0						+		
Y. enterocolitica	0	+	0	±	+	+	+		+	0	0	0	0	0	0	+	0	0
Legionella sp.		+	+	+	+	+	+	0	0	0						+		+
P. multocida				+	+	+	+		+	+	0	0	0	+	+	0	0	0
H. ducreyi					+	+	+		+	+			+	+	+	+		+
ANAEROBES:																		
Actinomyces		±ᵃ		0	0	0	+ 0	0	0	0	0	0						
Bacteroides fragilis		+	+	0	0	±	0	0	0	0			0	0	0	0	0	
P. melaninogenica		+	+	+	+	+	+		+	+			+	+	+			+
Clostridium difficile																		
Clostridium (not difficile)		+	+	+	+	+	+		+	+								
Fusobacterium necrophorum																		
Peptostreptococcus sp.		+	+	+	+	+	+		+	+		+	+	+	+	+		+

ᵃ Cefotetan is less active against B. ovatus, B. distasonis, B. thetaiotaomicron.

+ = **usually susceptible**; ± = **variably susceptible/resistant**; 0 = **usually resistant**; blank = **no data**
* A 1-carbacephem best classified as a cephalosporin

TABLE 4 (5)

Organisms	AMINO-GLYCOSIDES Gentamicin	AMINO-GLYCOSIDES Tobramycin	AMINO-GLYCOSIDES Amikacin	Chloramphenicol	Clindamycin	MACROLIDES Erythro	MACROLIDES Azithromycin	MACROLIDES Clarithromycin	KETOLIDE Telithromycin	TETRA-CYCLINES Doxycycline	TETRA-CYCLINES Minocycline	GLYCYL-CYCLINE Tigecycline	Daptomycin	GLYCO-/LIPOGLYCO-/LIPO-PEPTIDES Vancomycin	GLYCO-/LIPOGLYCO-/LIPO-PEPTIDES Teicoplanin[NUS]	GLYCO-/LIPOGLYCO-/LIPO-PEPTIDES Telavancin	Fusidic Acid[NUS]	Trimethoprim	TMP-SMX	AGENTS URINARY TRACT Nitrofurantoin	AGENTS URINARY TRACT Fosfomycin	MISCELLANEOUS Rifampin	MISCELLANEOUS Metronidazole	MISCELLANEOUS Quinupristin-dalfopristin	MISCELLANEOUS Linezolid	MISCELLANEOUS Colistimethate (Colistin)
GRAM-POSITIVE:																										
Strep Group A, B, C, G	0	0	0	+	+	±	±	±	+	±	+	+	±	+	+	+	±	+	+[5]	+		+	0	+	+	0
Strep. pneumoniae	0	0	0	+	+	±	±	±	+	+	+	+	+	+	+	+	±	+	+	+	+	+	0	+	+	0
Enterococcus faecalis	S	S	S	±	0	0	0	0	±	0	0	+	+	+	+	+	+	0	0	+	±	0	0	0	+	0
Enterococcus faecium	S	S	S	±	0	0	0	0	0	0	0	+	+	±	±	+	+	±	±	+	±	0	0	+	+	0
Staph. aureus (MSSA)	+	+	+	+	+	±	±	±	+	±	±	+	+	+	+	+	+	±	+	+	±	+	0	+	+	0
Staph. aureus (MRSA)	0	0	0	±	0	0	0	0	0	+	+	+	+	+	+	+	+	+	+	+	±	+	0	+	+	0
Staph. aureus (CA-MRSA)	+	+	+	+	+	±	±	±	+	+	+	+	+	+	+	+	+	+	+	+	±	+	0	+	+	0
Staph. epidermidis	±	±	±	+	0	0	0	0	0	0	0	+	+	+	+	+	+	0	0	+		+	0	+	+	0
C. jeikeium												+	±	+	+	+			+			+	0	+	+	0
L. monocytogenes	+	+	+	+	0	+	+	+	+	+	+	+	0	0	0	0	0	+	+	0		+	0	+	+	0
GRAM-NEGATIVE:																										
N. gonorrhoeae	0	0	0	+	0	±	+	±	+	±	±	+	0	0	0	0	+	0	±			+	0	±	0	±
N. meningitidis	0	0	0	+	0	0	+	0	+	+	+	+	0	0	0	0	+	+	+			+	0	0	0	0
M. catarrhalis	+	+	+	+	0	+	+	+	+	+	+	+	0	0	0	0	0	+	+	+		0	0	0	0	+
H. influenzae	+	+	+	+	0	±	±	±	+	+	+	+	0	0	0	0	0	+	+	±	±	0	0	0	0	+
Aeromonas	+	+	+	+						±	±	+	0	0	0	0	0	+	+	±		0	0	0	0	+
E. coli	+	+	+	+						±	±	+	0	0	0	0	0	+	+	+	+	0	0	0	0	+
Klebsiella sp	+	+	+	+						±	±	+	0	0	0	0	0	±	±	±	±	0	0	0	0	+
E. coli/Klebs sp ESBL+	±	±	+	±						±	±	+	0	0	0	0	0	±	±	±	±	0	0	0	0	+
E. coli/Klebs sp KPC+	0	0	0	0						0	0	+	0	0	0	0	0	0	0			0	0	0	0	+
Enterobacter sp	+	+	+	±						±	±	+	0	0	0	0	0	±	±	±		0	0	0	0	+
Salmonella sp	+	+	+	+						±	±	+						±	±	±	±		0	0	0	
Shigella sp	+	+	+	+						±	±	+						±	±	+	+		0	0	0	

+ = **usually susceptible**; ± = **variably susceptible/resistant**; 0 = **usually resistant**; blank = **no data**
Antimicrobials such as azithromycin have high tissue penetration & some such as clarithromycin are metabolized to more active compounds, hence in vivo activity may exceed in vitro activity.
** Vancomycin, metronidazole given po active vs C. difficile. IV vancomycin not effective. S = Synergistic with cell wall-active antibiotics.

[5] Although active in vitro. TMP-SMX is not clinically effective for Group A strep pharyngitis or for infections due to E. faecalis.
[6] Although active in vitro, daptomycin is not clinically effective for pneumonia caused by strep pneumonia.

TABLE 4 (6)

Organisms	AMINO-GLYCOSIDES			MACROLIDES					KETOLIDE	TETRA-CYCLINES		GLYCYL-CYCLINE	GLYCO/LIPOGLYCO-/LIPO-PEPTIDES				MISC.:			AGENTS URINARY TRACT		MISCELLANEOUS				
	Gentamicin	Tobramycin	Amikacin	Chloramphenicol	Clindamycin	Erythro	Azithromycin	Clarithromycin	Telithromycin	Doxycycline	Minocycline	Tigecycline	Daptomycin	Vancomycin	Teicoplanin[NUS]	Telavancin	Fusidic Acid[NUS]	Trimethoprim	TMP-SMX	Nitrofurantoin	Fosfomycin	Rifampin	Metronidazole	Quinupristin-dalfopristin	Linezolid	Colistimethate (Colistin)
Serratia marcescens	+	+	+	o	o	o	o	o	o	o	o	+	o	o	o	o	o	o	+|	o	+|	o	o		o	o
Proteus vulgaris	+	+	+	+|	o	o	o	o	o	o	o	+|	o	o	o	o	o	o	o	o	+|	o	o		o	o
Ps. aeruginosa	+	+	+|	o	o	o	o	o	o	o	o	+|	o	o	o	o	o	o	+|	o		o	o		o	+
Acinetobacter sp.	o	o	o	o	o	o	o	o	o	o +|	o +|	o	o	o	o	o	o	o	o			o	o		o	+
S. (X.) maltophilia	+	o	o	+	o	o	o	+		+	+		o	o	o	o	o	+o	+	o		o	o		o	o
Y. enterocolitica	+	o	o	+	o	o	+			+	+		o	o	o	o		+	+	o		o	o		o	+|
F. tularensis	+	+								+	+		o	o	o	o			+				o		o	
Brucella sp.	+|	+|								+	+		o	o	o	o	+|		+			+	o		o	
Legionella sp.						o	+	+	+	+	+	+	o	o	o	o	o					+	o			
H. ducreyi						+	+	+					o	o	o	o							o			
V. vulnificus										+	+	+	o	o	o	o							o			
MISC.:																										
Chlamydophila sp.	o	o	o	o	+|	+	+	+ o	+ o	+++	+++	+++	o	+o		+o	+	o	o	o		+	o		+o	
M. pneumoniae	o	o	o	o	o	+	+	+	+	+++	+++	+++	o	o		o	+	+					o			
Mycobacterium avium	o	o	+o			+|	+|	+|			+|			o	o		o	+	+				+	o	+|	+|	o
ANAEROBES:																										
Actinomyces	o	o	o	+	+	+|	+|	+|		+|	+|	+|	o	+o	+o	+o	+	+	o				+	+|	+|	
Bacteroides fragilis	o	o	o	+	+	+|	+|	+|		+	+	+	o	o	o	o	+	o	o			o	+	+|	+|	
P. melaninogenica	o	o	o	+	+	+|	+|	+|		+	+	+	o	o	o	o	+	+	o			+	+	+|	+|	
Clostridium difficile				+	+++	+|	+|	+|		+	+	+++	o	+o		o	+	+	+			+	++	+++	+++	
Clostridium (not difficile)[**]	o	o	o	+	+	+|	+|	+|	+	+	+	+++	o	+o	+o	+o	+	+	+			+	+	+|	+|	
Fusobacterium necrophorum	o	o	o	+	+++	+|	+|	+|		+	+	+++	o	+o	+o	+o	+					+	+++	+|	+	
Peptostreptococcus sp.	o	o	o	+	+++	+|	+|	+|	+	+	+	+++	o	+	+	+	+					+	+++	+	+	

+ = usually susceptible; ± = variably susceptible/resistant; o = usually resistant; blank = no data
Antimicrobials such as azithromycin have high tissue penetration & some such as clarithromycin are metabolized to more active compounds, hence in vivo activity may exceed in vitro activity.
** Vancomycin, metronidazole given po active vs C. difficile; IV vancomycin not effective. S = Synergistic with cell wall-active antibiotics.
[NUS] not US

TABLE 5A – TREATMENT OPTIONS FOR SYSTEMIC INFECTION DUE TO SELECTED RESISTANT GRAM-POSITIVE BACTERIA

ORGANISM	RESISTANT TO	PRIMARY TREATMENT OPTIONS	ALTERNATIVE TREATMENT OPTIONS	COMMENTS
Enterococcus sp.	Vancomycin, Ampicillin, Penicillin, Gentamicin	No clearly effective therapy. Can try **Daptomycin** 8-12 mg/kg IV q24h but monitor for emergence of resistance (NEJM 365:892, 2011).	**Quinupristin-dalfopristin** 22.5 mg/kg/day IV divided q8h (see Comment for activity) OR **Linezolid** 600 mg IV/po q12h	Activity of quinupristin/dalfopristin is limited to E. faecium (CID 33:816, 2001). Linezolid bacteriostatic with 40% relapse rate in endocarditis (AnIM 138:133, 2003). Role of televancin unclear.
Staphylococcus aureus (See also Table 6 for more details)	Vancomycin (VISA or VRSA) and all beta lactams (except Ceftaroline)	**Daptomycin** 6-10 mg/kg IV q24h or **Quinupristin-dalfopristin** 7.5 mg/kg IV q8h	**Linezolid** 600 mg IV/po q12h	Confirm dapto susceptibility as VISA strains may be non-susceptible. If prior vanco therapy (or persistent infection on vanco) there is significant chance of developing resistance to dapto (AAC 66:1696, 2011). Addition of an anti-staphylococcal beta-lactam (ASBL) may restore susceptibility against Dapto-resistant MRSA (AAC 54:3161, 2010). Combination of Dapto + ASBL has been successful in clearing refractory MRSA bacteremia (CID 53:158, 2011). Other possibilities: televancin, ceftaroline.
Streptococcus pneumoniae	Penicillin G (MIC ≥ 4 μg/mL)	If no meningitis: **Ceftriaxone** 2 gm IV once daily OR **Ceftaroline** 600 mg IV q12h OR **Linezolid** 600 mg IV/po q12h	Meningitis: **Vancomycin** 15 mg/kg IV q8h OR **Meropenem** 2 gm IV q8h	Ceftriaxone 2 gm IV q12h should also work for meningitis.

TABLE 5B: TREATMENT OPTIONS FOR SYSTEMIC INFECTION DUE TO SELECTED MULTI-DRUG RESISTANT GRAM-NEGATIVE BACILLI

The suggested treatment options in this Table are usually not FDA-approved. Suggestions are variably based on in vitro data, animal studies, and/or limited clinical experience.

ORGANISM	RESISTANT TO	PRIMARY TREATMENT OPTIONS	ALTERNATIVE TREATMENT OPTIONS	COMMENTS
Acinetobacter baumannii	All Penicillins, All Cephalosporins, Aztreonam, Carbapenems, Aminoglycosides and Fluoroquinolones	**Polymyxin E (Colistin)** + (**Imipenem** or **Meropenem**) See Table 10A, page 101, for guidance on Colistin dosing.	**Polymyxin E (Colistin)** + **Rifampin** 300 mg IV q12h or 600 mg IV q24h. Another option (if active in vitro): **Minocycline** (IDCP 20:184, 2012) (in vitro synergy between minocycline and imipenem)	Refs: Int J Antimicrob Agts 37:244, 2011; BMC Inf Dis 11:109, 2011. Detergent effect of colistin reconstitutes antibiotic activity of carbapenems and other drugs. Do not use colistin as monotherapy.
E. coli, Klebsiella pneumoniae, or other Enterobacteriaceae producing extended spectrum beta-lactamase producing organisms (ESBLs)	All Cephalosporins, TMP-SMX, Fluoroquinolones, Aminoglycosides	**Imipenem** 500 mg IV q6h OR **Meropenem** 1 gm IV q8h OR **Doripenem** 500 mg IV q8h (CID 49:31, 2004; Note: **Dori** is not FDA approved for treatment of pneumonia).	Perhaps high dose **Cefepime** 2 gm IV q12h; **Polymyxin E (Colistin)** in combination with carbapenem. For dosing, see Table 10A, page 101.	For UTI: Fosfomycin, nitrofurantoin (AAC 53:1278, 2009). Resistant to cefdinir, but combination of cefdinir with amox-clav active in vitro (AAC 53:1278, 2009).
Carbapenemase producing gram-negative bacilli	All Penicillins, Cephalosporins, Aztreonam, Carbapenems, Aminoglycosides, Fluoroquinolones	**Polymyxin E (Colistin)** in combination with carbapenem. See Table 10A page 101, for guidance on Colistin dosing.	Combination of Colistin and Rifampin.	See Table 10A, page 101, for guidance on Colistin dosing.
Pseudomonas aeruginosa	All beta-lactams, Aminoglycosides, Fluoroquinolones	**Polymyxin E (Colistin)** in combination with carbapenem See Table 10A, page 101, for guidance on Colistin dosing.	Inhaled **Colistin**[NAI] 50-75 mg in 3-4 mL saline via nebulizer + **Colistin** IV + carbapenem.	See Table 10A, page 101, for guidance on Colistin dosing.
Stenotrophomonas maltophilia	All beta-lactams except Ticar-Clav, Aminoglycosides, Fluoroquinolones	**TMP-SMX**, 8-10 mg/kg/day IV divided q8h/q12h (based on TMP component)	**Ticar-Clav**, 3.1 gm IV q4-6h	

77

TABLE 6 – SUGGESTED MANAGEMENT OF SUSPECTED OR CULTURE-POSITIVE COMMUNITY-ASSOCIATED METHICILLIN-RESISTANT S. AUREUS INFECTIONS
(See footnote[1] for doses)

IDSA Guidelines: CID 52 (Feb 1):1, 2011. With the magnitude of the clinical problem and a number of new drugs, it is likely new data will require frequent revisions of the regimens suggested. (See page 2 for abbreviations).
NOTE: Distinction between community and hospital strains of MRSA blurring.

CLINICAL ILLNESS	ABSCESS, AFEBRILE & IMMUNOCOMPETENT; OUTPATIENT CARE	ABSCESS(ES) WITH FEVER; OUTPATIENT CARE	PNEUMONIA	BACTEREMIA OR POSSIBLE ENDOCARDITIS OR BACTEREMIC SHOCK	TREATMENT FAILURE (See footnote[2])
Management Drug doses in footnote.	TMP-SMX-DS or doxycycline or minocycline or clindamycin (CID 40:1429, 2005 & AAC 51:2628, 2007). NOTE: I&D alone may be sufficient	TMP-SMX-DS or clindamycin or doxycycline plus incision and drainage. Note: Hospital associated MRSA strains are often resistant to Clindamycin.	Vanco IV or linezolid IV	Vanco or dapto IV. Dapto not inferior to vanco in bacteremia trial (NEJM 355:653, 2006). No apparent benefit of adding RIF to VANCO, maybe more (AAC 52:2463, 2008).	Confirm adequate vanco troughs of 15-20 μg/mL and vancomycin susceptibility. Switch to alternative regimen if vanco MIC ≥ 2 μg/mL. Dapto resistance reported after vanco exposure & prior to dapto therapy (CID 45:601, 2007). Dapto appears safe at doses of up to 12 mg/kg/d (AAC 50:3245, 2006).
		Culture abscess & maybe blood! I&D. Hot packs. Close follow-up.		Target Vancomycin troughs of 15-20 μg/mL (CID 52:975, 2011). Vancomycin MICs ≥ 2 μg/mL associated with treatment failure in serious infections but whether this is mediated by insensitivity to factor unclear (JID 204:340, 2011).	Data extremely limited concerning salvage regimens for treatment failures. Addition of aminoglycoside or rifampin to vancomycin is not effective in one retrospective study (0% success), whereas linezolid with or without a carbapenem was effective (86% success) in patients with bacteremia due to pneumonia, vascular catheter or graft infection; no patient had endocarditis (CID 49:395, 2009).
Comments continue on next page				If patient has slow response to vancomycin and isolate has MIC = 2, consider alternative therapy. An agent other than vancomycin should be used for infections caused by isolates with MICs ≥ 4 μg/mL.	Options: For endocarditis or complicated bacteremia dapto 10 mg/kg IV once daily plus gentamicin 1 mg/kg IV every 8 hours or RIF 300-450 mg twice daily, linezolid + a second agent (JAC 58:273, 2006 & JAC 56:923, 2005); quinupristin-dalfopristin (Q-D) ± with vanco. Case reports of success with Telavancin for MRSA failure (JAC 65:1315, 2010; AAC 54:5376, 2010; JAC (Jun 8), 2011). Options: For endocarditis or complicated bacteremia dapto 10 mg/kg IV once daily plus gentamicin 1 mg/kg IV every 8 hours or RIF 300-450 mg twice daily. Case reports of success with Telavancin 10 mg/kg/d for MRSA failure (JAC 65:1315, 2010; AAC 54:5376, 2010; JAC 66:2186, 2011) Or ceftaroline 600 mg q8h (JAC 67:1267, 2012 and J Infect Chemother - online Jul 14, 2012).

[1] Clindamycin: 300 mg po tid. Daptomycin: 6 mg/kg IV q24h is the standard dose; higher doses (10 mg/kg) and use of combination therapy recommended for vancomycin treatment failures. Doxycycline or minocycline: 100 mg po bid. Linezolid: 600 mg po/IV bid. Quinupristin-dalfopristin (Q-D): 7.5 mg per kg IV q8h via central line. Rifampin: Long serum half-life justifies dosing 600 mg po q24h; however, frequency of nausea less with 300 mg po bid. TMP-SMX-DS: Standard dose 8-10 mg per kg po bid. For 70 kg person = 700 mg TMP component per day. TMP-SMX contains 160 mg TMP and 800 mg SMX. The dose for treatment of CA-MRSA skin and soft tissue infections (SSTI) is 1 DS tablet twice daily. Vancomycin: 1 gm IV q12h; up to 45-60 mg/kg/day in divided doses may be required to achieve target trough concentrations of 15-20 mcg/ml; recommended for serious infections.

[2] The median duration of bacteremia in endocarditis is 7-9 days in patients treated with vancomycin (AnIM 115:674, 1991). Longer duration of bacteremia, greater likelihood of endocarditis (JID 190:1140, 2004). Definition of failure unclear. Clinical response should be factored in. **Unsatisfactory clinical response especially if blood cultures remain positive beyond 5-7 days is an indication for change in therapy.**

TABLE 6 (2)

CLINICAL ILLNESS	ABSCESS, AFEBRILE; & IMMUNOCOMPETENT: OUTPATIENT CARE	ABSCESS(ES) WITH FEVER; OUTPATIENT CARE	PNEUMONIA	BACTEREMIA OR POSSIBLE ENDOCARDITIS OR BACTEREMIC SHOCK	TREATMENT FAILURE (See footnote²)
Comments	Effective dose of **TMP-SMX-DS** is unclear. IV dose is 8-10 mg/kg/d; roughly equivalent to 2 tabs po bid. Anecdotally, most pts respond to I&D and 1 tab bid although failures may occur (see footnote¹) particularly in obese patients and 2 DS tabs bid recommended for those with BMI > 40. **Fusidic acid** 500 mg tid (not available in the US) + **rifampin** also an option (*J Antimicrob Chemother 61*: 976, 2008 and *Can J Infect Dis Med Microbiol*; *17(Suppl C): 4C, 2006*); do not use rifampin alone as resistance rapidly emerges. One retrospective study (*Peds 123*: e059, 2009) in children reports increased risk of treatment failure with TMP-SMX, compared to other agents for undrained, uncultured skin and soft tissue infections; presumably these were mainly cellulitis, which could reflect less activity of this agent against Group A streptococcus.	Note: Increasing frequency of strains with inducible resistance to clindamycin. Some authorities recommend addition of rifampin to TMP-SMX; do not use rifampin alone as resistance rapidly emerges. Patients not responding after 2-3 days should be evaluated for complicated infection and switched to **vancomycin**.	Prospective study of **Linezolid** vs **Vanco** showed slightly higher cure rate with Linezolid, no difference in mortality (*CID 54*:621, 2012).	Efficacy of IV **TMP-SMX** vs CA-MRSA uncertain. IV **TMP-SMX** was inferior to **vanco** vs bacteremic MSSA (*AnIM 117*:390, 1992). **Dapto** failures associated with development of **dapto** resistance (*NEJM 355*:653, 2006)	Do not add **linezolid** to **vanco**: no benefit & may be antagonistic (*AAC 47*:3002, 2003). **Ceftaroline** is approved for MSSA pneumonia but not MRSA pneumonia. MRSA was an exclusion in the clinical trials (*CID 51*:1395, 2010).

TABLE 7 - DRUG DESENSITIZATION METHODS

Penicillin. Oral route (Pen VK) preferred. 1/3 pts develop transient reaction, usually mild. **Perform in ICU setting. Discontinue β-blockers. Have IV line, epinephrine, ECG, spirometer available.**
Desensitization works as long as pt is receiving Pen; allergy returns after discontinuance. History of Steven-Johnson, exfoliative dermatitis, erythroderma are contraindications. Skin testing for evaluation of Pen allergy: Testing with major determinant (benzyl Pen polylysine) and minor determinants has negative predictive value (97-99%). Risk of systemic reaction to skin testing <1% (*Ann Allergy Asth Immunol* 106:1, 2011). General refs: *CID* 35:26, 2002; *Am J Med* 121:572, 2008; *Curr Clin Topics ID* 13:131, 1993.

- **Method:** Prepare dilutions using **Pen-VK** oral soln. 250 mg/5mL. Administer each dose @ 15 min intervals in 30 mL water/flavored bev. After Step 14 observe pt for 30 min, then give full therapeutic dose by route of choice. Ref: *Allergy, Prin & Prac, Mosby*, 1993, p. 1726

Step	Dilution (mg/mL)	mL Administered	Dose/Step mg	Dose/Step units	Cumulative Dose Given mg	Cumulative Dose Given units
1	0.5	0.1	0.05	80	0.05	80
2	0.5	0.2	0.1	160	0.15	240
3	0.5	0.4	0.2	320	0.35	560
4	0.5	0.8	0.4	640	0.75	1,200
5	0.5	1.6	0.8	1,280	1.55	2,480
6	0.5	3.2	1.6	2,560	3.15	5,040
7	0.5	6.4	3.2	5,120	6.35	10,160
8	5	1.2	6	9,600	12.35	19,760
9	5	2.4	12	19,200	24.35	38,960
10	5	4.8	24	38,400	48.35	77,360
11	50	1	50	80,000	98.35	157,360
12	50	2	100	160,000	198.35	317,360
13	50	4	200	320,000	398.35	637,360
14	50	8	400	640,000	798.35	1,277,360

TMP-SMX. Perform in hospital/clinic. Refs: *CID* 20:849, 1995; *AIDS* 5:311, 1991.
- **Method:** Use **TMP-SMX** oral susp. (40 mg TMP/200 mg SMX)/5 mL. Take with 6 oz water after each dose. Corticosteroids, antihistaminics NOT used.

Hour	Dose (TMP/SMX) (mg)
0	0.004/0.02
1	0.04/0.2
2	0.4/2
3	4/20
4	40/200
5	160/800

Penicillin. Parenteral (Pen G) route. Follow procedures/notes under Oral (Pen-VK) route. Ref: *Allergy, Prin & Prac, Mosby*, 1993, p. 1726.
- **Method:** Administer **Pen G** IM, IV or sc as follows:

Step	Dilution (units/mL)	mL Administered	Dose/Step (units)	Cumulative Dose Given (units)
1	100	0.2	20	20
2	100	0.4	40	60
3	100	0.8	80	140
4	1,000	0.2	200	340
5	1,000	0.4	400	740
6	1,000	0.8	800	1,540
7	10,000	0.2	2,000	3,540
8	10,000	0.4	4,000	7,540
9	10,000	0.8	8,000	15,540
10	100,000	0.2	20,000	35,540
11	100,000	0.4	40,000	75,540
12	100,000	0.8	80,000	155,540
13	1,000,000	0.2	200,000	355,540
14	1,000,000	0.4	400,000	755,540
15	1,000,000	0.8	800,000	1,555,540

Ceftriaxone. Ref: *Allergol Immunopathol (Madr)* 37:105, 2009.
- **Method:** Infuse **Ceftriaxone** IV @ 20 min intervals as follows:

Day	Dose (mg)
1	0.001, then 0.01, then 0.1, then 1
2	1, then 5, then 10, then 50
3	100, then 250, then 500
4	1000

Desensitization Methods for Other Drugs (References)
- **Imipenem-Cilastatin.** See *Ann Pharmacother* 37:513, 2003.
- **Meropenem.** See *Ann Pharmacother* 37:1424, 2003.
- **Daptomycin.** See *Ann All Asthma Immun* 100:87, 2008.
- **Ceftazidime.** *Curr Opin All Clin Immunol* 6(6): 476, 2006.
- **Vancomycin.** *Intern Med* 45:317, 2006.

TABLE 8A – RISK CATEGORIES OF ANTIMICROBICS IN PREGNANCY

DRUG	FDA CATEGORIES*	DRUG	FDA CATEGORIES	DRUG	FDA CATEGORIES	DRUG	FDA CATEGORIES
Antibacterial Agents:		**Antifungal Agents:** (CID 27:1151, 1998)		**Antimycobacterial Agents:**		**Antiviral Agents:** (continued)	
Aminoglycosides:		Amphotericin B preparations	B	Quinine	X	Fosamprenavir	C
Amikacin, gentamicin, isepamicin[NUS]		Anidulafungin	C	Capreomycin	C	Foscarnet	C
netilmicin[NUS], streptomycin & tobramycin	D	Caspofungin	C	Clofazimine/cycloserine	"avoid"	Ganciclovir	C
Beta Lactams		Fluconazole (150 mg SD	C	Indinavir	C	Interferons	C
Penicillins; pens + BL;		for vaginal candidiasis)		Ethambutol	"safe"	Lamivudine	C
cephalosporins; aztreonam	B	Fluconazole (other regimens, uses)	D	Ethionamide	C	Lopinavir/ritonavir	C
Imipenem/cilastatin	C	Itraconazole, ketoconazole, flucytosine	C	INH, pyrazinamide	C	Maraviroc	B
Meropenem, ertapenem, doripenem	B	Micafungin	C	Rifabutin	B	Nelfinavir	B
Chloramphenicol	C	Posaconazole	C	Rifampin	C	Nevirapine	C
Ciprofloxacin, ofloxa, levo, gati,		Terbinafine	B	Thalidomide	X	Oseltamivir	C
gemi, moxi	C	Voriconazole	D	**Antiviral Agents:**		Raltegravir	C
Clindamycin	B	**Antiparasitic Agents:**		Abacavir	C	Ribavirin	X
Colistin	C	Albendazole/mebendazole	C	Acyclovir	B	Rilpivirine	B
Daptomycin	B	Artemether/lumefantrine	C	Adefovir	C	Rimantadine	C
Fosfomycin	B	Atovaquone/proguanil; atovaquone alone	C	Amantadine	C	Ritonavir	B
Fidaxomicin	B	Chloroquine	C	Atazanavir	B	Saquinavir	B
Fusidic acid[†]	See Footnote[†]	Dapsone	C	Cidofovir	C	Stavudine	C
Linezolid	C	Eflornithine	C	Cobicistat	C	Telbivudine	B
Macrolides:		Ivermectin	C	Danuravir	C	Tenofovir	B
Erythromycins/azithromycin	B	Mefloquine	C	Delavirdine	C	Tipranavir	C
Clarithromycin	C	Miltefosine	D	Didanosine (ddI)	B	Valacyclovir	B
Metronidazole	B	Nitazoxanide	B	Efavirenz	D	Valganciclovir	C
Nitrofurantoin	B	Pentamidine	C	Elvitegravir/cobicistat/		Zalcitabine	C
Polymyxin B	C	Praziquantel	B	emtricitabine/tenofovir	B	Zanamivir	C
Quinupristin–Dalfopristin	B	Proguanil	B	Emtricitabine	B	Zidovudine	C
Rifaximin	C	Pyrimethamine/pyrisulfadoxine	C	Enfuvirtide	B		
Sulfonamides/trimethoprim	C	Quinidine	C	Entecavir	C		
Telavancin	C			Etravirine	B		
Telithromycin	C			Famciclovir	B		
Tetracyclines, tigecycline	D						
Tinidazole	C						
Vancomycin	C						

* **FDA Pregnancy Categories: A**—studies in pregnant women, no risk; **B**—animal studies no risk, but human not adequate or animal toxicity but human studies no risk; **C**—animal studies show toxicity, human studies inadequate but benefit of use may exceed risk; **D**—evidence of human risk, but benefits may outweigh; **X**—fetal abnormalities in humans, risk > benefit
† **Fusidic acid**[NUS]: potential for neonatal kernicterus

TABLE 8B – ANTIMICROBIAL DOSING IN OBESITY

The number of obese patients is increasing. Intuitively, the standard doses of some drugs may not achieve effective serum concentrations. Pertinent data on anti-infective dosing in the obese patient is gradually emerging. Though some of the data needs further validation, the following table reflects what is currently known. **Obesity is defined as ≥ 20% over Ideal Body Weight (Ideal BW) or Body Mass Index (BMI) > 30. Dose** = suggested body weight (BW) for dose calculation in obese patient, or specific dose if applicable.

Drug	Dose	Comments
Acyclovir	Use **Ideal BW** Example: for HSV encephalitis, give 10 mg/kg of Ideal BW q8h	Unpublished data from 7 obese volunteers (Davis, et al., ICAAC abstract, 1991).
Aminoglycosides	Use **Adjusted BW** Example: Critically ill patient, Gentamicin or Tobramycin (not Amikacin) 7 mg/kg of Adjusted BW IV q24h (See Comment)	Adjusted BW = Ideal BW + 0.4(Actual BW – Ideal BW). Ref: *Pharmacother 27:1081, 2007*. Follow levels so as to lower dose once hemodynamics stabilize.
Cefazolin (surgical prophylaxis)	No dose adjustment needed: 2 gm x 1 dose (repeat in 3 hours?)	Conflicting data; unclear whether dose should be repeated, or if an even higher dose is required. Patients with BMI 40-80 studied. Refs: *Surg 136:738, 2004; Eur J Clin Pharmacol 67:985, 2011; Surg Infect 13:33, 2012*.
Cefepime	Modest dose increase: 2 gm IV q8h instead of the usual q12h	Data from 10 patients (mean BMI 48) undergoing bariatric surgery; regimen yields free T > MIC of 60% for MIC of 8ug/ml. Ref: *Obes Surg 22:465, 2012*.
Daptomycin	Use **Actual BW** Example: 4-12 mg/kg of Actual BW IV q24h	Data from a single-dose PK study in 7 obese volunteers. Ref: *Antimicrob Ag Chemother 51:2741, 2007*.
Flucytosine	Use **Ideal BW** Example: Crypto meningitis, give 25 mg/kg of Ideal BW po q6h	Date from one obese patient with cryptococcal disease. Ref: *Pharmacother 15:251, 1995*.
Levofloxacin	**No dose adjustment required** Example: 750 mg po/IV q24h	Data from 13 obese patients; variability in study findings renders conclusion uncertain. Refs: *Antimicrob Ag Chemother 55:3240, 2011; J Antimicrob Chemother 66:1653, 2011*.
Moxifloxacin	**No dose adjustment required** Example: 400 mg po/IV q24h	Data from 12 obese patients undergoing gastric bypass. Ref: *J Antimicrob Chemother 66:2330, 2011*.
Oseltamivir	**No dose adjustment required** Example: 75 mg po q12h	Data from 10 obese volunteers, unclear if applicable to patients >250 kg (OK to give 150 mg po q12h). Ref: *J Antimicrob Chemother 66:2083, 2011*.
Vancomycin	Use **Actual BW** Example: in critically ill patient give 25-30 mg/kg of Actual BW IV load, then 15-20 mg/kg of Actual BW IV q8h-12h (infuse over 1.5-2 hr). No single dose over 2 gm. Check trough levels.	Data from 24 obese patients; Vancomycin half-life appears to decrease with little change in Vd. Ref: *Eur J Clin Pharmacol 54:621, 1998*.
Voriconazole	**No dose adjustment required** Example: 400 mg po q12h x2 doses then 200 mg po q12h. Check trough concentrations (underdosing common with Voriconazole).	Data from a 2-way crossover study of oral voriconazole in 8 volunteers suggest no adjustment required, but data from one patient suggest use of adjusted BW. Recommended IV voriconazole dose based on actual BW (no supporting data). Refs: *Antimicrob Ag Chemother 55:2601, 2011; Clin Infect Dis 53:745, 2011*.

TABLE 9A – SELECTED PHARMACOLOGIC FEATURES OF ANTIMICROBIAL AGENTS

For pharmacodynamics, see Table 9B; for Cytochrome P450 interactions, see Table 9C. Table terminology key at bottom of each page. Additional footnotes at end of Table 9A, page 91.

DRUG	REFERENCE DOSE/ROUTE	PREG RISK	FOOD EFFECT (PO)[1]	ORAL %AB	PEAK SERUM LEVEL (μg/mL)	PROTEIN BINDING (%)	VOL OF DISTRIB (Vd)	AVER SERUM T½, hrs[2]	BILE PEN (%)[3]	CSF/BLOOD (%)	CSF PEN[5]	AUC (μg•hr/mL)	Tmax (hr)
PENICILLINS: Natural													
Benz Pen G	1.2 million units IM	B			0.15 (SD)								
Penicillin G	2 million units IV	B			20 (SD)	65	0.35 L/kg	0.5	500	5-10	Yes: Pen-sens S. pneumo		
Penicillin V	500 mg po	B	Tab/soln no food	60-73	5-6 (SD)	65		0.5					
PEN'ASE-RESISTANT PENICILLINS													
Cloxacillin[AUS]	500 mg	B	Cap no food	50	7.5-14 (SD)	95	0.1 L/kg	0.5	5-8				1-1.5
Dicloxacillin	500 mg	B	Cap no food	37	10-17 (SD)	98	0.1 L/kg	0.7	5-8				1-1.5
Nafcillin	500 mg	B			30 (SD)	90-94	27.1 Vss	0.5-1	>100	9-20	Yes		
Oxacillin	500 mg	B			43 (SD)	90-94	0.4 L/kg	0.7	25	10-15	Yes	18.1	
AMINOPENICILLINS													
Amoxicillin	500 mg po	B	± food	80	5.5-7.5 (SD)	17	0.36 L/kg	1.2	100-3000	13-14	Yes	22	1-2
Amoxicillin ER	775 mg po	B	Tab + food		6.6 (SD)	20		1.2-1.5				29.8	3.1
AM-CL	875/125 mg po	B	Cap/tab/susp ± food	80/30-98	11.6/2.2 (SD)	18/25		1.4/1.1	100-3000			AM: 26.8 - CL: 5.1	
AM-CL-ER	2 tabs [2000/125 mg]	B	Tab + food		17/2.1 (SD)	18/25		1.3/1.0				AM: 71.6 - CL: 5.3	
Ampicillin	2 gm IV	B			100 (SD)	18-22	0.29 L/kg	1.2	100-3000	13-14	Yes		
AM-SB	3 gm IV	B			109-150/48-88 (SD)	28/38		1.2				AM: 120 - SB: 71	
ANTIPSEUDOMONAL PENICILLINS													
PIP-TZ	3/.375 gm IV	B			242/24 (SD)	16-48	PIP: 0.24 L/kg	1.0	>100			PIP: 242 - TZ: 25	
TC-CL	3.1 gm IV	B			330/8 (SD)	45/25	TC: 9.7 Vss	1.2/1.0				TC: 485 - CL: 8.2	
CEPHALOSPORINS—1st Generation													
Cefadroxil	500 mg po	B	Cap/tab/susp ± food	90	16 (SD)	20	0.31 L/kg V/F	1.5	22			47.4	
Cefazolin	1 gm IV	B			188 (SD)	73-87	0.19 L/kg	1.9	29-300	1-4	No	236	
Cephalexin	500 mg po	B	Cap/tab/susp ±	90	18 (SD)	5-15	0.38 L/kg V/F	1.0	216			29	1

Preg Risk: FDA risk categories: A = no risk, **B** = No risk - human studies, **C** = toxicity in animals - inadequate human studies, **D** = human risk, but benefit may outweigh risk, **X** = fetal abnormalities – risk > benefit; **Food Effect (PO dosing): †** food = take with food, **no food** = take with or without food; **Oral % AB** = % absorbed; **Peak Serum Level: SD** = after single dose; **SS** = steady state after multiple doses; **Volume of Distribution (Vd): V/F** = Vd/oral bioavailability, **Vss** = Vd at steady state, **Vss/F** = Vd at steady state/oral bioavailability; **CSF Penetration:** therapeutic efficacy comment based on dose, usual susceptibility or target organism & penetration into CSF; **24hr** = AUC 0-24; **Tmax** = time to max plasma concentration.

83

TABLE 9A (2) (Footnotes at the end of table)

DRUG	REFERENCE DOSE/ROUTE	PREG RISK	FOOD EFFECT (PO)	ORAL %AB	PEAK SERUM LEVEL (μg/mL)	PROTEIN BINDING (%)	VOL OF DISTRIB (Vd)	AVER SERUM T½, hrs[1]	BILE PEN (%)[1]	CSF/BLOOD (%)	CSF PEN[6]	AUC (μg•hr/mL)	Tmax (hr)
CEPHALOSPORINS—2nd Generation													
Cefaclor	500 mg po	B	Cap/susp ± food	93	13 (SD)	22–25	0.33 L/kg V/F	0.8	≥60			20.5	0.5-1.0
Cefaclor–ER	500 mg po	B	Tab + food		8.4 (SD)	22–25		0.8	≥60			18.1	2.5
Cefotetan	1 gm IV	B			158 (SD)	78–91	10.3 L	4.2	2–21			504	
Cefoxitin	1 gm IV	B			110 (SD)	65–79	16.1 L Vss	0.8	280	3	No		
Cefprozil	500 mg po	B	Tab/susp ± food	95	10.5 (SD)	36	0.23 L/kg Vss/F	1.5				25.7	
Cefuroxime	1.5 gm IV	B			100 (SD)	33–50	0.19 L/kg Vss	1.5	35–80	17–88	Marginal	150	
Cefuroxime axetil	250 mg tabs IV	B	Susp + food; Tab ± food	52	4.1 (SD)	50	0.66 L/kg V/F	1.5				12.9	2.5
CEPHALOSPORINS—3rd Generation													
Cefdinir	300 mg po	B	Cap/susp ± food	25	1.6 (SD)	60–70	0.35 L/kg V/F	1.7				7.1	2.9
Cefditoren pivoxil	400 mg po	B	Tab + food	16	4 (SD)	88	9.3 L Vss/F	1.6				20	1.5-3.0
Cefixime	400 mg tabs po	B	Tab/susp ± food	50	3–5 (SD)	65	0.93 L/kg V/F	3.1	800			25.8	4
Cefotaxime	1 gm IV	B			100	30–51	0.28 L/kg	1.5	15–75	10	Yes	70	
Cefpodoxime proxetil	200 mg po	B	Tab + food Susp ± food	46	2.3 (SD)	40	0.7 L/kg V/F	2.3	115			14.5	2-3
Ceftazidime	1 gm IV	B			69 (SD)	<10	0.24 L/kg Vss	1.9	13–54	20–40	Yes	127	
Ceftibuten	400 mg po	B	Cap/susp no food	80	15 (SD)	65	0.21 L/kg V/F	2.4				73.7	2.6
Ceftizoxime	1 gm IV	B			60 (SD)	30	0.34 L/kg	1.7	34–82			85	
Ceftriaxone	1 gm IV	B			150 (SD), 172-204 (SS)	85–95	5.8-13.5 L	8	200–500	8–16	Yes	1006	
CEPHALOSPORINS—4th Generation and Anti-MRSA													
Cefepime	2 gm IV	B			164 (SD)	20	18 L Vss	2.0	10–20	10	Yes	284.8	
Ceftaroline	600 mg IV	B			21.3	20	20.3 Vss	2.7				56.3	
Ceftobiprole[NUS]	500 mg IV	B			33-34.2 (SD)	16	18 L Vss	2.9-3.3				116	
CARBAPENEMS													
Doripenem	500 mg IV	B			23	8.1	16.8 L Vss	1	117 (0–611)			36.3	
Ertapenem	1 gm IV	B			154	95	0.12 L Vss	4	10	8.5	+[6]	572.1	
Imipenem	500 mg IV	C			40	15–25	0.27 L/kg	1	minimal			42.2	
Meropenem	1 gm IV	B			49	2	0.29 L/kg	1	3–300	Approx. 2	+	72.5	

Preg. Risk: FDA risk categories: **A** = no risk, **B** = No risk - human studies, **C** = toxicity in animals - inadequate human studies, **D** = human risk, but benefit may outweigh risk, **X** = fetal abnormalities - risk > benefit; **Food Effect (PO dosing):** + **food** = take with food, **no food** = take without food; ± **food** = take with or without food; **Oral % AB** = % absorbed; **Peak Serum Level: SD** = after single dose, **SS** = steady state after multiple doses; **Volume of Distribution (Vd): V/F** = Vd/oral bioavailability, **Vss** = Vd at steady state/oral bioavailability; **CSF Penetration:** therapeutic efficacy comment based on dose, usual susceptibility of target organism & penetration into CSF; **24hr** = AUC 0-24; **Tmax** = time to max plasma concentration.

TABLE 9A (3) (Footnotes at the end of table)

DRUG	REFERENCE DOSE/ROUTE	PREG RISK	FOOD EFFECT (PO)	ORAL %AB	PEAK SERUM LEVEL (μg/mL)	PROTEIN BINDING (%)	VOL OF DISTRIB (Vd)	AVER SERUM T½, hrs[2]	BILE PEN (%)[3]	CSF/ BLOOD (%)	CSF PEN[4]	AUC (μg*hr/mL)	Tmax (hr)
MONOBACTAM													
Aztreonam	1 gm IV	B			90 (SD)	56	12.6 L Vss	2	115–405	3–52	±	271	
AMINOGLYCOSIDES													
Amikacin, gentamicin, kanamycin, tobramycin—see Table 10D, page 109, for dose & serum levels		D				0–10	0.26 L/kg	2.5	10–60	0–30	No; intrathecal dose: 5–10 mg		
Neomycin	po	D	Tab/soln ± food	<3	0								
FLUOROQUINOLONES[1]													
Ciprofloxacin	750 mg po q12h	C	± food	70	3.6 (SS)	20–40	2.4 L/kg	4	2800–4500		1 μg/mL Inadequate for Strep. sp. (CID 31:1131, 2000)	31.6 (24 hr) 25.4 (24 hr)	.1-2
	400 mg IV q12h	C			4.6 (SS)	20–40		4	2800–4500	26		8 (24 hr) 16 (24 hr)	
	500 mg ER po q24h	C	± food		1.6 (SS)	20–40		6.6					1.5
	1000 mg ER po q24h	C	± food		3.1 (SS)	20–40		6.3					2.0
Gemifloxacin	320 mg po q24h	C	Tab ± food	71	1.6 (SS)	55–73	2–12 L Vss/F	7		30–50		9.9 (24 hr)	0.5–2.0
Levofloxacin	500 mg po/IV q24h	C	Tab ± food	99	5.7/6.4 (SS)	24–38	74–112 L Vss	7				PO:47.5, IV 54.6 (24 hr)	PO: 1.3
	750 mg po/IV q24h	C	Tab ± food Oral soln: no food	99	8.6/12.1 (SS)	24–38	244 L Vss	7				PO 90.7, IV 108 (24 hr)	PO: 1.6
Moxifloxacin	400 mg po/IV q24h	C	Tab ± food	89	4.2–4.6/4.5 (SS)	30–50	2.2 L/kg	10–14		>50	Yes (CID 49:1080, 2009)	PO 48, IV 38 (24 hr)	PO: 1–3
Ofloxacin	400 mg po/IV q12h	C	Tab ± food	98	4.6/6.2 (SS)	32	1–2.5 L/kg	7				PO 82.4, IV 87 (24 hr)	PO: 1–2
MACROLIDES, AZALIDES, LINCOSAMIDES, KETOLIDES													
Azithromycin	500 mg po	B	Tab/Susp ± food	37	0.4 (SD)	7–51	31.1 L/kg F	68	High			4.3	2.5
	500 mg IV	B			3.6 (SD)	7–51		12/6				9.6 (24 hr, pre SS)	
Azithromycin-ER	2 gm po	B	Susp no food	≈ 30	0.8 (SD)	7–50		59	High				5.0
Clarithromycin	500 mg po q12h	C	Tab/Susp ± food	50	3–4 (SS)	65–70	4 L/kg	5–7	7000			20 (24 hr)	2.0–2.5
	1000 mg ER po q12h	C	Tab + food		2–3 (SS)	65–70							5–8

Preg. Risk: FDA risk categories: A = no risk, **B** = no risk in humans, **C** = toxicity in animals - inadequate human studies, **D** = human risk, but benefit may outweigh risk, **X** = fetal abnormalities - risk > benefit; **Food Effect (PO dosing): + food** = take with food, **no food** = take without food, **± food** = take with or without food; **Oral % AB** = % absorbed; **Peak Serum Level: SD** = after single dose; **SS** = steady state after multiple doses; **Volume of Distribution (Vd)**: **V/F** = Vd/oral bioavailability, **Vss** = Vd at steady state/oral bioavailability; **CSF Penetration**: therapeutic efficacy comment based on dose, usual susceptibility of target organism & penetration into CSF; **24hr** = AUC 0-24; **Tmax** = time to max plasma concentration.

TABLE 9A (4) (Footnotes at the end of table)

DRUG	REFERENCE DOSE/ROUTE	PREG RISK	FOOD EFFECT (PO)†	ORAL %AB	PEAK SERUM LEVEL (μg/mL)	PROTEIN BINDING (%)	VOL OF DISTRIB (Vd)	AVER SERUM T½, hrs‡	BILE PEN (%)³	CSF/ BLOOD (%)	CSF PEN⁴	AUC (μg*hr/mL)	Tmax (hr)
MACROLIDES, AZALIDES, LINCOSAMIDES, KETOLIDES													
Erythromycin Oral (various)	500 mg po	B	Tab/Susp no food DR Caps ± food	18–45	0.1–2 (SD)	70–74	0.6 L/kg	2–4		2–13	No		Delayed Rel: 3
Lacto/glucep	500 mg IV	B			3–4 (SD)	60–70		2–4					
Telithromycin	800 mg po q24h	C	Tab ± food	57	2.3 (SS)	60–70	2.9 L/kg	10	7			12.5 (24 hr)	1
Clindamycin	150 mg po	B	Cap ± food	90	2.5 (SD)	85-94	1.1 L/kg	2.4	250–300		No		0.75
	900 mg IV	B		90	14.1 (SS)	85-94		2.4	250–300		No		
MISCELLANEOUS ANTIBACTERIALS													
Chloramphenicol	1 gm po q6h	C	Cap ± food	High	18 (SS)	25–50	0.8 L/kg	4.1		45–89	Yes		
Colistin (Polymyxin E)	150 mg IV	C			5–7.5 (SD)		0.34 L/kg	2–3			No (AUC 53-4907, 2009)		
Daptomycin	4–6 mg/kg IV q24h	B			58–99 (SS)	92	0.1 L/kg Vss	8–9	0	0-8		494-632 (24 hr)	
Doxycycline	100 mg po	B	Tab/cap/susp ± food		1.5–2.1 (SD)	93	53–134 L Vss	18	200–3200		No (26%)	31.7	2
Fosfomycin	3 gm po	B	Sachet ± food		26 (SD)	<10	136.1 L Vss/F	5.7				150	
Fusidic acid^NUS	500 mg po	C	Tab + food	91	30 (SD)	95-99	0.3 L/kg	5–15	100–200			315	2-4
Linezolid	600 mg po/IV q12h	C	Tab/susp ± food	100	15–20 (SS)	31	40-50 L Vss	5		60-70	Yes (AUC 50:397:1, 2006)	PO: 276(V): 179 (24 hr)	PO: 1.3
Metronidazole	500 mg po/IV q6h	B	ER tab no food, Tab/cap ± food		20–25 (SS)	20	0.6-0.85 L/kg	6–14	100	45–89		560 (24 hr)	Imm Rel: 1.6 ER: 6.8
Minocycline	200 mg po	D	Cap/tab ± food		2.0–3.5 (SD)	76	80-114 L Vss	16	200–3200		No	48.3	2.1
Polymyxin B	2 mg/kg IV	C			1–8 (SD)	78-92	0.07–0.2 L/kg	4.3–6				Dai: 31.8 (24 hr)	
Quinu-Dalfo	7.5 mg/kg IV q8h	B			3.2/8 (SS)		0.45/0.24 L/kg Vss	1.5				58	
Rifampin	600 mg po	C	Cap no food		4-32 (SD)	80	0.65 L/kg Vss	2–5	10,000				1.5-2
Rifaximin	200 mg po	C	Tab ± food	<0.4	0.004–0.01 (SD)								
Tetracycline	250 mg po	D	Cap no food		1.5–2 (SD)		1.3 L/kg	6–12	200–3200		No (7%)	30	2-4
Telavancin	10 mg/kg/q24h	C			108 (SS)	90	0.13 L/kg	8.1	Low			780 (24 hr)	

Preg Risk: FDA risk categories: A = no risk, **B** = No risk - human studies, **C** = toxicity in animals - inadequate human studies, **D** = human risk, but benefit may outweigh risk - **X** = fetal abnormalities - risk > benefit. **Food Effect (PO dosing): ± food** = take with food, **no food** = take without food, **± food** = take with or without food. **Oral % AB** = % absorbed; **Peak Serum Level: SD** = after single dose, **SS** = steady state after multiple doses; **Volume of Distribution (Vd): V/F** = Vd/oral bioavailability, **Vss** = Vd at steady state/oral bioavailability. **CSF Penetration:** therapeutic efficacy comment based on dose, usual susceptibility of target organism & penetration into CSF; **AUC** = area under drug concentration curve; **24hr** = AUC 0-24; **Tmax** = time to max plasma concentration.

TABLE 9A (5) (Footnotes at the end of table)

DRUG	REFERENCE DOSE/ROUTE	PREG RISK	FOOD EFFECT (PO)[1]	ORAL %AB	PEAK SERUM LEVEL (μg/mL)	PROTEIN BINDING (%)	VOL OF DISTRIB (Vd)	AVER SERUM T½, hrs[2]	BILE PEN (%)[3]	CSF/ BLOOD (%)	CSF PEN[4]	AUC (μg*hr/mL)	Tmax (hr)
MISCELLANEOUS ANTIBACTERIALS (continued)													
Tigecycline	50 mg IV q12h	D			0.63 (SS)	71-89	7-9 L/kg	42	138		No	4.7 (24 hr)	
Trimethoprim (TMP)	100 mg po	C		80	1 (SD)		100-120 V/f	8-15					1-4
TMP-SMX-DS	160/800 mg po q12h	C	Tab/susp ± food	85	1-2/40-60 (SS) 9/105 (SS)		TM: 100-120 L SM: 12-18 L		100-200 40-70	50/40			TMP PO: 1-4 SMX IV: 1-4
Vancomycin	1 gm IV q12h	C			20-50 (SS)	<10-55	0.7 L/kg	4-6	50	7-14			
ANTIFUNGALS													
Amphotericin B: Standard	0.4-0.7 mg/kg IV	B			0.5-3.5 (SS)		4 L/kg	24		0-		17	
Lipid (ABLC)	5 mg/kg IV	B			1-2.5 (SS)		131 L/kg	173				1.4 (24 hr)	
Cholesteryl complex	4 mg/kg IV	B			2.9 (SS)		4.3 L/kg	39				36 (24 hr)	
Liposomal	5 mg/kg IV				83 (SS)		0.1-0.4 L/kg Vss	6.8 ± 2.1				555 (24 hr)	
Fluconazole	400 mg po/IV	D	Tab/susp ± food	90	6.7 (SD)	10	50 V/F	20-50		50-94	Yes.		PO: 1-2
	800 mg po/IV	D	Tab/susp ± food	90	Approx. 14 (SD)			20-50					
Itraconazole	200 mg po soln	C	Soln no food	Low	0.3-0.7 (SD)	99.8	796 L	35		0		29.3 (24 hr)	2.5 Hydroxy: 5.3
Ketoconazole	200 mg po	C	Tab ± food	75	1-4 (SD)	99	1.2 L/kg	6-9	ND	<10	No	12	1-2
Posaconazole	200 mg po	C	Susp + food		0.2-1.0 (SD)	98-99	1774 L	20-66			Yes (JAC 56:745, 2005)	15.1	3-5
Voriconazole	200 mg po q12h	D	Tab/susp no food	96	3 (SS)	58	4.6 L/kg Vss	6		22-100	Yes (CID 37:728, 2003)	39.8 (24 hr)	1-2
Anidulafungin	200 mg IV x 1, then 100 mg IV q24h	C			7.2 (SS)	>99	30-50 L	26.5			No	112 (24 hr)	
Caspofungin	70 mg IV x 1, then 50 mg IV qd	C			9.9 (SD)	97	9.7 L Vss	9-11			No	87.3 (24 hr)	
Flucytosine	2.5 gm po	C	Cap ± food	78-90	30-40 (SD)	4	0.6 L/kg	3-6		60-100	Yes		2
Micafungin	150 mg IV q24h	C			16.4 (SS)	>99	0.39 L/kg	15-17			No	167 (24 hr)	
ANTIMYCOBACTERIALS													
Bedaquiline	400 mg qd	ND	Tab + food	ND	3.3 (Wk 2)	>99	~60x total body water Vss	24-30	ND	ND	ND	22 (24hr)	5
Capreomycin	15 mg/kg IM	C			25-35 (SD)	ND	0.4 L/kg	2-5	ND	<10	No	ND	1-2
Cycloserine	250 mg po	C	Cap, no food	70-90	4-8 (SD)	<20	0.47 L/kg	10	ND	54-79	Yes	110	1-2
Ethambutol	25 mg/kg	Safe	Tab ± food	80	2-6 (SD)	10-30	6 L/kg Vss/F	4	ND	10-50	No	29.6	2-4

Preg Risk: FDA risk categories: **A** = no risk, **B** = No risk - human studies, **C** = toxicity in animals - inadequate human studies, **D** = human risk, benefit may outweigh risk, **X** = fetal abnormalities - risk > benefit; **Food Effect (PO dosing):** **+ food** = take with food, **no food** = take without food; **Oral % AB** = % absorbed; **Peak Serum Level: SD** = after single dose, **SS** = steady state after multiple doses; **Volume of Distribution (Vd): V/F** = Vd/oral bioavailability, **Vss** = Vd at steady state; **Vss/F** = Vd at steady state/oral bioavailability; **CSF Penetration:** therapeutic efficacy comment based on dose, usual susceptibility or target organism & penetration into CSF; **AUC** = area under drug concentration curve; **24hr** = AUC 0-24; **Tmax** = time to max plasma concentration.

TABLE 9A (6) *(Footnotes at the end of table)*

DRUG	REFERENCE DOSE/ROUTE	PREG RISK	FOOD EFFECT (PO)	ORAL %AB	PEAK SERUM LEVEL (μg/mL)	PROTEIN BINDING (%)	VOL OF DISTRIB (Vd)	AVER SERUM T½, hrs[2]	BILE PEN (%)[3]	CSF/BLOOD (%)	CSF PEN[5]	AUC (μg*hr/mL)	Tmax (hr)
ANTIMYCOBACTERIALS *(continued)*													
Ethionamide	500 mg po	C	Tab ± food	90	2.2 (SD)	10-30	80 L	1.9	ND	≈100	Yes	10.3	1.5
Isoniazid	300 mg po	C	Tab/syrup no food	100	3-5 (SD)		0.6-1.2 L/kg	0.7-4	ND	Up to 90	Yes	20.1	1-2
Para-aminosalicylic acid (PAS)	4 gm po	C	Gran + food	ND	20 (SD)	50-73	0.9-1.4 L/kg (V/F)	0.75-1.0	ND	10-50	Marg	108	8
Pyrazinamide	20-25 mg/kg po	C	Tab ± food	95	30-50 (SD)	5-10		10-16		100	Yes	500	2
Rifabutin	300 mg po	B	Cap + food	20	0.2-0.6 (SD)	85	9.3 L/kg (Vss)	32-67	300-500	30-70	ND	8.6	2.5-4.0
Rifampin	600 mg po	C	Cap no food	70-90	4-32 (SD)	80	0.65 L/kg Vss	2-5	10,000	7-56	Yes	58	1.5-2
Rifapentine	600 mg po q72h	C	Tab + food	ND	15 (SS)	98	70 L	13-14	ND	ND	ND	320 over 72hrs	4.8
Streptomycin	1 gm IV	D			25-50 (SD)	0-10	0.26 L/kg	2.5	10-60	0-30	No; Intrathecal: 5-10 mg		
ANTIPARASITICS													
Albendazole	400 mg po	C	Tab + food		0.5-1.6	70		Art: 1.6, D-Art: 1.6, Lum: 101					Sulfoxide: 2-5
Artemether/ Lumefantrine	4 tabs po: 80/480 mg	C	Tab + food		Art: 9 (SS), D-Art: 1, Lum: 5.6-9 (not SS)								Art: 1.5-2.0 Lum: 6-8
Atovaquone	750 mg po bid	C	Susp + food	47	24 (SS)	99.9	0.6 L/kg Vss	67		<1	No	801 (750 mg x1)	
Dapsone	100 mg po q24h	C	Tab ± food	100	1.1 (SS)		1.5 L/kg	10-50					
Ivermectin	12 mg po	C	Tab no food		0.05-0.08 (SD)	98	9.9 L/kg						4
Mefloquine	1.25 gm po	C	Tab + food		0.5-1.2 (SD)	98	20 L/kg	13-24 days					17
Miltefosine	50 mg po tid	X	Cap + food			95		7-31 (long) AAC 52:2855, 2008					
Nitazoxanide	500 mg po tab	B	Tab/susp + food		9-10 (SD)	99						41.9 Tizoxanide	Tizoxanide: 1-4
Proguanil[a]	100 mg	C	Tab + food	"High"	No data	75	1600-2000 L/F						
Pyrimethamine	25 mg po	C	Tab ± food		0.1-0.3 (SD)	87	3 L/kg	96					2-6
Praziquantel	20 mg per kg po	B	Tab + food	80	0.2-2.0 (SD)		8000 L V/F	0.8-1.5				1.51	1-3
Tinidazole	2 gm po	B	Tab + food	48	48 (SD)	12	50 L	13				902	1.6

Preg Risk: FDA risk categories: A = no risk, **B** = No risk - human studies, **C** = toxicity in animals - inadequate human studies, **D** = human risk, but benefit may outweigh risk, **X** = fetal abnormalities – risk > benefit; **Food Effect (PO dosing): + food** = take with food, **no food** = take with or without food, **± food** = take with or without food, **% absorbed; Oral % AB** = % absorbed; **Peak Serum Level; SD** = after single dose; **SS** = steady state after multiple doses; **Volume of Distribution (Vd); V/F** = Vd/oral bioavailability, **Vss** = Vd at steady state; **Vss/F** = Vd at steady state/oral bioavailability, **CSF Penetration:** therapeutic efficacy comment based on dose, usual susceptibility or target organism & penetration into CSF.; **24hr** = AUC 0-24; **Tmax** = time to max plasma concentration.

TABLE 9A (7) (Footnotes at the end of table)

DRUG	REFERENCE DOSE/ROUTE	PREG RISK	FOOD EFFECT (PO)[1]	ORAL %AB	PEAK SERUM LEVEL (μg/mL)	PROTEIN BINDING (%)	VOL OF DISTRIB (Vd)	AVER SERUM T½, hrs[2]	BILE PEN (%)[3]	CSF/ BLOOD (%)	CSF PEN[6]	AUC (μg*hr/mL)	Tmax (hr)
ANTIVIRAL DRUGS—NOT HIV													
Acyclovir	400 mg po bid	B	Tab/cap/susp ± food	10–20	1.21 (SS)	9–33	0.7 L/kg	2.5–3.5				7.4 (24 hr)	
Adefovir	10 mg po	C	Tab ± food	59	0.02 (SD)	≤4	0.37 L/kg Vss	7.5				0.22	1.75
Boceprevir	800 mg po q8h	B	Cap + food		1.7 (SS)	75	772L (Vss/F)	3.4	ND	ND	ND	5.41 (8 hr)	
Cidofovir w/Probenecid	5 mg/kg IV	C			19.6 (SD)	<6	0.41 L/kg (VSS)	2.2	ND	0	No	40.8	1.1
Entecavir	0.5 mg po q24h	C	Tab/soln no food	100	4.2 ng/mL (SS)	13	>0.6 L/kg V/F	128–149				0.14	0.5–1.5
Famciclovir	500 mg po	B	Tab ± food	77	3–4 (SD)	<20	1.1 L/kg*	2–3				8.9 Penciclovir	Penciclovir: 0.9
Foscarnet	60 mg/kg IV	C			155 (SD)	4	0.46 L/kg	3				2195 μM*hr	
Ganciclovir	5 mg/kg IV	C			8.3 (SD)	1–2	0.7 L/kg Vss	<1	No			24.5	
Oseltamivir	75 mg po bid	C	Cap/susp ± food	75	0.065/0.35§ (SS)	3	23–26 L/kg Vss*	1–3				5.4 (24 hr) Carboxylate	
Peramivir	600 mg IV	C			35–45 (SD)	<30	ND	7.7–20.8	ND	ND	ND	90–95	ND
Ribavirin	600 mg po	X	Tab/cap/soln + food	64	0.8 (SD)	44	2825 L V/F	44				25.4	2
Rimantadine	100 mg po	C	Tab ± food		0.05–0.1 (SD)		17–19 L/kg	25				3.5	6
Telaprevir	750 mg po q8h	B	Tab+ food (high fat)		3.51 (SS)	59–76	252L (V/F)	4.0–4.7 (SD)	ND	ND	ND	22.3 (8 hr)	
Telbivudine	600 mg po q24h	B	Tab/soln ± food		3.7 (SS)	3.3	>0.6 L/kg V/F	40–49				26.1 (24 hr)	2
Valacyclovir	1000 mg po	B	Tab ± food	55	5.6 (SD)	13–18	0.7 L/kg	3				19.5 Acyclovir	
Valganciclovir	900 mg po q24h	C	Tab/soln + food	59	5.6 (SS)	1–2	0.7 L/kg	4				29.1 Ganciclovir	Ganciclovir: 1–3

Preg Risk: FDA risk categories: **A** = no risk, **B** = No risk - human studies, **C** = toxicity in animals - inadequate human studies, **D** = human risk, but benefit may outweigh risk, **X** = fetal abnormalities - risk > benefit; **Food Effect (PO dosing):** ± **food** = take with food, **no food** = take without food, ± **food** = take with or without food; **Oral % AB** = % absorbed; **Peak Serum Level; SD** = after single dose, **SS** = steady state after multiple doses; **Volume of Distribution (Vd)**: **V/F** = Vd/oral bioavailability; **Vss** = Vd at steady state; **Vss/F** = Vd at steady state/oral bioavailability; **CSF Penetration:** therapeutic efficacy comment based on dose, usual susceptibility of target organism & penetration into CSF; **AUC** = area under drug concentration curve; **24hr** = AUC 0–24; **Tmax** = time to max plasma concentration.

89

TABLE 9A (8) (Footnotes at the end of table)

DRUG	REFERENCE DOSE/ROUTE	PREG RISK	FOOD EFFECT (PO Prep)	ORAL %AB	PEAK SERUM LEVEL (μg/mL)	PROT BIND (%)	VOL DISTRIB (Vd)	AVER SERUM T½, hrs²	INTRA CELL T½, HOURS	CSF/ BLOOD (%)	CSF PEN⁶	AUC (μg•hr/mL)	Tmax (hr)
ANTI-HIV VIRAL DRUGS													
Abacavir (ABC)	600 mg po q24h	C	Tab/soln ± food	83	4.3 (SS)	50	0.86 L/kg	1.5	12-26	Low	No	12 (24 hr)	
Atazanavir (ATV)	400 mg po q24h	B	Cap + food	Good	2.3 (SS)	86	88.3 L V/F	7		Intermed	?	22.3 (24 hr)	2.5
Darunavir (DRV)	600 mg + 100 mg RTV bid		Tab ± food	82	3.5 (SS)	95	2 L/kg	15		Intermed	?	116.8 (24 hr)	2.5-4.0
Delavirdine (DLV)	400 mg po bid	C	Tab ± food	85	19 ± 11 (SS)	98		5.8				180 μM*hr	1
Didanosine (ddI)	400 mg EC® po	B	Cap no food	30-40	?	<5	308-363 L	1.4	25-40	Intermed	?	2.6	2
Efavirenz (EFV)	600 mg po q24h	D	Cap/tab no food	42	4.1 (SS)	99	252 L V/F	52-76				184 μM*hr (24 hr)	3-5
Elvitegravir (with cobicistat, TDF and FTC, as Stribild)	150 mg	B	Tab + Food		1.7	98-99		12.9				23	4
Emtricitabine (FTC)	200 mg po q24h	B	Cap/soln ± food	93	1.8 (SS)	<4		10	39	Intermed	?	10 (24 hr)	1-2
Enfuvirtide (ENF)	90 mg sc bid	B		84	5 (SS)	92	5.5 L	4				97.4 (24 hr)	
Etravirine (ETR)	200 mg po bid	B	Tab + food		0.3 (SS)	99.9		41	No data	Intermed	?	9 (24 hr)	2.5-4.0
Fosamprenavir (FPV)	(700 mg po + 100 mg RTV) bid	C	Boosted ped susp + food Adult susp no food	No data	6 (SS)	90		7.7				79.2 (24 hr)	2.5
Indinavir (IDV)	800 mg po bid	C	Boosted cap + food, Cap alone no food	65	9 (SS)	60		1.2-2		High	Yes	92.1 μM*hr (24 hr)	0.8
Lamivudine (3TC)	300 mg po	C	Tab/soln ± food	86	2.6 (SS)	<36	1.3 L/kg	5-7	18-22	Intermed	?	11	
Lopinavir/RTV (LPV/r)	400 mg po bid	C	Soln + food	No data	9.6 (SS)	98-99		5-6 (LPV)		Intermed	?	186 LPV	LPV: 4
Maraviroc (MVC)	300 mg po bid	B	Tab ± food	33	0.3-0.9 (SS)	76	194 L	14-18		Intermed	?	3 (24 hr)	0.5-4.0
Nelfinavir (NFV)	1250 mg po bid	B	Tab/powd + food	20-80	3-4 (SS)	98	2-7 L/kg V/F	3.5-5		Low	No	53 (24 hr)	
Nevirapine (NVP)	200 mg po	B	Tab ± food	>90	2 (SD)	60	1.2 L/kg Vss	25-30		High	Yes	110 (24 hr)	
Raltegravir (RAL)	400 mg po bid	C	Tab ± food	?	5.4 (SD)	83	287 L Vss/F	9		Intermed	?	28.6 μM*hr (24 hr)	3
Rilpivirine	25 mg po	B	Tab + food	?	0.1-0.2 (SD)	99.7	152L	45-50		-	-	2.4 (24 hr)	-
Ritonavir (RTV)	600 mg po bid	B	Cap/soln + food	65	11.2 (SS)	98-99	0.41 L/kg V/F	3-5		Low	No		Soln: 2-4
Saquinavir (SQV)	(1000 + 100 RTV) po	B	Tab/cap + food	4	0.37 nM (SS conc)	97	700 L Vss	1-2		Low	No	29.2	

Preg Risk: FDA risk categories: A = no risk, **B** = No risk - human studies, **C** = toxicity in animals - inadequate human studies, **D** = human risk, but benefit may outweigh risk, **X** = fetal abnormalities – risk > benefit. **Food Effect (PO dosing): + food** = take with food, **no food** = take without food, **± food** = take with or without food. **Oral % AB** = % absorbed; **Peak Serum Level: SD** = after single dose, **SS** = steady state after multiple doses; **Volume of Distribution (Vd): V/F** = Vd/oral bioavailability, **Vss** = Vd at steady state/oral bioavailability. **CSF Penetration:** therapeutic efficacy comment based on dose, usual susceptibility of target organism & penetration into CSF; **24hr** = AUC 0-24; **Tmax** = time to max plasma concentration.

TABLE 9 (9) (Footnotes at the end of table)

DRUG	REFERENCE DOSE/ROUTE	PREG RISK	FOOD EFFECT (PO Prep)	ORAL %AB	PEAK SERUM LEVEL (µg/mL)	PROT BIND (%)	VOL DISTRIB (Vd)	AVER SERUM T½, hrs[2]	INTRA CELL T½, HOURS	CSF/BLOOD (%)	CSF PEN[6]	AUC (µg*hr/mL)	Tmax (hr)
ANTI-HIV VIRAL DRUGS (continued)													
Stavudine (d4T)	40 mg bid	C	Cap/soln ± food	86	0.54 (SS)	<5	46L	1	7.5			2.6 (24 hr)	1
Tenofovir (TDF)	300 mg po	B	Tab ± food	25	0.3 (SD)	<1-7	1.3 L/kg Vss	17	>60	Low	No	2.3	1
Tipranavir (TPV)	(500 + 200 RTV) mg po bid	C	Cap/soln + food	60	47–57 (SS)	99.9	7.7–10 L	5.5–6		Low	No	1600 µM*hr (24 hr)	3
Zidovudine (ZDV)	300 mg po	C	Tab/cap/syrup ± food		1–2	<38	1.6 L/kg	0.5–3	11	High	Yes	2.1	0.5–1.5

1. Food decreases rate and/or extent of absorption. For adult oral preps; not applicable for peds suspensions.
2. Assumes CrCl >80 mL per min.
3. Peak concentration in bile/peak concentration in serum x 100. If blank, no data.
4. CSF levels with inflammation
5. Judgment based on drug dose & organism susceptibility. CSF concentration ideally ≥10 above MIC.
6. Concern over seizure potential; see Table 10B.
7. Take all po FQs 2–4 hours before sucralfate or any multivalent cations: Ca^{++}, Fe^{++}, Zn^{++}
8. Given with atovaquone as Malarone for malaria prophylaxis.
9. Oseltamivir/oseltamivir carboxylate.
10. EC = enteric coated.

Preg. Risk: FDA risk categories: A = no risk, **B** = No risk, **C** = toxicity in animals - inadequate human studies, **D** = human risk, but benefit may outweigh risk, **X** = fetal abnormalities - risk > benefit. **Food Effect (PO dosing): ±** = take with food, **no food** = take without food; **+ food** = take with or without food; **Oral % AB** = % absorbed; **Peak Serum Level: SD** = after single dose. **SS** = steady state after multiple doses; **Volume of Distribution (Vd): V/F** = Vd/oral bioavailability. **Vss** = Vd at steady state. **Vss/F** = Vd at steady state/oral bioavailability. **CSF Penetration:** therapeutic efficacy comment based on dose, usual susceptibility of target organism & penetration into CSF; **AUC** = area under drug concentration curve; **24hr** = AUC 0-24; **Tmax** = time to max plasma concentration.

TABLE 9B - PHARMACODYNAMICS OF ANTIBACTERIALS*

BACTERIAL KILLING/PERSISTENT EFFECT	DRUGS	THERAPY GOAL	PK/PD MEASUREMENT
Concentration-dependent/Prolonged persistent effect	Aminoglycosides; daptomycin; ketolides; quinolones, metro	High peak serum concentration	24-hr AUC/MIC
Time-dependent/No persistent effect	Penicillins; cephalosporins, carbapenems; monobactams	Long duration of exposure	Time above MIC
Time-dependent/Moderate to long persistent effect	Clindamycin; erythro/azithro/clarithro; ketolides; tetracyclines; vancomycin	Enhanced amount of drug	24-hr AUC/MIC

*Adapted from Craig, WA: IDC No. Amer 17:479, 2003 & Drusano, GL: CID 44:79, 2007

TABLE 9C - CYTOCHROME P450 INTERACTIONS OF ANTIMICROBIALS

Cytochrome P450 isoenzyme terminology:
e.g., 3A4. **3** = family, **A** = subfamily, **4** = gene; **PGP** = an intestinal drug transporter; **P** = glycoprotein; **UGT** = uridine diphosphate glucuronosyltransferase

DRUG	Cytochrome P450 Interactions			
	Substrate	Inhibits	Induces	
Antibacterials				
Azithromycin (all)	PGP	PGP (weak)		
Chloramphenicol		2C19, 3A4		
Ciprofloxacin (all)		1A2, 3A4 (minor)		
Clarithromycin (all)		3A4, PGP		
Erythromycin (all)	3A4, PGP	3A4, PGP		
Metronidazole		2C9		
Nafcillin			2C9 (?), 3A4	
Quinu-Dalfo		Quinu: 3A4		
Rifampin	PGP		1A2, 2C9, 2C19, 2D6 (Weak), 3A4, PGP	
Telithromycin		3A4, PGP		
TMP-SMX	SMX: 2C9 (major), 3A4	SMX: 2C9, TMP: 2C8		
Trimethoprim		2C8		
Antifungals				
Fluconazole (400 mg)	3A4 (minor), PGP	2C9, 2C19, 3A4, UGT		
Itraconazole	3A4, PGP	3A4, PGP		
Ketoconazole	3A4	3A4, PGP		
Posaconazole	PGP, UGT	3A4, PGP		
Terbinafine	2D6			
Voriconazole	2C9, 2C19, 3A4	2C9, 2C19 (major), 3A4		
Antimycobacterials (Also Rifampin, above)				
Bedaquiline	CYP3A4			
Ethionamide	3A4 (?)			
Isoniazid	2E1	3A4		
Rifabutin	3A4			
Rifapentine				
Dapsone	3A4		3A4, UGT	

TABLE 9C - CYTOCHROME P450 INTERACTIONS OF ANTIMICROBIALS

DRUG	Cytochrome P450 Interactions		
	Substrate	Inhibits	Induces
Antiparasitics			
Mefloquine	3A4, PGP	PGP	
Praziquantel	3A4		
Proguanil	2C19 (conversion to cycloguanil)		
Tindazole	3A4		
Antiretrovirals			
Atazanavir	3A4	1A2, 2C9, 3A4	
Cobicistat	CYP3A4, CYP2D6	CYP3A4, CYP2D6, PGP, BCRP OATP1B1, OATP1B3	
Darunavir	3A4	3A4	
Delavirdine	2D6, 3A4		
Efavirenz	2B6, 3A4	2C9, 2C19, 3A4	2C19, 3A4
Elvitegravir	CYP3A4		CYP2C9
Etravirine	2C9, 2C19, 3A4	2C19 (weak)	3A4
Fosamprenavir	3A4	2C19, 3A4	
Indinavir	3A4, PGP	3A4, PGP	
Lopinavir	3A4, PGP	3A4	
Maraviroc	3A4	2D6	
Nelfinavir	2C9, 2C19, 3A4, PGP	3A4, PGP	3A4
Nevirapine	2B6, 3A4		3A4
Raltegravir	UGT		
Ritonavir	2D6, 3A4, PGP	2B6, 2C9, 2C19, 2D6, 3A4, PGP	3A4, 1A2 (?), 2C9 (?), PGP (?)
Saquinavir	3A4, PGP	3A4, PGP	
Tipranavir	3A4, PGP	1A2, 2C9, 2C19, 2D6	3A4, PGP (weak)

Refs: Hansten PD, Horn JR. The top 100 drug interactions: a guide to patient management 2012; E. Freeland (WA): H&H Publications; 2010; and package inserts.

TABLE 10A – ANTIBIOTIC DOSAGE* AND SIDE-EFFECTS

CLASS, AGENT, GENERIC NAME (TRADE NAME)	USUAL ADULT DOSAGE*	ADVERSE REACTIONS, COMMENTS (See Table 10B for Summary)
NATURAL PENICILLINS		Allergic reactions a major issue. 10% of all hospital admissions give history of pen allergy, but only 10% have allergic reaction if given penicillin. Why? Possible reasons: inaccurate history, waning immunity with age, aberrant response during viral illness. If given **Bicillin C-R IM (procaine Pen + benzathine Pen)** could be reaction to procaine. **Most serious reactions: immediate IgE-mediated anaphylaxis**; incidence only 0.05% but 5-10% fatal. Other IgE-mediated reactions: urticaria, angioedema, laryngeal edema, bronchospasm, abdominal pain with emesis, or hypotension. All appear within 4 hrs. Can form IgE antibody against either the beta-lactam ring or the R-group side chain. Non IgE-mediated and not serious. **Serious late allergic reactions:** Coombs-positive hemolytic anemia, neutropenia, thrombocytopenia, serum sickness, interstitial nephritis, hepatitis, eosinophilia, drug fever. **Cross-allergy to cephalosporins and carbapenems** varies from 0-11%. One factor is similarity, or lack of similarity, of side chains. **For pen desensitization**, see Table 7. For skin testing, suggest referral to allergist. High **CSF** concentrations cause seizures. Reduce dosage with renal impairment, see Table 17. Allergy refs: AJM 121:572, 2008; NEJM 354:601, 2006.
Benzathine penicillin G (Bicillin L-A)	600,000-1.2 million units IM q2-4 wks	
Penicillin G	Low: 600,000-1.2 million units IM per day High: ≥20 million units IV q24h (12 gm) div q4h	
Penicillin V (250 & 500 mg caps)	0.25-0.5 gm po bid, tid, qid before meals & at bedtime. Pen V preferred over Pen G for oral therapy due to greater acid stability	
PENICILLINASE-RESISTANT PENICILLINS		Blood levels ~2 times greater than cloxacillin so preferred for po therapy. Acute hemorrhagic cystitis reported.
Dicloxacillin (Dynapen) (125 & 500 mg caps)	0.125-0.5 gm po q6h before meals	
Flucloxacillin (Floxapen, Lutropin, Staphcil)	0.25-0.5 gm po q6h 1-2 gm IV q4h	Acute abdominal pain heralding bleeding without antibiotic-associated colitis also reported. Cholestatic hepatitis occurs in 1 in 15,000 exposures, more frequently in age >55yrs, females and therapy >2 wks duration. Can appear wks after end of therapy and take wks to resolve (JAC 66:1431, 2011). **Recommendation: use only in severe infection**.
Nafcillin (Unipen, Nafcil)	1-2 gm IV/IM q4h. Due to >90% protein binding, need 12gm/day for bacteremia	Extravasation can result in tissue necrosis. With dosages of 200-300 mg per kg per day hypokalemia may occur. **Reversible neutropenia** (over 10% with ≥21-day rx, occasionally **WBC <1000 per mm³**).
Oxacillin (Prostaphlin)	1-2 gm IV/IM q4h. Due to >90% protein binding, need 12gm/day for bacteremia	**Hepatic dysfunction** with ≥12 gm per day. LFTs usually 1 2-24 days after start of rx, reversible. In children, more rash and liver toxicity with oxacillin as compared to nafcillin (CID 34:50, 2002).
AMINOPENICILLINS		
Amoxicillin (Amoxil, Polymox)	250 mg-1 gm po tid	IV available in UK & Europe. IV amoxicillin rapidly converted to ampicillin. Rash with infectious mono– see *Ampicillin*.
Amoxicillin extended release (Moxatag)	One 775 mg tab po once daily	Increased risk of cross-allergy with oral cephalosporins with identical side-chains: cefadroxil, cefprozil. Allergic reactions, C. difficile associated diarrhea, false positive test for urine glucose with clinitest.
Amoxicillin-clavulanate (Augmentin) AM-CL extra-strength peds suspension (ES-600) AM-CL-ER—extended release adult tabs	*See Comment for adult products* **Peds Extra-Strength susp.: 600/42.9 per 5 mL dose: 90/6.4 mg/kg div bid.** For adult formulations, see Comments IV amox-clav available in Europe	With bid regimen, less clavulanate & less diarrhea. In pts with immediate allergic reaction to AM-CL, ⅓ to Clav component (J Allergy Clin Immunol 125:502, 2010). Positive blood tests for 1,3-beta D-glucan with IV AM-CL (NEJM 354:2834, 2006). Hepatotoxicity linked to clavulanic acid; AM-CL causes 13-23% of drug-induced liver injury. Onset delayed. Usually mild; rare liver failure (JAC 66:1431, 2011). **Comparison adult Augmentin dosage regimens:** Augmentin 500/125 1 tab po tid Augmentin 875/125 1 tab po bid Augmentin 1000/62.5 2 tabs po bid Augmentin-XR 1000/62.5 2 tabs po bid
Ampicillin (Principen) (250 & 500 mg caps)	0.25-0.5 gm po q6h. 50-200 mg/kg IV/day.	A maculopapular rash occurs (not urticarial), **not true penicillin allergy**, in 65-100% pts with infectious mono, 90% with chronic lymphocytic leukemia, and 15-20% in pts taking allopurinol. EBV-associated rash does not indicate permanent allergy; post-EBV no rash when challenged. Increased risk of true cross-allergenicity with oral cephalosporins with identical side chains: cefaclor, cefadroxil, cephalexin, loracarbef.

* NOTE: all dosage recommendations are for adults (unless otherwise indicated) & assume normal renal function.
(See page 2 for abbreviations)

93

TABLE 10A (2)

CLASS, AGENT, GENERIC NAME (TRADE NAME)	USUAL ADULT DOSAGE*	ADVERSE REACTIONS, COMMENTS (See Table 10B for Summary)
AMINOPENICILLINS (continued)		
Ampicillin-sulbactam (Unasyn)	1.5–3 gm IV q6h; for Acinetobacter: 3 gm (Amp 2 gm/Sulb 1 gm) IV q4h	Supplied in vials: ampicillin 0.5 gm or amp 2 gm, sulbactam 1 gm. AM-SB is not active vs pseudomonas. Total daily dose sulbactam ≤4 gm. Increasing resistance of aerobic gram-negative bacilli. Sulbactam doses up to 9-12 gm/day evaluated (J Infect 54:432, 2006). See also CID 50:133, 2010.
EXTENDED SPECTRUM PENICILLINS. NOTE: Platelet dysfunction may occur with any of the antipseudomonal penicillins, esp. in renal failure patients.		
Piperacillin (Pipracil) (Hard to find, PIP alone; usually use PIP-TZ)	3–4 gm IV q4–6h (max 24 gm/day). For urinary tract infection: 2 gm IV q6h. See Comment	1.85 mEq Na+ per gm. See PIP-TZ comment on extended infusion. For P. aeruginosa infections: 3 gm IV q4h.
ANTIPSEUDOMONAL PENICILLINS		
Piperacillin-tazobactam (PIP-TZ) (Zosyn) Prolonged infusion dosing, see Comment and Table 10E.	**Formulations:** PIP/TZ: 2/0.25 gm (2.25 gm) PIP/TZ: 3/0.375 gm (3.375 gm) PIP/TZ: 4/0.5 gm (4.5 gm) **Standard Dose (no P. aeruginosa):** 3.375 gm IV q6h or 4.5 gm IV q8h **Standard Dose for P. aeruginosa:** 3.375 gm IV q4h or 4.5 gm IV q6h	Based on PK/PD studies, there is emerging evidence in support of **prolonged infusion** of PIP-TZ: Initial "loading" dose of 4.5gm over 30min, then 4 hrs later, start 3.375gm IV over 4hrs q 8h (CrCl>20) or 3.375gm IV over 4hrs q12h (CrCl<20) aerobic gram-negative bacilli. Source: www.eu.medica.be CID 44:357, 2007; AAC 54:460, 2010. • Cystic fibrosis + P. aeruginosa infection: 350-450 mg/kg/day div q4-6h • P. aeruginosa pneumonia. Combine PIP-TZ with CIP or Tobra. Misc: Assoc false-pos galactomannan test for aspergillus, thrombocytopenia 2.79 mEq Na+ per gram of PIP.
Temocillin[NUS]	1-2 gm IV q12h.	Semi-synthetic penicillin highly resistant to wide range of beta-lactamases; used to treat beta-lactamase producing aerobic gram-negative bacilli. Source: www.eu.medica.be Coagulation abnormalities common with large doses; interferes with platelet function, ↑ bleeding times; may be clinically significant in pts with renal failure. (4.5 mEq Na+ per gm)
Ticarcillin disodium (Ticar)	3 gm IV q4–6h.	Supplied in vials: ticarcillin 3 gm, clavulanate 0.1 gm per vial. 4.5–5 mEq Na+ per gm. Diarrhea due to clavulanate.
Ticarcillin-clavulanate (Timentin)	3.1 gm IV q4–6h.	Rare reversible cholestatic hepatitis secondary to clavulanate (AIM 156:1327, 1996). In vitro activity vs. Stenotrophomonas maltophilia.
CARBAPENEMS: Review: AAC 55:4943, 2011. **NOTE:** Cross allergenicity: In studies of pts with history of Pen-allergy but no confirmatory skin testing, 0–11% "had allergic reactions with cephalosporin therapy" (JAC 54:1155, 2004). In better studies, pts with positive skin tests for Pen allergy were given carbapenems: no reaction in 99% (Allergy 63:237, 2008; NEJM 354:2835, 2006; J Allergy Clin Immunol 124:167, 2009). Increasing reports of carbapenemase-producing aerobic gram-negative bacilli (JCM 48:1019, 2010; LnID 11:381, 2011; CID 53:49 & 60, 2011).		
Doripenem (Doribax) Ref: CID 49:291, 2009.	Intra-abdominal & complicated UTI: 500 mg IV q8h (1-hr infusion). For prolonged infusion, see Table 10E, page 110. Do not use for pneumonia	Most common adverse reactions ≥5%). Headache, nausea, diarrhea, rash & phlebitis. Seizure reported in post-marketing surveillance. Can lower serum valproic acid levels. Adjust dose if renal impairment. Somewhat more stable in solution than **IMP** or **MER** (JAC 65:1023, 2010; CID 49:291, 2009). FDA safety announcement (01/05/12): Trial of Dori for the treatment of VAP stopped early due to safety concerns. Compared to IMP, patients treated with Dori were observed to have excess mortality and poorer cure rate. **Dori is not approved to treat any type of pneumonia.** Dori dose for pts with BMI ≥30 may be inadequate in obesity (BMI ≥40)
Ertapenem (Invanz)	1 gm IV/IM q24h.	Lidocaine **Dori** = in vials not >500 mg q8h. Lidocaine diluent for IM use. Incidence of drug rash eosinophilia systemic symptoms) Syndrome. Visual hallucinations reported (NZ Med J 122:78, 2009). No predictable activity vs. P. aeruginosa.
Imipenem + cilastatin (Primaxin) Ref: JAC 58:916, 2006	0.5 gm IV q6h, for P. aeruginosa: 1 gm q6-8h (see Comment)	For infection due to P. aeruginosa, increase dosage to 3 or 4 gm per day div. q6h or q8h. Continuous infusion of carbapenems may be more efficacious & safer (AAC 49:1881, 2005). Seizure comment, see footnote[a], Table 10B, page 105. Cilastatin blocks enzymatic degradation of Imipenem in lumen of renal proximal tubule & also prevents tubular toxicity.

* NOTE: all dosage recommendations are for adults (unless otherwise indicated) & assume normal renal function.

(See page 2 for abbreviations)

TABLE 10A (3)

CLASS, AGENT GENERIC NAME (TRADE NAME)	USUAL ADULT DOSAGE*	ADVERSE REACTIONS, COMMENTS (See Table 10B for Summary)
CARBAPENEMS (continued)		
Meropenem (Merrem)	0.5-1 gm IV q8h. Up to 2 gm IV q8h for meningitis. Prolonged infusion in critically ill: If CrCl 50-2 gm (over 3hr) q8h If CrCl 30-49: 1 gm (over 3hr) q8h If CrCl 10-29: 1 gm (over 3hr) q12h (Inten Care Med 37:632, 2011)	For seizure incidence comment, see Table 10B, page 105. Comments: Does not require a dehydropeptidase inhibitor (cilastatin). Activity vs aerobic gm-neg. slightly ↑ over IMP, activity vs staph & strep slightly ↓; anaerobes: B. ovatus, B. distasonis more resistant to meropenem.
MONOBACTAMS		
Aztreonam (Azactam)	1 gm q8h-2 gm IV q6h.	Can be used in pts with allergy to penicillins/cephalosporins. Animal data and a letter raise concern about cross-reactivity with ceftazidime (Rev Infect Dis 7(Suppl4):S613, 1985; Allergy 53:624, 1998); **side-chains of aztreonam and ceftazidime are identical.**
Aztreonam for inhalation (Cayston)	75 mg inhaled tid/x 28 days. Use bronchodilator before each inhalation.	Improves respiratory symptoms in CF pts colonized with P. aeruginosa. Alternative to inhaled Tobra. AEs: bronchospasm, cough, wheezing. So far, no emergence of other resistant pathogens. Ref: Chest 135:1223, 2009.
CEPHALOSPORINS (1st parenteral, then oral drugs). NOTE: Prospective data demonstrate correlation between use of cephalosporins (esp. 3rd generation) and ↑ risk of C. difficile toxin-induced diarrhea. May also ↑ risk of colonization with vancomycin-resistant enterococci. See Oral Cephalosporins, page 96, **for important note on cross-allergenicity.**		
1st Generation, Parenteral		
Cefazolin (Ancef, Kefzol)	1-1.5 gm IV/IM q8h, occasionally 2 gm IV q8h for serious infections, e.g., MSSA bacteremia (max. 12 gm/day).	Do not give into lateral ventricles—seizures! No activity vs. community-associated MRSA. Rare failures if ceftazolin treatment of MSSA bacteremia due to hyperproduction of type A beta lactamase (AAC 53:3437, 2009).
2nd Generation, Parenteral (Cephamycins): May be safe in vitro vs. ESBL-producing aerobic gram-negative bacilli. **Do not use as there are no clinical data for efficacy.**		
Cefotetan (Cefotan)	1-3 gm IV/IM q12h. (max. dose not > 6 gm q24h).	Increasing resistance of B. fragilis, Prevotella bivia, Prevotella disiens (most common in pelvic infections); do not use for intra-abdominal infections. Methylthiotetrazole (MTT) side chain can inhibit vitamin K activation. Avoid alcohol-disulfiram reaction.
Cefoxitin (Mefoxin)	1 gm q8h-2 gm IV/IM q6-8h.	Increasing resistance of B. fragilis isolates.
Cefuroxime (Kefurox, Ceftin, Zinacef)	0.75-1.5 gm IV/IM q8h.	↑ improved activity against H. influenzae compared with 1st generation cephalosporins. See Cefuroxime axetil oral preparation.
3rd Generation, Parenteral—Use correlates with incidence of C. difficile toxin diarrhea; all are inactivated by ESBLs and amp C cephalosporinase from aerobic gram-negative bacilli.		
Cefoperazone-sulbactam[NUS] (Sulperazon)	Cefoperazone component 1-2 gm IV q12h. If larger doses, do not exceed 4 gm/day of sulbactam.	In SE Asia & elsewhere, used to treat intra-abdominal, biliary, & gyn. infections. Other uses due to broad spectrum of activity. Possible clotting problem due to side-chain.
Cefotaxime (Claforan) Ceftazidime (Fortaz, Tazicef)	1 gm q8-12h to 2 gm IV q4h. Usual dose: 1-2 gm IV/IM q8-12h. **Prolonged infusion dosing:** Initial dose: 15 mg/kg over 30 min, then immediately begin: If CrCl > 50: 6 gm (over 24 hr) daily If CrCl 31-50: 4 gm (over 24 hr) daily If CrCl 10-30: 2 gm (over 24 hr) daily (AAC 49:3550, 2005; Inf Dis Clin NA 23:791, 2009).	Maximum daily dose: 12 gm. Can give as 4 gm IV q8h. Similar to ceftriaxone but requires multiple daily doses. Often used in healthcare-associated infections, where P. aeruginosa is a consideration. Use may result in ↑ incidence of C. difficile-assoc. diarrhea and/or selection of vancomycin-resistant E. faecium. (same side chain) as aztreonam.
Ceftizoxime (Cefizox) Ceftriaxone (Rocephin)	From 1-2 gm IV q8-12h up to 2 gm IV q4h. Ceftriaxone dosage in adults: 1-2 gm once daily. Purulent meningitis: 2 gm q12h. Can give IM in 1% lidocaine.	Maximum daily dose: 12 gm, can give as 4 gm IV q8h. **Pseudocholelithiasis**: 2° to sludge in gallbladder by ultrasound (50%), symptomatic (9%) (NEJM 322:1821, 1990). More likely with ≥2 gm/day with or without total parenteral nutrition and not eating (AJM 115:172, 1991). Clinical significance unclear but has led to pancreatitis (JID 77:356, 1995) and gallstones (Ln 352:1325, 1998; AAC 43:662, 1998). In pilot study: 2 gm once daily by continuous infusion superior to 2 gm bolus once daily (JAC 59:285, 2007). For Ceftriaxone Desensitization, see Table 7, page 80.

*NOTE: all dosage recommendations are for adults (unless otherwise indicated) & assume normal renal function.

(See page 2 for abbreviations)

95

TABLE 10A (4)

CLASS, AGENT, GENERIC NAME (TRADE NAME)	USUAL ADULT DOSAGE*	ADVERSE REACTIONS, COMMENTS (See Table 10B for Summary)
CEPHALOSPORINS (1st parenteral, then oral drugs) (continued)	All are substrates for ESBLs & amp C cephalosporins.	
Other Generation, Parenteral:		
Cefepime (Maxipime)	Usual dose: 1–2 gm IV q8–12h. **Prolonged infusion dosing:** Initial dose: 15 mg/kg over 30 min, then immediately begin: If CrCl >60: 6 gm (over 24 hr) daily. If CrCl 30–60: 4 gm (over 24 hr) daily. If CrCl 11–29: 2 gm (over 24 hr) daily.	**Cefepime penetrates to target faster than other cephalosporins.** Active vs P. aeruginosa and many strains of ceftazidime, cefotaxime, aztreonam (LnID 7:338, 2007). More active vs MSSA than 3rd generation cephalosporins. Neutropenia after 14 days rx (Scand J Infect Dis 42:156, 2010). Prolonged infusion: JAC 57:1017, 2006; Am J Health Syst Pharm 68:319, 2011. Case of red man syndrome reported (AAC 56:6387, 2012).
Cefpirome[NUS] (HR 810)	1–2 gm IV q12h	Similar to cefepime; ↑ activity vs enterobacteriaceae; P. aeruginosa, Gm + organisms. Anaerobes: less active than cefoxitin, more active than cefotax or ceftaz.
Ceftaroline fosamil (Teflaro)	600 mg IV q12h (1-hr infusion)	Avid binding to PBP 2a; active vs MRSA. Inactivated by Amp C & ESBL enzymes. Approved for MRSA skin and skin structure infections, but not for other MRSA infections. Active in vitro: VISA, VRSA. Refs: CID 52:1156, 2011; Med Lett 53:5, 2011.
Ceftobiprole[NUS]	0.5 gm IV q8h for mixed gm- neg & gm-pos infections. 0.5 gm IV q12h for gm-pos infections	Infuse over 2 hrs for q8h dosing, over 1 hr for q12h dosing. Associated with caramel-like taste disturbance. Ref.: Clin Microbiol Infections 13(Suppl 2):17 & 25, 2007. Active vs. MRSA.
Oral Cephalosporins		**Cross-Allergenicity:** Patients with a history of IgE-mediated allergic reactions to penicillin (e.g., bronchospasm anaphylaxis, angioneurotic edema, immediate urticaria) should not receive a cephalosporin. If the history is a "measles-like" rash to penicillin, available data suggest a 5–10% rate of rash in such patients: there is no enhanced risk of anaphylaxis.
1st Generation, Oral		
Cefadroxil (Duricef)	0.5–1 gm po q12h.	In pts with history of Pen reaction and no skin testing, 0.2–8.4% react to a cephalosporin (Aller Asthma Proc 26:135, 2006). If positive Pen G skin test, only 2% given a cephalosporin will react. Can predict with cephalosporin skin testing, but not easily without it (Ann IM 141:16, 2004; AJM 125:572, 2008).
Cephalexin (Keflex) (500 mg caps, 1 gm tabs)	0.25–1 gm po q6h (max 4 gm/day).	IgE antibodies against either ring structure or side chains; 80% pts lose IgE over 10 yrs post-reaction (J Aller Clin Immunol 103:918, 1999). Amox. Cefadroxil. Cefprozil have similar side chains; Amp. Cefaclor. Cephalexin. Cephradine have similar side chains.
2nd Generation, Oral		
Cefaclor (Ceclor, Raniclor) (250 & 500 mg tabs)	0.25–0.5 gm po q8h.	If Pen/Ceph skin testing not available or clinically no time, proceed with cephalosporin if history does not suggest IgE-mediated reaction; prior reaction more than 10 yrs ago or cephalosporin side chain differs from implicated Pen. Any of the cephalosporins can result in C. difficile toxin-mediated diarrhea/enterocolitis.
Cefprozil (Cefzil) (250 & 500 mg tabs)	0.25–0.5 gm po q12h.	The reported frequency of nausea/vomiting and non-C. difficile toxin diarrhea is summarized in Table 10B.
Cefuroxime axetil (Ceftin)	0.125–0.5 gm po q12h.	**Other side effects, usually drug-specific, include, e.g.,:**
3rd Generation, Oral		Cefaclor: Serum sickness-like reaction 0.1–0.5%. Arthralgia, rash, erythema multiforme but no adenopathy, proteinuria or demonstrable immune complexes. Appear due to mixture of drug biotransformation and genetic susceptibility (Ped Pharm & Therap 125:805, 1994).
Cefdinir (Omnicef) (300 mg cap)	300 mg po q12h or 600 mg q24h.	Cefdinir: Drug-iron complex causes red stools in roughly 1% of pts.
Cefditoren pivoxil (Spectracef) (400 mg tab)	400 mg po bid.	Cefditoren pivoxil: Hydrolysis yields pivalate. Pivalate absorbed (70%), becomes pivaloyl-carnitine which is renally excreted; 33–63% ↓ in serum carnitine. Concern in fatty acid (FA) metabolism & FA transport. Contraindicated in patients with carnitine deficiency or those in whom inborn errors of metabolism might result in clinically significant carnitine deficiency. Also contains caseinate (milk protein); **avoid if milk allergy** (not same as lactose intolerance). Need gastric acid for optimal absorption.
Cefixime (Suprax) (400 mg tab)	0.4 gm po q12–24h.	
Cefpodoxime proxetil (Vantin)	0.1–0.2 gm po q12h.	Cephalexin: There are rare reports of acute liver injury, bloody diarrhea, pulmonary infiltrates with eosinophilia.
Ceftibuten (Cedax) (400 mg tab)	0.4 gm po q24h.	Can cause false-neg. urine dipstick test for leukocytes.

(See page 2 for abbreviations)

* NOTE: all dosage recommendations are for adults (unless otherwise indicated) & assume normal renal function.

TABLE 10A (5)

CLASS, AGENT, GENERIC NAME (TRADE NAME)	USUAL ADULT DOSAGE*	ADVERSE REACTIONS, COMMENTS (See Table 10B for Summary)
AMINOGLYCOSIDES AND RELATED ANTIBIOTICS—See Table 10D, page 109, and Table 17A, page 205		
GLYCOPEPTIDES, LIPOGLYCOPEPTIDES, LIPOPEPTIDES		
Teicoplanin[NUS] (Targocid)	For septic arthritis—maintenance dose 12 mg/kg per day; S. aureus endocarditis required trough serum levels >20 mcg/mL (CID 55:1192, 2012), often 3 loading dose, then 12 mg/kg q24h	Hypersensitivity, fever (at 3 mg/kg 2.2%, at 24 mg per kg 8.2%), skin reactions 2.4%. Marked ↓ platelets (high dose ≥15 mg per kg per day). Red man syndrome less common than with vancomycin.
Telavancin (Vibativ) Lipoglycopeptide Ref: CID 49:1908, 2009	Skin/soft tissue: 10 mg/kg IV q24h if CrCl > 50 mL/min. Infuse each dose over 1 hr. Adjust dose if wt ≥30% over IBW, see Table 10D	Avoid during pregnancy: teratogenic in animals. Do pregnancy test before therapy. Adverse events: dysgeusia (taste) 33%, nausea 27%, vomiting 14%, headache 14%, ↑ creatinine (3.1%), foamy urine; flushing if infused rapidly. In clin trials, evidence or renal injury in 3% telavancin vs. 1% vanco. In practice, renal injury reported in 1/3 of 21 complicated pts (AAC 67:723, 2013).
Vancomycin (Vancocin) Med Let 52:1, 2010; Guidelines Ref: CID 49:325, 2009. See Comments for po dose.	Initial doses based on actual wt, including for obese pts. Subsequent doses adjusted based on measured trough serum levels. For critically ill pts, give loading dose of 25–30 mg/kg IV then 15–20 mg/kg q8–12h. Target trough level is 15–20 μg/mL. For individual doses over 1 gm, infuse over 1.5–2 hrs. **Dosing for morbid obesity (BMI ≥40 kg/m²):** If CrCl ≥50 mL/min, 6 gm/day divided q8–12h; 30 mg/kg per day q8–12h—no dose over 2 gm. Infuse doses over 1 gm or more over 1.5–2 hrs. Check trough levels. Limit maximal single dose to 2 gm. Oral tabs for C. difficile colitis: 125 mg po q6h. Generic drug now available	Vanco treatment failure of MRSA bacteremia associated with Vanco trough concentration <15 μg/mL & MIC > 1 μg/mL (CID 52:975, 2011). IDSA Guideline supports target trough of AUC/MIC > 400 (CID 52:975, 2011). Pertinent issues: • Max Vanco effect vs. MRSA when ratio of AUC/MIC > 400 (CID 49:260, 2011) • MIC values vary with method used, so hard to be sure re compatible (JCM 49:269, 2011) • With MRSA Vanco MIC = 1.8, Vanco clinical success rate > 3 gm/day IV, AUC/MIC > 400 in 80% with est. risk of nephrotoxicity of 25%. With MIC = 2 & 4 gm/day IV, AUC/MIC > 400 in only 57% (nephrotoxicity risk 35%) (CID 52:969, 2011). • Higher Vanco doses assoc with nephrotoxicity; causal relation unproven; other factors: renal disease, other nephrotoxic drugs, shock/vasopressors, radiographic contrast (AJM 123:182e1, 2010; AAC 55:3278, 2011; AJM 123:182e1, 2010). • If pt clinically failing Vanco (regardless of MIC or AUC/MIC), consider other drugs active vs. MRSA: ceftaroline, daptomycin, linezolid, televancin. **PO vanco for C. difficile colitis: 125 mg po q6h.** Commercial po formulation very expensive. Can compound po vanco from IV formulation: 5 g, IV vanco powder + 47.5 mL sterile H₂O, 0.2 gm saccharin, 0.05 gm stevia powder, 40 mL glycerin and then enough cherry syrup to yield 100 mL = 50 mg vanco/mL. Oral dose = 2.5 mL q6h po. **Intrathecal dose:** 5–10 mg/day (infants); 10–20 mg/day (children & adults) for meningitis to target CSF concentration of 10–20 μg/mL. **Nephrotoxicity:** with dosing at or above 4 gm/day (AAC 52:1330, 2008); see also CID 49:507, 2009). Concomitant hypertension causing renal insult (AAC 55:5475, 2009). Nausea, vomiting, rash with rapid infusion (red man syndrome). **Other adverse effects:** rash, immune thrombocytopenia (NEJM 356:904, 2007), fever, neutropenia, initial dose-dependent decrease in platelet count (AAC 57:727, 2012). For CrCl calculation for morbidly obese patients see Table 10D or Am J Health Sys Pharm 66:642, 2009.
Daptomycin (Cubicin) (Ref on resistance: CID 50:S10, 2010)	Skin/soft tissue: 4 mg per kg IV over 2 or 30 minutes q24h Bacteremia/right-sided endocarditis: 6 mg per kg IV q24h or 30 min q24h; up to 12 mg/kg IV q24h under study Morbid obesity (BMI 540 kg/m²): base dose on total body weight (J Clin Pharm 45:48, 2005)	**Pneumonia:** Dapto failed to eradicate S. pneumo with a trend toward failure to eradicate S. aureus in trials of CAP (CID 46:1142, 2008). In animal models Dapto failed vs. S. pneumo because lung surfactant with necrotizing S. aureus pneumonia, S. pneumo rarely eradicated. Dapto not efficacious vs. S. aureus pneumonia, dapto also failed in S. aureus right-sided endocarditis (NEJM 355:653, 2006). Disturbing case report of deoxy US S. aureus while on dapto (CID 49:1286, 2009). **Dapto Resistance:** Can occur de novo, after or during Vanco therapy, or after or during Dapto therapy (CID 50(Suppl 1):S10, 2010). As Dapto MIC increases, MRSA more susceptible to TMP-SMX, ceftaroline (AAC 54:5187, 2010) and Nafcillin (CID 53:158, 2011). Concomitant Oxacillin restores Dapto activity (CID 53:158, 2011). **Potential muscle toxicity:** At 4 mg per kg per day, 1 CPK in 2.8% dapto pts & 1.8% comparator-treated pts. Risk increases if min conc ≥24.3 mg/L (CID 50:1568, 2010). Suggest weekly CPK. DC dapto if CPK exceeds 10x normal if level or symptoms of myopathy occur. CPK can ↑ later in course of therapy. Selected reports of rhabdomyolysis (CID 50:177, 2009), rare (1/1 pt). Selected reports of rhabdomyolysis with dapto rx (AAC 53:1538, 2009). Occasional eosinophilic pneumonia reported (AAC 50:3245, 2006) and in pts given mean dose of 8 mg/kg/day (CID 49:177, 2009). Immune thrombocytopenia reported (AAC 56:6430, 2012). **Eosinophilic pneumonia** reported (CID 50:e63, 2010).

*NOTE: all dosage recommendations are for adults (unless otherwise indicated) & assume normal renal function.

(See page 2 for abbreviations)

TABLE 10A (6)

CLASS, AGENT, GENERIC NAME (TRADE NAME)	USUAL ADULT DOSAGE*	ADVERSE REACTIONS, COMMENTS (See Table 10B for Summary)
CHLORAMPHENICOL, CLINDAMYCIN(S), ERYTHROMYCIN GROUP, KETOLIDES, OXAZOLIDINONES, QUINUPRISTIN-DALFOPRISTIN		
Chloramphenicol (Chloromycetin)	50-100 mg/kg/day po/IV q6h (max 4 gm/day)	No oral drug distrib in U.S. Hematologic (↓ RBC –1/3 pts, aplastic anemia 1:21,600 courses). Gray baby syndrome in premature infants, anaphylactoid reactions, optic atrophy or neuropathy (very rare), digital paresthesias, minor disulfiram-like reactions.
Clindamycin (Cleocin)	0.15-0.45 gm po q6h, 600-900 mg IV/IM q8h.	Based on number of exposed pts, these drugs are the most frequent cause of **C. difficile toxin-mediated diarrhea.** In most severe form can cause pseudomembranous colitis/toxic megacolon. Available as caps, IV sol'n, topical (for acne) & intravaginal suppositories & cream. Used to inhibit synthesis of toxic shock syndrome toxins.
Lincomycin (Lincocin)	0.6 gm IV/IM q8h.	Risk of C. difficile colitis. Rarely used.
Erythromycin Group (Review drug interactions before use)		**Motilin:** activates gastroduodenal motilin receptors to initiate peristalsis. Erythro (E) and E esters activate motilin receptors and cause uncoordinated peristalsis with resultant anorexia, nausea or vomiting. Less binding and GI distress with azithromycin/clarithromycin. No peristalsis benefit (JAC 59:347, 2007).
Azithromycin (Zithromax) Azithromycin ER (Zmax)	po preps: Tabs 250 & 500 mg. Peds suspension 100 & 200 mg per 5 ml. Adult ER suspension: 2 gm. Dose varies with indication, see Table 1; Acute otitis media (page 11); acute exac. chronic bronchitis (page 37), Comm-acq. pneumonia (pages 39-40) & sinusitis (page 50) IV 0.5 gm per day.	Systemic erythro in 1st 2 wks of life associated with **infantile hypertrophic pyloric stenosis** (J Ped 139:380, 2001). **Frequent drug-drug interactions:** see Table 22, page 217. Major concern is prolonged QTc interval on EKG. **Prolonged QTc:** Erythro, clarithro & azithro all increase risk of ventricular tachycardia via increase in QTc interval. Can be congenital or acquired (NEJM 358:169, 2008). 5 days azithro assoc w/ increased risk of cardiovascular death (hazard ratio 2.88) compared to amoxicillin or no antimicrobial, 47 additional cardio-vascular deaths per 1 million courses (NEJM 366:1881, 2012).
Erythromycin Base and esters (Erythrocin) (V,llone E. Es, llosone) or clarithro extended release (Biaxin XL)	0.25 gm q6h-0.5 gm po/IV q6h; 15-20 mg/kg/day up to 4 gm q24h. Infuse over 30-60 min. **Extended release: Two 0.5 gm tabs po per day.**	**↑ risk QTc > 500 msec: Risk amplified by other drugs** (macrolides, antiarrhythmics, & drug-drug interactions (see FQs page 100 for list)). Prolonged QTc can result in torsades de pointes (ventricular tachycardia) and/or cardiac arrest. Refs: CID 43:1603, 2006; www.qtdrugs.org & www.torsades.org. Cholestatic hepatitis in approx. 1:1000 adults (not children) given E. estolate. **Transient reversible tinnitus or deafness** with 24 gm per day of erythro IV in pts with renal or hepatic impairment. Reversible sensorineural hearing loss with erythro (AnIM 121:649, 1994). Oral/IV with food: up to 60% absorbed after IV. Dosage of erythro refers to erythro base; other forms dosed as base equivalents. With differences in absorption/biotransformation, variable amounts of erythro esters required to achieve same free erythro serum level, e.g., 400 mg Erythro ethyl succinate = 250 mg Erythro base. **Azithromycin** reported to exacerbate symptoms of myasthenia gravis.
Fidaxomicin (Dificid) (200 mg tab)	One 200 mg tab po bid x 10 days with or without food	Approved for treatment of C. difficile toxin-mediated diarrhea. Patent activity vs. C. diff., including hypervirulent NAP1/B1/027 strains. Minimal GI absorption; high fecal concentrations. Limited activity vs. normal bowel flora. In trial vs. oral Vanco, lower relapse rate vs. non NAP1 strains than Vanco (NEJM 364:422, 2011). Cohort study reported slight ↑ in cardiovascular mortality during 5 days of therapy with azithromycin (NEJM 366:1881, 2012), leading to a warning statement by FDA (http://www.fda.gov/Drugs/DrugSafety/ucm304372.htm); N=100 WHI trial of azithro vs. placebo did not show difference in mortality.
Ketolide: Telithromycin (Ketek) (Med Lett 46:66, 2004; Drug Safety 31:561, 2008)	Two 400 mg tabs po q24h. 300 mg tabs available.	Drug safety issues: acute liver failure & serious liver injury post treatment (AnIM 144:415, 447, 2006). **Uncommon: blurred vision 2° slow accommodation, may cause exacerbation of myasthenia gravis (Black Box Warning: Contraindicated in this disorder)** 2° inhibition of nicotinic acetylcholine receptor at neuromuscular junction (AAC 54:5399, 2010). Potential QTc prolongation. Several **drug-drug interactions** (Table 22, pages 217-218) (NEJM 355:2260, 2006).

* NOTE: all dosage recommendations are for adults (unless otherwise indicated) & assume normal renal function.

(See page 2 for abbreviations)

TABLE 10A (7)

CHLORAMPHENICOL, CLINDAMYCIN(S), ERYTHROMYCIN GROUP, KETOLIDES, OXAZOLIDINONES, QUINUPRISTIN-DALFOPRISTIN (See Table 10B for Summary)

CLASS, AGENT, GENERIC NAME (TRADE NAME)	USUAL ADULT DOSAGE*	ADVERSE REACTIONS, COMMENTS (See Table 10B for Summary)
Linezolid (Zyvox) (600 mg tab) Review: JAC 66(Suppl4):i3, 2011	PO or IV dose: 600 mg q12h. (100 mg per 5 mL 3.8% solution. Special populations Refs: Renal insufficiency (J Infect Chemother 17:70, 2011); Liver transplant (CID 42:434, 2006); Cystic fibrosis (AAC 48:281, 2004); Burns (J Burn Care Res 31:207, 2010).	**Reversible myelosuppression:** thrombocytopenia, anemia, & neutropenia reported. Most often after >2 wks of therapy. Platelets <50% baseline in wk 2, 5% of pts; wk 3, 7%; wk 4, 15%. Monitor wkly CBC, esp. if >2 wks therapy in pts with ESRD (AAC 50:2042, 2006). Refs: Clin Pharmacokinet 42:1411, 2003 & 38:1058 & 985, 2000. Increased risk in pts with ESRD (AAC 50:2042, 2006). **Lactic acidosis; peripheral neuropathy, optic neuropathy:** After 4 or more wks of therapy. Data consistent with time and dose-dependent inhibition of intramitochondrial protein synthesis (CID 42:1111, 2006; AAC 50:2042, 2006; Pharmacotherapy 27:771, 2007). **Inhibitor of monoamine oxidase:** risk of severe hypertension if taken with foods rich in tyramine. Avoid concomitant pseudoephedrine, phenylpropanolamine, and caution with SSRIs. **Serotonin syndrome** (fever, agitation, mental status changes, tremors, rhythmic muscle jerks) reported with coadmin of SSRIs: (CID 42:1578 and 43:180, 2006). Other adverse effects: black hairy tongue and acute interstitial nephritis (IDCP 17:61, 2009). **Rhabdomyolysis:** a case of this entity, probably related to linezolid, was reported in a patient receiving linezolid as a component of therapy for XDR tuberculosis (CID 50:821, 2010). Resistance due, primarily to mutation of the 23S rRNA binding site (AAC 56:603, 2012).
Quinupristin + dalfopristin (Synercid) (CID 36:473, 2003)	7.5 mg per kg IV q8h via central line	Venous irritation (5%); none with central venous line. Asymptomatic ↑ in unconjugated bilirubin. **Arthralgia** 2%–50% (CID 36:476, 2003). **Note:** E. faecium susceptible; E. faecalis resistant. **Drug-drug interactions:** Cyclosporine, nifedipine, midazolam, many more—see Table 22.

TETRACYCLINES

Doxycycline (Vibramycin, Doryx, Monodox, Adoxa, Periostat) (20, 50, 75, 100 mg tab)	0.1 gm po/IV q12h	Similar to other tetracyclines. ↑ nausea on empty stomach. Erosive esophagitis, **take with lots of water.** Photosensitivity & photo-onychoiysis occur but less than with tetracycline. Deposition in teeth less. Can be used in patients with renal failure. Comments: Effective in treatment and prophylaxis for malaria, leptospirosis, typhus fevers.
Minocycline (Minocin, Dynacin) (50, 75, 100 mg cap; 45, 90, 135 mg ext rel tab; IV prep)	200 mg po/IV loading dose, then 100 mg po/IV q12h IV minocycline no longer available.	Vestibular symptoms (30–90% in some groups, none in others); vertigo 33%, ataxia 43%, nausea 50%, vomiting 3%, women more frequently than men. Hypersensitivity pneumonitis, reversible, ~34 cases reported (BMJ 310:1520, 1995). Can increase **pigmentation** of the skin with long-term use. Comments: More effective than other tetracyclines vs staph and in prophylaxis of meningococcal disease. P. acnes: many resistant to other tetracyclines, not to mino. Induced autoimmunity reported in children treated for acne (J Ped 153:314, 2008). Active vs Nocardia asteroides, Mycobacterium marinum.
Tetracycline, Oxytetracycline (Sumycin) (250, 500 mg cap) (CID 36:462, 2003)	0.25–0.5 gm po q6h, 0.5–1 gm IV q12h	GI (oxy 19%, tetra 4), anaphylactoid reaction (rare), deposition in teeth, negative N balance, hepatotoxicity, enamel ageneisis, pseudotumor cerebri, esophageal ulcerations, Outdated drug: Fanconi syndrome. See drug-drug interactions, Table 22. **Contraindicated in pregnancy: hepatotoxicity in the mother, fatal to fetus.** Comments: **Pregnancy:** IV dosage over 2 gm per day may be associated with fatal hepatotoxicity. (Ref. JAC 66:1431, 2011).
Tigecycline (Tygacil) Meta-analysis & editorial: Ln ID 11:804 & 834, 2011. Also CID 54:1699 & 1707, 2012. Increased mortality in serious infections compared with comparative therapies. Use with caution in serious infections.	100 mg IV initially, then 50 mg IV q12h with food, if possible to decrease risk of nausea.	**If severe liver dis. (Child Pugh C):** 100 mg IV initially, then 25 mg IV q12h. Derivative of tetracycline. High incidence of nausea (25%) & vomiting (20%) but only 1% of pts discontinued therapy due to an adverse event. Details on AEs in JAC 62 (Suppl 1): i17, 2008. Pregnancy Category D. Do not use in children under age 18. Like other tetracyclines, may cause photosensitivity, pseudotumor cerebri, pancreatitis, a catabolic state (elevated BUN) and maybe hyperpigmentation (Int J Antimicrob Agents, 34:486, 2009). **Tetracycline, minocycline & tigecycline** associated with acute pancreatitis (Int J Antimicrob Agents, 34:486, 2009). Dear Doctor Letter (4/27/09): lower cure rate and higher mortality in pts with VAP treated with tigecycline. Ref: Diag Micro Infect Dis 68:140, 2010. FDA drug safety communication: http://www.fda.gov/Drugs/DrugSafety/ucm224370.htm

[1] **SSRI** = selective serotonin reuptake inhibitors, e.g., fluoxetine (Prozac).
(See page 2 for abbreviations)   * NOTE: all dosage recommendations are for adults (unless otherwise indicated) & assume normal renal function.

TABLE 10A (8)

CLASS, AGENT, GENERIC NAME (TRADE NAME)	USUAL ADULT DOSAGE*	ADVERSE REACTIONS, COMMENTS (See Table 10B for Summary)
FLUOROQUINOLONES (FQs): All can cause false-positive urine drug screen for opiates (*Pharmacother 26:435, 2006*). Toxicity review: *Drugs Aging 27:193, 2010.*		
Ciprofloxacin (Cipro) and **Ciprofloxacin-extended release** (Cipro XR, Proquin XR) (100, 250, 500, 750 mg tab; 500 mg ext rel tab)	Usual Parenteral Dose: **400 mg IV q12h** For P. aeruginosa: **400 mg IV q8h** Uncomplicated Urethritis/cystitis (Oral) Dose: **250 mg bid or CIP XR 500 mg po once daily** Other Indications (Oral): **500-750 mg po bid**	FQs are a common precipitant of C. difficile toxin-mediated diarrhea. **Children:** No FDA approved for use under age 18 based on joint cartilage injury in immature animals. Articular SEs in children est. at 2–3% (*LnID 3:537, 2003*). The exception is anthrax. Pathogenesis believed to involve FQ chelation of Mg++ & damaging chondrocyte mitochondria (*Sci Transl Med 4:135, 2012; AAC 56:4940, 2012*). **CNS toxicity:** Poorly understood and idiosyncratic. Varies from mild (lightheadedness) to moderate (confusion) to severe (seizures). May be aggravated by NSAIDs.
Gatifloxacin (Tequin) See comments	**200–400 mg IV/po q24h** (See comment)	Gemi skin rash: Macular rash after 8–10 days of rx. Incidence of rash with ≤5 days of therapy only 1.5%. Frequency highest females, < age 40, treated 14 days (22.6%). In men, < age 40, treated 14 days, frequency 7.7%. Mechanism unclear. Indication to D/C therapy. Ref: *Diag Micro Infect Dis 68:140, 2010.*
Gemifloxacin (Factive) (320 mg tab)	**320 mg po q24h**	Ophthalmic solution (1x/m/l) **Hypoglycemia/hyperglycemia:** Due to documented hypo- and hyperglycemic reactions (*NEJM 354:1352, 2006; AnIM 146:82, 2006*), US distribution of Gati in its oral & ophthalmic solution remains available. **Opiate screen false-positives:** FQs can cause false-positive urine assay for opiates (*JAMA 296:3115, 2001; Arm Pharmacotherapy 38:1525, 2004*). **Photosensitivity:** See Table 10C, page 108. Rarely, retinal detachment (*JAMA 307:1414, 2012*).
Levofloxacin (Levaquin) (250, 500, 750 mg tab)	**250–750 mg po/IV q24h.** For most indications, 750 mg is preferred dose. PO therapy: avoid concomitant dairy products, multivitamins, iron, antacids due to chelation by multivalent cations & interference with absorption.	**QT_c (corrected QT) interval prolongation:** ↑ QT_c (>500 msec or >60 msec from baseline) is considered possible with any FQ. ↑ QT_c can lead to torsades de pointes and ventricular fibrillation. Risk for ↑ with current marketed drugs. Risk ↑ in women, ↓ K⁺, ↓ mg⁺⁺, bradycardia. (Refs. *CID 43:1603, 2006*). Major problem is ↑ risk with concomitant drugs.
		Avoid concomitant drugs with potential to prolong QTc such as:
		Antiarrhythmics: Amiodarone, Disopyramide, Dofetilide, Ibutilide, Flecainide, Procainamide, Quinidine, quinine, Sotalol
		Anti-Infectives: Azoles (not posa), Clarithro/erythro, FQs (not CIP), Halofantrine, NNRTIs, Protease Inhibitors, Pentamidine, Telavancin, Telithromycin
		CNS Drugs: Fluoxetine, Haloperidol, Phenothiazines, Pimozide, Quetiapine, Risperidone, Sertraline, Tricyclics, Venlafaxine, Ziprasidone
		Misc: Dolasetron, Droperidol, Fosphenytoin, Indapamide, Methadone, Naratriptan, Salmeterol, Sumatriptan, Tamoxifen, Tizanidine
		Anti-Hypertensives: Bepridil, Isradipine, Nicardipine, Moexipril
		Updates online: www.qtdrugs.org; www.torsades.org
Moxifloxacin (Avelox)	**400 mg po/IV q24h.** Note: no need to increase dose for morbid obesity (*AAC 66:2330, 2011*). Ophthalmic solution (Vigamox)	**Tendinopathy:** Over age 60, approx. 2–6% of all Achilles tendon ruptures attributable to use of FQ (*AdM 163:1801, 2003*); ↑ risk with concomitant steroid, renal disease or post-transplant (heart, lung, kidney) (*CID 36:1404, 2003*). Overall incidence is low (*Eur J Clin Pharm 63:499, 2007*); **Chelation:** Risk of chelation of oral FQs by multivalent cations (Ca++, Mg++, Fe++, Zn++) with dairy products; multivitamins (*Clin Pharmacother 40 (Suppl1) 33:2001*). Avoid dairy products, multivitamins with Moxi. 3 pts
Ofloxacin (Floxin)	**200–400 mg po bid** Ophthalmic solution (Ocuflox)	**Allergic Reactions:** Rare (1:50,000); IgE-mediated: urticaria, anaphylaxis. May be more common with Moxi. 3 pts with Moxi immediate reactions tolerated CIP (*Am J Pharmacother 44:740, 2010*). **Myasthenia gravis:** Any of the FQs can cause increased weakness in pts with myasthenia gravis. **Retinal detachment:** A case-control study from Canada described an association between current (but not recent or past) use of fluoroquinolones and occurrence of retinal detachment (*JAMA 307:1414, 2012*).

*NOTE: all dosage recommendations are for adults (unless otherwise indicated) & assume normal renal function.

(See page 2 for abbreviations)

TABLE 10A (9)

CLASS, AGENT, GENERIC NAME (TRADE NAME)	USUAL ADULT DOSAGE*	ADVERSE REACTIONS, COMMENTS (See Table 10B for Summary)
POLYMYXINS (POLYPEPTIDES)	**Note: Proteus sp., Providencia sp, Serratia sp., B. cepacia are intrinsically resistant to polymyxins.**	
Polymyxin B (Poly-Rx) 1 mg = 10,000 units Avoid monotherapy, see Colistin.	Standard Dose: 15,000-25,000 units/kg/day IV divided q12h 50,000 units/dose into CSF daily x 3-4 days, then qod x 2 or more wks	**Adverse effects: Neurologic:** rare but serious is neuromuscular blockade; other: circumoral paresthesias, extremity numbness, blurred vision, drowsy, irritable, ataxia. **Renal:** reversible acute tubular necrosis. PK study in septic pts: no need to reduce dose in renal insufficiency (CID 57:1298, 2008). Efficacy correlates with AUC/MIC & need maximal daily dose to optimize AUC (JAC 65:2231, 2010).
Colistin, Polymyxin E (Colymycin) All doses based on mg of Colistin base. Calculated doses are higher than the package insert dosing; need to avoid underdosage in the critically ill. Do not use as monotherapy (combine with carbapenem or rifampin) Dosing formula based on PK study of 105 pts (AAC 55:3284, 2011) Loading dose (AAC 53:3430, 2009), PK/PD studies (AAC 54:3783, 2010 (in vitro), JAC 65:1984, 2010 (in vivo)).	**Severe Systemic infection:** **LOADING DOSE**: 3.5 (targeted average serum steady state level) x 2 x body weight in kg (lower of ideal or actual weight) IV. This will often result as a loading dose of over 300 mg; first maintenance dose is given 12 h later. **MAINTENANCE DOSE:** Formula for calculating the daily maintenance dosage: • 3.5 (the desired serum steady state concentration) x [(1.5 x CrCl) + 30] = total daily dose divide and give q8h or q12h. The maximum suggested daily dose is 475 mgs. • **NOTE:** CrCl is the Creatinine Clearance (CrCl) normalized (n) for Body Surface Area (BSA) such that the CrCl_n = CrCl x BSA in m²/1.73 m². Combination therapy is recommended for all pts: Colistin (as above) + {IMP or MER) or RIF} (based on IBW) • **intrathecal or intraventricular for meningitis:** 10 mg/day • **inhalation therapy:** 50-75 mg in 3-4 mL of Saline via nebulizer 2-3x/day	• **GNB Resistance:** Some sp. are intrinsically resistant: Serratia sp, Proteus sp, Providencia sp, B. cepacia. In vitro and in animal models, gram-negative bacilli quickly become resistant; concomitant Tigecycline or Minocycline may attenuate the rate of resistance (JAC 60:421, 2007). Synergy with Rifampin or Tigecycline unpredictable. The greater the resistance of GNB to Colistin, the greater the susceptibility to beta-lactams (AM-SB, PIP-TZ, extended spectrum Ceph, maybe carbapenems). • **Bactericidal activity concentration dependent** but no post-antibiotic effect; do not dose once daily. Pharmacokinetics of colistin (> 5 mg/kg of ideal body weight per day) are associated with increased risk of nephrotoxicity and should be reserved for critically ill patients (Clin Infect Dis 53:879, 2011). • **Nephrotoxic:** exact risk unclear, but increased by concomitant nephrotoxins (IV contrast), hypotension, maybe Rifampin. Reversible. • **Neurotoxicity.** Frequent: circumoral paresthesia, vertigo, abnormal vision, confusion, ataxia. Rare: neuromuscular blockade with respiratory failure. • **Caution:** Some international colistimethate products are expressed in IUs. To convert IUs to mg of colistin base: 30,000 IUs colistimethate = 2.4 mg colistimethate base = 1 mg colistin base.
MISCELLANEOUS AGENTS		
Fosfomycin (Monurol) (3 gm packet)	3 gm with water po times 1 dose. For emergency use as single patient IND for IV use. From FDA: 1-888-463-6332.	Diarrhea in 9% compared to 6% of pts given nitrofurantoin and 2.3% given TMP-SMX. Available outside U.S., IV & PO, for treatment of multi-drug resistant bacteria. For MDR-GNB: 6-12 gm/day IV divided q6-8h. Ref: Int J Antimicrob Ag 37:415, 2011.
Fusidic acid^{NUS} (Fucidin, Taksta)	500 mg po/IV tid (Denmark & Canada) US: loading dose of 1500 mg po bid x 1 day, then 60 mg po bid	Activity vs. MRSA of importance. Approved outside the U.S.; currently in U.S. clinical trials. Ref for proposed US regimen: CID 52 (Suppl 7):S520, 2011.
Methenamine hippurate (Hiprex, Urex) **Methenamine mandelate** (Mandelamine)	1 gm po bid 1 gm po qid	Nausea and vomiting, skin rash or dysuria. Overall ~3%. Methenamine requires acidic (pH ≤5) urine to liberate formaldehyde. Useful in suppressive therapy after infecting organisms cleared; do not use for pyelonephritis. **Comment:** Do not force fluids; may dilute formaldehyde. Of no value in pts with chronic Foley. If urine pH >5.0, co-administer ascorbic acid (1-2 gm q4h) to acidify the urine; cranberry juice (1200-4000 mL per day) has been used, results ±. Do not use concomitantly with sulfonamides (precipitate), or in presence of renal or severe hepatic dysfunction.

(See page 2 for abbreviations)   * NOTE: all dosage recommendations are for adults (unless otherwise indicated) & assume normal renal function.

TABLE 10A (10)

CLASS, AGENT, GENERIC NAME (TRADE NAME)	USUAL ADULT DOSAGE*	ADVERSE REACTIONS, COMMENTS (See Table 10B for Summary)
MISCELLANEOUS AGENTS (continued)		
Metronidazole (Flagyl) (250, 375, 500 mg tab/cap) Ref: Activity vs. *B. fragilis* Still drug of choice (*CID* 50 (Suppl 1):S16, 2010).	Anaerobic infections: usually IV, 7.5 mg per kg (~500 mg) q6h (not to exceed 4 gm q24h). With type 1%, can use IV at 15 mg per kg q12h. In life-threatening, use loading dose of IV 15 mg per kg. Oral dose: 500 mg qid; extended release tabs available 750 mg.	**Common AEs:** nausea (12%), metallic taste, "furry" tongue. Avoid alcohol during 48 hrs after last dose to avoid disulfiram reaction (N/V, flushing, tachycardia, dyspnea). Neurologic AEs with high dose/long Rx: peripheral, autonomic and optic neuropathy (*J Child Neurol* 21:429, 2006). Aseptic meningitis, encephalopathy, seizures & reversible cerebellar lesion reported (*NEJM* 346:68, 2002). Also topical & vaginal gels. Can use IV soln as enema for *C. difficile*. Resistant anaerobic organisms: *Actinomyces, Propionibacterium, Lactobacillus, Bifidobacterium*, non-*C. difficile Clostridium* sp. Pregnancy 1/2; standard in Europe; suggestive retrospective studies in adults with intra-abdominal infections (*JAC* 19:410, 2007).
Nitazoxanide See Table 13B, page 152		
Nitrofurantoin macrocrystals (Macrobid, Macrodantin (Furadantin/Macrodantin (25, 50, 100 mg caps)	Active UTI: Furadantin/Macrodantin 50-100 mg po qid x 7 days Macrobid 100 mg po bid x 7 days Dose for long-term UTI suppression: 50-100 mg at bedtime	Absorption ↑ with meals. Increased activity in acid urine, much reduced at pH 8 or over. Not effective in endstage renal disease. Nausea and vomiting, peripheral neuropathy, pancreatitis. **Pulmonary reactions** (with chronic rx): acute ARDS type or **chronic desquamative interstitial pneumonia with fibrosis**; intrahepatic cholestasis, & **hepatitis** similar to chronic active hepatitis. Hemolytic anemia in G6PD deficiency. Drug rash, eosinophilia, systemic symptoms (DRESS) hypersensitivity syndrome reported (*Neth J Med* 67:147, 2009). **Contraindicated in renal failure.** Should not be used in infants <1 month of age. Birth defects: increased risk reported (*Arch Ped Adolesc Med* 163:978, 2009).
Rifampin (Rimactane, Rifadin) (150, 300 mg cap)	300 mg po bid or 600 mg po once daily	Causes orange-brown discoloration of sweat, urine, tears, contact lens. **Many important drug-drug interactions,** see Table 22. Immune complex flu-like syndrome: fever, headache, myalgias, arthralgia—especially with intermittent rx. Thrombocytopenia, vasculitis reported (*C Ann Pharmacother* 42: 727, 2008). Can cause interstitial nephritis. Risk-benefit of looking to standard therapies for *S. aureus* endocarditis (*AAC* 52:2463, 2008). See also, *Antimycobacterial Agents*, Table 12B, page 138.
Rifaximin (Xifaxan) (200, 550 mg tab)	Traveler's diarrhea: 200 mg tab po tid times 3 days. Hepatic encephalopathy: 550 mg tab po bid. C. difficile diarrhea as "chaser": 400 mg po bid.	For traveler's diarrhea and hepatic encephalopathy (*AAC* 54:3618, 2010; *NEJM* 362:1071, 2010). In general, adverse events equal to or less than placebo.
Sulfonamides (e.g., sulfisoxazole (Gantrisin), sulfamethoxazole (Gantanol), (Truxazole), sulfadiazine)	Dose varies with indications. See Nocardia & Toxoplasmosis	**CNS:** fever, headache, dizziness. **Derm:** mild rash to life threatening Stevens-Johnson syndrome, toxic epidermal necrolysis, photosensitivity. **Hem:** agranulocytosis, aplastic anemia; **Cross-allergenicity:** other sulfa drugs, sulfonylureas, diuretics, crystalluria (esp. sulfadiazine-need ≥ 1500 mL po fluid/day); **Other:** serum sickness, hemolysis if G6PD def., polyarteritis, SLE reported.
Tinidazole (Tindamax)	Tabs 250, 500 mg. Dose for giardiasis: 2 gm po times 1 with food. 100 mg po q12h or 200 mg po q24h.	**Adverse reactions:** metallic taste 3.7%, nausea 3.2%, anorexia/vomiting 1.5%. All higher with multi-day dosing. Avoid alcohol during & for 3 days after last dose, cause disulfiram reaction, flushing, N/V, tachycardia. **CNS:** drug fever, aseptic meningitis; **Derm:** rash (3-7% at 200 mg/day), photosensitivity, Stevens-Johnson syndrome (rare), toxic epidermal necrolysis (rare); **Renal:** ↑ K⁺, ↓ Na⁺, ↓ Cl⁻; **Hem:** neutropenia, thrombocytopenia, methemoglobinemia.
Trimethoprim (Trimpex, Proloprim, and others) (100, 200 mg tab)	Standard rx: 1 DS tab bid. P. carinii (component): standard 8-10 mg per kg TMP per day divided q6h, q8h, or q12h. For shigellosis: 2.5 mg per kg po q6h.	Adverse reactions in 10%: GI, nausea, vomiting, anorexia; skin: rash, urticaria, photosensitivity. More serious (1-10%): **Stevens-Johnson syndrome** (*Ann Pharmacotherapy* 32:381, 1998). Daily ascorbic acid 0.5-1.0 gm may promote detoxification (*JAIDS* 36:1041, 2004). Rare hypoglycemia, esp. AIDS pts. (*LnID* 6:178, 2006). **Sweet's Syndrome** can occur. TMP competes with creatinine for tubular secretion, serum creatinine can ↑ . TMP also blocks distal renal tubule secretion of K⁺, ↑ serum K⁺ in 21% of pts (*AnIM* 124:316, 1996). Risk of hyperkalemia increased 7× if concomitant ACE inhibitor (*Arch Int Med* 170:1045, 2010). Discussion of renal injury (*AJKD* 77:27, 2011). TMP-SMX (1 DS tab) effective in prophylaxis/treatment of PCP (*MMWR* 58(RR-4):1-207, 2009). TMP-SMX contains sulfites and may trigger asthma in sulfite-sensitive pts. Frequent drug cause of thrombocytopenia, cross allergenicity with other sulfonamide non-antibiotic drugs (*NEJM* 349:1628, 2003). **For TMP-SMX desensitization, see Table 7, page 80.**
Trimethoprim-sulfamethoxazole (SMX) (Bactrim, Septra, Sulfatrim, Cotrimoxazole) Single-strength (SS) is 80 TMP/400 SMX, double-strength (DS) 160 TMP/800 SMX	See Table 14B, page 145. IV: 8-10 mg per kg (based on TMP component): standard 8-10 mg per kg TMP per day divided q6h, q8h, or q12h. For shigellosis: 2.5 mg per kg po q6h.	

*NOTE: all dosage recommendations are for adults (unless otherwise indicated) & assume normal renal function.

(See page 2 for abbreviations)

TABLE 10A (11)

CLASS, AGENT, GENERIC NAME (TRADE NAME)	USUAL ADULT DOSAGE*	ADVERSE REACTIONS, COMMENTS (See Table 10B for Summary)
Topical Antimicrobial Agents Active vs. S. aureus & Strep. pyogenes (CID 49:1541, 2009). **Review of topical antiseptics, antibiotics** (CID 49:1541, 2009).		
Bacitracin (Baciguent)	20% bacitracin zinc ointment, apply 1-5 x/day.	Active vs. staph, strep & clostridium. Contact dermatitis occurs. Available without prescription.
Fusidic acid[Aus] ointment	2% ointment, apply tid	Available in Canada and Europe (Leo Laboratories). Active vs. S. aureus & S. pyogenes.
Mupirocin (Bactroban)	Skin cream or ointment 2%: Apply tid times 10 days. Nasal ointment 2%: apply bid times 5 days.	Skin cream: itch, burning, stinging 1-1.5%. Nasal: headache 9%, rhinitis 6%, respiratory congestion 5%. Not active vs. enterococci or gm-neg bacteria. Summary of resistance: CID 49:935, 2009. If large amounts used in azotemic pts, can accumulate polyethylene glycol (CID 49:1541, 2009).
Polymyxin B—Bacitracin (Polysporin)	5000 units/gm; 400 units/gm: Apply 1-4x/day	Polymyxin active vs. some gm-neg bacteria but not Proteus sp., Serratia sp. or gm-pos bacteria. See Bacitracin comment above. Available without prescription.
Polymyxin B—Bacitracin—Neomycin (Neosporin, triple antibiotic ointment (TAO))	5000 units/gm; 400 units/gm; 3.5 mg/gm. Apply 1-3x/day.	See Bacitracin and polymyxin B comments above. Neomycin active vs. some gm-neg bacteria and staphylococci; not active vs. streptococci. Contact dermatitis incidence 1%; risk of nephro- & oto-toxicity if absorbed. TAO spectrum broader than mupirocin and active mupirocin-resistant strains (DMID 54:63, 2006). Available without prescription.
Retapamulin (Altabax)	1% ointment; apply bid. 5, 10 & 15 gm tubes.	Microbiologic success in 90% S. aureus infections and 97% of S. pyogenes infections (J Am Acad Derm 55:1003, 2006). Package insert says **do not use for MRSA** (not enough pts in clinical trials). Active vs. some mupirocin-resistant S. aureus strains.
Silver sulfadiazine	1% cream, apply once or twice daily.	A sulfonamide but the active ingredient is released silver ions. Activity vs. gram-pos & gram-neg bacteria (including P. aeruginosa). Often used to prevent infection in pts with 2nd/3rd degree burns. Rarely, may stain into the skin.

* NOTE: all dosage recommendations are for adults (unless otherwise indicated) & assume normal renal function.

(See page 2 for abbreviations)

TABLE 10B – SELECTED ANTIBACTERIAL AGENTS—ADVERSE REACTIONS—OVERVIEW

Adverse reactions in individual patients represent all-or-none occurrences, even if rare. After selection of an agent, the physician should read the manufacturer's package insert [statements in the product labeling (package insert) must be approved by the FDA].

Numbers = frequency of occurrence (%); **+** = occurs, incidence not available; **++** = significant adverse reaction; **0** = not reported; **R** = rare, defined as <1%.

NOTE: Important reactions in bold print. A blank means no data found.

ADVERSE REACTIONS	PENICILLINASE-RESISTANT ANTI-STAPH. PENICILLINS			PENICILLINS, CARBAPENEMS, MONOBACTAMS, AMINOGLYCOSIDES										CARBAPENEMS					AMINOGLYCO-SIDES Amikacin Gentamicin Kanamycin Netilmicin[NUS] Tobramycin	MISC.	
				AMINOPENICILLINS			AP PENS											
	Penicillin G, V	Dicloxacillin	Nafcillin	Oxacillin	Amoxicillin	Amox-Clav	Ampicillin	Amp-Sulb	Piperacillin	Pip-Taz	Ticarcillin	Ticar-Clav	Doripenem	Ertapenem	Imipenem	Meropenem	Aztreonam		Linezolid	Telithromycin
Rx stopped due to AE	+					2-4.4		3		3.2			3.4			1.2	<1			
Hypersensitivity																	4			
Fever	+	+	++	+	+	+	+	+	+	4	3	+	4-8	4	3	3				
Rash	**3**	**4**	**4**	**4**	**5**	**3**	**5**	**2**	**1**	**4**	**3**	**2**	R	4	3	+	2	+	**3/1**	7/2
Photosensitivity	0	0	0	0	0	0	0	0	0	0	0	0	**1-5**	+	+	+	**2**		4	10
Anaphylaxis	0	R	R	R	R	+	R	+	R	+	+	+	R	+	+	+	+		+	+
Serum sickness	4					+			+	+	+	+					+			
Hematologic																				
↑ Coombs	3	0	R	R	+	0	+	0	+	+	0	+		1	2	+	R		1.1	
Neutropenia	R	+	0	0	+	0	+	+	6	7	+	+	R	2	+	+	+			
Eosinophilia	R	+	22	22	2	+	22	22	+	11	+	+	+	+	+	+	8			
Thrombocytopenia	R	0	R	R	R	R	R	R	R	+	R	R	+	+	+	+	+		3-10 (see IDC)	
↑ PT/PTT	R	0	+[1]	0	+	+	+	0	+	+	+	+			R		R			
GI																				
Nausea/vomiting		+	0	0	+	3	+	+	+	7	+	1	4-12	3	2	4	R		3/1	7/2
Diarrhea	+	+	0	0	**5**	**9**	**10**	**2**	2	11	3	1	6-11	6	2	5	R		4	10
C. difficile colitis	R	R	R	R	R	R	R	R	R	R	R	R	R	R	R	R	R		R	+
Hepatic, ↑ LFTs	R	R	0	+	R	+	6	6	0	+	+	0	+	6	4	4	2		1.3	+
Hepatic failure	0	0	0	0	0	0	0	0	0	0	0	0	0	0	0	0	0			
Renal: ↑ BUN, Cr	R	R	R	R	0	0	R	R	R	R	R	R	4-16	2	+	3	0	5-25[2]		
CNS																				
Headache	R	0	R	R	+	0	R	R	R	R	R	R	R	R	R	R	+		2	2
Confusion	R	0	R	R	0	0	R	R	+	+	R	R			R		+		+	

[1] A case of antagonism of warfarin effect has been reported (*Pharmacother* 27:1467, 2007).
[2] Varies with criteria used.

TABLE 10B (1)

ADVERSE REACTIONS

	PENICILLINS, CARBAPENEMS, MONOBACTAMS, AMINOGLYCOSIDES																			MISC.
	PENICILLINASE-RESISTANT ANTI-STAPH. PENICILLINS			AMINOPENICILLINS				AP PENS			CARBAPENEMS				MONOBACTAM	AMINOGLYCOSIDES				
ADVERSE REACTIONS	Penicillin G, V	Dicloxacillin	Nafcillin	Oxacillin	Amoxicillin	Amox-Clav	Ampicillin	Amp-Sulb	Piperacillin	Pip-Taz	Ticarcillin	Ticar-Clav	Doripenem	Ertapenem	Imipenem	Meropenem	Aztreonam	Amikacin Gentamicin Kanamycin Netilmicin[NUS] Tobramycin	Linezolid	Telithromycin
CNS (continued)																				
Seizures	R	0	0	0	0	0	0	0	0	0	0	0	0	0	See footnote[3]	0	+			
Special Senses																				
Ototoxicity	0	0	0	0	0	0	0	0	0	0	0	0			R		0	3–14[4]		
Vestibular	0	0	0	0	0	0	0	0	0	0	0	0					0	4–6[4]		
Cardiac																				
Dysrhythmias	R																			
Miscellaneous, Unique (table 10A)	+	+		+	+	+	+	+	+	+				+	+	+	+	+	+	+
Drug/drug interactions, common (table 22)	0	0	0	0	0	0	0	0	0	+	0	0		0	+	0	0		+	+

	CEPHALOSPORINS/CEPHAMYCINS																			
ADVERSE REACTIONS	Cefazolin	Cefotetan	Cefoxitin	Cefuroxime	Cefotaxime	Ceftazidime	Ceftizoxime	Ceftriaxone	Cefepime	Ceftaroline	Ceftobiprole[NUS]	Piperacillin... Ceftobiprole	Cefaclor/Cef.ER[5]/Loracarbef[NUS]	Cefadroxil	Cefdinir	Cefixime	Cefpodoxime	Cefprozil	Ceftibuten	Cefditoren pivoxil	Cefuroxime axetil	Cephalexin
Rx stopped due to AE	+	+		2	1	2		2	1.5	2.7	4				3		2.7	2	2	2	2.2	
Local, phlebitis	5	1	R	R	1	2	4	2	1	2	1.9		2					+				
Hypersensitivity																						
Fever	+	+			2	2	+		+		1.3			+	R	R	R	+	R	R	R	
Rash	+	2	R	R	2	2	R	R	2	3	2.7		1	+	1	1	1	1	R	R	R	1
Photosensitivity	0	0	0	0	0	0	0	0														

[3] **All β-lactams in high concentration can cause seizures** (JAC 45:5, 2000). In rabbit, IMP 10x more neurotoxic than benzyl penicillin (JAC 22:687, 1988). In clinical trial of IMP for pediatric meningitis, trial stopped due to seizures in 7/25 IMP recipients; hard to interpret as purulent meningitis causes seizures (PIDJ 10:122, 1991). Risk with IMP ↓ with careful attention to dosage (Epilepsia 42:1590, 2001). **Postulated mechanism**: Drug binding to GABA₍ receptor. IMP binds with greater affinity than MER.
Package insert, percent seizures: ERTA 0.5, IMP 0.4, MER 0.7. However, in 3 clinical trials of MER for bacterial meningitis, no drug-related seizures (Scand J Inf Dis 31:3, 1999; Drug Safety 22:191, 2000). In febrile neutropenic cancer pts., IMP-related seizures reported at 2% (CID 32:381, 2001; Peds Hem Onc 17:585, 2000). Also reported for DORI.
[4] Varies with criteria used.
[5] Cefaclor extended release tablets.

TABLE 10B (2)

CEPHALOSPORINS/CEPHAMYCINS

ADVERSE REACTIONS	Cefazolin	Cefotetan	Cefoxitin	Cefuroxime	Cefotaxime	Ceftazidime	Ceftizoxime	Ceftriaxone	Cefepime	Ceftaroline	Ceftobiprole[NUS]	Cefaclor/Cef.ER[6]/Loracarbef[NUS]	Cefadroxil	Cefdinir	Cefixime	Cefpodoxime	Cefprozil	Ceftibuten	Cefditoren pivoxil	Cefuroxime axetil	Cephalexin
Hypersensitivity (continued)																					
Anaphylaxis	R	+		R		R					R	R								R	+
Serum sickness												≤0.5[5]	+						R	R	+
Hematologic																					
+ Coombs	3	+	2	R	6	4		R	14	9.8		R							R	R	+
Neutropenia	+		2	R	+	+	+	+	1		+	+	+	R	R	R	R	6	R	R	3
Eosinophilia		+	3	7	1	8	+	6	1		+	1-4		15	16	7	3	2	6/1	2	9
Thrombocytopenia	+		1			1	+	2	+		+	2			+	3	2	5	1,4	1	
↑ PT/PTT		++			+	+	+	+	+	4/2	+					+	+	R	R	R	2
GI																					
Nausea/vomiting		1		R	R	R		R	1	5	+	3		3	13	4	4	6	3	R	
Diarrhea		4	3	R	1	1		3	1	9,1/4,8	+	2	+	7		7	3	2	14	4	2
C. difficile colitis	+	+	1	+	+	+	+	+	+	<1	+	1-4	+	15	+	+	+	3	+	+	
Hepatic: ↑ LFTs	+	1	3	4	6	1	4	3	+	2	+	3	+	1	+	4	2	R	R	2	+
Renal: ↑ BUN, Cr	+	+	1		0	0	0	1	0		R							R	R		+
CNS																					
Headache	0	0	0	0	0			R	2		4.5	3		2	4	1	4	2	R	R	R
Confusion	0	0	0	0	0							+								+	+
Seizures	0			0	0	0		0	+[7]		R										
Special Senses																					
Ototoxicity	0	0	0	0	0	0	0	0				0	0		0	0	0	0	0	0	0
Vestibular	0	0	0	0	0	0	0	0				0	0		0	0	0	0	0	0	0
Cardiac																					
Dysrhythmias	0	0	0	0	0	0	0	0				0	0		0	0	0	0	0	0	0
Miscellaneous, Unique (table 10A)									+		+	+							+		
Drug/drug interactions, common (table 22)	0	0	0	0	0	0	0	0	0			0	0		0	0	0	0	0	0	0

[6] Serum sickness requires biotransformation of parent drug plus inherited defect in metabolism of reactive intermediates (Ped Pharm & Therap, 125:805, 1994).
[7] FDA warning of seizure risk when dose not adjusted for renal insufficiency.

TABLE 10B (3)

ADVERSE REACTIONS	MACROLIDES			QUINOLONES						OTHER AGENTS										
	Azithromycin, Reg. & ER[a]	Clarithromycin, Reg. & ER[a]	Erythromycin	Ciprofloxacin/Cipro XR	Gatifloxacin[NUS]	Gemifloxacin	Levofloxacin	Moxifloxacin	Ofloxacin	Chloramphenicol	Clindamycin	Colistimethate (Colistin)	Daptomycin	Metronidazole	Quinupristin-dalfopristin	Rifampin	Telavancin	Tetracycline/Doxy/Mino	Tigecycline	TMP-SMX	Vancomycin
Rx stopped due to AE		3		3.5	2.9	2.2	4.3	3.8	4				2.8				3		5		
Local, phlebitis			++		5		0.1-1						6		++		3.1	R	2	2	13
Hypersensitivity			25													1				++	8
Fever										+	+	+	2			+		+	7	+	1
Rash	R		+	3	R	1-22[a]	2	R	2	+	+	+	4	+	R	+	4	+	2.4	+	3
Photosensitivity	R			R	R	R	+	R	R		4		4					+	+	+	0
Anaphylaxis			+	R	R	+	+		R		+			R					+		R
Serum sickness											+							R			
Hematologic																					
Neutropenia	R	1		R	R				1	+	+			+				R			2
Eosinophilia				R			+				+					+		+		+	+
Thrombocytopenia	R	R				0.1-1				+				R				+		+	+
↑ PT/PTT		1																	4		0
GI			++																		
Nausea/vomiting	3	3[10]		5	8/<3	2.7	7/2	7/2	7	+	+	+	6.3	12	++	+	27/14	+	30/20	3	+
Diarrhea	5	3-6	8	2	4	3.6	5	5	4	+	7	+	5	+		+	7	+	13	3	+
C. difficile colitis		R		R	R	R	R	R	R		R					R	R	+		+	+
Hepatic, ↑ LFTs	R	R	R	2	R	1.5	0.1-1	R	2		++		+		2	+		+	4	+	0
Hepatic failure	0	R	R				+									+					0
Renal																					
↑ BUN, Cr	+	4		1					R		0	++	R			+	3		2	+	5
CNS													++								
Dizziness, light headedness				R	3	0.8	3	2	3								3.1		3.5		
Headache	R	2		1	4	1.2	6	2	2	+	+		5	+		+		+		+	
Confusion			+	+	R	R	R	R	R	+				+						+	
Seizures				+	+	0.1-1	0.1-1	0.1-1	R	+				+						+	

[a] Regular and extended-release formulations.
[9] **Highest frequency**: females <40 years of age after 14 days of rx; with 5 days or less of Gemi; incidence of rash <1.5%.
[10] Less GI upset/abnormal taste with ER formulation.

TABLE 10B (4)

ADVERSE REACTIONS	MACROLIDES			QUINOLONES					OTHER AGENTS											
	Azithromycin, Reg. & ER[a]	Clarithromycin, Reg. & ER[a]	Erythromycin	Ciprofloxacin/Cipro XR	Gatifloxacin[NUS]	Gemifloxacin	Levofloxacin	Moxifloxacin	Ofloxacin	Chloramphenicol	Clindamycin	Colistimethate (Colistin)	Daptomycin	Metronidazole	Quinupristin-dalfopristin	Rifampin	Telavancin	Tetracycline/Doxy/Mino	Tigecycline	TMP-SMX	Vancomycin
Special senses																					
Ototoxicity	+			0					0												R
Vestibular																		21[11]			0
Cardiac																					
Dysrhythmias	+	+	+	R	+[12]	+[12]	R[12]	+[12]	+[12]		R										+
Miscellaneous, Unique (Table 10A)	+	+	+	+	+	+	+	+	+	+	+	+	+	+	+	+	+	+	+	+	+
Drug/drug interactions, common (table 22)	+	+	+	+	+	+	+	+	+						++	++		+		+	+

TABLE 10C – ANTIMICROBIAL AGENTS ASSOCIATED WITH PHOTOSENSITIVITY

The following drugs are known to cause photosensitivity in some individuals. There is no intent to indicate relative frequency or severity of reactions.
Source: 2007 Red Book, Thomson Healthcare, Inc. Listed in alphabetical order:

Azithromycin, benznidazole, ciprofloxacin, dapsone, doxycycline, erythromycin ethyl succinate, flucytosine, ganciclovir, gatifloxacin, gemifloxacin, griseofulvin, interferons, lomefloxacin, ofloxacin, pyrazinamide, saquinavir, sulfonamides, tetracyclines, tigecycline, tretinoin, voriconazole

[11] Minocycline has 21% vestibular toxicity.
[12] Fluoroquinolones as class are associated **with QT$_c$ prolongation**. Ref.: *CID 34:861, 2002*.

TABLE 10D – AMINOGLYCOSIDE ONCE-DAILY AND MULTIPLE DAILY DOSING REGIMENS
(See Table 17, page 205, if estimated creatinine clearance <90 mL per min.)

- General Note: dosages are given as once daily dose (OD) and multiple daily doses (MDD).
- For **calculation of dosing weight in non-obese patients** use **Ideal Body Weight (IBW):**
  Female: 45.5 kg + 2.3 kg per inch over 60 inch height = dosing weight in kg
  Male: 50 kg + 2.3 kg per inch over 60 inch height = dosing weight in kg
- **Adjustment for calculation of dosing weight in obese patients** (actual body weight (ABW) is ≥ 30% above IBW): IBW + 0.4 (ABW minus IBW) = adjusted weight (*Pharmacotherapy 27:1081, 2007; CID 25:112, 1997*).
- If CrCl >90 mL/min, use doses in this table. If CrCl <90, use doses in Table 17, page 205.

- For non-obese patients, calculate estimated creatinine clearance (CrCl) as follows:
$$\frac{(140 - \text{age}) \times \text{IBW (in kg)}}{72 \times \text{serum creatinine}} = \begin{array}{l}\text{CrCl in mL/min for men.}\\ \text{Multiply answer by 0.85}\\ \text{for women (estimated)}\end{array}$$

- **For morbidly obese patients, calculate estimated creatinine clearance (CrCl)** as follows (*AJM 84:1053, 1988*):
$$\frac{(137 - \text{age}) \times [(0.285 \times \text{wt in kg}) + (12.1 \times \text{ht in meters}^2)]}{51 \times \text{serum creatinine}} = \text{CrCl (obese male)}$$
$$\frac{(146 - \text{age}) \times [(0.287 \times \text{wt in kg}) + (9.74 \times \text{ht in meters}^2)]}{60 \times \text{serum creatinine}} = \text{CrCl (obese female)}$$

DRUG	MDD AND OD IV REGIMENS/ TARGETED PEAK (P) AND TROUGH (T) SERUM LEVELS	COMMENTS For more data on once-daily dosing, see AAC 55:2528, 2011 and Table 17, page 204
Gentamicin (Garamycin), **Tobramycin** (Nebcin)	MDD: 2 mg per kg load, then 1.7 mg per kg q8h P 4–10 mcg/mL, T 1–2 mcg per mL OD: 5.1 (7 if critically ill) mg per kg q24h P 16–24 mcg per mL, T <1 mcg per mL	All aminoglycosides have potential to cause tubular necrosis and renal failure, deafness due to cochlear toxicity, vertigo due to damage to vestibular organs, and rarely neuromuscular blockade. Risk minimal with oral or topical application due to small % absorption unless tissues altered by disease. Risk of nephrotoxicity ↑ with concomitant administration of cyclosporine, vancomycin, amphotericin B, radiocontrast. Risk of nephrotoxicity ↓ by concomitant AP Pen and perhaps by once-daily dosing method (especially if baseline renal function normal). In general, same factors influence risk of ototoxicity. **NOTE: There is no known method to eliminate risk of aminoglycoside nephro/ototoxicity. Proper rx attempts to ↓ the % risk.** The clinical final data of OD aminoglycosides have been reviewed extensively by meta-analysis (*CID 24:816, 1997*). **Serum levels:** Collect peak serum level (PSL) exactly 1 hr after the start of the IV infusion of the 3rd dose. In critically ill pts, PSL after the 1st dose as volume of distribution and renal function may change rapidly. Other dosing methods and references: For once-daily 7 mg per kg per day of gentamicin—Hartford Hospital method (may under dose if <7 mg/kg/day dose), see *AAC 39:650, 1995*. One in 500 patients (Europe) have mitochondrial mutation that predicts cochlear toxicity (*NEJM 360:640 & 642, 2009*). Aspirin supplement (3 gm/day) attenuated risk of cochlear injury from gentamicin (*NEJM 354:1856, 2006*).
Kanamycin (Kantrex), **Amikacin** (Amikin), Streptomycin	MDD: 7.5 mg per kg q12h P 15–30 mcg per mL, T 5–10 mcg per mL OD: 15 mg per kg q24h P 56–64 mcg per mL, T <1 mcg per mL	
Netilmicin[NUS]	MDD: 2 mg per kg q8h P 4–10 mcg per mL, T 1–2 mcg per mL OD: 6.5 mg per kg q24h P 22–30 mcg per mL, T <1 mcg per mL	
Isepamicin[NUS]	Only OD: Severe infections 15 mg per kg q24h, less severe 8 mg per kg q24h	
Spectinomycin (Trobicin)[NUS]	2 gm IM times 1-gonococcal infections	
Neomycin—oral	Prophylaxis GI surgery: 1 gm po times 3 with erythro, see Table 15B, page 193 For hepatic coma: 4–12 gm per day po	
Tobramycin—inhaled (Tobi): See Cystic fibrosis, Table 1, page 43. Adverse effects few: transient voice alteration (13%) and transient tinnitus (3%)		
Paromomycin—oral: See *Entamoeba and Cryptosporidia*, Table 13A, page 141.		

TABLE 10E: PROLONGED OR CONTINUOUS INFUSION DOSING OF SELECTED BETA LACTAMS

Based on current and rapidly changing data, it appears that prolonged or continuous infusion of beta-lactams is at least as successful as intermittent dosing. Hence, this approach can be part of stewardship programs as supported by recent publications.

A meta-analysis of observational studies found reduced mortality among patients treated with extended or continuous infusion of carbapenems or piperacillin-tazobactam (pooled data) as compared to standard intermittent regimens. The results were similar for extended and continuous regimens when considered separately. There was a mortality benefit with piperacillin-tazobactam but not carbapenems (CID 56:272, 2013). The lower mortality could, at least in part, be due to closer professional supervision engendered by a study environment. On the other hand, a small prospective randomized controlled study of continuous vs. intermittent pip-tazo, ticar-clav, and meropenem found a higher clinical cure rate and a trend toward lower mortality in the continuous infusion patients (CID 56:236, 2013).

DRUG	MINIMUM STABILITY (AT ROOM TEMP)	RECOMMENDED DOSE	COMMENTS
Cefepime	24 hr (8 hr at 37°C)	Initial dose: 15 mg/kg over 30 min, then immediately begin: • If CrCl > 60: 6 gm (over 24 hr) daily • If CrCl 30-60: 4 gm (over 24 hr) daily • If CrCl 11-29: 2 gm (over 24 hr) daily	CrCl adjustments extrapolated from prescribing information, not clinical data. Refs: JAC 57:1017, 2006; Am. J. Health-Syst. Pharm. 68:319, 2011.
Ceftazidime	24 hr (8 hr at 37°C)	Initial dose: 15 mg/kg over 30 min, then immediately begin: • If CrCl > 50: 6 gm (over 24 hr) daily • If CrCl 31-50: 4 gm (over 24 hr) daily • If CrCl 10-30: 2 gm (over 24 hr) daily	CrCl adjustments extrapolated from prescribing information, not clinical data. Refs: Br J Clin Pharmacol 50:184, 2001; IJAA 17:497, 2001; AAC 49:3550, 2005; Infect 37: 418, 2009.
Doripenem	4 hr (in D5W) 12 hr (in NS)	• If CrCl ≥ 50: 500 mg (over 4 hr) q8h • If CrCl 30-49: 250 mg (over 4 hr) q8h • If CrCl 10-29:250 mg (over 4 hr) q12h	Based on a single study (Crit Care Med 36:1089, 2008).
Meropenem	4 hrs	• If CrCl ≥ 50: 2 gm (over 3 hr) q8h • If CrCl 30-49: 1 gm (over 3 hr) q8h • If CrCl 10-29: 1 gm (over 3 hr) q12h	Initial 1 gm dose reasonable but not used by most investigators. Ref: Intens Care Med 37:632, 2011.
Pip-Tazo	24 hr	Initial dose: 4.5 gm over 30 min, then 4 hrs later start: • If CrCl ≥ 20: 3.375 gm (over 4 hr) q8h • If CrCl < 20: 3.375 gm (over 4 hr) q12h	Reasonable to begin first infusion 4 hrs after initial dose. Refs: CID 44:357, 2007; AAC 54:460, 2010. See CID 56:236, 245 & 272, 2013.

TABLE 11A – TREATMENT OF FUNGAL INFECTIONS—ANTIMICROBIAL AGENTS OF CHOICE*

TYPE OF INFECTION/ORGANISM/ SITE OF INFECTION	ANTIMICROBIAL AGENTS OF CHOICE PRIMARY	ALTERNATIVE	COMMENTS
Aspergillosis (A. fumigatus most common, also A. flavus and others). (See NEJM 360:1870, 2009 for excellent review.)			
Allergic bronchopulmonary aspergillosis (ABPA) Clinical manifestations: wheezing, pulmonary infiltrates, bronchiectasis & fibrosis. Airway colonization assoc. with ↑ blood eosinophils, ↑ serum IgE, ↑ specific serum antibodies.	Acute asthma attacks associated Rx of ABPA: **Corticosteroids** with ABPA. **Corticosteroids**	**Itraconazole** 200 mg po bid times 16 wks or longer	Itra decreases number of exacerbations requiring corticosteroids with improved immunological markers improved lung function & exercise tolerance (IDSA Guidelines updated CID 46:327, 2008).
Allergic fungal sinusitis: relapsing chronic sinusitis; nasal polyps without bony invasion; asthma, eczema or allergic rhinitis; ↑ IgE levels and isolation of Aspergillus sp. or other dematiaceous sp. (Alternaria, Cladosporium, etc.)	**Rx controversial:** systemic corticosteroids + surgical debridement (relapse common).	For failures try Itra 200 mg po bid times 12 mos or flucon nasal spray.	Controversial area.
Aspergilloma (fungus ball)	No therapy or surgical resection. Efficacy of antimicrobial agents not proven.		Aspergillus may complicate pulmonary sequestration.
Invasive, pulmonary (IPA) or extrapulmonary: (See Am. J. Respir Crit Care Med 173:707, 2006). Good website:doctorfungus.org Post-transplantation and post-chemotherapy in neutropenic pts (PMN <500 per mm³) but may also present with neutrophil recovery. Most common pneumonia in transplant recipients. Usually a late (>10 days) complication in allogeneic bone marrow & liver transplantation. High mortality (CID 44:531, 2007). **Typical x-ray/CT lung lesions** (halo sign, cavitation, or macronodules) (CID 44:373, 2007). Initiation of antifungal Rx based on halo signs on CT associated with better response to Rx & improved outcome. **galactomannan** is available for dx of invasive aspergillosis (Lancet ID 4:349, 2005). Galactomannan detection in the blood relatively insensitive; antifungal rx may decrease sensitivity (CID 40:1762, 2005). One study suggests improved sensitivity when performed on BAL fluid (Am J Respir Crit Care Med 177:27, 2008). **False-positive** galactomannan test seen with use of **Pip-TZ & AM-CL**. Numerous other causes of false positive galactomannan tests reported. For strengths & weaknesses of the test see CID 42:1417, 2006. Posaconazole superior to Flu or Itra with fewer invasive fungal infections and improved survival in patients with hematologic malignancies undergoing induction chemotherapy (NEJM 356:348, 2007).	**Primary therapy** (See CID 46:327, 2008): **Voriconazole** 6 mg/kg IV q12h on day 1; then either (4 mg/kg IV q12h) or (200 mg po q12h for body weight ≥40 kg, but 100 mg po q12h for body weight <40 kg) **Alternative therapies:** **Liposomal ampho B** (L-AmB) 3-5 mg/kg/day IV; OR **Ampho B lipid complex** (ABLC) 5 mg/kg/d IV; OR **Caspofungin** 70 mg/day then 50 mg/day thereafter; OR **Micafungin**^NAI 100 mg bid (JAC 64:840, 2009- based on PK/PD study); OR **Posaconazole**^NAI 200 mg qid, then 400 mg bid after stabilization of disease; OR **Itraconazole** capsules 600 mg/day for 3 days, then 400 mg/day (or 2.5 mg/kg of oral solution once daily).		**Voriconazole** more effective than ampho B. Vori, both a substrate and an inhibitor of CYP2C19, CYP2C9, and CYP3A4, has potential for deleterious drug interactions (e.g., with protease inhibitors) and careful review of concomitant medications is mandatory. Measurement of serum concentrations advisable with prolonged therapy or for patients with possible drug-drug interactions. In patients with CrCl <50 mL/min, the drug should be given orally, not IV, since the intravenous vehicle (SBECD-sulfobutylether-B cyclodextrin) may accumulate. **Ampho B: not recommended except as a lipid formulation**, either L-AMB or ABLC. 10 mg/kg and 3 mg/kg doses of L-AmB are equally efficacious with greater toxicity of higher dose (CID 2007; 44:1289-97). One comparative trial found much greater toxicity with ABLC than with L-AMB: 34.6% vs 9.4% adverse events and 21.2% vs 2.8% nephrotoxicity (Cancer 112(1282, 2008). Vori preferred as primary therapy. **Caspo**—50% response rate in IPA. Licensed for salvage therapy. Efavirenz, nelfinavir, nevirapine, phenytoin, rifampin, dexamethasone, and carbamazepine, may reduce caspofungin concentrations. **Micafungin:** Favorable responses to micafungin as a single agent in 6/12 patients in primary therapy group and 9/22 in the salvage therapy group of an open-label, non-comparative trial (J Infect 53: 337, 2006). Outcomes no better with combination therapy. Few significant drug-drug interactions. (Continued on next page)

* Oral solution preferred to tablets because of ↑ absorption (see Table 11B, page 124).

See page 2 for abbreviations. All dosage recommendations are for adults (unless otherwise indicated) and assume normal renal function

TABLE 11A (2)

TYPE OF INFECTION/ORGANISM/ SITE OF INFECTION	ANTIMICROBIAL AGENTS OF CHOICE		COMMENTS
	PRIMARY	ALTERNATIVE	
Aspergillosis (continued from previous page)			(Continued from previous page)
			Itraconazole: Licensed for treatment of invasive aspergillosis in patients refractory to or intolerant of standard antifungal therapy. Itraconazole formulated as capsules, oral solution in hydroxypropyl-beta-cyclodextrin (HPCD), and parenteral solution with HPCD as a solubilizer; oral solution and parenteral formulation not licensed for treatment of invasive aspergillosis. 2.5 mg/kg oral solution provides dose equivalent to 400 mg capsules. Parenteral HPCD formulation dosage is 200 mg every 12h IV for 2 days, followed by 200 mg daily thereafter. Oral absorption of capsules enhanced by low gastric pH, erratic in fasting state and with hypochlorhydria, measurements of plasma concentrations recommended during oral therapy of invasive aspergillosis; target troughs concentrations > 0.25 mcg/mL. Itraconazole is a substrate of CYP3A4 and non-competitive inhibitor of CYP3A4 with potential for significant drug-drug interactions. Do not use for azole-non-responders. **Combo therapy:** Uncertain role and not routinely recommended for primary therapy; consider for treatment of refractory disease, although benefit unproven. A typical combo regimen would be an echinocandin in combination with either an azole or a lipid formulation of ampho B.
Blastomycosis (CID 46: 1801; 2008) (Blastomyces dermatitidis) Cutaneous, pulmonary or extrapulmonary	**LAB,** 3-5 mg/kg per day, OR **Ampho B,** 0.7-1 mg/kg per day, for 1-2 weeks, **then Itra** 200 mg tid for 3 days followed by Itra 200 mg bid for 6-12 months **LAB** 5 mg/kg per day for 4-6 weeks, followed by **Flu** 800 mg per day	**Itra** 200 mg tid for 3 days then once or twice per day for 6-12 months for mild to moderate disease; OR **Flu** 400-800 mg per day for those intolerant to Itra	Serum levels of **Itra** should be determined after 2 weeks to ensure adequate drug exposure. Flu less effective than itra; role of vori or posa unclear but active in vitro.
Blastomycosis: CNS disease (CID 50:797, 2010)		**Itra** 200 mg tid or tid; OR **Vori** 200-400 mg q12h	Flu and vori have excellent CNS penetration, perhaps counterbalance their slightly reduced activity compared to Itra. Treat for at least 12 months and until CSF has normalized. Document serum Itra levels to assure adequate drug concentrations. Recent study suggests more favorable outcome with Voriconazole (CID 50:797, 2010).

[a] **Oral solution preferred to tablets because of ↑ absorption** (see Table 11B, page 124).

See page 2 for abbreviations. All dosage recommendations are for adults (unless otherwise indicated) and assume normal renal function

112

TABLE 11A (3)

TYPE OF INFECTION/ORGANISM/ SITE OF INFECTION	ANTIMICROBIAL AGENTS OF CHOICE		COMMENTS
	PRIMARY	ALTERNATIVE	
Candidiasis: Candida is a common cause of nosocomial bloodstream infection. A decrease in C. albicans & increase in non-albicans species show ↓ susceptibility among candida species to antifungal agents (esp. fluconazole). These changes have predominantly affected immunocompromised pts in environments where antifungal prophylaxis (esp. fluconazole) is widely used. Oral, esophageal, or vaginal candidiasis is a major manifestation of advanced HIV & represents one of the most common AIDS-defining diagnoses. See CID 48:503, 2009 for updated IDSA Guidelines.			
Candidiasis: Bloodstream infection			
Bloodstream: non-neutropenic patient Remove all intravascular catheters (if possible; replace catheters at a new site (not over a wire). Higher mortality associated with delay in therapy (CID 43:25, 2006).	**Caspofungin** 70 mg IV loading dose, then 50 mg IV daily, OR **Micafungin** 100 mg IV daily, OR **Anidulafungin** 200 mg IV loading dose then 100 mg IV daily.	**Fluconazole** 800 mg (12 mg/kg) loading dose, then 400 mg daily PO OR **PO Lipid-based ampho B** 3-5 mg/kg IV daily, OR **Ampho B** 0.7 mg/kg IV daily, OR **Voriconazole** 400 mg (6 mg/kg) twice daily for 2 doses then 200 mg q12h.	**Fluconazole** recommended for patients with mild-to-moderate illness, hemodynamically stable, with no recent azole exposure. Fluconazole not recommended for treatment of documented C. krusei; use an echinocandin or voriconazole or posaconazole (note: echinocandins have better in vitro activity than either vori or posa against C. glabrata). Fluconazole recommended for treatment of Candida parapsilosis because of reduced susceptibility of this species to echinocandins. Transition from echinocandin to fluconazole for stable patients with Candida albicans or other azole-susceptible species. **Echinocandin** for patients with recent azole exposure or with moderately severe or severe illness, hemodynamic instability. An echinocandin should be used for treatment of Candida glabrata unless susceptibility to fluconazole or voriconazole has been confirmed. Echinocandin may be preferred empirical therapy in centers with high prevalence of non-albicans candida species. A double-blind randomized trial of anidulafungin (n=127) and fluconazole (n=118) showed an 88% microbiologic response rate (119/135 candida species) with anidulafungin vs a 76% (95/130 candida species) with fluconazole (p=0.02) (NEJM 356: 2472, 2007). **Voriconazole** with little advantage over fluconazole (more drug-drug interactions) except for oral step-down therapy of Candida krusei or voriconazole-susceptible Candida glabrata. Recommended **duration of therapy** is 14 days after last positive blood culture. Duration of systemic therapy should be extended to 4-6 weeks for eye involvement. **Funduscopic examination** within first week of therapy to exclude ophthalmic involvement. Ocular findings present in ~15% of patients with candidemia, but endophthalmitis is uncommon (~2%) (CID 53:262, 2011). Intraocular injections of ampho B may be required for endophthalmitis; echinocandins have poor penetration into the eye. For **septic thrombophlebitis**, catheter removal and incision and drainage and resection of the vein, as needed, are recommended; duration of therapy at least 2 weeks after last positive blood culture.

See page 2 for abbreviations. All dosage recommendations are for adults (unless otherwise indicated) and assume normal renal function

TABLE 11A (4)

TYPE OF INFECTION/ORGANISM/ SITE OF INFECTION	ANTIMICROBIAL AGENTS OF CHOICE PRIMARY	ALTERNATIVE	COMMENTS
Candidiasis: Bloodstream Infection (continued)			
Bloodstream: neutropenic patient Remove all intravascular catheters if possible; replace catheters at a new site (not over a wire)	**Caspofungin** 70 mg IV loading dose, then 50 mg IV daily, 35 mg for moderate hepatic insufficiency; OR **Micafungin** 100 mg IV daily; OR **Anidulafungin** 200 mg IV loading dose then 100 mg daily; OR **Lipid-based ampho B** 3-5 mg/kg IV daily.	**Fluconazole** 800 mg IV loading dose, then 400 mg daily IV or PO, OR **Voriconazole** 400 mg (6 mg/kg) twice daily for 2 doses then 200 mg (3 mg/kg) q12h.	Fluconazole may be considered for less critically ill patients without recent azole exposure. Duration of therapy in absence of metastatic complications is for 2 weeks after last positive blood culture, resolution of signs, and resolution of neutropenia. Perform fundoscopic examination after recovery of white count as signs of ophthalmic involvement may not be seen during neutropenia. See comments above for recommendations concerning choice of specific agents.
Candidiasis: Bone and Joint Infections			
Osteomyelitis	**Fluconazole** 400 mg (6 mg/kg) daily IV or PO; OR **Lipid-based ampho B** 3-5 mg/kg daily for several weeks, then oral fluconazole.	An **echinocandin** (as above) or **ampho B** 0.5-1 mg/kg daily for several weeks then oral **fluconazole**.	Treat for a total of 6-12 months. **Surgical debridement** often necessary; **remove hardware** whenever possible.
Septic arthritis	**Fluconazole** 400 mg (6 mg/kg) daily IV or PO; OR **Lipid-based ampho B** 3-5 mg/kg daily for several weeks, then oral fluconazole.	An **echinocandin** or **ampho B** 0.5-1 mg/kg daily for several weeks then oral **fluconazole**.	**Surgical debridement** in all cases; removal of prosthetic joints whenever possible. Treat for at least 6 weeks and indefinitely if retained hardware.
Candidiasis: Cardiovascular Infections			
Endocarditis (See Eur J Clin Microbiol Infect Dis 27;519, 2008)	An **echinocandin**: **Caspofungin** 50-150 mg/day; OR **Micafungin** 100-150 mg/day; OR **Anidulafungin** 100-200 mg/day; OR **Lipid-based ampho B** 3-5 mg/kg daily + **5-FC** 25 mg/kg qid	**Ampho B** 0.6-1 mg/kg daily + **5-FC** 25 mg/kg qid	Consider use of higher doses of echinocandins for endocarditis or other endovascular infections. Can switch to **fluconazole 400-800 mg orally in stable patients** with negative blood cultures and fluconazole susceptible organism. See Med 90:237, 2011 for review of Fluconazole for Candida endocarditis. Valve replacement strongly recommended, particularly in those with prosthetic valve endocarditis. Duration of therapy not well defined, but treat for at least 6 weeks after valve replacement and longer in those with complications (e.g., perivalvular or myocardial abscess, extensive disease, delayed resolution of candidemia). Long-term (life-long?) suppression with fluconazole 400-800 mg daily for native valve endocarditis and no valve replacement; life-long suppression for prosthetic valve endocarditis if no valve replacement.
Myocarditis	**Lipid-based ampho B** 3-5 mg/kg daily; OR **Fluconazole** 400-800 mg (6-12 mg/kg) daily IV or PO; OR **An echinocandin** (see endocarditis).		Can switch to **fluconazole 400-800 mg orally in stable patients** with negative blood cultures and fluconazole susceptible organism. Recommended duration of therapy is for several months.

See page 2 for abbreviations. All dosage recommendations are for adults (unless otherwise indicated) and assume normal renal function

TABLE 11A (5)

TYPE OF INFECTION/ORGANISM/ SITE OF INFECTION	ANTIMICROBIAL AGENTS OF CHOICE — PRIMARY	ALTERNATIVE	COMMENTS
Candidiasis: Cardiovascular infections *(continued)*			
Pericarditis	**Lipid-based ampho B** 3–5 mg/kg daily, OR **Fluconazole** 400–800 mg (6–12 mg/kg) daily IV or PO; OR **An echinocandin** (see endocarditis)		**Pericardial window or pericardiectomy** also is recommended. Can switch to **fluconazole 400-800 mg orally in stable patients** with negative blood cultures and fluconazole susceptible organism. Recommended duration of therapy is for several months.
Candidiasis: Mucosal, esophageal, and oropharyngeal			
Candida esophagitis Primarily encountered in HIV-positive patients	**Fluconazole** 200–400 (3-6 mg/kg) mg daily, OR **An echinocandin (caspofungin** 50 mg IV daily, OR **micafungin** 150 mg IV daily, OR **anidulafungin** 200 mg IV loading dose then 100 mg IV daily); OR **Ampho B** 0.5-0.7 mg/kg daily.	An azole (**itraconazole** solution 200 mg daily, or **posaconazole** suspension 400 mg bid for 3 days then 400 mg daily, or **voriconazole** 200 mg q12h.	**Duration of therapy** 14-21 days. IV echinocandin or ampho B for patients unable to tolerate oral therapy. For fluconazole refractory disease, itra (80% will respond), posa, vori, an echinocandin, or ampho B. Echinocandins associated with higher relapse rate than fluconazole. ARV therapy recommended. Suppressive therapy with fluconazole 200 mg 3x/wk for recurrent infections. Suppressive therapy may be discontinued once CD4 > 200/mm³.
Oropharyngeal candidiasis Non-AIDS patient	**Clotrimazole troches** 10 mg 5 times daily; OR **Nystatin suspension** or pastilles qid; OR **Fluconazole** 100-200 mg daily.	**Itraconazole** solution 200 mg daily OR **posaconazole** suspension 400 mg bid for 3 days then 400 mg daily; or **voriconazole** 200 mg q12h; OR an echinocandin (**caspofungin** 70 mg IV loading dose then 50 mg IV daily, or **micafungin** 100 mg IV daily, or **anidulafungin** 200 mg IV loading dose then 100 mg IV daily); OR **Ampho B** 0.3 mg/kg daily.	**Duration of therapy** 7-14 days. Clotrimazole or nystatin recommended for mild disease; fluconazole preferred for moderate-to-severe disease. Alternative agents reserved for refractory disease.
AIDS patient	**Fluconazole** 100-200 mg daily for 7-14 days.	Same as for non-AIDS patient, above, for 7-14 days.	Antiretroviral therapy (ARV) recommended in HIV-positive patients to prevent recurrent disease. Suppressive therapy not necessary, especially with ARV therapy and CD4 > 200/mm³, but if required fluconazole 100 mg thrice weekly recommended. Itra, posa, or vori for 28 days for fluconazole-refractory disease. IV echinocandin also an option. Dysphagia or odynophagia predictive of esophageal candidiasis.

See page 2 for abbreviations. All dosage recommendations are for adults (unless otherwise indicated) and assume normal renal function

TABLE 11A (6)

TYPE OF INFECTION/ORGANISM/ SITE OF INFECTION	ANTIMICROBIAL AGENTS OF CHOICE		COMMENTS
	PRIMARY	ALTERNATIVE	
Candidiasis: Mucosal, esophageal, and oropharyngeal *(continued)*			
Vulvovaginitis Non-AIDS Patient	**Topical azole therapy: Butoconazole 2% cream** (5 gm) q24h at bedtime x 3 days or 2% cream SR 5 gm x 1; OR **Clotrimazole 100 mg vaginal tabs** (2 at bedtime x 3 days) or 1% cream (5 gm) at bedtime times 7 days (14 days may ↑ cure rate) or 100 mg vaginal tab x 7 days or 500 mg vaginal tab x 1; OR **Miconazole 200 mg vaginal suppos** (1 at bedtime x 3 days) or 100 mg vaginal suppos. q24h x 7 days or 2% cream (5 gm) at bedtime x 7 days; OR **Terconazole 80 mg vaginal tab** (1 at bedtime x 3 days) or 0.4% cream (5 gm) at bedtime x 7 days or 0.8% cream 5 gm intravaginal q24h x 3 days; or tioconazole 6.5% vag. ointment x 1 dose **Oral therapy: Fluconazole 150 mg po x 1**; OR **Itraconazole 200 mg po q24h x 1 day**.		**Recurrent vulvovaginal candidiasis:** fluconazole 150 mg weekly for 6 months.
AIDS Patient	Topical **azoles** (clotrimazole, buto, mico, tico, or tercon) x3-7d; OR Topical **nystatin** 100,000 units/day as vaginal tablet x14d; OR Oral **flu** 150 mg x1 dose.	**Fluconazole 200 mg po q24h x 14 days**	For recurrent disease 10-14 days of topical azole or oral flu 150 mg, then flu 150 mg weekly for 6 mos.
Candidiasis: Other infections CNS Infection	Lipid-based ampho B 3-5 mg/kg daily ± 5-FC 25 mg/kg qid.	Fluconazole 400-800 mg (6-12 mg/kg) IV or PO.	Removal of **intraventricular devices** recommended. Flu 400-800 mg as step-down therapy in the stabile patient and in patient intolerant of ampho B. Experience too limited to recommend echinocandins at this time. **Treatment duration** for several weeks until resolution of CSF, radiographic, and clinical abnormalities.
Cutaneous *(including paronychia, Table 1, page 28)*	Apply topical ampho B, clotrimazole, econazole, miconazole, or nystatin 3-4 x daily for 7-14 days or ketoconazole 400 mg po once daily x 14 days. Ciclopirox olamine 1% cream/lotion, apply topically bid x 7-14 days.		
Disseminated candidiasis	Fluconazole 400 mg (6 mg/kg) daily IV or PO; OR Lipid-based ampho B 3-5 mg/kg daily; OR echinocandin (as for bloodstream infection)	Ampho B 0.5-0.7 mg/kg daily.	Ampho B recommended for **unstable patients;** flu in stabile patients. **Step-down** to oral flu once patient is stabilized. Other azoles may also be effective. Treatment, usually for several months, should be continued until lesions have resolved and during periods of immunosuppression.
Endophthalmitis • Occurs in 10% of candidemia, thus ophthalmological consult for all pts • Diagnosis: typical white exudates on retinal exam and/or isolation by vitrectomy	Ampho B 0.7-1 mg/kg daily + Flucytosine 25 mg/kg qid; OR Fluconazole 6-12 mg/kg daily.	Lipid-based ampho B 3-5 mg/kg daily, OR voriconazole 6 mg/kg q12h for 2 doses, then 3-4 mg/kg q12h	**Duration of therapy**: 4-6 weeks or longer, based on resolution determined by repeated examinations. Patients with chorioretinitis only often respond to systemically administered antifungals. Intravitreal amphotericin and/or vitrectomy may be necessary for those with vitritis or endophthalmitis (*Br J Ophthalmol* 92:466, 2008; *Pharmacotherapy* 27:1711, 2007).

See page 2 for abbreviations. All dosage recommendations are for adults (unless otherwise indicated) and assume normal renal function

TABLE 11A (7)

TYPE OF INFECTION/ORGANISM/ SITE OF INFECTION	ANTIMICROBIAL AGENTS OF CHOICE PRIMARY	ALTERNATIVE	COMMENTS
Candidiasis: Other infections *(continued)*			
Neonatal candidiasis	Ampho B 1 mg/kg daily; OR Fluconazole 12 mg/kg daily.	Lipid-based ampho B 3-5 mg/kg daily.	**Lumbar puncture** to rule out CNS disease, **dilated retinal examination**, and **intravascular catheter removal** strongly recommended. Lipid-based ampho B used only if there is no renal involvement. Echinocandins considered 3rd line therapy. Duration of therapy is at least 3 weeks.
Peritonitis (Chronic Ambulatory Peritoneal Dialysis) See *Table 19, page 213*.	Fluconazole 400 mg po q24h x 2-3 wks, or **caspofungin** 70 mg IV on day 1 followed by 50 mg IV q24h for 14 days; or **micafungin** 100 mg q24h for 14 days.	**Ampho B**, continuous intraperitoneal dosing at 1.5 mg/L of dialysis fluid times 4-6 wks.	Remove cath immediately or if no clinical improvement in 4-7 days.
Candidiasis: Urinary tract infections			
Cystitis Asymptomatic See *CID 52:s427, 2011; CID 52:s452, 2011*.	If possible, remove catheter or stent. No therapy indicated except in patients at high risk for dissemination or undergoing a urologic procedure.		**High risk** patients include neonates and neutropenic patients; these patients should be managed as outlined for treatment of bloodstream infection. For patients undergoing urologic procedures, flu 200 mg (3 mg/kg) daily or ampho B 0.5 mg/kg daily (for flu-resistant organisms) for several days pre- and post-procedure.
Symptomatic	Fluconazole 200 mg (3 mg/kg) daily for 14 days.	Ampho B 0.5 mg/kg daily (for fluconazole resistant organisms) for 7-10 days.	Concentration of echinocandins in urine is low: case reports of efficacy versus azole resistant organisms (*Can J Infect Dis Med Microbiol 18:149, 2007; CID 44:e46, 2007*).
Pyelonephritis	Fluconazole 200-400 mg (3-6 mg/kg) once daily orally.	Ampho B 0.5 mg/kg daily IV ± 5-FC 25 mg/kg orally qid.	Persistent candiduria in immunocompromised pt warrants ultrasound or CT of kidneys to rule out fungus ball. Treat for **2 weeks**. For suspected disseminated disease treat as if bloodstream infection is present.
Chromoblastomycosis (*Clin Exp Dermatol, 34:849, 2009*) (Cladophialophora, Phialophora, or Fonsecaea). Cutaneous (usually feet, legs): raised scaly lesions, most common in tropical areas	If lesions small & few, **surgical excision or cryosurgery with liquid nitrogen**. If lesions chronic, extensive, burrowing: **itraconazole**.		**Terbinafine**[NAI] 500-1000 mg once daily alone or in combination with itraconazole 200-400 mg; or **posaconazole** (800 mg/d) also may be effective.

See page 2 for abbreviations. All dosage recommendations are for adults (unless otherwise indicated) and assume normal renal function

TABLE 11A (8)

TYPE OF INFECTION/ORGANISM/ SITE OF INFECTION	ANTIMICROBIAL AGENTS OF CHOICE PRIMARY	ALTERNATIVE	COMMENTS
Coccidioidomycosis (Coccidioides immitis) *IDSA Guidelines 2005: CID 41:1217, 2005; see also Mayo Clin Proc 83:343, 2008)* **Primary pulmonary** (San Joaquin or Valley Fever): Pts low risk persistence/complication • Primary pulmonary in pts with ↑ risk for complications or dissemination. Rx indicated: — Immunosuppressive disease, post-transplantation, TNF-α antagonists) • Pregnancy in 3rd trimester. • Diabetes • CF antibody >1:16 • Pulmonary infiltrates • Dissemination (identification of spherules or culture of organism from ulcer, joint effusion, pus from subcutaneous abscess or bone biopsy, etc.)	Antifungal rx not generally indicated. Treat if fever, wt loss and/or fatigue do not resolve within several wks to 2 mos (see below). Itraconazole solution 200 mg po bid, OR Fluconazole 400 mg po q24h for 3–12 mos **Locally severe or disseminated disease**: **Ampho B** 0.6–1 mg/kg per day x 7 days then 0.8 mg/kg every other day, or **liposomal ampho B** 3–5 mg/kg IV, until clinical improvement (usually several wks or longer in disseminated disease), followed by **itra** or **flu** for at least 1 year. Some use combination of Ampho B & Flu for progressive severe disease; controlled series lacking. Consultation with specialist recommended; surgery may be required. Lifetime suppression in HIV+ patients or until CD4 ≥ 250 & infection controlled (flu 200 mg po q24h or itra 200 mg po bid *(MMWR 46:42, 2009)*).		Uncomplicated pulmonary is most common in endemic areas *(Emerg Infect Dis 12:958, 2006)*. Influenza-like illness of 1–2 wks duration. **Ampho B** cure rate ~50–70%. Response to azoles slow, but ultra after rx 40%. Relapse rate 1 if CF titer ≥1:256. Following CF titers after completion of rx important; rising titers warrant retreatment. **Posaconazole** reported successful in 73% of pts with refractory non-meningeal cocci *(Chest 132:952, 2007)*. Not frontline therapy.
Meningitis: occurs in 1/3 to 1/2 of pts with disseminated coccidioidomycosis Adult *(CID 42:103, 2006)*	**Fluconazole** 400–1,000 mg po q24h indefinitely	**Ampho B** IV as for pulmonary (above) + 0.1–0.3 mg daily intrathecal (intraventricular) via reservoir device. OR **itra** 400–600 mg q24h OR **voriconazole** (see Comment)	80% relapse rate, continue flucon indefinitely. **Voriconazole** successful in high doses (6 mg/kg IV q12h) followed by oral suppression (200 mg q12h).
Child	**Fluconazole** 400–1,000 mg po q24h indefinitely. Pediatric dose not established, 6 mg per kg q24h course		
Cryptococcosis *(IDSA Guideline: CID 30:710, 2000)*. New Guidelines *CID 50:291, 2010*. Excellent review: *Brit Med Bull 72:99, 2005* Risk 57% in organ transplant & those receiving other forms of immunosuppressive agents *(EID 13:953, 2007)*.			
Non-meningitis (non-AIDS)	**Fluconazole** 400 mg po per day for 8 wks to 6 mos For more severe disease: **Ampho B** 0.5–0.8 mg/kg per day (± flucytosine) until clinical improvement, then change to **fluconazole** 400 mg po q24h for 8–10 wks course	**Itraconazole** *(CID 36:291, 2003)* 200 mg po q12h x 6-12 mos OR **Ampho B** 0.3 mg/kg per day IV + **flucytosine** 37.5 mg/kg po qid times 6 wks	
Meningitis (non-AIDS)	**Ampho B** 0.5–0.8 mg/kg per day (+ flucytosine) until afebrile & cultures neg (~6 wks), start **fluconazole** 200 mg po q24h *(AnIM 113:183, 1990)*, OR **Fluconazole** 400 mg po q24h x 8–10 wks (Some recommend flu for 2 yrs to reduce relapse rate *(CID 28:297, 1999)*. Some recommend AMB plus fluconazole as induction Rx. Studies underway.		**Flucon alone 90% effective for meningeal and non-meningeal forms.** Fluconazole as effective as ampho B. Addition of **Interferon-γ** (IFN-γ-1b 50 mcg per M² subcut, 3x per wk x 9 wks) to liposomal ampho B assoc. with response rise in failing antifungal rx *(CID 40:1686, 2005)*. Posaconazole 400-800 mg also effective in a small series of patients *(CID 45:562, 2007; Chest 132:952, 2007)*. If CSF opening pressure >25 cm H₂O, repeat LP to drain fluid to control pressure. Outbreaks of C. gattii meningitis have been reported in the Pacific Northwest *(EID 13:42, 2007)*; severity of disease and prognosis appear to be worse than with C. neoformans. Initial therapy with ampho B + flucytosine recommended. C. gattii less susceptible to flucon than C. neoformans *(Clin Microbiol Inf 14:727, 2008)*. Outcomes in both AIDS and non-AIDS cryptococcal meningitis improved with Ampho B + 5FC induction therapy for 14 days in those with neurological abnormalities or high organism burden *(PLoS ONE 3:e2870, 2008)*.

[a] Some experts would reduce to 25 mg per kg q6h

See page 2 for abbreviations. All dosage recommendations are for adults (unless otherwise indicated) and assume normal renal function

TABLE 11A (9)

TYPE OF INFECTION/ORGANISM/ SITE OF INFECTION	ANTIMICROBIAL AGENTS OF CHOICE PRIMARY	ALTERNATIVE	COMMENTS
Cryptococcosis (continued)			
HIV+/AIDS: Cryptococcemia and/or Meningitis			
Treatment See *Clin Infect Dis 50:291, 2010* (IDSA Guidelines). ↓ with ARV but still common presenting OI in newly diagnosed AIDS pts. Cryptococcal infection may be manifested by positive blood culture or positive serum cryptococcal antigen (CRAG; >96% sens). CRAG no help in monitoring response to therapy. With AIDS, symptoms >14 days or more, may return: immune reconstitution inflammatory syndrome (IRIS). ↑ CSF pressure (> 250 mm H₂O) associated with high mortality, lower with CSF removal. If frequent LPs not possible, ventriculoperitoneal shunts are an option (*Surg Neurol 63:529 & 531, 2005*).	**Ampho B** 0.7 mg/kg IV q24h + **flucytosine**[a] 25 mg/kg po q6h for at least two weeks or longer until CSF is sterilized. See *Comment*. **Then** **Consolidation therapy**: **Fluconazole** 400-800 mg po to complete a 10-wks course then suppression (see below). Start Antiretroviral Therapy (ARV) if possible.	**Amphotericin B** or **liposomal ampho B plus fluconazole** 400 mg po IV daily. **OR** **Amphotericin B** 0.7 mg/kg **or liposomal ampho B** 4 mg/kg IV q24h alone; **OR Fluconazole** ≥ 800 mg/day (1200 mg preferred if amp B + 5FC not used) + flu cytosine 25 mg/kg po q6h for 4-6 weeks.	Outcome of treatment: treatment failure associated with dissemination of infection, high serum antigen titer, indicative of high burden of organisms and lack of 5FC use during induction Rx, abnormal neurological evaluation & underlying hematological malignancy. Mortality rates still high, particularly in those with concomitant pneumonia (*PLOS Medicine 4:e47, 2007*). Ampho B + 5FC treatment ↓ crypto CFUs more rapidly than ampho + flu or ampho B + flu. Ampo B 1 mg/kg/d alone which more rapidly fungicidal in vivo than flu 400 mg/d. (*CID 45:76&81, 2007*). Use lipid-based ampho B associated with lower mortality compared to ampho B deoxycholate in solid organ transplant recipients (*CID 48:1566, 2009*). Monitor 5-FC levels: peak 70-80 mg/L, trough 30-40 mg/L. Higher levels assoc. with bone marrow toxicity. No difference in outcome of given IV or po (*AAC 51:1038, 2007*). Failure of flu may rarely be due to resistant organism, especially, if burden of organism high at initiation of Rx. Although 200 mg qd → 400 mg qd of flu: median survival 76 & 82 days respectively, authors prefer 400 mg po qd (*BMC Infect Dis 6:118, 2006*). Trend toward improved outcomes with fluconazole 400-800 mg combined with ampho B versus ampho B alone in AIDS patients (*CID 48:1775, 2009*). Role of other azoles uncertain: successful outcomes were observed in 14/29 (48%) subjects treated with voriconazole, and in 11/25 (44%) with posaconazole (*JAC 56:745, 2005*). Voriconazole also may be effective. Survival probably improved with ART but IRIS may complicate its use. There is considerable controversy as to the timing of initiation of ART (see *CID 50:1532, 2010* and *CID 51: 984, 985, 986, 987, 2010*). One study suggests higher mortality with initiation of ART within 72 hrs of diagnosis (*CID 50:1532, 2010*), but the generalization of this study is an issue. Among most authorities continue to recommend ART within 2-6 wks of diagnosis.
Suppression (chronic maintenance therapy) Discontinuation of antifungal rx can be considered among pts who remain asymptomatic, with CD4 >100-200/mm³ for ≥6 months. Some perform lumbar puncture before discontinuation to demonstrate negative CSF culture. See www.hivatis.org. Authorities would do suppressive rx. See www.hivatis.org. Reappearance of pos. serum CRAG may predict relapse	**Fluconazole** 200 mg/day po [If CD4 count rises to > 100/mm³ with effective antiretroviral rx, some authorities recommend do suppressive rx. See www.hivatis.org. Authorities would only do if CSF culture negative.]	**Itraconazole** 200 mg po q12h if flu intolerant or failure. No data on Vori for maintenance.	Itraconazole less effective than fluconazole & not recommended because of higher relapse rate (23% vs 4%) Recurrence rate of 0.4 to 3.9 per 100 patient-years with discontinuation of suppressive therapy in 100 patients on ARV with CD4 >100 cells/mm³

[a] Flucytosine = 5-FC

See page 2 for abbreviations. All dosage recommendations are for adults (unless otherwise indicated) and assume normal renal function

119

TABLE 11A (10)

TYPE OF INFECTION/ORGANISM/ SITE OF INFECTION	ANTIMICROBIAL AGENTS OF CHOICE — PRIMARY	ALTERNATIVE	COMMENTS
Dermatophytosis (See *Mycopathologia* 166:353, 2008) **Onychomycosis** (*NEJM* 360:2108, 2009) Ciclopirox olamine 8% lacquer daily for 48 weeks; best suited for superficial and distal infections (overall cure rates approx 30%).	**Fingernail Rx Options:** **Terbinafine**[a] 250 mg po q24h x 6 wks (79% effective) OR **Itraconazole**[a] 200 mg po q24h x 3 mos[NAI] OR **Itraconazole**[a] 200 mg po bid x 1 wk/mo x 2 mos[NAI] OR **Fluconazole**[a] 150–300 mg po q wk x 3–6 mos.[NAI] **Terbinafine**[a] 250 mg po q24h x 6 wks (children)		**Toenail Rx Options:** **Terbinafine**[a] 250 mg po q24h (children <20 kg: 67.5 mg/day, 20–40 kg: 125 mg/day, >40 kg: 250 mg/day) x 12 wks (76% effective) OR **Itraconazole**[a] 200 mg po q24h x 3 mos (59% effective)[NAI] OR **Itraconazole**[a] 200 mg po bid x 1 wk/mo x 3–4 mos (63% effective)[NAI] OR **Fluconazole**[a] 150–300 mg po q wk x 6–12 mos (48% effective)[NAI]
Tinea capitis ("ringworm") (*Trichophyton tonsurans*, N. America; other sp. elsewhere) *Microsporum canis* (*PIDJ* 18:191, 1999)	**Terbinafine**[a] 250 mg po q24h x 2–4 wks OR **Itraconazole**[a] 5 mg/kg per day x 4 wks[NAI/a]	**Fluconazole** 6 mg/kg q wk x 8–12 wks. **Griseofulvin**[NAI] Cap at 150 mg po q wk for adults. **Griseofulvin**: adults 500 mg po q24h x 6–8 wks, children 10–20 mg/kg per day until hair regrows.	Durations of therapy are for T. tonsurans; treat for approx. twice as long for M. canis. All agents with similar cure rates (60–100%) in clinical studies. Addition of topical ketoconazole or selenium sulfate shampoo reduces transmissibility (*Int J Dermatol* 39:261, 2000)
Tinea corporis, cruris, or pedis (*Trichophyton rubrum*, *T. mentagrophytes*, *Epidermophyton floccosum*) "Athlete's foot, jock itch," and ringworm	**Topical rx:** Generally applied 2x/day. Available as creams, ointments, sprays, by prescription & over the counter. Apply 2x/day x 2–4 wks. Recommend: Lotrimin Ultra or Lamisil AT; contain butenafine & terbinafine — both are fungicidal	**Terbinafine** 250 mg po q24h x 2 wks[NAI] OR **ketoconazole** 200 mg po q24h x 4 wks OR **fluconazole** 150 mg po 1x/wk for 2–4 wks **Griseofulvin**: adults 500 mg po q24h times 4–6 wks, children 10–20 mg/kg per day. Duration: 2–4 wks for corporis, 4–8 wks for pedis.	Keto po often effective in severe recalcitrant infection. Follow for hepatotoxicity; many drug-drug interactions.
Tinea versicolor (*Malassezia furfur* or *Pityrosporum orbiculare*) Rule out erythrasma — see Table 1, page 54	**Ketoconazole** 400 mg po single dose[NAI] or (2% cream 1x q24h x 7 days) or (2% cream 1x q24h x 2 wks)	**Fluconazole** 400 mg po single dose or **Itraconazole** 400 mg po q24h x 3–7 days	Keto (po) times 1 dose was 97% effective in 1 study. Another alternative: Selenium sulfide (Selsun), 2.5% lotion; apply as lather, leave on 10 min then wash off. 1/day x 7 day or 3–4/wk times 2–4 wks
Fusariosis Third most common cause of invasive mould infections, after Aspergillus and Mucorales and related molds, in patients with hematologic malignancies. (*Mycoses* 52:197, 2009). Pneumonia, skin infections, bone and joint infections, and disseminated disease occur in severely immunocompromised patients. In contrast to other moulds, blood cultures are frequently positive. *Fusarium solani*, *F. oxysporum*, *F. verticillioides* and *F. moniliforme* account for approx 90% of isolates (*Clin Micro Rev* 20: 695, 2007). Frequently fatal, outcome depends on decreasing the level of immunosuppression.	**Lipid-based ampho B** 5–10 mg/kg/d. OR **Ampho B** 1–1.5 mg/kg/d.	**Posaconazole** 400 mg bid with meals (if not taking meals, 200 mg qid); OR **Voriconazole** IV: 6 mg per kg q12h times 1 day, then 4 mg per kg q12h; PO: 400 mg q12h, then 200 mg q12h. See Comments.	**Surgical debridement** for localized disease. *Fusarium* spp. resistance to most antifungal agents, including echinocandins. *F. solani* and *F. verticillioides* typically are resistant to azoles. *F. oxysporum* and *F. moniliforme* may be susceptible to voriconazole and posaconazole. Role of combination therapy not well defined but outcome depends on response. (*Mycoses* 50: 227, 2007). Outcome dependent on reduction or discontinuation of immuno-suppression. Duration of therapy depends on response; long-term suppressive therapy for patients continuing on immunosuppressive therapy.

[a] **Serious but rare cases of hepatic failure** have been reported in pts receiving terbinafine & should not be used in those with chronic or active liver disease (see Table 11B, page 126).
[b] Use of itraconazole has been associated with myocardial dysfunction and with onset of congestive heart failure.

See page 2 for abbreviations. All dosage recommendations are for adults (unless otherwise indicated) and assume normal renal function

TABLE 11A (11)

TYPE OF INFECTION/ORGANISM/ SITE OF INFECTION	ANTIMICROBIAL AGENTS OF CHOICE		COMMENTS
	PRIMARY	**ALTERNATIVE**	
Histoplasmosis (Histoplasma capsulatum): See IDSA Guideline: *CID* 45:807, 2007. Best diagnostic test is urinary, serum, or CSF histoplasma antigen: MiraVista Diagnostics (1-866-647-2847)			
Acute pulmonary histoplasmosis	**Mild to moderate disease, symptoms <4 wks:** No rx; If symptoms last over one month: **Itraconazole** 200 mg po tid for 3 days then once or twice daily for 6-12 wks.	Ampho B for patients at low risk of nephrotoxicity.	
	Moderately severe or severe: Liposomal ampho B, 3-5 mg/kg/d or **ABLC** 5 mg/kg/d IV or ampho B 0.7-1.0 mg/kg/d for 1-2 wks, then itra 200 mg po tid for 3 days, then bid for 12 wks. + **methylprednisolone** 0.5-1 mg/kg/d for 1-2 wks.		
Chronic cavitary pulmonary histoplasmosis	**Itra** 200 mg po tid for 3 days then once or twice daily for at least 12 mos (some prefer 18-24 mos).		Document therapeutic itraconazole blood levels at 2 wks. Relapses occur in 9-15% of patients.
Mediastinal lymphadenitis, mediastinal granuloma, pericarditis; and rheumatologic syndromes	**Mild Cases:** Anti-fungal therapy not indicated. Nonsteroidal anti-inflammatory drug for pericarditis or rheumatologic syndromes. If no response to non-steroidals, **Prednisone** 0.5-1.0 mg/kg/d tapered over 1-2 weeks for 1) pericarditis with hemodynamic compromise, 2) lymphadenitis with obstruction or compression syndromes, or 3) severe rheumatologic syndromes. In severe cases, or if prednisone is administered, use **itra** 200 mg po once or twice daily for 6-12 wks for moderately severe to severe cases.		
	Mild to moderate disease: Itra 200 mg po tid for 3 days then bid for at least 12 wks.		Check itra blood levels to document therapeutic concentrations.
Progressive disseminated histoplasmosis	**Moderately severe to severe disease: Liposomal ampho B,** 3 mg/kg/d or **ABLC** 5 mg/kg/d for 1-2 weeks then **itra** 200 mg tid for 3 days, then bid for at least 12 mos.		**Ampho B** 0.7-1.0 mg/kg/d may be used for patients at low risk of nephrotoxicity. Confirm therapeutic itra blood levels. Azoles are teratogenic; itra should be avoided in pregnancy; use a lipid ampho formulation. Urinary antigen levels useful for monitoring response to therapy and relapse
CNS histoplasmosis	**Liposomal ampho B,** 5 mg/kg/d, for a total of 175 mg/kg over 4-6 wks, then **itra** 200 mg 2-3x a day for at least 12 mos. Vori likely effective for CNS disease or itra failures. (*Arch Neurology* 57:1235, 2006).		Monitor CNS histo antigen. Monitor itra blood levels. PCR may be better for Dx than histo antigen. Absorption of itra (check levels) and CNS penetration may be an issue; case reports of success with Fluconazole (*Baz J Infect Dis* 12:555, 2008) and Posaconazole (*Drugs* 65:1553, 2005) following Ampho B therapy.
Prophylaxis (immunocompromised patients)	**Itra** 200 mg po daily		Consider primary **prophylaxis in HIV-infected** patients with < 150 CD4 cells/mm³ in high prevalence areas. Secondary prophylaxis (i.e. suppressive therapy) indicated in HIV-infected patients with < 150 CD4 cells/mm³ and other immunocompromised patients in who immunosuppression cannot be reversed

See page 2 for abbreviations. All dosage recommendations are for adults (unless otherwise indicated) and assume normal renal function

TABLE 11A (12)

TYPE OF INFECTION/ORGANISM/ SITE OF INFECTION	ANTIMICROBIAL AGENTS OF CHOICE PRIMARY	ALTERNATIVE	COMMENTS
Madura foot (See Nocardia & Scedosporium)			
Mucormycosis & other related species—Rhizopus, Rhizomucor, Lichtheimia (CID 54:1629, 2012), Rhinocerebral, pulmonary invasive. Key to successful rx: early dx with symptoms suggestive of sinusitis (or lateral facial pain or numbness); think mucor with palatal ulcers, &/or black eschars, onset unilateral blindness in pt with DKA, or leukemia (x-Ray, total WBC, blood sugar). Dx by culture of tissue or stain: wide ribbon-like, non-septated with variation in diameter & right angle branching.	**Liposomal ampho B** 5-10 mg/kg/day; OR **Ampho B** 1-1.5 mg/kg/day.	**Posaconazole** 400 mg po bid with meals (if not taking meals, 200 mg po qid)[NAI]	**Combination therapy** of ampho B or a lipid-based ampho B plus caspofungin associated with improved cure rates (100% vs 45%) in one small retrospective study; (6 combo therapy patients, 31 monotherapy historical controls); ampho B lipid complex (ABLC) monotherapy relatively ineffective with 20% success rate vs 69% for other polyenes (CID 39:584, 2008). Complete or partial response rates of 60-80% in posaconazole salvage protocols (JAC 61: Suppl 1:i35, 2008). Resistant to voriconazole: prolonged use of voriconazole prophylaxis predisposes to mucormycosis infections. Total duration of therapy based on response: continue therapy until 1) resolution of clinical signs and symptoms of infection, 2) resolution or stabilization of radiographic abnormalities; and 3) resolution of underlying immunosuppression. Posaconazole for secondary prophylaxis for those on immunosuppressive therapy (CID 48:1743, 2009).
Paracoccidioidomycosis (South American blastomycosis) P. brasiliensis (Dermatol Clin 26:257, 2008; Expert Rev Anti Infect Ther 6:251, 2008). Important cause of death from fungal infection in HIV-infected patients in Brazil (Mem Inst Oswaldo Cruz 104:513, 2009).	**TMP/SMX** 800/160 mg bid-tid for 30 days, then 400/80 mg/day indefinitely (up to 3-5 years); OR **itraconazole** (100 or 200 mg orally daily)	**Ketoconazole** 200-400 mg daily for 6-18 months; OR **Ampho B** total dose > 30 mg/kg	Improvement in >90% pts with itra or keto.[NAI] **Ampho B** reserved for severe cases and for those intolerant to other agents. TMP-SMX suppression life-long in HIV+.
Lobomycosis (keloidal blastomycosis) P. loboi	Surgical excision, clofazimine or itraconazole		
Penicilliosis (Penicillium marneffei). Commonly disseminated fungal infection in AIDS pts in SE Asia (esp. Thailand & Vietnam).	**Ampho B** 0.5-1 mg/kg per day for 2 weeks followed by **itraconazole** 400 mg/day for 10 wks followed by 200 mg/day po for **indefinitely for HIV-infected pts.**	For less sick patients **itra** 200 mg po tid x 3 days, then 200 mg po bid x 12 wks, then 200 mg po q24h. (IV if unable to take po)	3rd most common OI in AIDS pts in SE Asia following TBc and cryptococcal meningitis. Prolonged fever, lymphadenopathy, hepatomegaly. Skin nodules are umbilicated, mimic cryptococcal infection or molluscum contagiosum). Preliminary data suggests vori effective (CID 43:1060, 2006.
Phaeohyphomycosis, Black molds, Dematiaceous fungi (See CID 48:1033, 2009) Sinuses, skin, bone & joint, brain abscess, endocarditis, disseminated especially in HSCT pts with disseminated disease. **Scedosporium prolificans,** Bipolaris, Wangiella, Curvularia, Exophiala, Phialemonium, Scytalidium, Alternaria.	Surgery + **Itraconazole** 400 mg/day po, duration not defined, probably 6 mo[NAI]	Case report of success with **voriconazole + terbinafine** (Scand J Infect Dis 39:87, 2007); OR **itraconazole + terbinafine** synergistic against S. prolificans. No clinical data & combination could show ↑ toxicity (see Table 11B, page 124)	**Posaconazole** successful in case of brain abscess (CID 34:1648, 2002) and refractory infection (Mycosis: 519, 2006). **Notoriously resistant to antifungal rx including amphotericin & azoles.** 44% of patients in compassionate use/salvage therapy study responded to voriconazole (AAC 52:1743, 2008). >80% mortality in immunocompromised hosts.

[7] Oral solution preferred to tablets because of ↑ absorption (see Table 11B, page 124).

See page 2 for abbreviations. All dosage recommendations are for adults (unless otherwise indicated) and assume normal renal function

TABLE 11A (13)

TYPE OF INFECTION/ORGANISM/ SITE OF INFECTION	ANTIMICROBIAL AGENTS OF CHOICE PRIMARY	ALTERNATIVE	COMMENTS
Madura foot (continued)			
Scedosporium apiospermum (Pseudallescheria boydii) (not considered a true dematiaceous mold) (Medicine 81:333, 2002) Skin, subcut. (Madura foot), brain abscess, recurrent meningitis. May appear after near-drowning incidents. Also emerging especially in hematopoietic stem cell transplant (HSCT) pts with disseminated disease	Voriconazole 6 mg/kg IV q12h on day 1, then either (4 mg/kg IV q12h) or (200 mg po q12h for body weight ≥40 kg, but 100 mg po q12h for body weight <40 kg) (AAC 52:1743, 2008). 300 mg bid if serum concentrations are subtherapeutic, i.e., <1 mcg/mL (CID 46:201, 2008).	Surgery + **Itraconazole** 200 mg po bid until clinically well^NAI (Many species now resistant or refractory to Itra); OR **Posa** 400 mg po bid with meals (if not taking meals, 200 mg po qid).	**Resistant to many antifungal drugs including amphotericin.** In vitro voriconazole more active than Itra and posaconazole in vitro (Clin Microbiol Rev 21:157, 2008). Case reports of successful rx of disseminated and CNS disease with voriconazole (AAC 52:1743, 2008). Posaconazole active in vitro and successful in several case reports.
Sporotrichosis IDSA Guideline: CID 45:1255, 2007. Cutaneous/Lymphocutaneous	Itraconazole po 200 mg/day for 2-4 wks after all lesions resolved, usually 3-6 mos.	If no response, **Itra** 200 mg po bid or **terbinafine** 500 mg po bid or **SSKI** 5 drops (eye drops) tid & increase to 40-50 drops tid	Fluconazole 400-800 mg daily only if no response to primary or alternative suggestions. Pregnancy or nursing: local hyperthermia (see below).
Osteoarticular	Itra 200 mg po bid x 12 mos.	**Liposomal ampho B** 3-5 mg/kg/d IV or **ABLC** 5 mg/kg/d IV or **ampho B deoxycholate** 0.7-1 mg/kg IV daily. If response, change to **Itra** 200 mg po bid x total 12 mos.	After 2 wks of therapy, document adequate serum levels of itraconazole.
Pulmonary	If severe, **lipid ampho B** 3-5 mg/kg IV or **standard ampho B** 0.7-1 mg/kg IV once daily until response, then **itra** 200 mg po bid x 4-6 wks, then—if better—**itra** 200 mg po bid for total of 12 mos.	Less severe: **Itraconazole** 200 mg po bid x 12 mos.	After 2 weeks of therapy document adequate serum levels of Itra. Surgical resection plus ampho B for localized pulmonary disease.
Meningeal or Disseminated	**Lipid ampho B** 5 mg/kg IV once daily x 4-6 wks, then—if better—**itra** 200 mg po bid for total of 12 mos.	AIDS/Other immunosuppressed pts: chronic therapy with **Itra** 200 mg po once daily.	After 2 weeks, document adequate serum levels of Itra.
Pregnancy and children	**Pregnancy**: Cutaneous—local hyperthermia. Severe: **lipid ampho B** 3-5 mg/kg IV once daily. **Avoid itraconazole.**	**Children**: **Itra** 6-10 mg/kg (max of 400 mg) daily. Alternative is **SSKI** 1 drop tid increasing to max of 1 drop/kg or 40-50 drops tid/day, whichever is lowest.	For children with disseminated sporotrichosis: Standard ampho B 0.7 mg/kg IV once daily & after response, **Itra** 6-10 mg/kg po (max 400 mg) once daily.

See page 2 for abbreviations. All dosage recommendations are for adults (unless otherwise indicated) and assume normal renal function.

123

TABLE 11B – ANTIFUNGAL DRUGS: DOSAGE, ADVERSE EFFECTS, COMMENTS

DRUG NAME, GENERIC (TRADE)/USUAL DOSAGE	ADVERSE EFFECTS/COMMENTS
Non-lipid amphotericin B deoxycholate (Fungizone): 0.3–1.5 mg/kg per day as single infusion **Ampho B predictably not active vs** *C. lusitaniae, C. guilliermondii, Aspergillus terreus* (TABLE 11C, page 127)	**Admin:** Ampho B is a colloidal suspension that must be prepared in electrolyte-free D5W at 0.1 mg/mL to avoid precipitation. No need to protect suspensions from light. Infusions cause chills/fever, myalgia, anorexia, nausea, rarely hemodynamic collapse/hypotension. Postulated to be histamine release (*Pharmacol* 23:966, 2003). Infusion duration usu. 4+ hrs. No difference found in 1 vs 4 hr infus. except chills/fever occurred sooner with 1 hr infus. Febrile rigors **respond to meperidine (25–50 mg IV)**. Rare pulmonary rxns (severe dyspnea & focal infiltrates suggest pulmonary edema) assoc with rapid infus. Premedication with acetaminophen, diphenhydramine, hydrocortisone (25–50 mg) and heparin (1000 units) had no influence on rigors/fever or cytokine production. Use of high-dose steroids may be efficacious but their use may risk worsening infection under rx. **Severe rigors respond to meperidine (25–50 mg IV)**. **Toxicity:** Major concern is nephrotoxicity. Manifest initially by kaliuresis and hypokalemia, then fall in serum bicarbonate, rising BUN/serum creatinine. Hypomagnesemia may occur. ↓ in renal erythropoietin and anemia, and rising BUN/serum creatinine. Hypomagnesemia may occur. Can reduce risk of renal injury by **(a) pre- & post-infusion hydration with 500 ml saline (if clinical status allows salt load), (b)** avoidance of other nephrotoxins, eg, radiocontrast, aminoglycosides, cis-platinum, **(c)** use of lipid prep of ampho B.
Lipid-based ampho B products: **Amphotericin B lipid complex (ABLC)** (Abelcet): 5 mg/kg per day as single infusion	**Admin:** Consists of ampho B complexed with 2 lipid bilayer ribbons. Compared to standard ampho B, larger volume of distribution, rapid blood clearance and high tissue concentrations (liver, spleen, lung). Dosage: **5 mg/kg once daily;** infuse at 2.5 mg/kg per hr. adult and ped. dose the same. Do NOT use an in-line filter. Do not dilute with saline or mix with other drugs or electrolytes. **Toxicity:** Fever and chills 14–18%, nausea 9%, vomiting 8%, serum creatinine ↑ in 11%, renal failure 5%, anemia 4%; ↓ K 5%, rash 4%. A fatal case of fat embolism reported following ABLC infusion (*Exp Mol Path* 77:246, 2004).
Liposomal ampho B (LAB, AmBisome): 1–5 mg/kg per day as single infusion.	**Admin:** Consists of a vesicular bilayer liposome with ampho B intercalated within the membrane. Dosage: **3–5 mg/kg per day** IV as single dose infused over a period of approx. 120 min. If well tolerated, infusion time can be reduced to 60 min. (see footnote[2]) Tolerated with elderly pts (*J Inf* 50:277, 2005). **Major toxicity:** Gen less than ampho B. Nephrotoxicity: liposome with ampho B result in creatinine ↑ 33.7% or ampho B 78.7%, nausea 39.7% vs 38.7%, vomiting 31.8% vs 43.9%, rash 24% for both, ↑ Liver 18.4% vs 20.9%, ↓ K 20.4% vs 25.6%, ↑ mg 20.4% vs 25.6%. Acute infusion-related reactions common with liposomal ampho B, 20–40%. 86% occur within 5 min of infusion. Include chest pain, dyspnea, hypoxia or severe abdom, flank or leg pain; 14% dev flushing & urticaria near end of 4 hr infusion. All responded to diphenhydramine (1 mg/kg) & interruption of infusion. Rxns may be due to complement activation by liposome (*CID* 36:1213, 2003).
Caspofungin (Cancidas): 70 mg IV on day 1, followed by 50 mg IV q24h reduce to 35 mg IV q24h with moderate hepatic insufficiency)	An echinocandin that inhibits synthesis of β-(1,3)-D-glucan. Fungicidal against candida (MIC <0.2 mcg/mL) including those resistant to other antifungals & active against aspergillus (MIC 0.4–2.7 mcg/mL). Approved indications for caspo incl: empirical rx for febrile, neutropenic pts, rx of candidemia, candida intraabdominal abscesses, peritonitis, & pleural space infections, esophageal candidiasis, invasive aspergillosis in pts refractory to or intolerant of other therapies. Serum levels on rec. dosages = peak 12 mcg/mL (1 hr after inf), mid-dosage interval 1.3 mcg/mL, trough 1.3 (24 hrs) mcg/mL. **Toxicity:** remarkably non-toxic. Most common adverse effect: pruritus at infusion site & headache, fever, chills, vomiting, & diarrhea assoc with infusion. In pts on caspo vs 21% short-course ampho B in 422 pts with candidemia (*Ln*, Oct. 12, 2005, *online*). Drug metab in liver & dosage ↓ to 35 mg in moderate to severe hepatic failure. Class C for preg (embryotoxic in rats & rabbits). *See Table 22, page 217 for drug-drug interactions, esp. cyclosporine (hepatic toxicity) & tacrolimus (drug level monitoring recommended)*. Reversible thrombocytopenia reported (*Pharmacother* 24:1408, 2004). **No drug in CSF or urine.**
Micafungin (Mycamine): 50 mg/day prophylaxis post-bone marrow stem cell trans; 100 mg candidemia, 150 mg candida esophagitis.	The 2nd echinocandin approved by FDA for rx of esophageal candidiasis & prophylaxis against candida infections in HSCT[3] recipients. Active against most strains of candida sp. & aspergillus sp. **Not** consistently fungicidal. Approved in Japan for rx of candidemia, some data of benefit with other antifungal drugs. No dosage adjust with severe renal or hepatic failure. No interactions with cyclosporine, tacrolimus. Worse tolerated than others: Micafungin well tolerated with common adverse events incl nausea 2.8%, vomiting 2.4%, & headache 2.4%. Transient ↑ LFTs, BUN, creatinine reported; rare cases of significant hepatitis & renal insufficiency. *See CID* 42:1171, 2006. **No drug in CSF or urine.**

[1] Published data from patients intolerant of or refractory to conventional ampho B deoxycholate (Amp B d). **None of the lipid ampho B preps have shown superior efficacy compared to ampho B in prospective trials (except liposomal ampho B was more effective vs ampho B in rx of disseminated histoplasmosis at 2 wks). Dosage equivalency has not been established** (*CID* 36:1500, 2003). Nephrotoxicity ↓ with all lipid ampho B preps.

[2] Comparative trials of AmBisome vs Abelcet suggest higher frequency of mild hepatic toxicity with AmBisome (59% vs 38%, p=0.05). Mild elevations in serum creatinine were observed in 1/3 of both (*BJ Hemat* 103:198, 1998; *Focus on Fungal Inf #9*, 1999; *Bone Marrow Tx* 20:39, 1997; *CID* 26:1383, 1998).

[3] HSCT = hematopoietic stem cell transplant.

See page 2 for abbreviations. All dosage recommendations are for adults (unless otherwise indicated) and assume normal renal function

125

TABLE 11B (2)

DRUG NAME, GENERIC (TRADE)/USUAL DOSAGE	ADVERSE EFFECTS/COMMENTS
Anidulafungin (Eraxis) For Candidemia: 200 mg IV on day 1 followed by 100 mg/day IV). Rx for EC: 100 mg IV x 1, then 50 mg IV once/d.	An echinocandin with antifungal activity (cidal) against candida sp. including ampho B- & triazole-resistant strains. FDA approved for treatment of esophageal candidiasis (EC), candidemia, and other complicated Candida infections. Effective in clinical trials of esophageal candidiasis & in 1 trial was superior to fluconazole in rx of invasive candidiasis/candidemia in 245 pts (75.6% vs 60.2%). Like other echinocandins, remarkably non-toxic; most common side-effects: nausea, vomiting, ↓ mg, ↓ K & headache in 11–13% of pts. No dose adjustments for renal or hepatic insufficiency. See CID 43:215, 2006. **No drug in CSF or urine.**
Fluconazole (Diflucan) 50 mg tabs 100 mg tabs 150 mg tabs 200 mg tabs 400 mg IV Oral suspension: 50 mg per 5 mL	IV-oral dose because of excellent bioavailability. **Pharmacology:** absorbed po, water solubility enables IV. For peak serum levels (see Table 9A, page 87). T½ 30hr (range 20–50 hr), 12% protein bound. **CSF levels 50–90% of serum in normals**, slightly less in meningitis. No effect on mammalian steroids. **Drug-drug interactions common, often fatal:** See Table 22. Side-effects overall 16% (more common in HIV+ pts (21%)). Nausea 3.7%, headache 1.9%, skin rash 1.8%, abdominal pain 1.7%, diarrhea 1.5%, ↑ SGOT 20%. Alopecia (scalp, pubic crest) in 12–20% pts on ≥400 mg po q24h after median of 3 mos (reversible in approx. 6mo). Rare: severe hepatotoxicity (CID 41:301, 2005), exfoliative dermatitis. **Note: Candida krusei and Candida glabrata resistant to Flu.**
Flucytosine (Ancobon) 500 mg cap	AEs: Overall 30%, GI 6% (diarrhea, anorexia, nausea, vomiting); hematologic 22% (leukopenia, thrombocytopenia, when serum level >100 mcg/mL (esp. in azotemic pts)); hepatotoxicity (asymptomatic ↑ SGOT, reversible), skin rash 7%, aplastic anemia (rare—2 or 3 cases). False ↑ on serum creatinine on EKTACHEM analyzer.
Griseofulvin (Fulvicin, Grifulvin, Grisactin) 500 mg, susp 125 mg/mL	Photosensitivity, urticaria, GI upset, fatigue, leukopenia (rare). Interferes with warfarin drugs. Increases blood and urine porphyrins, should not be used in patients with porphyria. Minor disulfiram-like reactions. Exacerbation of systemic lupus erythematosus.
Miconazole 2% For vaginal and/or skin use	Not recommended in 1st trimester of pregnancy. Local reactions: 0.5-1.5%: dyspareunia, mild vaginal or vulvar erythema, burning, pruritus, urticaria, rash. Rarely similar symptoms in sexual partner
Itraconazole (Sporanox) 100 mg cap 10 mg/mL oral solution IV usual dose 200 mg bid x 4 doses followed by 200 mg q24h for a max. of 14 days	**Itraconazole tablet & solution forms not interchangeable, solution preferred.** Many authorities recommend measuring drug serum concentration after 2 wks to ensure satisfactory absorption. To obtain highest plasma concentration, tablet is given with food & acidic drinks (e.g., cola) while solution is taken in fasted state; under these conditions, the peak conc. of capsule is approx. 3 mcg/mL & of solution 5.4 mcg/mL. Peak levels reached faster (2.2 vs 5 hrs) with solution. **Peak plasma concentrations after IV injection (200 mg) compared to oral capsule (200 mg): 2.8 mcg/mL (on day 7 of rx) vs 2 mcg/mL (on day 36 of rx).** Protein-binding for both preparations is over 99%, which explains virtual absence of penetration into CSF **(do not use to treat meningitis)**. Adverse effects: dose-related nausea 10%, diarrhea 8%, vomiting 6%, & abdominal discomfort 5.7%. Allergic rash 8.6%, ↑ bilirubin 6%, edema 3.5%, & hepatitis 2.7% reported. 7 doses may produce hypokalemia, 8% ↑ blood pressure 3.2%. Delirium, peripheral neuropathy & tremor reported (J Neur Neurosurg Psych 81:327, 2010). **Reported to produce impairment in cardiac function.** Severe liver failure reported, including pulse rx from transplant in pts receiving drug for onychomycosis. FDA reports 24 cases with 11 deaths out of 50 mill people who received the drug prior to 2001. Other concern, as with fluconazole and ketoconazole, is **drug-drug interactions**; see Table 22. Some can be life-threatening.
Ketoconazole (Nizoral) 200 mg tab	Gastric acid required for absorption - cimetidine, omeprazole, antacids block absorption. In achlorhydria, dissolve tablet in 4 mL 0.2N HCl, drink with a straw. Coca-Cola ↑ absorption by 65%. CSF levels "none". **Drug-drug interactions important, see Table 22. Some interactions can be life-threatening. Dose-dependent nausea and vomiting.** Liver toxicity of hepatocellular type reported in about 1:110,000 exposed pts—usually after several days to weeks of exposure. With high doses, adrenal (Addisonian) crisis reported. Decreases in serum testosterone and plasma cortisol levels fall. With high doses, adrenal (Addisonian) crisis reported.
Miconazole (Monistat IV) 200 mg, not available in U.S.	IV miconazole indicated in patient critically ill with Scedosporium (Pseudallescheria boydii) infection. Very toxic due to vehicle needed to get drug into solution.
Nystatin (Mycostatin) 30 gm cream 500,000 units oral tab	Topical: virtually no adverse effects. Less effective than imidazoles and triazoles. PO: large doses give occasional GI distress and diarrhea.

See page 2 for abbreviations. All dosage recommendations are for adults (unless otherwise indicated) and assume normal renal function

TABLE 11B (3)

DRUG NAME, GENERIC (TRADE)/USUAL DOSAGE	ADVERSE EFFECTS/COMMENTS
Posaconazole (Noxafil) 400 mg bid with meals (200 mg qid if not taking meals, 200 mg qid); for prophylaxis: 40 mg/mL suspension. Takes 7-10 days to achieve steady state. No IV formulation.	An oral triazole with activity against a wide range of fungi refractory to other antifungal rx including aspergillosis, mucormycosis (variability by species), fusariosis, Scedosporium (Pseudallescheria), phaeohyphomycosis, histoplasmosis, refractory coccidioidomycosis, refractory cryptococcosis, refractory chromoblastomycosis. **Should be taken with high fat meal for maximum absorption.** Approved for prophylaxis (NEJM 356:348, 2007). Clinical response in 75% of 176 AIDS pts with azole-refractory oral/esophageal candidiasis. Posaconazole has similar toxicities as other triazoles: nausea 9%, vomiting 6%, abd. pain 5%, headache 5%, diarrhea, ↑ ALT, AST, & rash (3% each). In pts rx for >6 mos, serious side-effects have included adrenal insufficiency, neurotoxicity, & QTc interval prolongation. Significant drug-drug interactions; inhibits CYP3A4 (see Table 22). Consider monitoring serum concentrations (AAC 53:24, 2009) (See Drugs 65:1552, 2005).
Terbinafine (Lamisil) 250 mg tab	In pts given terbinafine for onychomycosis, rare cases (8) of idiosyncratic & symptomatic hepatic injury & more rarely liver failure leading to death or liver transplant. The drug is **not recommended** for pts with **chronic or active liver disease**; hepatotoxicity may occur in pts with or without pre-existing disease. Pretreatment serum transaminases (ALT & AST) advised & alternate rx used for those with abnormal levels. Pts started on terbinafine should be warned about symptoms suggesting liver dysfunction (persistent nausea, anorexia, fatigue, vomiting, RUQ pain, jaundice, dark urine or pale stools). If symptoms develop, drug should be discontinued & liver function immediately evaluated. In controlled trials, complete cure rates of onychomycosis 38-59%—clinical significance unknown. Major drug-drug interaction is 100% ↑ in rate of clearance by rifampin. AEs: usually mild, transient and rarely caused discontinuation of rx; % with AE, terbinafine vs placebo: nausea/diarrhea 2.6-5.6 vs 2.9, rash 5.6 vs 2.2, taste abnormality 2.8 vs 0.7. Inhibits CYP2D6 enzymes (see Table 22). An acute generalized exanthematous pustulosis and subacute cutaneous lupus erythematosus reported.
Voriconazole (Vfend) IV: Loading dose 6 mg per kg q12h times 1 day, then 4 mg per kg q12h for invasive aspergillus & serious mold infections. **3 mg per kg IV q12h** for other serious candida infections. **Oral: ≥40 kg body weight:** 400 mg po q12h, then 200 mg po q12h. **<40 kg body weight:** 200 mg po q12h, then 100 mg po q12h. **Take oral dose 1 hour before or 1 hour after eating.** Oral suspension (40 mg per mL). Oral suspension dosing: Same as for oral tabs. Reduce to ½ maintenance dose for moderate hepatic insufficiency	A triazole with activity against Aspergillus sp., **including Ampho resistant strains of A. terreus.** Active vs Candida sp. (including krusei), Fusarium sp., & various molds. Steady state serum levels reach 2.5-4 mcg per mL. Up to 20% of patients with subtherapeutic levels with oral administration: check levels for suspected treatment failure, life threatening infections. 300 mg bid oral dose or 8 mg/kg IV dose may be required to achieve target steady-state drug concentrations in 1-6 exp/mL. Toxicity similar to other azoles/triazoles including uncommon serious hepatic toxicity (hepatitis, cholestasis & fulminant hepatic failure. Liver function tests should be monitored during rx & drug dc'd if LFT abnormalities develop. Rash reported in up to 20%, occ. photosensitivity & rare Stevens-Johnson, hyperpigmentation & anaphylactoid infusion reactions with fever and hypertension. 1 case of QT prolongation with ventricular tachycardia in a 15 y/o pt with ALL reported. **Approx. 21%** of patients on IV or po rx experience transient visual disturbances (blurring of vision, altered/enhanced visual perception, blurred or colored visual change or photophobia) within 30-60 minutes. Persistent visual changes occur rarely. Cause unknown. In patients with CrCl < 50 mL per min., the intravenous vehicle (SBECD-sulfobutylether-B cyclodextrin) may accumulate and lead to drug concentrations. Potential for drug-drug interactions high—see Table 22. electrolyte disturbance & pneumonitis attributed to 7 drug concentrations. Potential for drug-drug interactions high—see Table 22. **NOTE: Not in urine in active form. No activity vs. mucormycosis.**

See page 2 for abbreviations. All dosage recommendations are for adults (unless otherwise indicated) and assume normal renal function

TABLE 11C – AT A GLANCE SUMMARY OF SUGGESTED ANTIFUNGAL DRUGS AGAINST TREATABLE PATHOGENIC FUNGI

Microorganism	Fluconazole	Itraconazole	Voriconazole	Posaconazole	Echinocandin[4]	Polyenes
Candida albicans	+++	+++	+++	+++	+++	+++
Candida dubliniensis	+++	+++	+++	+++	+++	+++
Candida glabrata	±	+	+	+	+++	++
Candida tropicalis	+++	+++	+++	+++	+++	++
Candida parapsilosis[5]	+++	+++	+++	+++	++ (higher MIC)	+++
Candida krusei		+	+++	+++	+++	++
Candida guilliermondii	+++	+++	+++	+++	++ (higher MIC)	+++
Candida lusitaniae	+	+	++	++	+	-
Cryptococcus neoformans	+++	+++	+++	+++	-	++
Aspergillus fumigatus[3]	-	++	+++	+++	++	++
Aspergillus flavus[3]	-	-	+++	+++	++	++
Aspergillus terreus	-	++	+++	+++	+++	++ (higher MIC)
Fusarium sp	-	±	+++	++	-	
Scedosporium apiospermum (Pseudallescheria boydii)	-	±	++	++	-	++ (lipid formulations)
Scedosporium prolificans[10]	-	-	±	±	-	-
Trichosporon spp.	±	±	++	++	-	-
Mucormycosis (e.g. Mucor, Rhizopus, Lichtheimia)	-	-	-	+++	-	+++ (lipid formulations)
Dematiaceous molds[11] (e.g. Alternaria, Bipolaris, Curvularia, Exophiala)	-	++	+++	+++	+	++
Dimorphic Fungi						
Blastomyces dermatitidis	++	+++	++	++	-	+++
Coccidioides immitis/posadasii	+++	+++	+++	+++	-	+++
Histoplasma capsulatum	++	+++	++	++	-	+++
Sporothrix schenckii	-	++	-	+	-	+++

- = no activity; ± = possibly activity; + = active; ++ = Active, 2nd line therapy (less active clinically); +++ = Active, 1st line therapy (usually active clinically).

[1] Minimum inhibitory concentration values do not always predict clinical outcome.
[2] Echinocandins, voriconazole, posaconazole and polyenes have poor urine penetration.
[3] During severe immune suppression, success requires immune reconstitution.
[4] **Flucytosine** has activity against Candida sp, Cryptococcus sp, and dematiaceous molds, but is primarily used in combination therapy.
[5] For infections secondary to Candida sp, patients with prior triazole therapy have higher likelihood of triazole resistance.
[6] Echinocandin pharmacodynamics, see JAC 65:1108, 2010.
[7] Successful treatment of infections from Candida parapsilosis requires removal of foreign body or intravascular device.
[8] Treatment failures reported, even for susceptible strains.
[9] Lipid formulations of amphotericin may have greater activity against A. fumigatus and A. flavus (+++).
[10] Scedosporium prolificans is poorly susceptible to single agents and may require combination therapy (e.g., addition of terbinafine).
[11] Infections from mucormycosis, some Aspergillus sp., and dematiaceous molds often require surgical debridement.

TABLE 12A – TREATMENT OF MYCOBACTERIAL INFECTIONS*

Tuberculin skin test (TST), Same as PPD *(Chest 138:1456, 2010).*

Criteria for positive TST after 5 tuberculin units (intermediate PPD) read at 48-72 hours:
- ≥5 mm induration: + HIV, immunosuppressed, ≥15 mg prednisone per day, recent close contact
- ≥10 mm induration: foreign-born, countries with high prevalence; IVD Users; low income; NH residents; chronic illness; silicosis
- ≥15 mm induration: otherwise healthy

Two-stage to detect sluggish positivity: If 1st PPD + but <10 mm, repeat intermediate PPD in 1 wk. Response to 2nd PPD can also happen in pt if received BCG in childhood.

BCG vaccine as child: if ≥10 mm induration, & from country with TBc, should be attributed to M. tuberculosis. In areas of low TB prevalence, TST reactions of ≤18 mm more likely from BCG than TB *(CID 40:211, 2005).* Prior BCG may result in booster effect in 2-stage TST *(AJM 161:1760, 2001; Clin Micro Int 10:980, 2005)*

Routine anergy testing no longer recommended in HIV+ or HIV-negative patients *(JAMA 283:2003, 2000).*

Interferon Gamma Release Assays (IGRAs): IGRAs detect sensitivities to M. TBc by measuring IFN-8 release in response to M. TBc antigens. May be used in place of TST in all situations in which TST may be used *(MMWR 59 (RR-5), 2010).* Four such tests have now been approved by the U.S. FDA.
- QuantiFERON-TB (QFT) (approved 2001, but discontinued in 2005)
- QuantiFERON-TB Gold (QFT-G) (approved 2005)
- QuantiFERON-TB Gold In-Tube Test (QFT-GIT) (approved 2007)
- T-Spot (approved 2008)

QFT-G, QFT-GIT & T-Spot each measures different aspects of immune response so test results are not always interchangeable. IGRAs are relatively specific for M. TBc and should not cross-react with BCG or most nontuberculous mycobacteria. CDC recommends IGRA over TST for persons unlikely to return for reading TST & for persons who have received BCG. TST is preferred in children age < 5 yrs (IGRA is acceptable). IGRA or TST may be used without preference for recent contacts of TB with special utility for follow-up testing since IGRAs do not produce 'booster effect'. May also be used without preference over TBc for occupational exposures. As with TST, testing with IGRAs in low prevalence populations will result in false-positive results *(CID 53:234, 2011).* For detailed discussion of IGRAs, see *MMWR 59 (RR-5), 2010* and *JAMA 308:241, 2012*.

Nucleic acid amplification tests (NAAT) can reliably detect M. tuberculosis in clinical specimens 1 or more weeks earlier than conventional cultures. They are particularly useful in detecting M.TBc from smear-positive specimens. Sensitivity lower in smear-negative or extrapulmonary specimens *(CID 49:46, 2009; PLoS Medicine 5:e156, 2008).* CDC currently recommends that NAA testing be performed on at least one respiratory specimen from each patient for whom diagnosis of TB is being considered but has not yet been established, and for whom the test result would alter case management or TB control activities *(MMWR 58:7, 2009).*

Rapid (24-hr or less) diagnostic tests for M. tuberculosis: (1) the Amplified Mycobacterium tuberculosis Direct Test amplifies and detects M. tuberculosis ribosomal RNA; (2) the AMPLICOR Mycobacterium tuberculosis Test amplifies and detects M. tuberculosis DNA. Both tests have sensitivities & specificities >95% in sputum samples that are AFB-positive, & specificity remains >95% but sensitivity is 40-77% *(MMWR 58:7, 2009; CID 49:46, 2009).*

Xpert MTB/RIF is a rapid test (2 hrs) for M. TBc in sputum samples for M. TBc also detects RIF resistance with specificity of 99.2%, sensitivity of 72.5% in smear negative patients *(NEJM 363:1005, 2010).* The test may be effectively used in low resource settings *(Lancet online, accessed 4/19/2011).* Current antibody-based and ELISA-based rapid tests for TBc not recommended by WHO because they are less accurate than microscopy ± culture *(Lancet ID 11:736, 2011).*

CAUSATIVE AGENT/DISEASE	MODIFYING CIRCUMSTANCES	SUGGESTED REGIMENS	
		INITIAL THERAPY	CONTINUATION PHASE OF THERAPY
I. **Mycobacterium tuberculosis**, pulmonary, adult (household members & other close contacts of potentially infectious cases) **TST negative**	Neonate—Rx essential	INH¹ (10 mg/kg/day to 9 mos)	Repeat tuberculin skin test (TST) in 3 mos. If mother's smear neg & infant's TST neg & chest x-ray (CXR) normal, stop INH. In UK, BCG is then given at 3 mos, repeat HIV+ to mother's TST +&/or CXR abnormal (hilar adenopathy &/or infiltrate), INH + RIF (10-20 mg/kg/day) (or SM). Total rx 6 mos. If mother is being rx, continue INH for total of 9 mos. If INH not given initially, repeat TST at 3 mos.
	Children <5 years of age—Rx indicated	As for neonate for 1st 3 mos	**If + rx** with INH for 9 mos. (see Category II below).
	Older children & adults—Risk 2-4% 1st yr		No rx if repeat TST negative

See page 2 for abbreviations, page 137 for footnotes * Dosages are for adults (unless otherwise indicated) and assume normal renal function ¹ **DOT** = directly observed therapy

TABLE 12A (2)

CAUSATIVE AGENT/DISEASE	MODIFYING CIRCUMSTANCES	SUGGESTED REGIMENS INITIAL THERAPY	ALTERNATIVE
II. Treatment of latent infection with M. tuberculosis (formerly known as TB prophylaxis) (NEJM 364:1441, 2011) **A. INH indicated due to high-risk** Assumes INH susceptibility. INH pre-98% effective in 5–86% effective in preventing active TB for ≥20 yrs.	(1) + tuberculin reactor & HIV+ /risk of active disease 10% per yr; AIDS 170 times ↑, HIV+ 113 times ↑). (2) Newly infected persons (TST conversion in past 2 yrs—risk 3.3% 1 yr). (3) Past history of TB, not rx with adequate chemotherapy (INH, RIF, or alternatives) (4) + tuberculin reactors with CXR consistent with non-progressive tuberculous disease (risk 0.5–5.0% per yr) (5) + tuberculin reactors with specific predisposing conditions: illicit IV drug use (MMWR 38:236, 1989), silicosis, diabetes mellitus, prolonged adrenocorticosteroid or immunosuppressive therapy, hematologic diseases (Hodgkin's, leukemia), endstage renal disease, clinical condition with rapid substantial weight loss or chronic under-nutrition, previous gastrectomy (CID 45:428, 2007) (6) + tuberculin reactors due to start anti-TNF (alpha) therapy (CID 46:1738, 2008). For management algorithm see Thorax 60:800, 2005. **NOTE: For HIV+ see Sanford Guide to HIV/AIDS Therapy &/or JID 196:S35, 2007**	**INH** (5 mg/kg/day, max 300 mg/day for adults; 10 mg/kg/day not to exceed 300 mg/day for children) May use DOT with INH 900 mg (15 mg/kg) 2x/wk. Optimal duration 9 mos. (includes HIV+, children, some cases, 6 mos. may be given for cost-effectiveness (AJRCCM 161:S221, 2000). Do not use 6 mos. regimen in HIV+ persons <18 yrs. or those with fibrotic lesions on chest film (NEJM 345:189, 2001). For current recommendations for monitoring, see hepatotoxicity, etc., AJRCCM 174:935, 2006. **Rifapentine (wt-based dose)**, 10–14 kg: 300 mg; 14.1–25 kg: 450 mg; 25.1–32 kg: 600 mg; 32.1–49.9 kg: 750 mg; ≥50 kg: 900 mg. Not recommended for children age < 2 yrs, pts with HIV/AIDS on ART, pregnant women, or pts presumed infected with INH- or RIF-resistant M. Tb. (MMWR 60:1650, 2011).	If compliance problem: **INH** by DOT 15 mg/kg 2x/wk (max 900 mg) times 9 mos. **RIF** 600 mg/day po for 4 mos. (HIV– and HIV+) as effective as 9 mos. of INH (MMWR 52:735, 2003) Meta-analysis suggests 4 mos of INH + RIF equiv to "standard" (6–12 mos) INH therapy (CID 40:670, 2005); 3–4 month INH + RIF regimens also as safe and effective as 9 months INH in children (CID 45:715, 2007).
B. TST positive (organisms likely to be INH-susceptible	Age no longer considered modifying factor (see Comments)	**INH** (5 mg per kg per day, max 300 mg per day for adults; 10 mg per kg per day not to exceed 300 mg per day for children). Results with 6 mos. rx as effective as 12 mos. (65% vs 75% reduction in disease), 9 mos. is current recommendation. See II. A above for details and alternate rx.	Reanalyses of earlier studies favors **INH** prophylaxis (if INH related, hepatitis case fatality rate <1% and TB case fatality ≥6.7%, which appears to be the case) (AVM 150:2517, 1990). Recent data suggest INH prophylaxis has positive risk-benefit ratio in ≥35. If monitored closely for hepatotoxicity (AJVM 127:1051, 1997) Overall risk of hepatotoxicity 0.1–0.15% (JAMA 281:1014, 1999).
	Pregnancy—Any risk factors (II.A above)	Treat with **INH** as above. For women at risk for progression to active disease, esp. those who are HIV+ or who have been recently infected, rx should not be delayed even during the first trimester	
	Pregnancy—No risk factors	No viral rx (see Comment)	Delay rx until delivery
C. TST positive & drug resistance likely (For data on worldwide prevalence of drug resistance, see: NEJM 344:1294, 2001; JID 185:1197, 2002; JID 194:479, 2006; EID 13:380, 2007)	INH-resistant (or adverse reaction to INH); RIF-sensitive organisms likely	**RIF** 600 mg per day po for 4 mos. (HIV+ or HIV–)	Rifabutin 300 mg daily is an alternative. Estimate RIF alone has protective effect of 56%; 26% of pts reported adverse effects (only 2/157 did not complete 4 mos. rx, 4 months therapy with RIF (10 mg/kg) produced fewer adverse effects than 9 months of INH (AJM 149:689, 2008).
	INH- and RIF-resistant organisms likely	Efficacy of all regimens unproven. **PZA** 25–30 mg per kg per day to max. of 2 gm per day + **ETB** 15–25 mg per kg per day po times 12 mos.	**PZA** 25 mg per kg per day to max. of 2 gm per day) + (**levo** 500 mg per day), all po, times 6–12 mos.

See page 2 for abbreviations, page 137 for footnotes   * Dosages are for adults (unless otherwise indicated) and assume normal renal function   † **DOT** = directly observed therapy

TABLE 12A (3)

CAUSATIVE AGENT/DISEASE	MODIFYING CIRCUM-STANCES	SUGGESTED REGIMENS					COMMENTS
		INITIAL THERAPY[4]		**CONTINUATION PHASE OF THERAPY[1] AND DIRECTLY OBSERVED THERAPY[1] (DOT) REGIMENS** (in vitro susceptibility known)			
		Regimen: in order of preference	Drugs	Interval/Doses[1,2] (min. duration)	Regimen	Drugs	Interval/Doses[1,2] (min. duration)	Range of Total Doses (min. duration)
III. **Mycobacterium tuberculosis** A. Pulmonary TB General reference on rx in adults & children: *Ln* 362: 887, 2003; *MMWR* 52/(RR-11):1, 2003; *CID* 40(Suppl.1):S1, 2005. Reference on transplant & other immuno-compromised pts: *CID* 48:1276, 2009; *CID* 38:1229, 2004. In pts with newly diagnosed HIV and TB, rx for both should be started as soon as possible (*NEJM* 362:697, 2010). **Isolation essential!** Pts with active TB should be isolated in single rooms, not cohorted (*MMWR* 54(RR-17), 2005). Older observations on infectivity of susceptible & resistant M. TBc before and after rx (*ARRD* 85:5111, 1962) may not be applicable to MDR M. TBc or to the HIV+ individual. Extended isolation may be appropriate. 10% of immunocompromised cultures at day 60 (*CID* 51:371, 2010). See footnotes, page 137 **USE DOT REGIMENS IF POSSIBLE** (continued on next page)	Rate of INH resistance known to be <4% (drug-susceptible organisms) [Modified from *MMWR* 52(RR-11):1, 2003]	1 (See Figure 1, page 133)	INH RIF PZA ETB	7 days per wk times 56 doses (8 wks) or 5 days per wk times 40 doses (8 wks)[3]	1a	INH[5] RIF[5]	7 days per wk times 126 doses (18 wks) or 5 days per wk times 90 doses (18 wks)[3]	182–130 (26 wks)
					1b	INH[5] RIF	Fixed dose combination of INH, RIF, PZA & ETB currently being evaluated (*JAMA* 305:1415, 2011). 36 doses (18 wks)	92–76 (26 wks)
					1c[3]	INH[5] RFP	1 time per wk times 18 doses (18 wks)	74–58 (26 wks)
		2 (See Figure 1, page 133)	INH RIF PZA ETB	7 days per wk times 14 doses (2 wks), then 2 times per wk times 12 doses (6 wks) or 5 days per wk times 10 doses (2 wks) then 2 times per wk times 12 doses (6 wks)	2a	INH[5] RIF	2 times per wk times 36 doses (18 wks)	62–58 (26 wks)[4]
					2b[3]	INH[5] RFP	1 time per wk times 18 doses (18 wks)	44–40 (26 wks)
		3 (See Figure 1, page 133)	INH RIF PZA ETB	3 times per wk times 24 doses (8 wks)	3a	INH[5] RIF	3 times per wk times 54 doses (18 wks)	78 (26 wks)
		4 (See Figure 1, page 133)	INH RIF ETB	7 days per wk times 56 doses (8 wks) or 5 days per wk times 40 doses (8 wks)[3]	4a	INH[5] RIF[5]	7 days per wk times 217 doses (31 wks) or 5 days per wk times 155 doses (31 wks)	273–195 (39 wks)
					4b	INH[5] RIF	2 times per wk times 62 doses (31 wks)	118–102 (39 wks)

COMMENTS

Regimen* Q24h:	Dose in mg per kg (max. q24h dose)				
	INH	RIF	PZA	ETB	SM	RFB
Adult	5 (300)	10 (600)	15–30 (2000)	15–25	15 (1000)	5 (300)
Child	10–20 (300)	10–20 (600)	15–30 (2000)	15–25	20–40 (1000)	5 (300)
2 times per wk (DOT):						
Adult	15 (900)	10 (600)	50–70 (4000)	50	25–30 (1500)	5 (300)
Child	20–40 (900)	10–20 (600)	50–70 (4000)	50	25–30 (1500)	10–20 (300)
3 times per wk (DOT):						
Adult	15 (900)	10 (600)	50–70 (3000)	25–30	25–30 (1500)	NA
Child	20–40 (900)	10–20 (600)	50–70 (4000)	25–30	25–30 (1500)	NA

Second-line anti-TB agents can be dosed as follows to facilitate DOT: Cycloserine 500–750 mg po q24h (5 times per wk)
Ethionamide 500–750 mg po q24h (5 times per wk)
Kanamycin or capreomycin 15 mg per kg IM/IV q24h (3–5 times per wk)
Ciprofloxacin 750 mg po q24h (5 times per wk)
Ofloxacin 600–800 mg po q24h (5 times per wk)
Levofloxacin 750 mg po q24h (5 times per wk)
(*CID* 21:1245, 1995)

Risk factors for drug-resistant (MDR) TB: Recent immigration from Latin America or Asia or living in area of ↑ resistance (≥4%) or previous rx without RIF; exposure to known MDR TB. Incidence of primary drug resistance is particularly high (>25%) including countries like Russia, Estonia & Latvia. ~80% of US MDR cases in foreign born.

(continued on next page)

See page 2 for abbreviations, page 137 for footnotes   * Dosages are for adults (unless otherwise indicated) and assume normal renal function   † **DOT** = directly observed therapy

TABLE 12A (4)

CAUSATIVE AGENT/DISEASE	MODIFYING CIRCUMSTANCES	SUGGESTED REGIMEN[*]	DURATION OF TREATMENT (mos.)[a]	SPECIFIC COMMENTS[†]	COMMENTS
III. Mycobacterium tuberculosis A. Pulmonary TB (continued from previous page)	INH (± SM) resistance	RIF, PZA, ETB (a FQ may strengthen the regimen for pts with extensive disease). Emergence of FQ resistance a concern (AJRCCM 3:1201, 2003; AAC 49:3178, 2005)	6		(continued from previous page) Note that CIP not as effective as PZA + ETB in multidrug regimen for susceptible TB (CID 22:287, 1996). **Moxifloxacin, and levofloxacin have enhanced activity compared with CIP** against M. tuberculosis. FQ resistance may be seen in pts previously treated with FQ (CID 37:1448, 2003). WHO recommends using moxifloxacin (if MIC ≤ 2) if resistant to earlier generation FQs (AAC 54:4765, 2010). **Linezolid has excellent in vitro activity, including MDR strains** and effective in selected cases of MDR TB and XDR TB, but watch for toxicity (JAC 64:1119, 2009; CID 50:49, 2010). **Bedaquiline** recently FDA approved for treatment of MDR TB based on efficacy in Phase 2 trials (NEJM 360:2397, 2009; AAC 53:3271, 2012). Dose is 400 mg once daily for 2 weeks then 200 mg tiw for 22 weeks administered as directly observed therapy (DOT), taken with food, and always in combination with other anti-TB meds. Consultation with an expert in MDR-TB management strongly advised before use of this agent.
Multidrug-Resistant Tuberculosis (MDR TB): Defined as resistant to at least 2 drugs including INH & RIF. Pt clusters with high mortality (MMWR 363:1050, 2006)	Resistance to INH & RIF (± SM)	FQ, PZA, ETB, IA, ± alternative agent	18–24	In such cases, extended rx is needed to ↓ the risk of relapse. In cases with extensive disease, the use of an additional agent (alternative agents) may be prudent to ↓ the risk of failure & additional acquired drug resistance. Resectional surgery may be appropriate.	
	Resistance to INH, RIF (± SM), & ETB	FQ (ETB or PZA if active), IA, & 2 alternative agents[*]	24	Use the first-line agents to which there is susceptibility. Add 2 or more alternative agents in case of extensive disease. Surgery should be considered for survival in pts receiving active FQ & surgical intervention (AJRCCM 169:1103, 2004).	
Extensively Drug-Resistant TB (XDR-TB): Defined as resistant to INH & RIF plus any FQ and at least 1 of the 3 second-line drugs: capreomycin, kanamycin or amikacin (MMWR 56:250, 2007; Ln 370:19, 2009; CID 51:379, 2010).	Resistance to RIF or PZA	INH, ETB, FQ supplemented with PZA for the first 2 mos (an IA may be included for pts 2–3 mos. for pts with extensive disease)	12–18	C24h 3 times per wk regimens of INH, PZA & SM given for 9 mos. were effective in a BMRC trial (AJRCD 115:727, 1977). However, extended use of an IA may not be feasible. It is not known if ETB would be as effective as SM in these regimens. An all-oral regimen times 12–18 mos. should be effective. But for more extensive disease &/or to shorten duration (e.g., to 12 mos.), an IA may be added in the initial 2 mos. of rx.	
	XDR-TB	See Comments	18–24	Therapy requires administration of 4-6 drugs to which infecting organism is susceptible, including multiple second-line drugs (MMWR 56:250, 2007). Increased mortality seen primarily in HIV+ patients. Cure with outpatient therapy likely in non-HIV+ patients when regimens of 4 or 5 or more drugs to which organism is susceptible are employed (NEJM 359:563, 2008; Ln 375:1798, 2009). Successful sputum culture conversion correlates to initial susceptibility to FQs and kanamycin (CID 46:42, 2008). Addition of "later generation" FQ (Levo, Moxi) beneficial on meta-analysis of XDR-TB (CID 51:6, 2010).	
See footnotes, page 137 Reviews of therapy for MDR-TB: JAC 54:593, 2004; Med Lett 7:75, 2009; For XDR-TB see MMWR 55:250, 2007; NEJM 359:563, 2008					

See page 2 for abbreviations, page 137 for footnotes * Dosages are for adults (unless otherwise indicated) and assume normal renal function † **DOT** = directly observed therapy

131

TABLE 12A (5)

CAUSATIVE AGENT/DISEASE; MODIFYING CIRCUMSTANCES	SUGGESTED REGIMENS		COMMENTS
	INITIAL THERAPY	CONTINUATION PHASE OF THERAPY (In vitro susceptibility known)	
III. Mycobacterium tuberculosis *(continued)*			
B. Extrapulmonary TB	INH + RIF (or RFB) + PZA q24h times 2 months. Authors add **pyridoxine** 25–50 mg po q24h to regimens that include INH.	INH + RIF (or RFB) 25–50 mg po q24h to regimens	6 mos regimens with 9–12 mo regimens. Most experience with 9–12 mos regimens. Am Acad Ped (1994) recommends 6 mos rx for isolated cervical adenitis, renal and 12 mos for meningitis, miliary, bone/joint. DOT useful here as well as for pulmonary tuberculosis. IDSA recommends 6 mos for lymph node, pleural, pericarditis, disseminated disease, genitourinary & peritoneal TBc; 6–9 mos for bone & joint; 9–12 mos for CNS (including meningeal) TBc. Corticosteroids "strongly rec'" only for pericarditis & meningeal TBc (MMWR 52(RR-11):1, 2003).
C. Tuberculous meningitis Excellent summary of clinical aspects and therapy (incl. steroids). See CMR 21:243, 2008. Also J Infect 59:167, 2009.	INH + RIF + ETB + PZA		3 drugs often nec for initial rx; we prefer 4 (J Infect 59:167, 2009). May sub ethionamide for ETB. Infection with MDR-TB ↑ mortality & morbidity (CID 38:851, 2004; JID 192:79, 2005). Treatment worked in 2 HIV+ children with MDR-TB (PIDJ 22:1142, 2003). In adults (AAC 50:1051, 2006). PCR of CSF (marked↓ diagnostic sensitivity and ↑ specificity) aided dx but considerable variability, even in patients with INH resistant organisms (JID 192:2134, 2005). FQs: (Levo, Gati, CIP) may be useful if started early (AAC 55:3244, 2011).
D. Tuberculosis during pregnancy	INH + RIF + ETB for 9 mos		PZA not recommended: teratogenicity data inadequate. Because of potential ototoxicity to fetus throughout gestation (16%), SM should not be used unless other drugs contraindicated. Add pyridoxine 25 mg per day for pregnant women on INH. Breast-feeding should not be discouraged in pts on first-line drugs (MMWR 52(RR-11):1, 2003).
E. Treatment failure or relapse. Usually due to poor compliance and evolution of resistant organisms, or subtherapeutic drug levels (CID 55:169, 2012).	Directly observed therapy (DOT); check susceptibilities. (See section III/A, page 130 & above)	Pts whose sputum has not converted after 5–6 mos. = treatment failures. Failures may be due to non-compliance or resistant organisms. Check for current isolates. Non-compliance is common, therefore institute DOT. If isolates show resistance, modify regimen to include at least 2 effective agents, preferably ones which pt has not received. Surgery may be necessary. In HIV+ patients, reinfection vs relapse as a possible explanation for "failure." NB, patients with MDR-TB usually convert sputum within 12 weeks of successful therapy and TB progression (JID 204:358, 2011). Early deaths associated with depressed innate responses, bacterial infection and TB progression (JID 204:358, 2011).
F. HIV infection or AIDS—extrapulmonary (NOTE: 60–70% of HIV+ pts with TB have extrapulmonary disease)	INH + RIF (or RFB) q24h times 2 months	INH + RIF (or RFB) q24h times total mos. May need longer (9 mos) in pts with delayed response. (Authors add **pyridoxine** 25–50 mg po q24h to regimens that include INH.)	1. Because of possibility of developing resistance to RIF in pts with low CD4 cell counts who were getting RFB once weekly, CDC recommends at least 2x/wk dosing in initiation phase rx (MMWR 51:214, 2002) (or min 3x/wk) doses of RFB for initiation rx. 2. Clinical & microbiologic response same as in HIV-neg patient although there is considerable variability in outcomes among currently available studies (CID 32:623, 2001). 3. Post-treatment suppression not necessary for drug-susceptible strains. 4. Rate of INH resistance known to be 4% (ref) rates of resistance, see Section III/A. 5. Adequate response of tx of TB in HIV+ patients with CD4 counts >200 (JID 190:1856, 2004); MDR-TB + HIV: pleurisy (JID 190:869, 2004).
Concomitant protease inhibitor (PI) therapy (Modified from MMWR 49:185, 2000; AJRCCM 162:7, 2001)	**Initial & cont. therapy:** INH 300 mg (per dose) + PZA 25 mg per kg + ETB 15 mg per kg q24h times 2 mos; then INH + RFB times 4 mos. (up to 7 mos). **PI Regimen**	**RFB dose** Nelfinavir 1250 mg q12h or indinavir 1000 mg q8h or amprenavir 1200 mg q12h.. 150 mg q24h or 300 mg intermittently Saquinavir standard dose.... 300 mg q24h or intermittently Ritonavir standard dose........ 150 mg 2x weekly Lopinavir/ritonavir—standard dose 150 mg 3x per wk	**Comments:** Rifamycins induce cytochrome CYP450 enzymes (RIF > RFB > RFB) & reduce serum levels of concomitantly administered PIs. Conversely, PIs (ritonavir > amprenavir > indinavir not induced, toxicity ↑. RFB/PI combinations are therapeutically effective (CID 30:779, 2000). **Effavirenz is preferred over Nevirapine for pts on regimens containing RFB**. Rifabutin can be used for active TB in pts on ritonavir + saquinavir because of drug-induced hepatitis with markedly transaminase elevations has been seen in the few volunteers receiving this regimen (www.fda.gov). Monitor plasma levels of RFB when given with Lopinavir/Ritonavir (CID 49:1305, 2009). ART regimens containing Efavirenz for TB seems to increase Stavudine toxicity (CID 48:1672, 2009; CMR 24:351, 2011). **Effavirenz less compromised by concomitant RIF than Nevirapine** (CID 48:1752, 2009; CMR 24:351, 2011).

See page 2 for abbreviations, page 137 for footnotes * Dosages are for adults (unless otherwise indicated) and assume normal renal function † **DOT** = directly observed therapy

TABLE 12A (6)
FIGURE 1 [Modified from MMWR 52(RR-11):1, 2003]

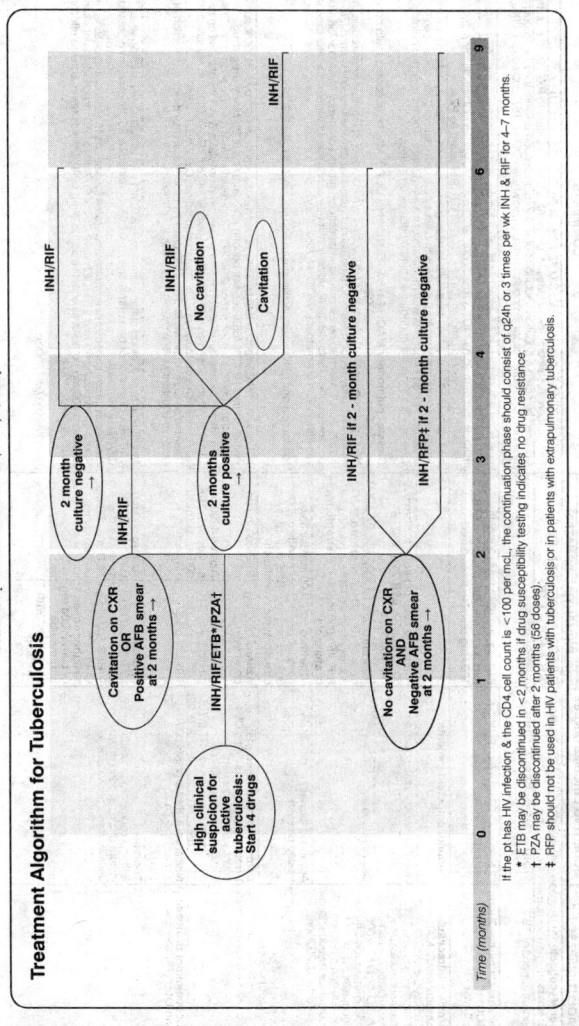

Treatment Algorithm for Tuberculosis

High clinical suspicion for active tuberculosis: Start 4 drugs

Cavitation on CXR OR Positive AFB smear at 2 months → INH/RIF/ETB*/PZA†

- 2 month culture negative → INH/RIF → INH/RIF (through month 6)
- 2 months culture positive ↑ → INH/RIF →
  - No cavitation → INH/RIF (through month 6)
  - Cavitation → INH/RIF (through month 9)

No cavitation on CXR AND Negative AFB smear at 2 months → INH/RIF/ETB*/PZA†
- INH/RIF‡ if 2-month culture negative
- INH/RPF‡ if 2-month culture negative

Time (months): 0 1 2 3 4 6 9

If the pt has HIV infection & the CD4 cell count is <100 per mcL, the continuation phase should consist of q24h or 3 times per wk INH & RIF for 4–7 months.

* ETB may be discontinued in <2 months if drug susceptibility testing indicates no drug resistance.
† PZA may be discontinued after 2 months (56 doses).
‡ RFP should not be used in HIV patients with tuberculosis or in patients with extrapulmonary tuberculosis.

See page 2 for abbreviations.

TABLE 12A (7)

CAUSATIVE AGENT/DISEASE	MODIFYING CIRCUMSTANCES	SUGGESTED REGIMENS PRIMARY/ALTERNATIVE		COMMENTS
IV. Other Mycobacterial Disease ("Atypical") (See ATS Consensus: *AJRCCM 175:367, 2007; IDC No. Amer 16:187, 2002; CMR 15:716, 2002; CID 42:1756, 2006; EID 17:506, 2011*)		INH + RIF + ETB		
A. M. bovis				The M. tuberculosis complex includes M. bovis. All isolates resistant to PZA. 9-12 months of rx used by some authorities. Isolation not required. Increased prevalence of extrapulmonary disease in U.S. born Hispanic populations and elsewhere (*CID 47:168, 2008; EID 17:457, 2011*).
B. Bacillus Calmette-Guerin (BCG) (derived from M. bovis)	Only fever (>38.5°C) for 12–24 hrs. Systemic illness or sepsis	INH 300 mg q24h times 3 months INH 300 mg + RIF 600 mg + ETB 1200 mg po q24h times 6 mos.		Intravesical BCG effective in superficial bladder tumors and carcinoma in situ. With sepsis, consider initial adjunctive prednisone. Also susceptible to RIF, cipro, oflox, streptomycin, amikacin, capreomycin (*AAC 53:316, 2009*). BCG may cause regional adenitis or pulmonary disease in HIV-infected children (*CID 37:1226, 2003*). **Resistant to PZA**.
C. M. avium-intracellulare complex (MAC, MAI, or Battey bacillus) ATS/IDSA Consensus Statement: *AJRCCM 175:367, 2007; alternative ref. CID 42:1756, 2006*. Anti-tumor necrosis factor-α increases risk of infection with MAI and other non-tuberculous mycobacteria (*EID 15:1556, 2009*).	**Immunocompetent patients**			See *AJRCCM 175:367, 2007* for details on dosing and duration of therapy.
	Nodular/Bronchiectatic disease	Clarithro 1000 mg tiw or azithro 500-600 mg tiw) + ETB 25 mg/kg tiw + RIF 600 mg tiw		Although no controlled trial data, many clinicians prefer intermittent (tiw) therapy for non-cavitary disease. Patients with moderate or severe disease, or those who have been previously treated or patients with moderate of severe disease. The primary microbiologic goal of therapy is 12 months of negative sputum cultures on therapy.
	Cavitary disease	Clarithro 500-1000 mg/day (lower dose for wt <50 kg) or azithro 250-300 mg/day) + ETB 15 mg/kg/day + RIF 450-600 mg/day ± streptomycin or amikacin		"Classic" pulmonary MAC. Men 50-75, smokers, COPD. May be associated with hot tub use (*Clin Chest Med 23:675, 2002*). "Hot tub lung" extract: *Vgw Chest*. Women >70, scoliosis, mitral valve prolapse, (bronchiectasis), pectus excavatum ("Lady Windermere syndrome") and fibronodular disease in elderly women (*EID 16:1576, 2010*). May also be associated with interferon gamma deficiency (*AJM 113:756, 2002*). For cervicofacial lymphadenitis (localized) in immunocompetent children, surgical excision is as effective as chemotherapy (*CID 44:1057, 2007*).
	Advanced (severe) or previously treated disease	Clarithro 500-1000 mg/day (lower dose for wt <50 kg) or azithro 250-300 mg/day) + ETB 15 mg/kg/day ± streptomycin or amikacin		Moxifloxacin and gatifloxacin, active in vitro & in vivo (*AAC 51:4071, 2007*).
	Immunocompromised pts: Primary prophylaxis—Pt's CD4 count <50-100 per mm³ Discontinue when CD4 count >100 per mm³ in response to ART (*NEJM 342:1085, 2000; CID 34:662, 2002*). Guideline: *AnIM 137:435, 2002*	Azithro 1200 mg po q24h OR Clarithro 500 mg po bid	RFB 300 mg po q24h OR Azithro 1200 mg po weekly + RIF 300 mg q24h	RFB reduces MAC infection rate by 55% (no survival benefit); clarithro by 69% (30% survival benefit); azithro by 59% (68% survival benefit) (*CID 26:611, 1998*). **Many drug-drug interactions, see Table 22, pages 219, 222**. Drug-resistant MAI disease seen in 29-58% of pts in whom breakthrough develops while taking clarithro prophylaxis & in 11% of those on azithro but has not been observed with RFB prophylaxis (*JID 38:6, 1999*). Clarithro resistance more likely than azithro (*AAC 42:1766, 1998*). Need to be sure no active M. TBc; RFB used for prophylaxis may promote selection of rifamycin-resistant M. TBc (*NEJM 335:384 & 428, 1996*).
	Treatment Either presumptive dx or after + culture of blood, bone marrow, or usually, sterile body fluids, eg liver	(Clarithro 500 mg* po bid + ETB 15 mg/kg/day + RIF 300 mg q24h) *Higher doses of clari (1000 mg bid) may be associated with ↑ mortality (*CID 29:125, 1999*)	Azithro 500 mg po/day + ETB 15 mg/kg/day +/- RFB 300-450 mg po/day	Median time to neg. blood culture: clarithro + ETB 4.4 wks vs azithro + ETB >16 wks. At 16 wks, clearance of bacteremia with 46% of azithro- & 85.7% of clarithro-treated pts (*CID 27:1278, 1998*). More recent study suggests similar clearance rates for azithro (46%) vs clarithro (56%) at 24 wks when combined with ETB (*CID 37:1245, 2000*). Azithro 250 mg po q24h not effective, but azithro 600 mg po q24h as effective as 1200 mg po q24h & yields fewer adverse effects (*AAC 43: 2869, 1999*). (*continued on next page*)

See page 2 for abbreviations, page 137 for footnotes * Dosages are for adults (unless otherwise indicated) and assume normal renal function † **DOT** = directly observed therapy

TABLE 12A (8)

CAUSATIVE AGENT/DISEASE	MODIFYING CIRCUMSTANCES	SUGGESTED REGIMENS PRIMARY/ALTERNATIVE		COMMENTS
IV. Other Mycobacterial Disease ("Atypical") *(continued)*				
C. M. avium-intracellulare complex *(continued)*				*(continued from previous page)* Addition of RFB to clarithro + ETB ↓ emergence of resistance to clari, ↓ relapse rate & improves survival (CID 37:1234, 2003). Clofazimine not recommended for MAI in HIV+ pts. Drug toxicity: With clarithro, 23% had to stop drug 2° to dose-limiting adverse reaction. Combination of clarithro, ETB and RFB led to uveitis and pseudojaundice; result is reduction in max. dose of RFB to 300 mg. Treatment failure rate is high. Reasons: drug toxicity, development of drug resistance, & inadequate serum levels. Serum levels of clarithro ↓ in pts also given RIF or RFB (JID 171:747, 1995). if pt not responding to initial regimen after 2–4 weeks, add one or more drugs.
	Chronic post-treatment suppression—secondary prophylaxis	**Always necessary.** (Clarithro or azithro) + ETB 15 mg/kg/day (dosage above)	Clarithro or azithro or RFB (dosage above)	Recurrences almost universal without chronic suppression. However, in patients on ART with robust CD4 cell response, it is possible to discontinue chronic suppression (JID 178:1446, 1998; NEJM 340:1301, 1999).
D. Mycobacterium celatum	Treatment; optimal regimen not defined	May be susceptible to **clarithro**, FQ (Clin Micro Inf 3:582, 1997). Suggest rx "like MAI" but often resistant to RIF (Int J 38:157, 1999). Most reported cases received 3 or 4 drugs, usually clarithro + ETB + RFB (EID 9:399, 2003).		Isolated from pulmonary lesions and blood in AIDS patients confused with M. xenopi (and MAC). Susceptibilities similar to MAC, but highly resistant to RIF (CID 24:140, 1997).
E. Mycobacterium abscessus Mycobacterium chelonae	Treatment; Surgical excision may facilitate clarithro rx in subcutaneous abscess and is important adjunct to rx. For role of surgery in M. abscessus pulmonary disease, see CID 52:565, 2011.	**Clarithro** 500 mg po bid times 6 mos. Azithro may also be effective. For serious disseminated infections add amikacin + IMP or cefoxitin 2–4 wks. (Clin Micro Rev 15:716, AJRCCM 175:367, 2007) or add Moxi or Levo (CID 49:1365, 2009).		M. abscessus susceptible to AMK (70%), clarithro (95%), cefoxitin (70%), CLO, cefmetazole, RFB, FQ, IMP, azithro, cipro, doxy, mino, tigecycline (CID 42:1756, 2006; JIC 15:46, 2009). Single isolates of M. abscessus often not associated with disease. Clarithro-resistant strains have described (Clin Micro Rev 15:716, 2002). M. chelonae susceptible to AMK (80%), clarithro, azithro, tobramycin (100%), IMP (60%), moxifloxacin (AAC 46:3283, 2002), cipro, mino, doxy, linezolid (94%) (CID 42:1756, 2006). Resistant to cefoxitin, FQ (CID 24:1147, 1997; AJRCCM 156:S1, 1997). Tigecycline highly active in vitro (AAC 52:4184, 2008; CID 49:1358, 2009).
F. Mycobacterium fortuitum	Treatment; optimal regimen not defined. Surgical excision of infected areas.	**AMK + cefoxitin + probenecid** 2–6 wks., then po **TMP-SMX**, or **doxy** 2–6 mos. Usually responds to 6–12 mos of oral rx with drugs to which susceptible (AAC 46:3283, 2002; Clin Micro Rev 15:716, 2002). Nail salon-acquired infections respond to 4–6 mos of minocycline, doxy, or CIP (CID 38:38, 2004).		**Resistant to all standard anti-TBc drugs.** Sensitive in vitro to doxycycline, minocycline, cefoxitin, IMP, AMK, TMP-SMX, CIP, ofiox, azithro, clarithro, linezolid, tigecycline (Clin Micro Rev 15:716, 2002), but some strains resistant to azithromycin, rifabutin (AAC 39:567, 1997; AAC 55:775, 2002). Acceptable to treat with susceptible agents active in vitro until sputum cultures negative for 12 months (AJRCCM 175:367, 2007).

See page 2 for abbreviations, page 137 for footnotes * Dosages are for adults (unless otherwise indicated) and assume normal renal function † **DOT** = directly observed therapy

TABLE 12A (9)

CAUSATIVE AGENT/DISEASE; MODIFYING CIRCUMSTANCES	SUGGESTED REGIMENS PRIMARY	SUGGESTED REGIMENS ALTERNATIVE	COMMENTS
IV. Other Mycobacterium Disease ("Atypical") (continued)			
G. Mycobacterium haemophilum	Regimen(s) not defined. In animal model, **clarithro** + **rifabutin** effective (CID 41:1569, 2005). Associates with extent cytokine or inhibitors (CID 52:488, 2011). Limited clinical experience limited (Clin Micro Rev 9:435, 1996; CID 52:488, 2011). Surgical debridement may be necessary (CID 26:505, 1998).	**CIP** + **RIF** + **clarithro**. Requires supplemented media to isolate. Sensitive in vitro to: INH, RIF, ETB, PZA, (AnIM 120:118, 1994). For localized cervicofacial lymphadenitis in immunocompetent children, surgical excision as effective as chemotherapy (CID 44:1057, 2007) or "watchful waiting" (CID 52:180, 2011).	Clinical: Ulcerating skin lesions, synovitis, osteomyelitis, cervicofacial lymphadenitis in children.
H. Mycobacterium genavense	Regimens should include 22 drugs: **ETB**, **RIF**, **RFB**, **CLO**, **clarithro**. In animal model, **clarithro** + **RFB** (& to lesser extent amikacin & **ETB**) shown effective in reducing bacterial counts. CIP not effective (JAC 42:483, 1998).		Clinical: CD4 <50. Symptoms of fever, weight loss, diarrhea. Lab: Growth in BACTEC vials slow (mean 42 days). Subcultures grow only on Middlebrook 7H11 agar containing 2 mg per mL mycobactin J. Growth still insufficient for in vitro sensitivity testing (JI 340:76, 1992; AnIM 117:586, 1992). Survival 1 from 81 to 263 days in pts n.kr at least 1 month with 22 drugs (AnIM 155:400, 1995).
I. Mycobacterium gordonae	Regimen(s) not defined, but consider **RIF** + **ETB** + **KM** or **CIP** (J Inf 38:157, 1999) or **linezolid** (AJRCCM 175:367, 2007).		Frequent colonizer, not associated with disease. In vitro: sensitive to ETB, RIF, AMK, CIP, clarithro, linezolid (AAC 47:1736, 2003). Resistant to INH (CID 14:1229, 1992). Surgical excision.
J. Mycobacterium kansasii	(Q24h po: **INH** (300 mg) + **RIF** (600 mg) + **ETB** (25 mg per kg) times 2 mos. then 15 mg per kg) Rx for 18 mos. (until culture-neg. times sputum times 12 mos.; 15 mos. if HIV+) (See Comment)	If RIF-resistant, (q24h po): **INH** (900 mg) + **pyridoxine** (50 mg) + **ETB** (25 mg per kg) + **sulfamethoxazole** (1 gm tid). Rx until all cultures-neg. times 12-15 mos. (See Comment). **Clari** + **ETB** + **RIF** also effective in small study (CID 37:1178, 2003).	All isolates are resistant to PZA. Highly susceptible to clarithro and moxi (AAC 47:1736, 2003) and to clarithro and moxifloxacin (AAC 55:950, 2006). INH + rifalling or protease inhibitor, substitute either clarithro (500 mg bid) or RFB (150 mg per day) for RIF. Because of variable susceptibility to INH, some substitute clarithro 500-750 mg q24h for INH. Resistance to clarithro reported, but most strains susceptible to clarithro as well as moxifloxacin (JAC 55:950, 2005) & levofloxacin (AAC 48:4562, 2004). Prognosis related to level of immunosuppression (CID 37:584, 2003).
K. Mycobacterium marinum	(**Clarithro** 500 mg bid) or **doxycycline** (100-200 mg q24h) or (**TMP-SMX** 160/800 mg bid) or (**RIF** + **ETB** (Am R Resp Dis 156:S1, 1997; Eur J Clin Microbiol ID 25:609, 2006)). Surgical excision.	**minocycline** 100-200 mg q24h or (**doxycycline** 100-200 mg q24h) or (**TMP-SMX** 160/800 mg bid) or (**RIF** + **ETB** (Am R Resp Dis 156:S1, 1997; Eur J Clin Microbiol ID 25:609, 2006)). Surgical excision.	Resistant to INH & PZA. Also susceptible to linezolid (AAC 47:1736, 2003). CIP, moxifloxacin also show moderate in vitro activity (AAC 46:1114, 2002).
L. Mycobacterium scrofulaceum	Regimen(s) not defined. Surgical excision. Chemotherapy seldom indicated. Although regimens not defined, **clarithro** + **CLO** with or without **ETB** + **INH** + **RIF** + **strep** + **cycloserine** have also been tried.		In vitro resistant to INH, RIF, ETB, PZA, AMK, CIP (CID 20: 549, 1995). Susceptible to clarithro, strep, erythromycin.
M. Mycobacterium ulcerans (Buruli ulcer)	Regimen(s) not defined. Start 4 drugs as for disseminated MAI. WHO recommends **RIF** + **SM** for 8 weeks (Lancet Infection 6:288, 2006; Lancet 367:1849, 2006; AAC 51:645, 2007). **RIF** + **SM** resulted in 47% cure rate (AAC 51:4029, 2007). **RIF** + **cipro** recommended as alternatives by WHO (CMAJ 31:119, 2009). Recent small studies document similar effectiveness of oral therapy followed by 4 weeks of **RIF** + **clarithro** (Lancet 375:664, 2010) and a regimen of 8 wks of **RIF** + **clarithro** (No relapse in 30 pts) (CID 52:94, 2011).		Most isolates resistant to all 1st line anti-tbc drugs. Isolates often not clinically significant (CID 26:625, 1998). Susceptible to most fluoroquinolones in vitro: RIF, strep, CLO, clarithro, CIP, oflox, amikacin, moxi, linezolid. Monotherapy with RIF selects resistant mutants in mice (AAC 47:1228, 2003). RIF + moxi; RIF + clarithro; moxi + clarithro similar to RIF + SM in mice (AAC 51:3737, 2007).
O. Mycobacterium xenopi	Regimen(s) not defined: (**RIF** or **rifabutin**) + **ETB** + **macrolide** + (**RIF** or **rifabutin**) (AAC 36:2841, 1992) and rifabutin (JAC 39:567, 1997). Some recommend a macrolide + (**RIF** or **rifabutin**) (AAC 156:S1, 1997) or **RIF** + **INH** + **ETB** (Resp Med 97:439, 2003) but recent study suggests no need to treat in most pts with HIV (CID 37:1250, 2003).		In vitro: sensitive to clarithro (AAC 36:2841, 1992) and rifabutin (JAC 39:567, 1997). Clarithro-containing regimens more effective than RIF/INH/ETB regimens in mice (AAC 45:3229, 2001). FQs, linezolid also active in vitro.
Mycobacterium leprae (leprosy) Classification: Clin ID 44:1096, 2007. Clinical mgmt of lep. reactions: IDCP 18:235, 2010. Overview: Lancet ID 11:464, 2011.	There are 2 sets of therapeutic recommendations here: one from USA (National Hansen's Disease Programs [N-HDP], Baton Rouge, LA) and one from WHO. Both are based on expert recommendations and neither has been subjected to controlled clinical trial (P. Joyce & D. Scollard, Corrs Current Therapy 2004; J Am Acad Dermatol 51:417, 2004).		

See page 2 for abbreviations, page 137 for footnotes. * Dosages are for adults (unless otherwise indicated) and assume normal renal function † **DOT** = directly observed therapy

TABLE 12A (10)

Type of Disease	NHDP Regimen	WHO Regimen	COMMENTS
Paucibacillary Forms: (Intermediate, Tuberculoid, Borderline tuberculoid)	(**Dapsone** 100 mg/day + **RIF** 600 mg po/daily for 12 months	(**Dapsone** 100 mg/day (unsupervised) + **RIF** 600 mg 1x/mo (supervised)) for 6 mos	Side effects overall 0.4%
Single lesion paucibacillary	Treat as paucibacillary leprosy for 12 months.	Single dose ROM therapy: (RIF 600 mg + Oflox 400 mg + Mino 100 mg). (*Ln* 353:655, 1999).	
Multibacillary forms: Borderline Borderline-lepromatous Lepromatous *See Comment for erythema nodosum leprosum* Rev.: *Lancet* 363:1209, 2004	(**Dapsone** 100 mg/day + **CLO** 50 mg/day + **RIF** 600 mg/day) for 24 mos **Alternative regimen:** (**Dapsone** 100 mg/day + **RIF** 600 mg/day + **Minocycline** 100 mg/day) for 24 mos if CLO is refused or unavailable.	(**Dapsone** 100 mg/day + **CLO** 50 mg/day (both unsupervised) + **RIF** 600 mg + **CLO** 300 mg once monthly (supervised)). Continue regimen for 12 months.	Side-effects overall 5.1%. For **erythema nodosum leprosum:** prednisone 60-80 mg/day or thalidomide 100-400 mg/day (*BMJ* 44: 775, 1988; *AJM* 108:487, 2000). Thalidomide available in US at 1-800-4-CELGENE. Altho thalidomide effective, WHO no longer rec because of potential toxicity (*JID* 193:I-S63, 2006) however the major exports lent naturally occur in young women. Alternatives for ENL include clofazimine and pentoxifylline. **CLO (Clofazimine)** available from NHDP under IND protocol, contact at 1-800-642-2477. **Ethionamide** (250 mg q24h) or **prothionamide** (375 mg q24h) may be subbed for CLO. Etanercept effective in one case refractory to above standard therapy (*CID* 52:e133, 2011). Regimens incorporating clarithro, minocycline, RIF, moxifloxacin, and/or oflox also show promise (*AAC* 44:2919, 2000; *AAC* 50:1558, 2006). Dapsone monotherapy has been abandoned due to emergence of resistance (*CID* 52:e127, 2011), but older patients previously treated with dapsone monotherapy may remain on lifelong maintenance therapy. Dapsone (or azadapsone)[4,6] effective for prophylaxis in one study (*IJnf* 41:137, 2000). Moxifloxacin highly active in vitro and produces rapid clinical response (*AAC* 52:3113, 2008).

FOOTNOTES:

1. When DOT is used, drugs may be given 5 days/wk & necessary number of doses adjusted accordingly. Although no studies compare 5 with 7 q24h doses, extensive experience indicates this would be an effective practice.
2. Patients with cavitation on initial chest x-ray & positive cultures at completion of 2 mos of rx should receive a 7 mos (31 wks; either 217 doses [q24h] or 62 doses [2x/wk] continuation phase.
3. 5 day/wk admin is always given by DOT.
4. Not recommended for HIV-infected pts with CD4 cell counts <100 cells/mcL.
5. Options 1c & 2b should be used only in HIV-neg. pts who have neg. sputum smears at the time of completion of 2 mos rx & do not have cavitation on initial chest x-ray. For pts started on this regimen & found to have a + culture from the 2 mos specimen, rx should be extended extra 3 mos.
6. Options 4a & 4b should be considered only when options 1-3 cannot be given.
7. Alternative agents = ethionamide, cycloserine, p-aminosalicylic acid, clarithromycin, AM-CL, linezolid.
8. Modified from *MMWR* 52(RR-11):1, 2003. See also *IDCP* 11:329, 2002
9. Continuation regimen with INH/ETB less effective than INH/RIF (*Lancet* 364:1244, 2004).

See page 2 for abbreviations. * Dosages are for adults (unless otherwise indicated) and assume normal renal function † **DOT** = directly observed therapy

TABLE 12B – DOSAGE AND ADVERSE EFFECTS OF ANTIMYCOBACTERIAL DRUGS

AGENT (TRADE NAME)[1]	USUAL DOSAGE*	ROUTE/[1] DRUG RESISTANCE (RES) US[2],[1]	SIDE-EFFECTS, TOXICITY AND PRECAUTIONS	SURVEILLANCE
FIRST LINE DRUGS				
Ethambutol (Myambutol) (100, 400 mg tab)	25 mg/kg/day for 2 mos then 15 mg/kg/day q24h as 1 dose (<10% protein binding) [Bacteriostatic to both extracellular & intracellular organisms]	RES: 0.3% (0–0.7%) po 400 mg tab	**Optic neuritis** with decreased visual acuity, central scotomata, and loss of green and red perception; peripheral neuropathy and headache (~1%), rashes (rare), arthralgia (rare), hyperuricemia (rare). Anaphylactoid reaction (rare). *Comment:* Primarily used to inhibit resistance. Disrupts outer cell membrane in M. avium with rx activity to other drugs.	Monthly visual acuity & red/green with dose >15 mg/kg/day; ≥10% loss considered significant. Usually reversible if drug discontinued.
Isoniazid (INH) (Nydrazid, Laniazid, Teebaconin) (50, 100, 300 mg tab)	Q24h dose: 5–10 mg/kg/day up to 300 mg. Twice wkly dose: 15 mg/kg (900 mg max dose) (<10% protein binding) [Bactericidal to both extracellular and intracellular organisms] Add pyridoxine in alcoholic, pregnant, or malnourished pts.	RES: 4.1% (2.6–8.5%) (No prior tx cases) 25.3% rare, 20.3% yrs (2% also in AIDS) IM 100 mg/ml in 10 ml (IV route not FDA-approved but has been used, esp. in AIDS)	Overall ~1%. **Liver. Hep** children 10% mild	SGOT normalizes with continued rx, age <20; rate 2.3%, 34 yrs 2%, also >50 yrs (2.3%) also 1 with alcohol & previous exposure to Hep C (usually asymptomatic if SGOT <3–5xnormal). May be fatal. With prodromal sx, dark urine do LFTs; discontinue if SGOT >3–5xnormal. **Peripheral neuropathy** (17% on 6 mg/kg per day, less on 300 mg, incidence ↑ in slow acetylators); **pyridoxine 10 mg q24h will decrease incidence**; other neurologic sequelae, convulsions, optic neuritis, toxic encephalopathy, psychosis, muscle twitching, dizziness, coma (all rare); allergic skin rashes, fever, minor disulfiram-like reaction; flushing after Swiss cheese; blood dyscrasias (rare); + antinuclear antibody (20%). **Drug-drug interactions common: see Table 22.**	Pre-rx liver functions. Repeat if symptoms (fatigue, weakness, malaise, anorexia, nausea or vomiting); >3 days AJRCCM 152:1705, 1995). Some recommend SGOT at 2, 4, 6 mos esp. if age >50 yrs. Clinical evaluation every mo.
Pyrazinamide (500 mg tab)	25 mg per kg per day (maximum 2.5 gm per day) q24h as 1 dose [Bactericidal for intracellular organisms]	po 500 mg tab	**Arthralgia; hyperuricemia** (with or without symptoms). Hepatitis (not over 2% if recommended dose not exceeded); gastric irritation, photosensitivity (rare).	Pre-rx liver functions. Monthly serum uric acid if symptomatic gouty attack occurs.
Rifamate — combination tablet	2 tablets single dose q24h	po (1 hr before meal)	1 tablet contains 150 mg INH, 300 mg RIF	As with individual drugs
Rifampin (Rifadin, Rimactane, Rifocin) (150, 300, 450, 600 mg cap)	10.0 mg per kg per day up to 600 mg per day q24h as 1 dose (60–90% protein binding) [Bactericidal to all populations of organisms]	RES: 0.2% (0–0.3%) po 300 mg cap (IV available, Merrell-Dow)	INH/RIF dc'd in ~3% for toxicity; gastrointestinal irritation, antibiotic-associated colitis, drug fever (1%), pruritus with or without skin rash (1–5%), anaphylactoid reactions in HIV+ pts, mental confusion, thrombocytopenia (1%), leukopenia (1%), hemolytic anemia, transient **abnormalities in liver function**, "flu syndrome" (fever, chills, headache, bone pain, shortness of breath) seen if RIF taken irregularly or if q24h dose restarted after an interval of no rx. May cause drug-induced lupus erythematosus (Ln 349:1521, 1977). **Discolors urine, tears, sweat, contact lens an orange-brownish color. Multiple significant drug-drug interactions, see Table 22.**	Pre-rx liver function. Repeat if symptoms. **Multiple significant drug-drug interactions, see Table 22.**
Rifater* — combination tablet (See Side-Effects)	Wt ≥55 kg, 6 tablets single dose q24h	po (1 hr before meal)	1 tablet contains 50 mg INH, 120 mg RIF, 300 mg PZA. Used in 1* 2 months of rx (PZA 25 mg per kg). Purpose is convenience in dosing, ↑ compliance (AnIM 122: 951, 1995) but cost 1.58 more. Side-effects = individual drugs.	As with individual drugs. PZA 25 mg per kg
Streptomycin (IV/IM soln)	15 mg per kg IM q24h, 0.75–1.0 gm per day initially for 60–90 days, then 1.0 gm 2–3 times per week (15 mg per kg per day q24h as 1 dose	RES: 3.9% (2.7–7.6%) IM (or IV)	Overall 8%. **Ototoxicity:** vestibular dysfunction (vertigo); paresthesias; dizziness & nausea (all less in pts receiving 2–3 doses per week); tinnitus and high frequency loss (1%); nephrotoxicity (rarely); peripheral neuropathy (rare); allergic skin rashes (4–5%); drug fever. Available from X-Gen Pharmaceuticals, 607-732-4411. Ref. re: N—CID 179:150, 1994. Toxicity similar with qd vs td dosing (CID 38:1538, 2004).	Monthly audiogram. In older pts, serum creatinine and BUN at start of rx and weekly if pt stable

* Note: Malabsorption of antimycobacterial drugs may occur in patients with AIDS enteropathy. For review of adverse effects, see AJRCCM 167:1472, 2003.

[1] **RES** = % resistance of M. tuberculosis [1] **DOT** = directly observed therapy
See page 2 for abbreviations. § Dosages are for adults (unless otherwise indicated) and assume normal renal function
* Mean (range) (higher in Hispanics, Asians, and patients <10 years old)

TABLE 12B (2)

AGENT (TRADE NAME)[1]	USUAL DOSAGE[*]	ROUTE/[1] DRUG RESISTANCE (RES) US[*][4]	SIDE-EFFECTS, TOXICITY AND PRECAUTIONS	SURVEILLANCE
SECOND LINE DRUGS (more difficult to use and/or less effective than first line drugs)				
Amikacin (Amikin) (IV soln)	7.5–10.0 mg per kg q24h [Bactericidal for extracellular organisms]	RES: (est. 0.1%) IM/IV 500 mg vial	See Table 10B, pages 104 & 109	Monthly audiogram. Serum creatinine or BUN weekly if pt stable
Bedaquiline (Sirturo) (100 mg tab)	Directly observed therapy (DOT): 400 mg once daily for 2 weeks, then 200 mg 3 times weekly for 22 weeks. Taken with food and always used in combination with other anti-TB medications.	Does not exhibit cross-resistance to other TB drugs; always use in combination with other TB drugs to prevent selection of resistant mutants	Most common: nausea, vomiting, arthralgia, headache, hyperuricemia. Elevated transaminases. Bedaquiline in clinical trials was administered as one component of a multiple drug regimen, so side-effects were common, yet difficult to assign to a particular drug.	Moderate QTc increases (average of 0.16 ms over the 24 weeks of therapy. Potential risks of pancreatitis, myopathy, myocardial injury, severe hepatotoxicity)
Capreomycin sulfate (Capastat sulfate)	1 gm per day (15 mg per kg per day) q24h as 1 dose	RES: 0.1% (0–0.9%) IM/IV	Nephrotoxicity (36%), ototoxicity (auditory 11%), eosinophilia, leukopenia, skin rash, fever, hypokalemia, neuromuscular blockade.	Monthly audiogram, biweekly serum creatinine or BUN
Ciprofloxacin (Cipro) (250, 500, 750 mg tab)	750 mg bid	po 500 mg or 750 mg ER requires median dose 800 mg IV 200–400 mg vial	CIP not a FDA-approved indication for CIP. Desired CIP serum levels 4-6 mcg per mL requires median dose 800 mg (AJRCCM 151:2006, 1995). Discontinuation rates 6–7%. CIP well tolerated (AJRCCM 151:2006, 1995). FQ-resistant M. Tb identified in New York (Ln 345:1148, 1995). See Table 10B, pages 107 & 100 for adverse effects.	None
Clofazimine (Lamprene) (50, 100 mg cap)	50 mg per day (unsupervised) + 300 mg 1 time per month supervised or 100 mg per day	po 50 mg (with meals)	Skin: **pigmentation (pink-brownish black)** 75–100%, dryness 20%, pruritus 5%. GI: abdominal pain 50% (rarely severe leading to exploratory laparoscopy), splenic infarction (VR), bowel obstruction (VR), GI bleeding (VR). Eye: conjunctival irritation, retinal crystal deposits.	None
Cycloserine (Seromycin) (250 mg tab)	750–1000 mg per day (15 mg per kg per day) 2–4 doses per day [Bacteriostatic for both extra-cellular & intracellular organisms]	RES: 0.1% (0–0.3%) po 250 mg cap	Convulsions, **psychoses** (5–10% of those receiving 1.0 gm per day), headache; somnolence, hyperreflexia; increased CSF protein and pressure, **peripheral neuropathy.** 100 mg pyridoxine (or more) q24h should be given concomitantly. Contraindicated in epileptics.	None
Dapsone (25, 100 mg tab)	100 mg per day	po 100 mg tab	Blood: ↓ hemoglobin (1–2 gm) & ↑ retics (2–12%), in most pts. Hemolysis in G6PD deficiency, ↑ hemolysis due to concomitant atazanavir (AAC 56:1081, 2012). **Methemoglobinemia.** CNS: peripheral neuropathy (rare). GI: nausea, vomiting. Renal: albuminuria, nephrotic syndrome. Erythema nodosum leprosum in pts rx for leprosy (½ pts 1st year)	None
Ethionamide (Trecator-SC) (120, 250 mg tab)	500–1000 mg per day (15–20 mg per kg per day) 1–3 doses per day [Bacteriostatic for extracellular organisms only]	RES: 0.8% (0–1.5%) po 250 mg tab	**Gastrointestinal irritation** (up to 50% on large dose); goiter; peripheral neuropathy (rare); convulsions; changes in affect (rare); difficulty in diabetes control; rashes; hepatitis; purpura, stomatitis; gynecomastia; menstrual irregularity. Give drug with meals or antacids; 50–100 mg pyridoxine per day concomitantly; SGOT monthly. Possibly teratogenic.	
Moxifloxacin (Avelox) (400 mg tab)	400 mg qd	po 400 mg cap IV	Not FDA-approved indication. Concomitant administration of rifampin reduces serum levels of moxi (CID 45:1001, 2007).	None
Ofloxacin (200, 300, 400 mg tab)	400 mg bid	po 400 mg cap IV	Not FDA-approved indication. Overall adverse effects 11%, 4% discontinued due to side-effects. GI: nausea 3%, diarrhea 1%. **CNS:** Insomnia 3%, headache 1%, dizziness 1%.	None

See page 2 for abbreviations. * Dosages are for adults (unless otherwise indicated) and assume normal renal function. † **DOT** = directly observed therapy
§ Mean (range) (higher in Hispanics, Asians, and patients <10 years old)

TABLE 12B (3)

AGENT (TRADE NAME)[1]	USUAL DOSAGE*	ROUTE(1° DRUG RESISTANCE (RES) US)[§]	SIDE-EFFECTS, TOXICITY AND PRECAUTIONS	SURVEILLANCE
SECOND LINE DRUGS (continued)				
Para-aminosalicylic acid (PAS, Paser) (Na⁺ or K⁺ salt) (4 gm cap)	4-6 gm bid (200 mg per kg per day) (Bacteriostatic for extracellular organisms only)	RES: 0.8% (0-1.5%) po 450 mg tab (see Comment)	**Gastrointestinal irritation** (10-15%); goitrogenic action (rare); depressed prothrombin activity (rare); G6PD-mediated hemolytic anemia (rare), drug fever, rashes, hepatitis, myalgia, arthralgia. Retards hepatic enzyme induction, may ↓ INH hepatotoxicity. Available from CDC. (404) 639-3670, Jacobus Pharm. Co. (609) 921-7447	None
Rifabutin (Mycobutin) (150 mg cap)	300 mg per day (prophylaxis or treatment)	po 150 mg tab	Polymyalgia, polyarthralgia, leukopenia, granulocytopenia. Anterior uveitis when given with concomitant clarithromycin; avoid 600 mg dose (*NEJM* 330:438, 1994). Uveitis reported with 300 mg per day (*AnIM* 12:510, 1994). Reddish urine, orange skin (pseudojaundice).	None
Rifapentine (Priftin) (150 mg tab)	600 mg twice weekly for 1ˢᵗ 2 mos., then 600 mg q week	po 150 mg tab	Similar to other rifabutins. (See *RIF, RFB*). Hyperuricemia seen in 21%. Causes red-orange discoloration of body fluids. Note ↑ prevalence of RIF resistance in pts on weekly rx (*Ln* 353:1843, 1999)	None
Thalidomide (Thalomid) (50, 100, 200 mg cap)	100-300 mg po q24h (may use up to 400 mg po q24h for severe erythema nodosum leprosum)	po 50 mg tab	**Contraindicated in pregnancy. Causes severe life-threatening birth defects. Both male and female patients must use barrier contraceptive methods (Pregnancy Category X). Frequently causes drowsiness or somnolence. May cause peripheral neuropathy.** (*AJM* 108:487, 2000) For review, see *Ln* 363:1803, 2004.	Available only through pharmacists participating in System for Thalidomide Education and Prescribing Safety (S.T.E.P.S).

See page 2 for abbreviations. * Dosages are for adults (unless otherwise indicated) and assume normal renal function [†] **DOT** = directly observed therapy [§] Mean (range) (higher in Hispanics, Asians, and patients <10 years old)

TABLE 13A – TREATMENT OF PARASITIC INFECTIONS

- Artesunate, Diethylcarbamazine (DEC), Melarsoprol, Nifurtimox, Sodium stibogluconate, Quinacrine, Suramin are available from the CDC Drug Service. Quinacrine, Iodoquinol, Niclosamide, Paromomycin, Diloxanide, Fumagillin, Triclabendazole, Spiramycin are available from compounding pharmacies and specialty labs. **See Table 13D for complete contact information for these antiparasitic drugs.**
- The following resources are available through the Centers for Disease Control and Prevention (CDC) in Atlanta. Website is www.cdc.gov. General advice for parasitic diseases other than malaria: (+1) (770) 488-7775 (day), (+1) (770) 488-7100 (after hours). CDC Drug Service 8:00 a.m. – 4:30 p.m. EST: (+1) (404) 639-3670; fax: (+1) (404) 639-3717. See www.cdc.gov/laboratory/drugservice/index.html
- **Malaria**: Prophylaxis advice (+1) (770) 488-7788; treatment (+1) (770) 488-7788, toll-free (US) 1-855-856-4713; website: www.cdc.gov/malaria
- **NOTE**: All dosages are for adults unless otherwise stated. Many of the suggested regimens are not FDA approved.
- For licensed drugs, suggest checking package inserts to verify dosing and side-effects. Occasionally, post-licensure data may alter dosage as compared to package inserts.
- **Reference with peds dosages: Treat Guide Med Lett 5 (Supp) 5):1, 2007.**

INFECTING ORGANISM	SUGGESTED REGIMENS PRIMARY	ALTERNATIVE	COMMENTS
PROTOZOA—INTESTINAL (non-pathogenic: E. hartmanni, E. coli, Iodamoeba bütschlii, Endolimax nana, Chilomastix mesnili)			
Balantidium coli	Tetracycline 500 mg qid x 10 days	Metronidazole 750 mg tid times 5 days	Another alternative: Iodoquinol 650 mg tid x 20 days.
Blastocystis hominis Need to treat dubious (See Comment). Ref.: J Clin Gastro 44:85, 2010	Metronidazole 1.5 gm po 1x/day x 10 days (placebo-controlled trial in J Travel Med 10:128, 2003)	Alternatives: Iodoquinol 650 mg po tid x 20 days or TMP-SMX-DS, one bid x 7 days or Nitazoxanide 500 mg po bid x 3 days	Role as pathogen unclear; may serve as marker of exposure to contaminated food/water.
Cryptosporidium parvum & hominis Treatment is unsatisfactory Ref.: Curr Opin Infect Dis 23:494, 2010	Immunocompetent—No HIV: **Nitazoxanide** 500 mg po bid x 3 days (expensive)	HIV with immunodeficiency: Effective antiretroviral therapy best therapy. **Nitazoxanide** no clinical or parasite response compared to placebo. Salvage regimen (azithro 600 mg po once daily + paromomycin 1 gm po bid) decrease sx; continue paromomycin for 8 wks (JID 178:900, 1998).	**Nitazoxanide**: Approved in liquid formulation for x of children & 500 mg tabs for adults who are immunocompetent. Ref: CID 40:1173, 2005. **C. hominis** assoc. with ↑ in post-infection eye pain, joint pain, recurrent headache, & dizzy spells (CID 39:504, 2004).
Cyclospora cayetanensis; cyclosporiasis (Clin Micro Rev 23:218, 2010)	Immunocompetent pts: TMP-SMX-DS 1 po bid x 7-10 days. Other options: see Comments. AIDS pts: CIP 500 mg po bid x 7 days but results inconsistent. Anecdotal success with nitazoxanide. Biliary disease described in HIV pts.		If sulfa-allergic: CIP 500 mg po bid x 7 days but results inconsistent. Anecdotal success with nitazoxanide. Biliary disease described in HIV pts.
Dientamoeba fragilis See AJTMH 82:614, 2010; Clin Micro 14:601, 2008	Iodoquinol 650 mg tid x 20 days or Paromomycin 25-35 mg/kg/day po in 3 div doses x 7 days.	For treatment failures: Tetracycline 500 mg po qid x 10 days + Iodoquinol 650 mg po tid x 10 days OR (Iodoquinol + Paromomycin*)	Metronidazole associated with high failure rates.
Entamoeba histolytica; amebiasis. Reviews: Ln 361:1025, 2003; NEJM 348:1563, 2003.			
Asymptomatic cyst passer	Paromomycin* (aminosidine in U.K.) 25-35 mg/kg/day po in 3 divided doses x 7 days OR Iodoquinol 650 mg po tid x 20 days	Diloxanide furoate* (Furamide) 500 mg po tid x 10 days.	Note: E. hartmanni and E. dispar are non-pathogenic.
Patient with diarrhea/dysentery; mild/moderate disease. Oral therapy possible	Metronidazole 500-750 mg po tid x 7-10 days or tinidazole 2 gm po daily x 3 days, followed by Either paromomycin 25-35 mg/kg/day divided in 3 doses x 7 days] or [iodoquinol 650 mg po tid x 20 days] to clear intestinal cysts. See comment.		Colitis can mimic ulcerative colitis; ameboma can mimic adenocarcinoma of colon. **Nitazoxanide** 500 mg po bid x 3 days may be effective (JID 184:381, 2001 & Tran R Soc Trop Med & Hyg 101:1025, 2007).
Severe or extraintestinal infection, e.g. hepatic abscess	Metronidazole 750 mg IV to PO tid x 10 days or tinidazole 2 gm 1x/day x 5 days) followed by paromomycin* 25-35 mg/kg/day po divided in 3 doses x 7 days or iodoquinol 650 mg po tid x 20 days.		Serology positive (antibody present) with extraintestinal disease.
Giardia lamblia (Giardia duodenalis); giardiasis	Tinidazole 2 gm (x 1) OR Nitazoxanide (400 mg po bid x 3 days), Albendazole (400 mg po once daily with food x 5 days), Metro & Paromomycin are alternatives	Metronidazole 250 mg po tid x 5 days (high frequency of GI side-effects). See Comment. Pregnancy: Paromomycin* 25-35 mg/kg/day po in 3 divided doses x 5-10 days.	Refractory pts: (metro 750 mg po + quinacrine 100 mg po) — both 3x/day x 3 wks (CID 33:22, 2001) or furazolidone 100 mg po qid x 7 days. **Nitazoxanide** ref: CID 40:1173, 2005.

* For source of drug, see Table 13D, page 155.

TABLE 13A (2)

INFECTING ORGANISM	SUGGESTED REGIMENS PRIMARY	ALTERNATIVE	COMMENTS
PROTOZOA—INTESTINAL (continued)			
Cystoisospora belli (formerly *Isospora belli*) (AIDS ref: MMWR 58 (RR-4):1, 2009)	**Immunocompetent:** TMP-SMX-DS tab 1 po bid x 7-10 days. **Immunocompromised:** TMP-SMX-DS qid to tid x 10 days, then bid x 3 wks. If CD4 <200 may not respond; need APT.	CIP 500 mg po bid x 7 days is second-line alternative (AnIM 132:885, 2000) OR **Pyrimethamine** 50-75 mg/day po + **Folinic acid** 10-25 mg/day (po).	**Chronic suppression in AIDS pts:** either **TMP-SMX-DS** 3x/wk OR **TMP-SMX-DS** 1x daily OR **pyrimethamine** 25 mg/day po + **folinic acid** 10 mg/day po) OR as 2nd-line alternative: CIP 500 mg po 3x/wk.
Microsporidiosis			
Ocular: Encephalitozoon hellum or cuniculi, Vittaforma corneae, Nosema ocularum	For HIV pts: antiretroviral therapy key **Albendazole** 400 mg po bid x 3 wks plus fumagillin eye drops (see Comment)	In HIV+ pts, reports of response of E. hellum to **fumagillin** eyedrops (see Comment) For V. corneae, may need keratoplasty	To obtain fumagillin: 800-292-6773 or www.leiterrx.com. Neutropenia & thrombocytopenia serious adverse events. Dx: Most labs use modified trichrome stain. Need electron micrographs for species identification. FA and PCR methods in development.
Intestinal (diarrhea): Enterocytozoon bieneusi, Encephalitozoon (Septata) intestinalis	**Albendazole** 400 mg po bid into 2 daily doses x 7 days for E. intestinalis. Fumagillin equally effective.	Oral **fumagillin** 20 mg po bid reported effective for E. bieneusi (NEJM 346:1963, 2002) — see Comment	Peds dose ref.: PIDJ 23:915, 2004
Disseminated: E. hellum, cuniculi, intestinalis; Pleistophora sp.; others in Comment	**Albendazole** 400 mg po x 3 wks	No established rx for Pleistophora sp.	For Trachipleistophora sp., try itraconazole + albendazole (NEJM 351:42, 2004). Other pathogens: Brachiola vesicularum & algerae (NEJM 351:42, 2004)
PROTOZOA—EXTRAINTESTINAL			
Amebic meningoencephalitis (Clin Infect Dis 51 e7, 2010 Balamuthia)			
Acanthamoeba sp.—no proven rx Rev. FEMS Immunol Med Micro 50:1, 2007 Balamuthia mandrillaris	Success with IV **pentamidine** + **sulfadiazine** + **flucytosine** + (either **fluconazole** or **itraconazole**) (FEMS Immunol Med Micro 50:1, 2007); 2 cultures children responded to rx: **TMP-SMX** + **rifampin** + **keto** (PIDJ 20:623, 2001).		For Acanthamoeba keratitis, miltefosine or voriconazole. Anecdotal response to miltefosine.
Naegleria fowleri. >95% mortality. Ref. MMWR 57:573, 2008.	**Pentamidine** + **Albendazole** + (**Fluconazole** or **Itraconazole**) or **Liposomal Ampho B** + **Sulfadiazine** + (**Azithro** or **Clarithro**). See CID 51:e7, 2010. **Ampho B** 1.5 mg/kg per day in 2 div. doses x 3 days; then 1 mg/kg/day x 6 days plus 1.5 mg/kg intrathecal x 2 days, then 1 mg/kg intrathecal qod x 8 days.		For Naegleria: Ampho B + azithro synergistic in vitro & in mouse model (AAC 50:4126, 2006). Ampho B + fluconazole + rifampin may work (Arch Med Res 36:83, 2005).
Sappinia diploidea	**Azithro** + **pentamidine** + **itra** + **flucytosine** (JAMA 285:2450, 2001)		
Babesia microti (US) and **Babesia divergens** (EU) (NEJM 366:2397, 2012)	For mild/moderate disease: **Atovaquone** 750 mg po bid + **Azithro** 500 mg po on day 1, then 250-1000 mg po daily for total of 7-10 days. If relapse, treat x 6 wks & until blood smear neg x 2 wks.	For **severe babesiosis**: **Clindamycin** 600 mg po tid) + (**quinine** 650 mg po qid) x 7-10 days For adults, can give **clinda** IV as 1.2 gm bid.	Overwhelming infection in asplenic patients. In immunocompromised patients, treat for 6 or more weeks (CID 46:370, 2008). **Consider exchange transfusion if ≥10% parasitemia** (Trans Med Rev 16:239, 2002)
Leishmaniasis (Suggest consultation – CDC (+1) 770 488 7775; see LnID 7:581, 2007; CID 43:1089, 2006)			
Cutaneous: Mild Disease (< 4 lesions, none > 5 cm diameter, no lesions in cosmetically sensitive area, none over joints). Otherwise, consider Moderate Disease	**Mild Disease** (< 4 lesions, none > 5 cm): **Paromomycin**[1] ointment bid x 20 days (investigational); cryotherapy (freeze up to 3x with liq nitrogen); intralesional Antimony 20 mg/kg into lesion (CID 43:1089, 2006). Spontaneous resolution in > 50% but may take 6 months (PLoS Negl Trop Dis 4:e628, 2010). Heat therapy ref: see www.thermosurgery.com.	**Moderate Disease:** **Sodium stibogluconate**[1] (Pentostam) or **Meglumine antimoniate** (Glucantime) 20 mg/kg/day IV/IM x 20 days. Dilute in 120 mL D5W & infuse over 2 hrs. Alternative: **Fluconazole** 200 mg po daily x 6 weeks (for L. mexicanus, L. panamensis, L. major) or **Ketoconazole** 600 mg po daily x 30 days (L. mexicana)	Oral therapy, Topical paromomycin[1] & other topical treatment only when low potential for mucosal spread; never use for L. brasiliensis or L. guyanensis (mucocutaneous focus lesions). Generic pentavalent antimony varies in quality and safety.

[1] For source of drug, see Table 13D, page 155.

TABLE 13A (3)

INFECTING ORGANISM	SUGGESTED REGIMENS PRIMARY	SUGGESTED REGIMENS ALTERNATIVE	COMMENTS
PROTOZOA—EXTRAINTESTINAL (continued)			
Leishmaniasis, Mucosal (Espundia). Usually due to L. braziliensis.	**Pentavalent antimony (Sb)*** 20 mg/kg/day IV or IM x 28 days or **liposomal amphotericin B** (regimens vary), with total cumulative dose of 20-60 mg/kg or **amphotericin B** 0.5-1 mg/kg IV daily or qod to total dose of 20-40 mg/kg.	No good alternative: variable efficacy of oral Miltefosine: **Miltefosine*** 2.5 mg/kg/day (to maximum of 150 mg/day) po divided tid x 28 days (AJTMH 81:387, 2009)	Antimony available from CDC drug service; miltefosine available from Paladin Labs. See Table 13D for contact information.
Visceral leishmaniasis – Kala-Azar – New World & Old World L. donovani: India, Africa L. infantum: Mediterranean L. chagasi: New World	**Liposomal ampho B** FDA-approved in immunocompetent hosts: 3 mg/kg once daily days 1-5 & days 14, 21. Alternative regimens: 3 mg/kg IV daily on days 1-5 and day 10 or 10 mg/kg IV daily x 2 days.	**Standard Ampho B** 1 mg/kg IV daily x 15-20 days for qod x 8 wks (to total of 15-20 mg/kg) **OR** **Miltefosine*** 2.5 mg/kg/day (max 150 mg/day) po x 28 days OR **pentavalent antimony*** 20 mg/kg/day IV/IM x 28 days.	In HIV patients, may need lifelong suppression with Amphotericin B q 2-4 wks
Malaria (Plasmodia species). —NOTE: CDC Malaria info — prophylaxis/treatment (770) 488-7788. After hours: 770-488-7100. US toll-free 1-855-856-4713. CDC offers species confirmation and drug resistance testing. Refs: *JAMA 297:2251, 2264 & 2285, 2007*. Websites: www.cdc.gov/malaria; www.who.int/health-topics/malaria.htm. Review of rapid diagnostic tests: *CID 54:1637, 2012*.			
Prophylaxis—Drugs plus personal protection: screens, nets, 30-35% DEET skin repellent (avoid > 50% DEET) on clothing and mosquito nets. Country risk in CDC Yellow Book.			
For areas free of chloroquine (CQ)-resistant P. falciparum: Central America (west of Panama Canal), Caribbean, Korea, Middle East (most)	**CQ** phosphate 500 mg (300 mg base) po per wk, starting 1-2 wks before travel, during travel, & 4 wks post-travel. **Pediatric CQ: 8.3 mg/kg (5 mg/kg of base)** once per day (1 day prior to, during, & 7 days post-travel). Another option for P. vivax only countries: **primaquine (PQ)** 30 mg base po daily in non-pregnant, G6PD-neg. travelers; >92% effective vs P. vivax (CID 33:1990, 2001). Note: CQ may exacerbate psoriasis.	**CQ Peds dose:** 8.3 mg/kg (5 mg/kg of base) po 1x/wk up to 300 mg (base) max. dose **or AP** by weight: peds tabs: 5-8 kg, 1/2 tab; 9-10 kg, 3/4 tab; 11-20 kg, 1 tab; 21-30 kg, 2 tabs; 31-40 kg, 3 tabs; >40 kg, 1 adult tab per day. **Adults: Doxy or MQ** as below	CQ safe during pregnancy. **The areas free of CQ-resistant falciparum malaria continue to shrink**. See CDC or WHO maps for most current information on CQ vs CQ-resistant areas. **Doxy AEs:** photosensitivity, candida vaginitis, gastritis.
For areas with CQ-resistant P. falciparum. CDC info on prophylaxis (770) 488-7788 or website: www.cdc.gov/malaria & LnID 6:139, 2006	**Atovaquone** 250 mg + **proguanil** 100 mg **(Malarone)** combo. tablet. 1 tab per day with food 1-2 days prior to, during, & 7 days post-travel. Peds dose in footnote[1]. **Not in pregnancy.** Malarone preferred for trips of a week or less; expense may preclude use for longer trips. Native population: intermittent pregnancy prophylaxis/treatment programs in a few countries. Fansidar 1 tab 3 times during pregnancy (*Expert Op Anti Infect Ther 8:569, 2010*).	**Doxycycline** 100 mg po daily for adults & children > 8 yrs of age[1]. Take 1-2 days before, during, & for 4 wks after travel **OR** **Mefloquine (MQ)** 250 mg (228 mg base) po once per wk, 1-2 wks before, during, & for 4 wks after travel (see Comment). Peds dose in footnote[1] **Doxy AEs:** photosensitivity, candida vaginitis, gastritis.	**Pregnancy: MQ current best option. Insufficient data with Malarone. Avoid doxycycline and primaquine. Primaquine:** Can cause hemolytic anemia if G6PD deficiency present. **MQ not recommended** if cardiac conduction abnormalities, seizures, or psychiatric disorders, e.g., depression, psychosis. MQ outside US: 275 mg tab, contains 250 mg of base. If used, can start 3 wks before travel to assure tolerability.

[1] **Peds prophylaxis dosages** (Ref.: *CID 34:493, 2002*): **Mefloquine** weekly dose by **weight** in kg: <15 = 5 mg/kg; 15-19 = ¼ adult dose; 20-30 = ½ adult dose; 31-45 = ¾ adult dose; >45 = adult dose. **Atovaquone/proguanil** by **weight** in kg, single daily dose using peds tab (62.5 mg atovaquone + 25 mg proguanil): 5-8 kg, 1/2 tab; 9-10 kg, 3/4 tab; 11-20 kg, 1 tab; 21-30 kg, 2 tabs; 31-40 kg, 3 tabs; 241 kg, one adult tab. **Doxycycline**, ages >8-12 yrs: 2 mg per kg per day up to 100 mg/day. Continue daily x 4 wks after leaving risk area. Side effects: photosensitivity, nausea, yeast vaginitis

* For source of drug, see *Table 13D*, page 155.

TABLE 13A (4)

PROTOZOA—EXTRAINTESTINAL/Malaria (Plasmodia species)

Treatment of Malaria. Diagnosis is by microscopy. Alternative: rapid antigen detection test (Binax NOW); detects 96-100% of P. falciparum and 50% of other plasmodia (CID 49:908, 2009; CID 54:1637, 2012). Need microscopy to speciate. Can stay positive for over a month after successful treatment.

INFECTING ORGANISM	PRIMARY	SUGGESTED REGIMENS ALTERNATIVE		COMMENTS
Clinical Severity/ Plasmodium sp.	Region Acquired	Suggested Treatment Regimens (Drug)		
		Adults	Peds	Comments
Uncomplicated/ P. falciparum (or species not identified) Malaria rapid diagnostic test (Binax NOW) CID 54:1637, 2012	Gen. Amer. west of Panama Canal; Haiti; Dom. Repub. & most of Mid-East **CQ-sensitive** CQ-resistant or unknown resistance. Note: If >5% parasitemia or Hb <7, treat as severe malaria.	**CQ phosphate** 1 gm salt (600 mg base) po, then 0.5 gm in 6 hrs, then 0.5 gm daily x 2 days. Total: 25 mg/kg base **Adults: Atovaquone-proguanil** 1 gm–400 mg (4 adult tabs) po 1x/day x 3 days w/ food **OR [QS** 650 mg po tid x 3 days (7 days if SE Asia)] + **[doxy** 100 mg po bid or **(tetra** 250 mg po qid or **clinda** 20 mg/kg/d divided tid) x 7 days] **OR Artemether-lumefantrine*** tabs 20(120 mg: 4 tabs po (at 0, 8 hrs) then bid x 2 days (total 6 doses); take with food **OR** a less desirable adult alternative, **mefloquine** 750 mg po x 1 dose, then 500 mg po x 1 dose 6-12 hr later. **MQ** is 2nd line alternative due to neuropsychiatric reaction. Also, resistance in SE Asia.	**Peds: CQ** 10 mg/kg of base po; then 5 mg/kg of base at 6, 24, & 48 hrs. Total: 25 mg/kg base **Peds: (QS** 10 mg/kg po tid x 3 days) + **clinda** 20 mg/kg per day div tid)—both x 7 days. **MQ Salt:** 15 mg/kg x 1, then 6-12 hrs later, 10 mg/kg. Avoid in 1st trimester. **Peds atovaquone-proguanil dose** (all once daily x 3 d) by weight: 5-8 kg: 2 peds tabs; 9-10 kg: 3 peds tabs; 11-20 kg: 1 adult tab; 21-30 kg: 2 adult tabs; 31-40 kg: 3 adult tabs; >40 kg: 4 adult tabs. **Note: Oral Artemether-lumefantrine tabs FDA-approved.** IV Artesunate available from CDC Drug Service, see Table 13D, page 155. **Artemether-lumefantrine*** • 5 kg to < 15 kg: 1 tablet (20 mg/ 120 mg) as a single dose, then 1 tablet again after 8 hours, then 1 tablet every 12 hours for 2 days • 15 kg to < 25 kg: 2 tablets (40 mg/ 240 mg) as a single dose, then 2 tablets again after 8 hours, then 2 tablets every 12 hours for 2 days • 25 kg to < 35 kg: 3 tablets (60 mg/ 360 mg) as a single dose, then 3 tablets again after 8 hours, then 3 tablets every 12 hours for 2 days • > 35 kg: as per adult dose **Atovaquone-proguanil** (1000/400 mg) 4 adult tabs po daily x 3 days	Peds dose should never exceed adult dose. **CQ + MQ prolong QTc.** **Pregnancy & children:** Can substitute clinda for doxy/tetra. 20 mg/kg per day po div. tid x 7 days. In U.S., QS only available as quinacrine 324 mg capsule, thus hard to use to treat children. **Pregnancy:** Artemether-lumefantrine
Uncomplicated/ P. malariae or P. knowlesi AJID 199: 1107 & 1143, 2009)	All regions – **CQ-sensitive**	**CQ** as above adults & peds in South Pacific, New Guinea; looks like P. malariae, but behaves like P. falciparum (CID 46:165, 2007).		
Uncomplicated/ P. vivax or P. ovale	**CQ-sensitive** (except Papua, New Guinea and Indonesia which are CQ-resistant-see below)	**CQ** as above + **PQ** base: 30 mg po once daily x 14 days Each primaquine phosphate tab is 26.3 mg base and 15 mg of base. 30 mg of base = 2 26.3 mg tabs prim. phos.	**Peds: CQ** as above. **Peds** (<8 yrs old): **QS** alone x 7 days or **MQ** alone. If either fail, **add doxy,** if <8 yrs.	PQ added to eradicate latent parasites in liver. **Screen for G6PD def. before starting PQ:** If G6PD deficient dose PQ as 45 mg po once weekly x 8 wks. **Note: rare severe reactions.** Avoid PQ in pregnancy.
Uncomplicated/ P. vivax	**CQ-resistant:** Papua, New Guinea & Indonesia	**QS + (doxy / tetra) + PQ**) as above or **Artemether-Lumefantrine** (same dose as for P. falciparum)	**MQ + PQ** as above. **Peds** (<8 yrs old): **QS** alone x 7 days or **MQ** alone. If either fail, **add doxy,** if <8 yrs.	Rarely acute. Lung injury and other serious complications. LnID 8:449, 2008.

* For source of drug, see Table 13D, page 155.

TABLE 13A (5)

PROTOZOA—EXTRAINTESTINAL/Malaria (Plasmodia species) /Treatment of Malaria (continued)

INFECTING ORGANISM	SUGGESTED REGIMENS			COMMENTS
	PRIMARY		ALTERNATIVE	
	Region Acquired	Suggested Treatment Regimens (Drug)		Comments
		Primary—Adults	Alternative & Peds	

Clinical Severity/ Plasmodia sp.

Uncomplicated Malaria/Alternatives for Pregnancy
Ref: *LnID 7:118 & 136, 2007*

Region Acquired	Primary—Adults	Alternative & Peds	Comments
CQ-sensitive areas	CQ as above	If failing or intolerant, **QS** + **doxy**	Doxy or tetra used if benefits outweigh risks. No controlled studies of AP in pregnancy. If P. vivax or P. ovale, after pregnancy check for G6PD deficiency & give PQ 30 mg po daily times 14 days.
CQ-resistant P. falciparum	**QS** + **clinda** as above		
CQ-resistant P. vivax	**QS** 650 mg po tid x 7 days		
CQ-resistant P. vivax. Intermittent pregnancy treatment (empiric)	Give treatment dose of [Sulfadoxine 500 mg + Pyrimethamine 25 mg (Fansidar) po] at 3 times during pregnancy to decrease maternal & fetal morbidity & mortality		

Severe malaria, i.e., impaired consciousness, severe anemia, renal failure, pulmonary edema, ARDS, DIC, jaundice, acidosis, seizures, parasitemia >5%. One or more of latter. **Almost always P. falciparum.**
Ref: *NEJM 358:1829, 2008; Science 320:30, 2008.*

| All regions | **Quinidine gluconate** (salt) 10 mg/kg (salt) IV over 1 hr then 0.02 mg/kg/min by constant infusion OR 24 mg/kg IV over 4 hrs & then 12 mg/kg over 4 hrs q8h. Continue until parasite density <1% & can take po OS. **QS** 650 mg po tid x 3 days (7 days if SE Asia) + **Doxy** 100 mg IV q12h x 7-14 days OR **clinda** 10 mg/kg IV load & then 5 mg/kg IV q8h x 7 days)] | **Peds: Quinidine gluconate** IV—same mg/kg dose as for adults **PLUS** [**Doxy**: if <45 kg, 4 mg per kg IV q12h; if ≥45 kg, same mg/kg dose as for adults) OR **Clinda**, same mg/kg dose as for adults Artesunate* 2.4 mg/kg IV at 0, 12, 24, 48 hrs, then **Doxy** 100 mg IV q12h x 7 days (see Comment) | During quinidine IV, monitor BP, EKG (prolongation of QT), & blood glucose (hypoglycemia). Consider exchange transfusion if parasitemia >10%. Switch to QS po + (Doxy or Clinda) when patient able to take oral drugs. **Steroids not recommended for cerebral malaria.** If quinidine not available, or patient intolerant or has high level parasitemia, **IV artesunate*** available from CDC Malaria Branch (B/N transport time post-approval), see Table 13D (Ref: CID 44:1067 & 1075, 2007). Substitute Clinda for Doxy in pregnancy. |

Malaria—self-initiated treatment: Only for people at high risk. Carry a reliable supply of recommended drug (to avoid counterfeit meds). Use only if malaria is lab-diagnosed and no available reliable meds.

| | **Artemether-lumefantrine** (20/120 mg tab) 4 tabs po x 1 dose, repeat in 8 hrs, then repeat (20/120 mg x 2 days (take with food) OR **Atovaquone-proguanil** (AP) 4 adult tabs (1 gm/400 mg) po daily x 3 days | **Peds:** Using adult **AP** tabs for 3 consecutive days: 11–20 kg, 1 tab; 21–30 kg, 2 tabs; 31–40 kg, 3 tabs; >41 kg, 4 tabs. For Peds dosing of Artemether-lumefantrine, see *Uncomplicated/P. falciparum*, page 144. | Do not use for renal insufficiency pts. Do not use if weight <11 kg, pregnant, or breast-feeding. **Artemether-lumefantrine:** sold as Riamet (EU) and Coartem (US & elsewhere). |

Pneumocystis carinii pneumonia (PCP).
Revised name is **Pneumocystis jiroveci** (yee-row-vee). Ref: *JAMA 301:2578, 2009*
Not acutely ill, able to take po meds. PaO₂ >70 mm Hg
Serum 1,3 B-D Glucan assay has high diagnostic accuracy for PCP (*JCM 50:7, 2012*).

| | (**TMP-SMX-DS**, 2 tabs po q8h) x 21 days] OR (**Dapsone** 100 mg po q24h + **trimethoprim** 5 mg/kg po tid) x 21 days
NOTE: Concomitant use of corticosteroids usually reserved for sicker pts with PaO₂ <70 (see below) | (**Clindamycin** 300–450 mg po q6h + **primaquine** 15 mg base po q24h) x 21 days OR **Atovaquone** suspension 750 mg po bid with food x 21 days | Mutations in gene of the enzyme target (dihydropteroate synthetase) of sulfamethoxazole identified. Unclear whether mutations result in resist to TMP-SMX or dapsone – TMP / EID 10:1721, 2004). Dapsone ref: CID 27:191, 1998. **After 21 days, chronic suppression in AIDS pts** (see below—post-treatment suppression). |

*For source of drug, see Table 13D, page 155.

TABLE 13A (6)

INFECTING ORGANISM	SUGGESTED REGIMENS PRIMARY	SUGGESTED REGIMENS ALTERNATIVE	COMMENTS
PROTOZOA—EXTRAINTESTINAL Malaria (Plasmodia species) /Treatment of Malaria *(continued)*			
Acutely ill, po rx not possible; PaO₂ <70 mmHg. Still unclear whether adjunctive corticosteroids should be started during treatment of PCP (CID 46: 634, 2008).	**Prednisone** (15-30 min. before TMP-SMX) 40 mg po bid times 5 days, then 40 mg q24h times 5 days, then 20 mg q24h times 11 days + **TMP-SMX** (15 mg of TMP component per kg per day) IV div. q6-8h times 21 days	**Prednisone** as in primary rx **PLUS** **Clinda** 600 mg IV q8h) + (**primaquine** 30 mg po q24h) times 21 days **OR** **Pentamidine** 4 mg per kg per day IV times 21 days Caspofungin active in animal models (*CID 36:1445, 2003*)	**After 21 days, chronic suppression in AIDS pts** (see post-treatment suppression). PCP can occur in absence of HIV infection & steroids (*CID 25:215 & 219, 1997*). Wait 4-8 days before declaring treatment failure & switching to clinda + primaquine or pentamidine (*AIDS 48:63, 2008*), or adding caspofungin
	Can substitute IV prednisolone (reduce dose 25%) for po prednisone		
Primary prophylaxis and post-treatment suppression	**TMP-SMX-DS or -SS,** 1 tab po q24h or 1 DS 3x/wk) **OR** (**dapsone** 100 mg po q24h). DC when CD4 >200 x3 mos (*NEJM 344:159, 2001*).	**Pentamidine** 300 in 6 mL sterile water by aerosol (Respirgard II) q4 wks **OR** (**dapsone** 200 mg po q24h) + **pyrimethamine** 75 mg) **OR** + **folinic acid** 25 mg po – **all once a week,** or **atovaquone** 1500 mg q24h with food.	TMP-SMX-DS regimen provides cross-protection vs toxo and other bacterial infections. Dapsone + pyrimethamine protects vs toxo. Atovaquone suspension 1500 mg once daily as effective as daily dapsone (*NEJM 339:1889, 1998*) or inhaled pentamidine (*JID 180:369, 1999*).
Toxoplasma gondii (Reference *Ln 363:1965, 2004*)			
Immunologically normal patients (For pediatric doses, see reference)			
Acute illness, lymphadenopathy (immunocompetent, no lab. sequelae)	No specific rx unless severe/persistent symptoms or evidence of vital organ damage		
Active chorioretinitis; meningitis, lowered resistance due to steroids or cytotoxic drugs	**Pyrimethamine** (pyri) 200 mg x 1 po, then 75 mg po q24h) + (**sulfadiazine** (see below) 1-1.5 gm po qid) + **leucovorin (folinic acid)** 5-20 mg 3x/wk; continue leucovorin 1 wk after stopping pyri. Treat 1-2 wks beyond resolution of signs/symptoms.	Clinda. **Pyrimethamine** (pyri) 50-75 mg q24h) + (**sulfadiazine** (see footnote²) 1-1.5 gm po qid) + **folinic acid** 5-20 mg 3x/wk)—see Comment.	For congenital toxo, toxo meningitis in adults, & chorioretinitis, **add pyrimethamine 1 mg/kg/day in 2 div. doses until CSF protein conc. falls or vision-threatening inflammation subsides.** Adjust folinic acid dose by following CBC results. Screen women with IgG/IgM for toxo. Commercial IgG- IgM neg. = remote past infection. IgG+/IgM+ = seroconversion. Suggest consultation with Palo Alto Medical Foundation Toxoplasma Serology Lab: 650-853-4828 or toxlab@pamf.org. Details in *Ln 363:1965, 2004*. **Consultation advisable.**
Acute in pregnant women. Ref: *CID 47:554, 2008.*	If <18 wks gestation at diagnosis: **Spiramycin** 1 gm po q8h until 16-18 wks. dc if amniotic fluid PCR is negative. Positive PCR or treat as below. If >18 wks gestation & documented fetal infection by positive amniotic fluid PCR: (**Pyrimethamine** 50 mg po q12h x 2 days, then 50 mg/kg po x 1 dose, then 50 mg/kg q12h (max 4 gm/day)) + **folinic acid** 10-20 mg po daily, for minimum of 4 wks or for duration of pregnancy.		
Fetal/congenital	Mgmt complex. Combo rx with pyrimethamine + sulfadiazine + leucovorin—see Comment		
AIDS			
Cerebral toxoplasmosis Ref: *MMWR 58(RR-4) 1, 2009.*	(**Pyrimethamine** (pyri) 200 mg x 1 po, then 75 mg/day po) + (**sulfadiazine** 1-1.5 gm po q6h (if <60 kg, use 1 gm q6h; if >60 kg, use 1.5 gm q6h)) + **folinic acid** (leucovorin) 10-25 mg/day po for minimum of 6 wks after resolution of signs/symptoms, and then suppressive rx (see below) **OR** TMP-SMX 10/50 mg/kg per day po or IV div q12h x 30 days (*AAC 42:1346, 1998*)	[**Pyri + folinic acid** (as in primary regimen)] + [(**clinda** 600 mg q6h po or IV) or (**atovaquone** 1.5 gm po bid) or (**azithro** 900-1200 mg po q24h)] **OR** TMP-SMX 5/25 mg/kg po or IV bid or (3) **atovaquone** 750 mg po q6h. Treat 4-6 wks after resolution of signs/symptoms.	Use alternative regimen for pts with severe sulfa allergy. CT or MRI: multiple enhancing brain lesions (CT or MRI), >85% of pts respond to 7-10 days of empiric rx. If no response, **suggest** brain biopsy. Pyri penetrates brain even if no inflammation. Folinic acid prevents pyrimethamine hematologic toxicity. Prophylactic TMP-SMX or dapsone effective vs toxo. Primary *MMWR 58(RR-4) 1, 2009.* **alternative:** (**Dapsone** 200 mg po + pyrimethamine 75 mg po + folinic acid 25 mg po) once weekly.
Primary prophylaxis: AIDS pts—IgG toxo antibody + CD4 count <100 per mcL	**TMP-SMX-DS,** 1 tab po q24h or 3x/wk) or **TMP-SMX-SS,** 1 tab q24h)	(**Dapsone** 50 mg po q24h) + (**pyri** 50 mg po q wk) + **folinic acid** 25 mg po q24h) **OR atovaquone** 1500 mg q24h	Treat 4-6 wks after resolution of signs/symptoms, then suppression.

² Sulfonamides for toxo. Sulfadiazine now commercially available. Sulfisoxazole much less effective.

* For source of drug, see *Table 13D, page 155*.

TABLE 13A (7)

INFECTING ORGANISM	SUGGESTED REGIMENS PRIMARY	ALTERNATIVE	COMMENTS
PROTOZOA—EXTRAINTESTINAL/Toxoplasma gondii/AIDS (continued)			
Suppression after rx of cerebral toxo	(Sulfadiazine 2-4 gm divided in 2-4 doses/day) + (pyri 25-50 mg po q24h) + (folinic acid 10-25 mg po q24h). DC if CD4 count >200 x 3 mos	((Clinda 600 mg po q8h) + (pyri 25-50 mg po q24h)) + (folinic acid 10-25 mg po q24h)) OR atovaquone 750 mg po q6-12h	(Pyri + sulfa) prevents PCP and toxo; (clinda + pyri) prevents toxo only. Additional drug needed to prevent PCP
Trichomonas vaginalis	See *Vaginitis*, Table 1, page 26.		
Trypanosomiasis. Ref.: *Ln* 362:1469, 2003. **Note: Drugs for African trypanosomiasis may be obtained free from WHO. See Table 13D, page 155, for source information.**			
West African sleeping sickness (T. brucei gambiense)			
Early: Blood/lymphatic—CNS OK	Pentamidine 4 mg/kg IV/IM daily x 7-10 days	Suramin: 100 mg IV (test dose), then 1 gm IV on days 1, 3, 7, 14, & 21	In US, free from CDC drug service
Late: Encephalitis	Eflornithine 100 mg/kg q6h IV x 14 days (*CID* 41:748, 2005). Obtain drug from WHO drug service (stmarroc@who.int or +41 22 791 1345). Combined with nifurtimox better, see Comment.	Melarsoprol 2.2 mg/kg per day IV x 10 days (melarsoprol/nifurtimox combination superior to melarsoprol alone (*JID* 195:311 & 322, 2007).	Combination of IV eflornithine, 400 mg/kg/day divided q12h x 7 days, plus nifurtimox, 15 mg/kg/day po divided q8h x 10 days more efficacious than standard dose eflornithine (*CID* 45:1435 & 1443, 2007; *Ln* 374:56, 2009)
East African sleeping sickness (T. brucei rhodesiense)			
Early: Blood/lymphatic	Suramin: 100 mg IV (test dose), then 1 gm IV on days 1, 3, 7, 14 & 21	Peds: Suramin: 10-15 mg/kg IV on days 1, 3, 7, 14 & 21	Suramin & Melarsoprol: CDC Drug Service or WHO (at no charge) (see Table 13D).
Late: Encephalitis (prednisone may prevent encephalitis)	Melarsoprol: From 2-3.6 mg/kg per day IV for 3 days; repeat 3.6 mg/kg per day after 7 days & for 3rd time at 10-21 days	Melarsoprol 2.2 mg/kg/day IV x 10 days (*PLoS NTD* 6:e1695, 2012)	Early illness: patient waiting for Suramin, use pentamidine 4 mg/kg/day IV/IM x 1-2 doses. Does not enter CSF.
T. cruzi—Chagas disease or acute American trypanosomiasis. For chronic disease: see Comment. Ref.: *Ln* 375:1388, 2010; *LnID* 10:556, 2010.	Benznidazole 5-7 mg/kg per day po div. 2x/day x 60 days. NOTE: Take with meals to reduce G-I side effects. Contraindicated in pregnancy.	Nifurtimox 8-10 mg/kg per day po div. 4x/day after meals x 120 days Ages 11-16 yrs: 12.5-15 mg/kg per day div. qid po x 90 days Children <11yrs: 15-20 mg/kg per day div. qid po x 90 days.	Immunosuppression for heart transplant can reactivate chronic Chagas disease (*J Card Failure* 15:249, 2009). Can transmit by organ/transfusions (*CID* 48:1534, 2009).
NEMATODES—INTESTINAL (Roundworms). Think Strongyloides, toxocaria and filariasis: *CID* 34:407, 2005; 42:1781 & 1655, 2006—See Table 13C.			
Anisakis simplex (anisakiasis) Anisakiasis differentiated from Anisakidosis (*CID* 51:806, 2010). Other: A. physalry, Pseudoterranova decipiens	Physical removal: endoscope or surgery IgE antibody test vs A. simplex may help diagnosis. No antimicrobial therapy.	Anecdotal reports of possible treatment benefit from albendazole (*Ln* 360:54, 2002; *CID* 41:1825, 2005)	Anisakiasis acquired by eating raw fish: herring, salmon, mackerel, cod, squid. Similar illness due to Pseudoterranova species acquired from cod, halibut, red snapper.
Ascaris lumbricoides (ascariasis)	Albendazole 400 mg po daily x 3 days or mebendazole 100 mg po bid x 3 days	Ivermectin 150-200 mcg/kg po x 1 dose	Review of efficacy of single dose: *JAMA* 299:1937, 2008.
Capillaria philippinensis (capillariasis)	Albendazole 400 mg po daily x 10 days	Mebendazole 200 mg po bid x 20 days	Albendazole preferred.
Enterobius vermicularis (pinworm)	Mebendazole 100 mg po x 1, repeat in 2 wks	Pyrantel pamoate 11 mg/kg (to max. dose of 1 gm) po x 1 dose, repeat in 2 wks OR Albendazole 400 mg po x 1 dose, repeat in 2 wks.	Side-effects in Table 13B, page 154.
Gongylonemiasis (adult worms in oral mucosa)	Surgical removal	Albendazole 400 mg/day po x 3 days	Ref: *CID* 32:1378, 2001; *J Helminth* 80:425, 2006.
Hookworm (Necator americanus and Ancylostoma duodenale)	Albendazole 400 mg po daily x 3 days	Mebendazole 100 mg po bid x 3 days OR Pyrantel pamoate 11 mg/kg (to max. dose of 1 gm) po daily x 3 days	NOTE: Ivermectin not effective. Eosinophilia may be absent but eggs in stool (*NEJM* 351:799, 2004).
Strongyloides stercoralis (strongyloidiasis) (Hyperinfection. See Comment)	Ivermectin 200 mcg/kg po x 2 days	Albendazole 400 mg po bid x 7 days. : less effective	For hyperinfections, repeat at 15 days. For hyperinfection: veterinary ivermectin given subcutaneously or rectally (*CID* 49:1411, 2009).

* For source of drug, see Table 13D, page 155.

TABLE 13A (8)

INFECTING ORGANISM	SUGGESTED REGIMENS — PRIMARY	ALTERNATIVE	COMMENTS
NEMATODES—INTESTINAL (Roundworms) *(continued)*			
Trichostrongylus orientalis, T. colubriformis	Pyrantel pamoate 11 mg/kg (max. 1 gm) po x 1	Albendazole 400 mg po x 1 dose	**Mebendazole** 100 mg po bid x 3 days
Trichuris trichuria (**whipworm**) (*Ln* 367:1521, 2006)	Albendazole 400 mg po 1x/day x 3 days. Often refractory; multiple courses may be necessary.	Mebendazole (100 mg po bid x 3 days or 500 mg once) or Ivermectin 200 mcg/kg daily x 3 days	Cure rate of 55% with one 500 mg dose of **Mebendazole** + one dose of **Ivermectin** 200 mcg/kg (*CID* 51:1420, 2010).
NEMATODES—EXTRAINTESTINAL (Roundworms)			
Ancylostoma braziliense & caninum: causes **cutaneous larva migrans** (Dog & cat hookworm)	Albendazole 400 mg po bid x 3-7 days (*Ln* 8:302, 2008)	Ivermectin 200 mcg/kg po x 1 dose/day x 1–2 days (not in children wt < 15 kg)	Also called "creeping eruption," dog and cat hookworm. Ivermectin cure rate 81–100% (1 dose) to 97% (2–3 doses) (*CID* 31:493, 2000).
Angiostrongylus cantonensis (**Angiostrongyliasis**) causes eosinophilic meningitis	Mild/moderate disease. Analgesics, serial LPs (if necessary). Prednisone 60 mg/day x 14 days reduces headache & need for LPs.	Adding **Albendazole** 15 mg/kg/day to prednisone 60 mg/day both for 14 days may reduce duration of headaches and need for repeat LPs.	**Do not use Albendazole without prednisone**, see *TRSMH* 102:990, 2008. Gnathostoma and Baylisascaris also cause eosinophilic meningitis.
Baylisascariasis (Raccoon roundworm); eosinophilic meningitis	No drug proven efficacious. Try po **albendazole**, corticosteroids. Treat for one month.	Peds: 25–50 mg/kg po; Adults: 400 mg po bid with	Steroids ref: *CID* 39:1484, 2004. Other causes of eosinophilic meningitis: Gnathostoma & Angiostrongylus.
Dracunculus medinensis: **Guinea worm** (*CMAJ* 170:495, 2004)	Slow extraction of pre-emergent worm over several days	No drugs effective. Oral analgesics, anti-inflammatory drugs, topical antiseptics/antibiotic ointments to alleviate symptoms and facilitate worm removal by gentle manual traction over several days.	
Filariasis. Wolbachia bacteria needed for filarial development. **Rx with doxy 100–200 mg/day x 6–8 wks** ; number of wolbachia & number of microfilaria decrease when **Doxy** used. No effect on adult worms.			
Lymphatic filariasis (**Elephantiasis**): Wuchereria bancrofti or Brugia malayi or B. timori. Ref: *Curr Opin Inf Dis* 21:673, 2008 (role of Wolbachia)	**Diethylcarbamazine** (DEC) 6 mg/kg/day x 12 days or in lymphatic or 14 days. For B. malayi 6 mg/kg as single po dose daily x 14 days OR gradual dose increase: day 1-50 mg po, day 2-50 mg po tid, day 3-100 mg po tid, day 4 through 12-6 mg/kg po divided tid + **Doxy** 200 mg/day x 6 wks.	Use in combination with DEC; in trials comparing combination vs. DEC alone. **Doxycycline** 200 mg/day x 6 wks PLUS DEC + albendazole reduced microfilaremia (*CID* 46:1385, 2008).	
Cutaneous			
Loiasis: **Loa loa**, eye worm disease	**Diethylcarbamazine (DEC)**[a]: Day 1, 50 mg; Day 2, 50 mg tid; Day 3, 100 mg tid; Days 4-21, 8-10 mg/kg/day in 3 divided doses. If eye worm, remove first.	**Albendazole** 200 mg bid x 21 days if still symptomatic after 2 courses of DEC.	If over 5,000 microfilaria/mL of blood, DEC can cause encephalopathy. Might start with albendazole x few days ± steroids, then DEC.
Onchocerca volvulus (**onchocerciasis**) — river blindness (*AJTMH* 81:702, 2009)	First give **doxy** 200 mg/day x 6 wks and then **ivermectin**: Single dose of 150 mcg/kg po; repeat every 3-6 months until asymptomatic.	DEC is contraindicated	Oncho & Loa loa may both be present. Check peripheral smear; if Loa loa microfilaria present, treat oncho first with ivermectin before DEC for Loa loa.
Mansonella perstans (dipetalonemiasis)	In randomized trial, doxy 200 mg once daily x 6 weeks cleared microfilaria from blood in 67 of 69 patients (*NEJM* 361:1448, 2009).	Albendazole in high dose x 3 weeks.	Efficacy of doxy believed to be due to inhibition of endosymbiont wolbachia; Ivermectin has no activity. Ref: *Trans R Soc Trop Med Hyg* 100:458, 2006.
Mansonella streptocerca	Ivermectin 150 mcg/kg x 1 dose.	May need antihistamine or corticosteroid for allergic reaction from disintegrating organisms that may be confused with leprosy. Can be asymptomatic.	

[a] May need antihistamine or corticosteroid for allergic reaction from disintegrating organisms
* For source of drug, see Table 13D, page 155.

TABLE 13A (9)

INFECTING ORGANISM	SUGGESTED REGIMENS PRIMARY	ALTERNATIVE	COMMENTS
NEMATODES—EXTRAINTESTINAL (Roundworms)/Filariasis (continued)			
Mansonella ozzardi	**Ivermectin** 200 μg/kg x 1 dose may be effective. Limited data but no other option.	Usually asymptomatic. Articular pain, pruritus, lymphadenopathy reported. May have allergic reaction from dying organisms.	
Dirofilariasis: **Heartworm** D. immitis, dog heartworm	No effective drugs; surgical removal only option		Can lodge in pulmonary artery → coin lesion. Eosinophilia rare.
D. tenuis (raccoon), D. ursi (bear), D. repens (dogs, cats)	No effective drugs		Worms migrate to conjunctivae, subcutaneous tissue, scrotum, breasts, extremities
Gnathostoma spinigerum Cutaneous larva migrans	**Albendazole** 400 mg po q24h or bid times 21 days	**Ivermectin** 200 μg/kg/day po x 2 days.	Other etiology of larva migrans: Ancyclostoma sp. see page 148
Eosinophilic meningitis	Supportive care; monitor for cerebral hemorrhage	Case reports of steroid use: both benefit and harm from Albendazole or Ivermectin (EIN 17:1174, 2011).	Other causes of eosinophilic meningitis: *Angiostrongylus* (see page 148) & *Baylisascaris* (see page 148)
Toxocariasis (Ann Trop Med Parasit 103:3, 2010) Visceral larval migrans	Rx directed at relief of symptoms as infection self-limited, e.g., steroids & antihistamines; use of anthelmintics controversial.		
	Albendazole 400 mg po bid x 5 days ± **Prednisone** 60 mg/day	**Mebendazole** 100–200 mg po bid times 5 days	Severe lung, heart or CNS disease may warrant steroids (Clin Micro Rev 16:265, 2003). Differential dx of larval migrans syndromes: Toxocara canis & catis, Ancylostoma spp., Gnathostoma spp., Spirometra spp.
Ocular larval migrans	First 4 wks of illness: (Oral **prednisone** 30–60 mg po q24h + subtenon **triamcinolone** 40 mg/wk) x 2 wks		No added benefit of anthelmintic drugs. Rx of little effect after 4 wks. Some use steroids (Clin Micro Rev 16:265, 2003).
	Concomitant **prednisone** 40–60 mg po q24h	then 400–500 mg po tid x 10 days	
	Albendazole 400 mg po bid x 1 day		
Trichinella spiralis (**Trichinellosis**)—muscle infection (Review: Clin Micro Rev 22:127, 2009)	**Albendazole** 400 mg po bid x 8–14 days		Use albendazole/mebendazole with caution during pregnancy. ↑ IgE, ↑ CPK, ESR 0, massive eosinophilia: >5000/μL
TREMATODES (Flukes) – Liver, Lung, Intestinal. All flukes have snail intermediate hosts; transmitted by injection of metacercariae on plants, fish or crustaceans.			
Clonorchis sinensis (liver fluke)	**Praziquantel** 25 mg/kg po tid x 2 days or **albendazole** 10 mg/kg per day po x 7 days		Same dose in children
Dicrocoelium dendriticum	**Praziquantel** 25 mg/kg po tid x 1 day		Ingestion of raw or undercooked sheep liver
Fasciola buski (intestinal fluke)	**Praziquantel** 25 mg/kg po tid x 1 day		Same dose in children
Fasciola hepatica (sheep liver fluke), Fasciola gigantica	**Triclabendazole** once, may repeat after 12–24 hrs. 10 mg/kg po x 1 dose. Single 10 mg/kg po dose effective in controlling endemic disease (PLoS Negl Trop Dis 6(8):e1720).	Alternative: **Bithionol*** Adults and children: 30–50 mg/kg (max. dose 2 gm/day) every other day times 10–15 doses. In CDC formulary, efficacy unclear.	
Heterophyes heterophyes (intestinal fluke), Metagonimus yokogawai (intestinal fluke), Metorchis conjunctus (No Amer liver fluke), Nanophyetus salmincola	**Praziquantel** 25 mg/kg po tid x 1 days		
Opisthorchis viverrini (liver fluke)	**Praziquantel** 25 mg/kg po tid x 2 days		
Paragonimus sp. (lung fluke)	**Praziquantel** 25 mg/kg po tid x 2 days or **Triclabendazole*** 10 mg/kg po x 2 doses over 12–24 hrs.		Same dose in children

* For source of drug, see *Table 13D, page 155*.

TABLE 13A (10)

INFECTING ORGANISM	SUGGESTED REGIMENS PRIMARY	ALTERNATIVE	COMMENTS
TREMATODES (Flukes) – Liver, Lung, Intestinal *(continued)*			
Schistosoma haematobium; GU bilharziasis. (*NEJM 346:1212, 2002*)	Praziquantel 40 mg/kg po on the same day (one dose of 40 mg/kg or two doses of 20 mg/kg)		Same dose in children.
Schistosoma intercalatum	Praziquantel 20 mg/kg po on the same day in 1 or 2 doses		Same dose in children.
Schistosoma japonicum, Oriental schisto. (*NEJM 346:1212, 2002*)	Praziquantel 60 mg/kg po on the same day (3 doses of 20 mg/kg)		Same dose in children. Cures 60-90% pts.
Schistosoma mansoni (intestinal bilharziasis) Possible praziquantel resistance (*JID 176:304, 1997*) (*NEJM 346:1212, 2002*)	Praziquantel 40 mg/kg po on the same day (one dose of 40 mg/kg or two doses of 20 mg/kg)		Praziquantel: Same dose for children and adults. Cures 60-90% pts. Report of success treating myeloradiculopathy with single po dose of praziquantel, 50 mg/kg, + prednisone for 6 mo. (*CID 39:1618, 2004*).
Schistosoma mekongi	Praziquantel 60 mg per kg po on the same day (3 doses of 20 mg/kg)		Same dose for children.
Toxemic schisto: Katayama fever	Praziquantel 20 mg per kg po bid with short course of high dose prednisone. Repeat Praziquantel in 4-6 wks (*Clin Micro Rev 16:225, 2010*).		Reaction to onset of egg laying 4-6 wks after infection exposure in fresh water.
CESTODES (Tapeworms)			
Echinococcus granulosus (hydatid disease) (*LnID 12:871, 2012; Int Dis Clin No Amer 26:421, 2012*)	Liver cysts: Meta-analysis supports percutaneous aspiration–injection-reaspiration (**PAIR**) + albendazole for uncomplicated single liver cysts. Before & after drainage: **albendazole** ≥60 kg, 400 mg bid or < 60 kg, 15 mg/kg per day div. bid, with meals. After 1-2 days puncture (P) & needle aspirate (A) cyst content. Instill (I) hypertonic saline (15-30%) or absolute alcohol. Wait 20-30 min, then re-aspirate (R) with final irrigation. **Continue albendazole for at least 30 days.** Cure in 96% as comp to 90% pts with surgical resection. Albendazole ref: *Acta Tropica 114:1, 2010*.		
Echinococcus multilocularis (alveolar cyst disease) (*CCID 16:437, 2003*)	Albendazole efficacy not clearly demonstrated, can try in dosages used for hydatid disease. Wide surgical resection only reliable rx; technique evolving. Post-surgical resection or if inoperable: Albendazole for several years (*Acta Tropic 114:1, 2010*).		
Intestinal tapeworms Diphyllobothrium latum (fish), Diphylidium caninum (dog), Taenia saginata (beef), & Taenia solium (pork)	Praziquantel 5-10 mg/kg po x 1 dose for children and adults.	Niclosamide[*] 2 gm po x 1 dose	Niclosamide from Expert Compounding Pharm, see Table 13D.
Hymenolepis diminuta (rats) and H. nana (humans)	Praziquantel 25 mg/kg po x 1 dose for children and adults.	Niclosamide[*] 2 gm po daily x 7 days	
	NOTE: Treat T. solium intestinal tapeworms, if present, with **praziquantel** 5-10 mg/kg po x 1 dose for children & adults.		
Neurocysticercosis (NCC): Larval form of T. solium Ref.: *AJTMH 72:3, 2005*			
Parenchymal NCC "Viable" cysts by CT/MRI Meta-analysis: Treatment assoc with cyst resolution, ↓ seizures, and ↓ seizure recurrence. Ref: *AIM 145:43, 2006*.	[**Albendazole** ≥60 kg 400 mg bid with meals or 60 kg 15 mg/kg per day in 2 div. doses (max. 800 mg/day) + **Dexamethasone** 0.1 mg/kg per day + Anti-seizure medication] — all x 10-30 days. May need anti-seizure therapy for 8 yr.	[**Praziquantel** 100 mg/kg per day in 3 div. doses po x 1 day, then 50 mg/kg/d in 3 doses plus **Dexamethasone** 0.1 mg/kg per day + Anti-seizure medication] — all x 29 days. See Comment	Albendazole assoc. with 46% ↓ in seizures (*NEJM 350:249, 2004*). Praziquantel less cysticidal activity. Steroids decrease serum levels of praziquantel. NIH reports methotrexate-sparing steroid use (*CID 44:549, 2007*). **Treatment improves prognosis of associated seizures.**
"Degenerating cysts"	Albendazole + dexamethasone as above		
Dead calcified cysts	No treatment indicated		
Subarachnoid NCC	Albendazole + steroids (as above) + shunting for hydrocephalus prior to drug therapy. Ref: *Expert Rev Anti Infect Ther 9:123, 2011.*		
Intraventricular NCC	Neuroendoscopic removal is treatment of choice with or without obstruction. If surgery not possible, **albendazole + dexamethasone; observe closely for evidence of obstruction of flow of CSF.**		

* For source of drug, see Table 13D, page 155

TABLE 13A (11)

CESTODES (Tapeworms)/Neurocysticercosis (NCC) (continued)

INFECTING ORGANISM	SUGGESTED REGIMENS PRIMARY	ALTERNATIVE	COMMENTS
Sparganosis (Spirometra mansonoides) Larval cysts: source—frogs/snakes	Surgical resection. No antiparasitic therapy. Can inject alcohol into subcutaneous masses.		

ECTOPARASITES. Ref.: CID 36:1355, 2003; Ln 363:889, 2004. NOTE: Due to potential neurotoxicity and risk of aplastic anemia, lindane not recommended.

DISEASE	INFECTING ORGANISM	PRIMARY	ALTERNATIVE	COMMENTS
Head lice Med Lett 51:57, 2009	Pediculus humanus, var. capitis	**Permethrin** 1% lotion: Apply to shampooed dried hair for 10 min; repeat in 9-10 days. **OR** **Malathion** 0.5% lotion (Ovide): Apply to dry hair for 8-12 hrs, then shampoo. 2 doses 7-9 days apart. **OR** **Spinosad** 0.9% suspension; wash off after 10 min (85% effective). Repeat in 7 days, if needed.	**Ivermectin** 200-400 µg/kg po once; 3 doses at 7 day intervals effective in 95% (IJD 193:474, 2006). Topical ivermectin 0.5% lotion, 75% effective. **Malathion:** Report that 1-2 20-min. applications 98% effective (Ped Derm 21:670, 2004). In alcohol—potentially flammable. **Benzyl alcohol:** 76% effective.	**Permethrin:** success in 78%. Extra combing of no benefit. Resistance increasing. No advantage to 5% permethrin. **Spinosad** is effective, but expensive. Refs: NEJM 367:1687 & 1750, 2012; Pediatrics 126:392, 2010.
Pubic lice (crabs)	Phthirus pubis	Pubic hair: **Permethrin OR malathion** as for head lice	**Eyelids: Petroleum jelly** applied qid x 10 days **OR** **yellow oxide of mercury** 1% qid x 14 days.	
Body lice	Pediculus humanus, var. corporis	No drugs for the patient. Organism lives in & deposits eggs in seams of clothing. Discard clothing; if not possible, treat clothing with 1% malathion powder or 0.5% permethrin powder. Success with ivermectin in homeless shelter: 12 mg po on days 0, 7, & 14 (IJD 193:474, 2006)		
Scabies Immunocompetent patients Refs: MMWR 59(RR-12):89, 2010; NEJM 362:717, 2010.	Sarcoptes scabiei	**Permethrin** 5% cream (ELIMITE) under nails (finger and toe). Apply entire skin from chin down to and including under fingernails and toenails. Leave on 8-14 hrs. Repeat in 1-2 wks. Safe for children age >2 mos.	**Ivermectin** 250 µg/kg po x 1. As above, second dose if persistent symptoms. **Less effective: Crotamiton** 10% cream, apply x 24 hr, rinse off, then reapply x 24 hr.	Trim fingernails. Reapply cream to hands after handwashing. Treat close contacts; wash and heat dry linens. Pruritus may persist times 2 wks after mites gone.
AIDS and HTLV-infected patients (CD4 <150 per mm³) debilitated or developmentally disabled patients (Norwegian scabies—see Comments)		For Norwegian scabies: **Permethrin** 5% cream daily x 7 days, then twice weekly until cured. Add **ivermectin** po (dose in Alternative)	**Ivermectin** 200 mcg/kg po on days 1, 2, 8, 9, 15 (and maybe 22, 29) + **Permethrin** cream.	Norwegian scabies in AIDS pts: Extensive, crusted. Can mimic psoriasis. Not pruritic. Highly contagious—isolate!
Myiasis Due to larvae of flies		Usually cutaneous/subcutaneous nodule with central punctum. Treatment: Occlude punctum to prevent gas exchange with petrolatum, fingernail polish, makeup cream or bacon. When larva migrates, manually remove.		

* For source of drug, see Table 13D, page 155.

151

TABLE 13B – DOSAGE AND SELECTED ADVERSE EFFECTS OF ANTIPARASITIC DRUGS

Doses vary with indication. For convenience, drugs divided by type of parasite; some drugs used for multiple types of parasites, e.g. albendazole.

CLASS, AGENT, GENERIC NAME (TRADE NAME)	USUAL ADULT DOSAGE	ADVERSE REACTIONS/COMMENTS
Antiprotozoan Drugs		
Intestinal Parasites		
Diloxanide furoate[NUS] (Furamide)	500 mg po tid x 10 days.	Source: See Table 13D, page 155. Flatulency, N/V, diarrhea.
Iodoquinol (Yodoxin)	Adults: 650 mg po tid (or 30-40 mg/kg/day div. tid); children: 40 mg/kg per day div. tid.	Rarely causes nausea, abdominal cramps, rash, acne. Contraindicated if iodine intolerance (contains 64% bound iodine). Can cause iododerma (papular or pustular rash) and/or thyroid enlargement.
Metronidazole	Side-effects similar for all. See metronidazole in Table 10B, page 107, & Table 10A, page 102.	
Nitazoxanide (Alinia)	Adults: 500 mg po q12h. Children 4-11: 200 mg susp. po q12h. Take with food. Expensive.	Abdominal pain 7.8%, diarrhea 2.1%. Rev. CID 40:1173, 2005; Expert Opin Pharmacother 7:953, 2006. Headaches; rarely yellow sclera (resolves after treatment).
Paromomycin (Humatin) Aminosidine IV in U.K.	Up to 750 mg qid (250 mg tabs). Source: See Table 13D.	Aminoglycoside similar to neomycin; if absorbed due to concomitant inflammatory bowel disease can result in oto/nephrotoxicity. Doses >3 gm daily are associated with nausea, abdominal cramps, diarrhea.
Quinacrine[NUS] (Atabrine, Mepacrine)	100 mg po tid. No longer available in U.S.: 2 pharmacies will prepare as a service: (1) Connecticut (+1)203-785-6818, [2] California 800-247-9767	Contraindicated for pts with history of psychosis or psoriasis. Yellow staining of skin. Dizziness, headache, vomiting, toxic psychosis (1.5%), hemolytic anemia, leukopenia, thrombocytopenia, urticaria, rash, fever, minor disulfiram-like reactions.
Tinidazole (Tindamax)	250-500 mg tabs, with food. Regimen varies with indication.	Chemical structure similar to metronidazole but better tolerated. Seizures/peripheral neuropathy reported. **Adverse effects:** Metallic taste 4-6%, nausea 3-5%, anorexia 2-3%.
Antiprotozoan Drugs: Non-Intestinal Protozoa		
Extraintestinal Parasites		
Antimony compounds[NUS] Stibogluconate sodium (Pentostam) from CDC or Meglumine antimoniate (Glucantime—French trade names)	For IV use: vials with 100 mg antimony/mL. Dilute selected dose in 50 mL of D5W shortly before use. Infuse over at least 10 minutes.	**AEs in 1st 10 days:** headache, fatigue, elevated lipase/amylase, clinical pancreatitis. After 10 days: elevated AST/ALT/ALK/PHOS. **Reversible T wave changes in 30-60%. Risk of QTc prolongation. NOTE:** Renal excretion; modify dose if renal insufficiency. Metabolized in liver; lower dose if hepatic insufficiency.
Artemether-Lumefantrine, po (Coartem, FDA-approved)	Tablets contain 20 mg Artemether and 120 mg Lumefantrine. Take with food. Can be crushed and mixed with a few teaspoons of water	Can prolong QTc; avoid in patients with congenital long QTc, family history of sudden death or long QTc, or been taking drugs known to prolong QTc (see list under *fluoroquinolones, Table 10A, page 100*). Artemether induces CYP3A4 and both Artemether & Lumefantrine are metabolized by CYP3A4 (see *drug-drug interactions, Table 22A, page 217*). Adverse effects experienced by >3% of adults: headache, anorexia, asthenia, arthralgia and dizziness.
Artesunate, IV Ref: NEJM 358:1829, 2008	Available from CDC Malaria Branch. 2.4 mg/kg IV at 0, 12, 24, & 48 hrs	More effective than quinine & safer than quinidine. Contact CDC at 770-488-7758 or 770-488-7100 after hours. No dosage adjustment for hepatic or renal insufficiency. No known drug interactions.
Atovaquone (Mepron) Ref: AAC 46:1163, 2002	Suspension: 1 tsp (750 mg) po bid 750 mg/5 mL	No pts stopping rx due to side-effects was 9%, rash 22%, GI 20%, headache 16%, insomnia 10%, fever 14%
Atovaquone and proguanil (Malarone) For prophylaxis of P. falciparum. The data on P. vivax. Generic available in US.	**Prophylaxis:** 1 tab po (250 mg + 100 mg) q24h with food **Treatment:** 4 tabs po (1000 mg + 400 mg) once daily with food x 3 days Adult tab: 250/100 mg; Peds tab: 62.5/25 mg; Peds dosage: *prophylaxis footnote 1 page 143*; *treatment see comment, page 144*.	Adverse effects in rx trials: Adults—abd. pain 17%, N/V 12%, headache 10%, dizziness 5%. Rx stopped in 1%. Asymptomatic, mild ↑ in ALT/AST. Children—cough, headache, anorexia, vomiting, abd. pain. See *drug interactions, Table 22*. Safe in G6PD-deficient pts. Can crush tabs for children and give with milk or other liquid nutrients. Renal insufficiency: contraindicated if CrCl <30 mL per min.

NOTE: Drugs available from CDC Drug Service indicated by "CDC." Call (+1) (404) 639-3670 (or -2888 (Fax)). **See Table 13D, page 155 for sources and contact information for hard-to-find antiparasitic drugs.**

TABLE 13B (2)

CLASS, AGENT, GENERIC NAME (TRADE NAME)	USUAL ADULT DOSAGE	ADVERSE REACTIONS/COMMENTS
Antiprotozoan Drugs: Non-Intestinal Protozoa/Extraintestinal Parasites *(continued)*		
Benznidazole (CDC Drug Service)	7.5 mg/kg per day po. 100 mg tabs	Photosensitivity in 50% of pts. GI: abdominal pain, nausea/vomiting/anorexia. CNS: disorientation, insomnia, twitching/seizures, paresthesias, polyneuritis. **Contraindicated in pregnancy**
Chloroquine phosphate (Aralen)	Dose varies—see *Malaria Prophylaxis and rx*, pages 143-151	Minor: anorexia/nausea/vomiting, headache, dizziness, blurred vision, pruritus in dark-skinned pts. Major: protracted rx in rheumatoid arthritis can lead to retinopathy. Can exacerbate psoriasis. Can block response to rabies vaccine. Contraindicated in pts with epilepsy.
Dapsone *See Comment re methemoglobinemia*	100 mg po q24h	Usually tolerated by pts with rash after TMP-SMX. Dapsone is common etiology of acquired methemoglobinemia (*NEJM 364:957, 2011*). Metabolite of dapsone converts heme iron to +3 chloride form (ferric 3+): reported level 11%; normal blood level 1%. Headache, insomnia, fatigue, tachycardia, dizziness at 30-40%, acidosis & coma at 60%, death at 70-80%. Low G6PD is a risk factor. Treatment: methylene blue 1-2 mg/kg IV over 5 min x 1 dose.
Eflornithine (Ornidyl) (WHO or CDC drug service)	200 mg/kg IV (slowly) q12h x 7 days for African trypanosomiasis	Diarrhea in ½ pts, vomiting, abdominal pain, anemia/leukopenia in ½ pts, seizures, alopecia, jaundice, ↓ hearing. Contraindicated in pregnancy.
Fumagillin	Eyedrops + po. 20 mg po tid. Leiter's: 800-292-6773.	Adverse events: Neutropenia & thrombocytopenia
Mefloquine	One 250 mg tab/wk for malaria prophylaxis: for rx: 1250 mg x 1 or 750 mg & then 500 mg in 6-8 hrs. In U.S., 250 mg base = 228 mg; outside U.S., 275 mg tab = 250 mg base	Side-effects in roughly 3%. Minor: headache, irritability, insomnia, weakness, diarrhea. Toxic psychosis, seizures can occur. Do not use with quinine, quinidine, or halofantrine. Rare: Prolonged QT interval and toxic epidermal necrolysis (*Ln 349:101, 1997*). Not used for self-rx due to neuropsychiatric side-effects.
Melarsoprol (Mel B, Arsobal) (CDC)	See Trypanosomiasis for adult dose Peds dose: 0.36 mg/kg IV initial ↑ to 3.6 mg/kg q1-5 days for total of 9-10 doses.	Post-rx encephalopathy (2-10%) with 50% mortality overall: risk of death 2° to rx 6-14%. Prednisolone (1 mg/kg per day) may prevent encephalopathy. Other: Heart damage, albuminuria, abdominal pain, vomiting, peripheral neuropathy. Herxheimer-like reaction, pruritus.
Miltefosine (Impavido) (*Expert Rev Anti Infect Ther 4:177, 2006*)	100-150 mg (approx. 2.25 mg/kg per day) po divided tid x 28 days Cutaneous leishmaniasis 2.25 mg/kg po q24h x 6 wks	Source: See Table 13D, page 155. **Pregnancy—No;** teratogenic. Side-effects vary; kala-azar pts, vomiting in up to 40%, diarrhea in 17%, "motion sickness," headache & ↑ increased creatinine. Daily dose >150 mg can cause severe GI side effects (*Ln 352:1821, 1998*).
Nifurtimox (Lampit) (CDC) (Manufactured in Germany by Bayer)	8-10 mg/kg per day po div. 4 x per day for 90-120 days	Side-effects in 40-70% of pts. GI: abdominal pain, nausea/vomiting. CNS: polyneuritis (1/3), disorientation, insomnia, twitching, seizures. Skin rash. Hemolysis with G6PD deficiency.
Pentamidine (NebuPent)	300 mg via aerosol q month. Also used IM.	Hypotension, hypocalcemia, hypoglycemia followed by hyperglycemia, pancreatitis. Neutropenia (15%), thrombocytopenia. Nephrotoxicity. Others: nausea/vomiting, ↑ liver tests, rash.
Primaquine phosphate	26.3 mg (= 15 mg base). Adult dose is 30 mg of base po daily.	In G6PD def, can cause hemolytic anemia, esp. African, Asian peoples. Methemoglobinemia. Nausea/abdominal pain if pt. fasting. (*CID 39:1336, 2004*). **Pregnancy: No.**
Pyrimethamine (Daraprim, Malocide) Also combined with sulfadoxine as **Fansidar** (25-500 mg)	100 mg po, then 25 mg/day. Cost of folinic acid (leucovorin)	Major problem is hematologic: megaloblastic anemia, ↓ WBC, ↓ platelets. Can give 5 mg folinic acid per day to ↓ bone marrow depression and not interfere with antitoxoplasmosis effect. If high-dose pyrimethamine, ↑ folinic acid to 10-50 mg/day. Pyrimethamine + sulfadiazine can cause mental changes due to carnitine deficiency (*AJM 95:112, 1993*). Other: Rash, vomiting, diarrhea, xerostomia.
Quinidine gluconate Cardiotoxicity ref: *LnID 7:549, 2007*	Loading dose of 10 mg (equiv to 6.2 mg of quinidine base)/kg IV over 1-2 hr, then constant infusion of 0.02 mg/kg of quinidine gluconate / kg per minute. May be available for compassionate use from Lilly.	Adverse reactions of quinidine/quinine similar: (1) IV bolus injection can cause fatal hypotension, (2) ↓ rate of infusion if QT prolongs (>0.6 sec) or QRS widens (>25% of baseline), (3) insulin-induced hypoglycemia, esp. pregnancy, (4) reduce dose 30-50% after day 3 due to ↓ renal clearance and ↓ vol. of distribution.

NOTE: Drugs available from CDC Drug Service indicated by "CDC". Call (+1) (404) 639-3670 (or -2888 (Fax)). **See Table 13D, page 155 for sources and contact information for hard-to-find antiparasitic drugs.**

153

TABLE 13B (3)

CLASS, AGENT, GENERIC NAME (TRADE NAME)	USUAL ADULT DOSAGE	ADVERSE REACTIONS/COMMENTS
Antiprotozoan Drugs: Non-Intestinal Protozoa/Extraintestinal Parasites (continued)		
Quinine sulfate (Qualaquin) (300 mg salt = 250 mg base)	324 mg tabs. No IV prep. in US. Oral rx of chloroquine-resistant falciparum malaria: 624 mg po tid x 3 days, then (tetracycline 250 mg po qid or doxy 100 mg bid) x 7 days	Cinchonism: tinnitus, headache, nausea, abdominal pain, blurred vision. Rarely, blood dyscrasias, drug fever, asthma, hypoglycemia. Transient blindness in <1% of 500 pts (AnIM 136:339, 2002). **Contraindicated if prolonged QTc, myasthenia gravis, optic neuritis or G6PD deficiency.**
Spiramycin (Rovamycin)	1 gm po q8h (see Comment)	GI and allergic reactions have occurred. Available at no cost after consultation with Palo Alto Medical Foundation Toxoplasma Serology Lab: 650-853-4828 or from U.S. FDA 301-796-1600.
Sulfadiazine	1–1.5 gm po q6h.	See Table 10A, page 102, for sulfonamide side-effects
Sulfadoxine & pyrimethamine combination (Fansidar)	Contains 500 mg sulfadoxine & 25 mg pyrimethamine	Long half-life of both drugs: Sulfadoxine 169 hrs, pyrimethamine 111 hrs allows weekly dosage. In African, used empirically in pregnancy for intermittent preventative treatment (ITPp) against malaria; dosing at 3 set times during pregnancy. Reduces material and fetal mortality if HIV+. See Expert Rev AnfI Infect Ther 8:589, 2010. Fatalities reported due to Stevens-Johnson syndrome and toxic epidermal necrolysis. Renal excretion—caution if renal impairment.
DRUGS USED TO TREAT NEMATODES, TREMATODES, AND CESTODES		
Albendazole (Albenza)	Doses vary with indication. Take with food; fatty meal increases absorption.	**Pregnancy Cat. C;** give negative pregnancy test. Abdominal pain, nausea/vomiting, alopecia, ↑ serum transaminase. Rare leukopenia.
Bithionol (CDC)	Adults & children: 30–40 mg/kg (to max. of 2 gm/day) po every other day x 10-15 doses	Photosensitivity, skin reactions, urticaria, GI upset.
Diethylcarbamazine (CDC)	Used to treat filariasis.	Headache, dizziness, nausea, fever. Host may experience inflammatory reaction to death of adult worms; fever, urticaria, asthma. GI upset (Mazzotti reaction). **Pregnancy—No.**
Ivermectin (Stromectol, Mectizan) (3 mg tab & topical 0.5% lotion for head lice)	Strongyloidiasis dose: 200 µg/kg/day po x 2 days Onchocerciasis: 150 µg/kg x 1 po Scabies: 200 µg/kg po x 1; if AIDS, wait 14 days & repeat	Headache, bone/joint pain. Host may experience inflammatory reaction to death of adult worms; fever, urticaria, asthma. GI upset (Mazzotti reaction).
Mebendazole (Vermox)	Doses vary with indication.	Rarely causes abdominal pain, nausea, diarrhea. Contraindicated in pregnancy & children <2 yrs old.
Praziquantel (Biltricide)	Doses vary with parasite; see Table 13A.	Mild, dizziness/drowsiness; N/V, rash, fever. Only contraindication is ocular cysticercosis. Potential exacerbation of neurocysticercosis. Metab. induced by anticonvulsants and steroids; can negate effect w/ cimetidine 400 mg po tid. Reduce dose if advanced liver disease.
Pyrantel pamoate (over-the-counter)	Oral suspension. Dose for all ages: 11 mg/kg (to max. of 1 gm) x 1 dose.	Rare GI upset, headache, dizziness, rash
Suramin (Germanin) (CDC)	Drug powder mixed to 10% solution with 5 mL water and used within 30 min. First give test dose of 0.1 gm IV. Try to avoid during pregnancy.	Does not cross blood-brain barrier: no effect on CNS infection. Side-effects: vomiting, pruritus, urticaria, fever, paresthesias, albuminuria (discontinue drug if casts appear). Do not use if renal/liver disease present. Deaths from vascular collapse reported.
Triclabendazole (Egaten) (CDC)	Used for fasciola hepatica liver fluke infection: 10 mg/kg po x 1 dose. May repeat in 12-24 hrs. 250 mg tabs	AEs ≥10%: sweating and abdominal pain. AEs 1-10%: weakness, chest pain, fever, anorexia, nausea, vomiting. Note: use with caution if G6PD def. or impaired liver function.

NOTE: Drugs available from CDC Drug Service indicated by "CDC." Call (+1) (404) 639-3670 (or -2888 (Fax)). **See Table 13D, page 155 for sources and contact information for hard-to-find antiparasitic drugs.**

TABLE 13C – PARASITES THAT CAUSE EOSINOPHILIA (EOSINOPHILIA IN TRAVELERS)

Frequent and Intense (>5000 eos/mcL)	Moderate to Marked Early Infections	During Larval Migration; Absent or Mild During Chronic Infections	Other
Strongyloides (absent in compromised hosts); Lymphatic Filariasis; Toxocaria (cutaneous larva migrans)	Ascaris; Hookworm; Clonorchis; Paragonimis	Opisthorchis	Schistosomiasis; Cysticercosis; Trichuris; Angiostrongylus; Non-lymphatic filariasis; Gnathostoma; Capillaria; Trichostrongylus

TABLE 13D – SOURCES FOR HARD-TO-FIND ANTIPARASITIC DRUGS

Source	Drugs Available	Contact Information
CDC Drug Service	Artesunate, Benznidazole, Diethylcarbamazine (DEC), Eflornithine, Melarsoprol, Nifurtimox, Sodium stibogluconate, Suramin, Triclabendazole	www.cdc.gov/laboratory/drugservice/index.html (+1) 404-639-3670
WHO	Drugs for treatment of African trypanosomiasis	simarrop@who.int; (+41) 794-682-726; (+41) 227-911-345 franco@who.int; (+41) 796-198-535; (+41) 227-913-313
Compounding Pharmacies, Specialty Labs, Others		
Expert Compounding Pharmacy	Quinacrine, Iodoquinol, niclosamide	www.expertpharmacy.org 1-800-247-9767; (+1) 818-988-7979
Fagron Compounding Pharmacy (formerly Gallipot)	Quinacrine, Iodoquinol, Paromomycin, Diloxanide	www.fagron.com 1-800-423-6967; (+1) 651-681-9517
Leiter's Pharmacy		www.leiterrx.com 1-800-292-0773
Paladin Labs	Miltefosine	www.paladin-labs.com
Victoria Apotheke Zurich	Paromomycin (oral and topical), Triclabendazole	www.pharmaworld.com (+41) 43-344-6060
Fast Track Research	Miltefosine (may be free under treatment IND for cutaneous, mucocutaneous leishmaniasis)	jberman@fasttrackresearch.com
Palo Alto Medical Foundation, Toxoplasma Serology Lab	Spiramycin	(+1) 650-853-4828

TABLE 14A – ANTIVIRAL THERAPY**
For HIV, see Table 14D; for Hepatitis, see Table 14F and Table 14G

VIRUS/DISEASE	DRUG/DOSAGE	SIDE EFFECTS/COMMENTS
Adenovirus: Cause of RTIs resulting in fatal pneumonia in children & young adults and 60% mortality in transplant pts (CID 43:331, 2006). Frequent cause of cystitis in transplant patients. Adenovirus 14 associated with severe pneumonia in otherwise healthy adults (MMWR 56(45):1181, 2007). Other clinical manifestations include: fever, ↑ liver enzymes, leukopenia, thrombocytopenia, diarrhea, pneumonia, or hemorrhagic cystitis.	In severe cases of pneumonia or post HSCT[1]: **Cidofovir** • 5 mg/kg/wk x 2 wks, then q 2 wks + **probenecid** 1.25 gm/m² given 3 hrs before cidofovir and 3 & 9 hrs after cidofovir infusion • OR 1 mg/kg IV 3x/wk. For adenovirus hemorrhagic cystitis (CID 40:199, 2005; Transplantation. 2006; 81:1398). Intravesical **cidofovir** (5 mg/kg in 100 mL saline instilled into bladder).	Successful in 3/8 immunosuppressed children (CID 38:45, 2004 & 8 of 10 children with HSCT) (CID 41: 1812, 2005). ↓ in virus load predicted response to cidofovir. Ribavirin has had mixed activity, appears restricted to group C serotypes. Vidarabine and ganciclovir activity against human adenovirus is too low for clinical data. New adenovirus, "titi monkey adenovirus" (TMAdV) transmitted from a monkey to researcher and subsequently to members of his family. PLoS Pathog 2011 Jul 14; 7:e1002155.
Coronavirus—SARS-CoV (Severe Acute Respiratory Distress Syn.) A new coronavirus, isolated Spring 2003 (NEJM 348:1953 & 1967, 2003), emerged from southern China & spread to Hong Kong and over 24 countries. Bats appear to be a primary reservoir for SARS virus (PNAS 102: 14040, 2005).	Therapy remains predominantly supportive care. Therapy tried or under evaluation (see Comments): • Ribavirin—ineffective. • Interferon alfa ± steroids—small case series. • Pegylated IFN–α effective in monkeys. • Low dose steroids alone successful in one Beijing hospital. High dose steroids ↑ serious fungal infections. • Inhaled nitric oxide improved oxygenation & improved chest x-ray (CID 39:1531, 2004).	**Transmission by close contact:** effective infection control practices (mask [changed frequently], eye protection, gown, gloves) key to stopping transmission. Other coronaviruses (HCOV-229E, OC43, NL63, etc.) implicated as cause of croup, asthma exacerbations, & other RTIs in children (CID 40:1721, 2005; JID 191:492, 2005). May be associated with Kawasaki disease (JID 191:499, 2005).
Enterovirus—Meningitis: most common cause of aseptic meningitis. Rapid CSF PCR test is accurate; reduces costs and hospital stay for infants (Peds 109:469, 2007).	No rx currently recommended; however, **pleconaril** (VP 63843) still under investigation.	No clinical benefit demonstrated in double-blind placebo-controlled study in 21 infants with enteroviral aseptic meningitis (PIDJ 22:335, 2003). Failed to ameliorate symptoms but did have some improvement among those with severe headache (AAC 2006 50:2409-14).
Hemorrhagic Fever Virus infections: For excellent reviews, see Med Lab Observer, May 2005, p. 16, Lancet Infectious Disease Vol. 6 No 4. **Congo-Crimean Hemorrhagic Fever HF** (CID 52:284, 2004) Tick-borne, symptoms include N/V, fever, headache, myalgias, & stupor (1/3). Signs: conjunctival injection, hepatomegaly, petechiae (1/3). Lab: ↓ platelets, ↓ WBC; ↑ ALT, AST, LDH & CPK (100%).	Oral **ribavirin, 30 mg/kg** as initial loading dose &, 15 mg/kg q6h x 4 days then 7.5 mg/kg/day x 6 days (WHO recommendation) (see Comment). Reviewed Antiviral Res 78:125, 2008.	3/3 healthcare workers in Pakistan had complete recovery (Ln 346:472, 1995) & 61/69 (89%) with confirmed CCHF survived in Iran (CID 36:1613, 2003). Shorter time of hospitalization among ribavirin treated pts (7.7 vs. 10.3 days), but no difference in mortality or transfusion needs in study done in Turkey (J Infection 52: 207-215, 2006).
Ebola/Marburg HF (Central Africa) Severe outbreak of Ebola in Angola 308 cases with 277 deaths (NEJM 355:909, 2005; NEJM 371:2423, 2014; MMWR 54:308, 2005; LnID 5:331, 2005) Major epidemic of Marburg 1998-2000 in Congo & 2004-5 in Angola (NEJM 355:866, 2006)	No effective antiviral rx (J Virol 77: 9733, 2003).	Can infect gorillas & chimps that come in contact with other dead animal carcasses (Science 303:390, 2004). Marburg reported in African fruit bat, Rousettus aegyptiacus (PLoS Pathog 5:e1000536 2009). Study in Gabon revealed 15% seroprevalence among 4349 healthy volunteers from 220 randomly selected villages. None recalled any illness similar to Ebola. Seroprevalence among children rises until age 15, then plateaus. Seropositive status correlates to location of fruit bats. PLoS ONE (Feb 9); 5:e9126, 2010
With pulmonary syndrome: Hantavirus pulmonary syndrome, "sin nombre virus"	No benefit from ribavirin has been demonstrated (CID 39:1307, 2004). Early recognition of disease and supportive (usually ICU) care is key to successful outcome.	Acute onset of fever, headache, myalgias, non-productive cough, thrombocytopenia and non-cardiogenic pulmonary edema with respiratory insufficiency following exposure to rodents.
With renal syndrome: Lassa, Venezuelan, Korean, HF, Sabia, Argentinian HF, Bolivian HF, Junin, Machupo	Oral **ribavirin, 30 mg/kg** as initial loading dose & 15 mg/kg q6h x 4 days & then 7.5 mg/kg x 6 days (WHO recommendation) (see Comment)	Toxicity low, hemolysis reported but recovery when treatment stopped. No significant changes in WBC, platelets, hepatic or renal function. See CID 36:1254, 2003, for management of contacts.

[1] HSCT = Hematopoietic stem cell transplant
** See page 2 for abbreviations. NOTE: All dosage recommendations are for adults (unless otherwise indicated) and assume normal renal function.

TABLE 14A (2)

VIRUS/DISEASE	DRUG/DOSAGE	SIDE EFFECTS/COMMENTS
Hemorrhagic Fever Virus Infections (continued)		
Dengue and dengue hemorrhagic fever (DHF) www.cdc.gov/ncidod/dvbid/dengue/dengue-hcp.htm Think dengue in traveler to tropics or subtropics (incubation period usually 4-7 days) with fever, bleeding, thrombocytopenia, or hemoconcentration with shock. Dx by viral isolation or serology; serum to CDC (telephone 787-706-2399).	**No data on antiviral rx.** Fluid replacement with careful hemodynamic monitoring critical. Rx of **DHF** with colloids (dextran or starch), hydroxyethyl starch preferred in 1 study (*NEJM* 353:9, 2005). Review in *Semin Ped Infect Dis* 16: 60-65, 2005.	Of 77 cases dx at CDC (2001–2004), recent (2-wks) travel to Caribbean island 30%, Asia 17%, Central America 15%, S. America 15% (*MMWR* 54:556, *June 10*, 2005), 5 pts with severe **DHF** rx'd with dengue antibody-neg gamma globulin 500 mg per kg q24h IV for 3-5 days. IgM in platelet counts (*CID* 36:1623, 2003). New test approved by FDA in 2011: DENV Detect IgM Capture ELISA test. Has some cross-reactivity with West Nile Virus infection. Should only be used in pts with symptoms c/w Dengue Fever.
West Nile virus (see *AnIM* 104:545, 2004) A flavivirus transmitted by mosquitoes, blood transfusions, transplanted organs. (*NEJM* 348: 2196, 2003; *CID* 61:1257, 2004), & breast-feeding (*MMWR* 51:877, 2002). Birds (>200 species) are main host with humans & horses incidental hosts. The US epidemic continues.	**No proven rx to date.** 2 clinical trials in progress: (1) Interferon alfa-N3 (*CID* 40:764, 2005) (this option falling out of favor) (2) IV form: Israel with high titer antibody; West Nile IG (*JID* 188:5, 2003; *Transpl Inf Dis* 4:160, 2003). Contact NIH. 301-496-7453; see www.clinicaltrials.gov/show/NCT00068055. Reviewed in *Lancet Neurology* 6: 171-181, 2007.	Usually nonspecific febrile disease but 1/150 cases develops meningoencephalitis, aseptic meningitis or polio-like paralysis (*AnIM* 104:545, 2004; *JCI* 113: 1102, 2004). Long-term sequelae (neuromuscular weakness & psychiatric) common (*CID* 43:723, 2006). Dx by ↑ IgM in serum & CSF or ↑ PCR (contact state Health Dept/CDC). Blood supply now tested in U.S. ↑ serum lipase in 11/17 cases (*NEJM* 352:420, 2005).
Yellow fever	**No data on antiviral rx. Guidelines for use of preventative vaccine:** (*MMWR* 51: RR17, 2002)	Reemergence in Africa & S. Amer. due to urbanization of susceptible population (*Lancet Int* 15:604, 2005). Vaccination effective. (*JAMA* 276:1157, 1996). Vaccine safe and effective in HIV patients, especially in those with suppressed VL and higher CD4 counts (*CID* 46:659, 2008). A purified whole-virus, inactivated, cell-culture-derived vaccine (XRX-001) produced using the 17D strain has proven safe and resulted in neutralizing antibodies after 2 doses in a de-escalation, phase I study. (*N Engl J Med* 2011 Apr 7; 364:1326)
Chikungunya fever A self-limited arbovirus illness spread by Aedes mosquito. High epidemic potential.	**No antiviral therapy.** Mice given purified human polyvalent CHIKV immunoglobulins were therapeutic (*JID* 200: 516, 2009).	Clinical presentation: high fever, severe myalgias & headache, macular papular rash with occ. thrombocytopenia. Rarely hemorrhagic complications. Dx by increase in IgM antibody.
SFTSV (Severe fever with thrombocytopenia syndrome virus)	**No known therapy.**	New hemorrhagic fever in the Bunyaviridae family described in China. Initially thought to be anaplasma infection, serology showed new virus. Possibly transmitted by Haemaphysalis longicornis ticks. (*N Engl J Med* 2011; 364:1523-32)
Hepatitis Viral Infections	See Tables *Table 14F (Hepatitis A & B)*, *Table 14G (Hepatitis C)*	

* See page 2 for abbreviations. NOTE: All dosage recommendations are for adults (unless otherwise indicated) and assume normal renal function.

TABLE 14A (3)

VIRUS/DISEASE	DRUG/DOSAGE	SIDE EFFECTS/COMMENTS
Herpesvirus Infections **Cytomegalovirus (CMV)** Marked ↓ in HIV associated CMV infections & death with Highly Active Antiretroviral Therapy. Initial treatment should optimize ART.	Primary prophylaxis not generally recommended except in certain transplant populations (see below). Preemptive therapy in pts with ↑ CMV DNA titers in plasma & CD4 <100/mm³. Recommended is: **valganciclovir** 900 mg po q24h (CID 32: 783, 2001). Authors rec. primary prophylaxis be dc if response to ART with ↑ CD4 >100 for 6 mos. (MMWR 53:98, 2004).	Risk for developing CMV disease correlates with quantity of CMV DNA in plasma: each log₁₀ associated with 3.1-fold ↑ in disease (JCI 101:497, 1998; CID 28:759, 1999). Resistance demonstrated in 5% of transplant recipients receiving primary prophylaxis (J Antimicrob Chemother 65:2628, 2010).
Colitis, Esophagitis, Gastritis Dx: CMV IgG & biopsy based on endoscopic appearance (Clin Gastro Hepatol 2:564, 2004) with demonstration of CMV inclusions & other pathogen(s).	**Ganciclovir** as with retinitis except IV induction period extended to 3-6 wks. No agreement on use of maintenance, may not be necessary except after relapse. Responses less predictable than for retinitis. **Valganciclovir also likely effective**. Switch to oral valganciclovir when po tolerated & when symptoms not severe enough to interfere with absorption. Antiretroviral therapy is essential in long term suppression. Alternative: **Cidofovir** 5 mg/kg IV, qwk × 2 wks followed by administration q2 wks; MUST be administered with **probenecid** 2 gm po 3 hrs before each dose and further 1 gm doses 2 hrs and 8 hrs after completion of the cidofovir infusion. IV saline hydration is essential.	
Encephalitis, Ventriculitis: Treatment not defined, but should be considered the same as retinitis. Disease may develop while taking ganciclovir as suppressive therapy. See Herpes 11 (Suppl 12):95A, 2004. Lumbosacral polyradiculopathy: diagnosis by CMV DNA in CSF	**Ganciclovir**, as with retinitis. **Foscarnet** 40 mg/kg IV q12h another option. Switch to **valganciclovir** when possible. Suppression continued until CD4 remains >100-150/mm³ for 6 mos. Alternative: **Cidofovir** 5 mg/kg IV, qwk × 2 wks followed by administration q2 wks; MUST be administered with probenecid 2 gm po 3 hrs before each dose and further 1 gm doses 2 hrs and 8 hrs after completion of the cidofovir infusion. IV saline hydration is essential.	About 50% will respond; survival ↑ (5.4 wks to 14.6 wks) (CID 27:345, 1998). Resistance can be demonstrated genotypically.
Mononeuritis multiplex	Not defined	Due to vasculitis & may not be responsive to antiviral therapy
Pneumonia— Seen predominantly in transplants (esp. bone marrow), **rare in HIV**. Treat only when histological evidence present in AIDS & other pathogens not identified. High rate of CMV reactivation in immunocompetent ICU patients; prolonged hospitalizations and increased mortality (JAMA 300:413, 2008).	**Ganciclovir/valganciclovir**, as with retinitis. In bone marrow transplant pts, combination therapy with CMV immune globulin.	In bone marrow transplant pts, serial measure of pp65 antigen was useful in establishing early diagnosis of CMV interstitial pneumonia with good results if ganciclovir was initiated within 6 days of antigen positivity (Bone Marrow Transplant 26:413, 2000). For preventive therapy, see Table 15E.

* See page 2 for abbreviations. NOTE: All dosage recommendations are for adults (unless otherwise indicated) and assume normal renal function.

TABLE 14A (4)

VIRUS/DISEASE	DRUG/DOSAGE	SIDE EFFECTS/COMMENTS
Herpesvirus Infections (continued)		
CMV Retinitis Most common cause of blindness in AIDS patients with <50/mm3 CD4 counts. 19/30 pts (63%) with inactive CMV retinitis who responded to ART (↑ to ≥60 CD4 cells/mcL) developed immune recovery vitreitis (vision ↓ & floaters with posterior segment inflammation — vitreitis, papillitis & macular changes) an average of 43 wks after rx started (*JID* 179: 697, 1999). Corticosteroid rx ↓ inflammatory reaction of immune recovery vitreitis without reactivation of CMV retinitis, either periocular corticosteroids or short course of systemic steroid.	**For immediate sight-threatening lesions:** **Ganciclovir** intraocular implant & **valganciclovir** 900 mg po q24h. **For peripheral lesions:** **Valganciclovir** 900 mg po q12h x 14–21d, then 900 mg po q24h for maintenance therapy	Differential diagnosis: HIV retinopathy, herpes simplex retinitis, varicella-zoster retinitis (rare, hard to diagnose). **Ganciclovir:** 5 mg/kg IV q12h x 14–21d, then **valganciclovir** 900 mg po q24h **OR** **Foscarnet** 60 mg/kg IV q8h or 90 mg/kg IV q12h x 14–21d, then 90–120 mg/kg IV q24h **OR** **Cidofovir** 5 mg/kg IV q1 wk, then 5 mg/kg every other wk, IV saline hydration & oral probenecid **OR** Repeated intravitreal injections with **fomivirsen** (for relapses only, not as initial therapy).
Pts who discontinue suppression therapy should undergo regular eye examination for early detection of relapses!	**Post treatment suppression** (Prophylactic) if CD4 count <100/mm³: **Valganciclovir** 900 mg po q24h.	Discontinue if CD4 >100/mm³ x 6 mos on ART.
CMV in Transplant patients: See Table 15E. Use of **valganciclovir** to prevent infections in CMV seronegative recipients of organs from a seropositive donor & in seropositive receivers has been highly effective (*Ln* 365:2105, 2005); *Pharm Ther* 35:676, 2010. Extended prophylaxis for up to a year before prophylaxis than short term prophylaxis in lung transplant recipients (*Ann Intern Med* 152:761, 2010). CMV in pregnancy: Hyperimmune globulin 200 IU/kg maternal weight as single dose during pregnancy (early), administered IV reduced complications of CMV in infant at one year of life. (*CID* 55: 497, 2012).		
Epstein Barr Virus (EBV) — Mononucleosis (*Ln* 3:131, 2003)	No treatment. Corticosteroids for tonsillar obstruction, CNS complications, or threat of splenic rupture.	Etiology of atypical lymphocytes: EBV, CMV, Hep A, Hep B, toxo, measles, mumps, drugs (*Int Pediatr* 18:20, 2003)
HHV-6—Implicated as cause of roseola (exanthum subitum) & other febrile diseases of childhood (*NEJM* 352:768, 2005) Fever & rash documented in 47% of 110 U.S. hematopoetic stem cell transplant pts assoc. with delayed monocytes & platelet engraftment (*CID* 40:932, 2005). Recognized in assoc. with meningoencephalitis in immunocompetent adults. Diagnosis made by pos. PCR in CSF ↓ viral copies in response to **ganciclovir** rx (*CID* 40:890 & 894, 2005). Foscarnet therapy improved thrombotic microangiopathy (*Am J Hematol* 76:156, 2004)		
HHV-7—ubiquitous virus (>90% of the population is infected by age 3 yrs). No relationship to human disease. Infects CD4 lymphocytes via CD4 receptor; transmitted via saliva.		
HHV-8—The agent of Kaposi's sarcoma, Castleman's disease, & body cavity lymphoma. Associated with diabetes in sub-Saharan Africa (*JAMA* 299:2770, 2008).	No antiviral treatment. Effective anti-HIV therapy may help.	Localized lesions: radiotherapy, laser surgery or intralesional chemotherapy. Systemic chemotherapy, Castleman's disease responded to ganciclovir (*Blood* 103:1632, 2004) & valganciclovir (*JID* 2006).

* See page 2 for abbreviations. NOTE: All dosage recommendations are for adults (unless otherwise indicated) and assume normal renal function.

TABLE 14A (5)

VIRUS/DISEASE	DRUG/DOSAGE	SIDE EFFECTS/COMMENTS
Herpes simplex virus (HSV Types 1 & 2) Bell's palsy Bell's palsy: most implicated etiology. Other etiologic considerations: VZV, HHV-6, Lyme disease.	As soon as possible after onset of palsy: **Prednisone** 1 mg/kg po divided bid x 5 days then taper to 5 mg bid over the next 5 days (total of 10 days prednisone) Alternate: **Prednisone** (dose as above) + **Valacyclovir** 500 mg bid x 5 days	Prospective randomized double blind placebo controlled trial compared prednisolone vs acyclovir vs. (prednisolone + acyclovir) vs placebo. Best result with prednisolone: 85% recovery with placebo, 96% recovery with prednisolone, 93% with combination of acyclovir & prednisolone (NEJM 357:1598 & 1653, 2007). **Large meta-analysis confirms: Steroids alone, effective; antiviral drugs alone, not effective; steroids + antiviral drugs, no more effective than steroids alone** (JAMA 302:985, 2009).
Encephalitis UK experience reviews: CID 35: 254, 2002; Eur J Neurol 9:234, 2003; Antiviral Res. 71:141-148, 2006)	**Acyclovir** IV 10 mg/kg IV (infuse over 1 hr) q8h x 14-21 days Up to 20 mg/kg q8h in children <12 yrs. Dose calculation in obese patients uncertain. To lessen risk of nephrotoxicity with larger doses, seems reasonable to infuse each dose over more than 1 hour.	HSV is most common cause of sporadic encephalitis. Survival & recovery from neurological sequelae are related to mental status at time of initiation of rx. **Early dx and rx imperative.** Mortality risk reduced from >70% to 19% with acyclovir rx. PCR analysis of CSF (NEJM 357:1598 & 1653, 2007) is 100% specific & 75-98% sensitive. 8/33 (25%) CSF samples drawn before day 3 were neg. by PCR; neg. PCR assoc. with ↓ protein & <10 WBC per mm³ in CSF (CID 36:1335, 2003). All were + after 3 days. Relapse after successful rx reported in 7/27 (27%) children. Relapse was associated with a lower total dose of initial acyclovir rx (265 ± 82 mg/kg vs relapse group vs 482 ± 143 mg per kg, p <0.03) (CID 30:185, 2000; Neuropediatrics 35:371, 2004)
Genital Herpes: *Sexually Transmitted Guidelines 2010: MMWR 59 (RR-12), 2010.* Primary (initial episode)	**Acyclovir** (Zovirax or generic) 400 mg po tid x 7-10 days OR **Valacyclovir** (Valtrex) 1000 mg po bid x 7-10 days OR **Famciclovir** (Famvir) 250 mg po tid x 7-10 days	↓ by 2 days time to resolution of signs & symptoms, ↓ by 4 days time to healing of lesions, ↓ by 7 days duration of viral shedding. Does not prevent recurrences. For severe cases only: 5 mg per kg IV q8h times 5-7 days.
Episodic recurrences	**Acyclovir** 800 mg po bid x **2 days** or 400 mg po tid x **5 days** or **Famciclovir** 1000 mg bid x **1 day** or 125 mg po bid x 5 days or **Valacyclovir** 500 mg po bid x **3 days** or 1 gm po once daily x 5 days For HIV patients, see Comment	An ester of acyclovir, which is well absorbed, bioavailability 3-5 times greater than acyclovir. Metabolized to acyclovir, which is active component. Side effects and activity similar to acyclovir. Famciclovir 500 mg once daily is **equal to acyclovir** 200 mg 5 times per day. For episodic recurrences in HIV patients: **acyclovir** 400 mg po tid x 5-10 days or **famciclovir** 500 mg po bid x 5-10 days or **valacyclovir** 1 gm po bid x 5-10 days
Chronic daily suppression	Suppressive therapy reduces the frequency of genital herpes recurrences by 70-80% among pts who have frequent recurrences (i.e., >6 recurrences per yr) & many report no symptomatic outbreaks. **Acyclovir** 400 mg po bid, **or famciclovir** 250 mg po bid, **or valacyclovir** 1 gm po q24h; pts with <9 recurrences per yr could use 500 mg po q24h and then use valaciclovir 1 gm po q24h if breakthrough at 500 mg. For HIV patients, see Comment	For chronic suppression in HIV patients: **acyclovir** 400-800 mg po bid or tid or **famciclovir** 500 mg po bid or **valacyclovir** 500 mg po bid
Genital, immunocompetent Gingivostomatitis, primary (children)	**Acyclovir** 15 mg/kg po 5x/day x 7 days	Efficacy in randomized double-blind placebo-controlled trial (BMJ 314:1800, 1997).
Keratoconjunctivitis and recurrent epithelial keratitis	**Trifluridine** (Viroptic), 1 drop 1% solution q2h x 9 drops per day) for max. of 21 days (see Table 1, page 13)	Suppressive rx with acyclovir (400 mg bid) reduced recurrences of ocular HSV from 32% to 19% (NEJM 339:300, 1998).
Mollaret's recurrent "aseptic" meningitis (usually HSV-2) (LN 363:1772, 2004)	No controlled trials of antiviral rx & relapses spontaneously. If given, **acyclovir** 10 mg/kg IV q8h (5 mg/kg/day IV) or **valacyclovir** 1-2 gm po qd should be used.	Pos. PCR for HSV in CSF confirms dx (EJCMID 23:560, 2004). Acyclovir po rx might ↓ frequency of recurrence but no clinical trials. Oral Valacyclovir ref: JAC 47:855, 2001.

See page 2 for abbreviations. NOTE: All dosage recommendations are for adults (unless otherwise indicated) and assume normal renal function.

TABLE 14A (6)

VIRUS/DISEASE	DRUG/DOSAGE	SIDE EFFECTS/COMMENTS
Herpes simplex virus (HSV Types 1 & 2) *(continued)*		
Mucocutaneous *(for genital see previous page)*		
Oral labial, "fever blisters": **Normal host** See *Ann Pharmacotherapy* 38:705, 2004; *JAC* 53:703, 2004	Start rx with prodrome symptoms (tingling/burning) before lesions show. **Oral: Valacyclovir** — Dose: 2 gm po q12h x 1 day — Sx Decrease: ↓ 1 day **Famciclovir**[3] — 500 mg po bid x 7 days — ↓ 2 days **Acyclovir**[NFDA] — 400 mg po 5x per day — ↓ ½ day (q4h while awake) x 5 days) **Topical:** Penciclovir 1% cream — q2h during day x 4 days — ↓ 1 day Acyclovir 5% cream[3] — 5x/day (q3h) x 7 days — ↓ ½ day See Table 1, page 28	Penciclovir (*J Derm Treat* 13:67, 2002; *JAMA* 277:1374, 1997; *AAC* 46: 2848, 2002). Docosanol (*J Am Acad Derm* 45:222, 2001). Oral acyclovir 5% cream (*AAC* 46:2238, 2002). Oral famciclovir (*JID* 179:303, 1999). Topical fluocinonide (0.05%) + acyclovir with famciclovir 5 days in combination with famciclovir ↓ lesion size and pain when compared to famciclovir alone (*JID* 181:1906, 2000).
Herpes Whitlow		
Oral labial or genital: immunocompromised (CU includes pts with AIDS) and critically ill pts in ICU) may develop chronic ulcers in perineum or face. (See Comment)	**Acyclovir** 5 mg per kg IV (infused over 1 hr) q8h times 7 days (250 mg per M²) or 400 mg po 5 times per day times 14–21 days (see Comment if suspect acyclovir-resistant) OR **Famciclovir:** In HIV infected, 500 mg po bid for 7 days for recurrent episodes of genital herpes OR **Valacyclovir**[NFDA]: In HIV-infected, 500 mg po bid 5–10 days for recurrent episodes of genital herpes or 500 mg po bid for chronic suppressive rx.	**Acyclovir-resistant HSV: IV Foscarnet** 90 mg/kg IV q12h x 7 days. Suppressive therapy with famciclovir (500 mg po bid), valacyclovir (500 mg po bid) or acyclovir (400-800 mg po bid) reduces viral shedding and clinical recurrences.
Pregnancy and genital H. simplex	Acyclovir safe even in first trimester. No proof that acyclovir at delivery reduces risk/severity of neonatal Herpes. In contrast, C-section in women with active lesions reduces risk of transmission. Ref. *Obstet Gyn* 106:845, 2006.	
Herpes simiae (Herpes B virus): **Monkey bite** *CID* 35:1191, 2002	**Postexposure prophylaxis:** Valacyclovir 1 gm po q8h times 14 days or acyclovir 800 mg po 5 times per day times 14 days. **Treatment of disease:** (1) CNS symptoms absent: Acyclovir 12.5–15 mg per kg IV q8h or ganciclovir 5 mg per kg IV q12h. (2) CNS symptoms present: Ganciclovir 5 mg per kg IV q12h	Fatal human cases of myelitis and hemorrhagic encephalitis have been reported following bites, scratches, or eye inoculation of saliva from monkeys. Initial sx include fever, headache, myalgias and diffuse adenopathy, incubation period of 2–14 days (*EID* 9:246, 2003). In vitro ACV and ganciclovir less active than other nucleosides (penciclovir or 5-ethyldeoxyuridine may be more active; clinical data needed) (*AAC* 51:2028, 2007).

[2] FDA approved only for HIV pts
[3] Approved for immunocompromised pts
* See page 2 for abbreviations. NOTE: All dosage recommendations are for adults (unless otherwise indicated) and assume normal renal function.

TABLE 14A (7)

Herpesvirus Infections (continued)

Varicella-Zoster Virus (VZV)

Varicella: Vaccination has markedly ↓ incidence of varicella & morbidity (NEJM 352:450, 2005; NEJM 356:1338, 2007). Guidelines for VZV vaccine (MMWR 56(RR-4) 2007).

VIRUS/DISEASE	DRUG/DOSAGE	SIDE EFFECTS/COMMENTS
Normal host (chickenpox) Child (2-12 years)	**In general, treatment not recommended.** Might use oral **acyclovir** for healthy persons at ↑ risk for moderate to severe varicella, i.e., >12 yrs of age, chronic cutaneous or pulmonary diseases, chronic salicylate rx (↑ risk of Reye syndrome), **acyclovir dose:** 20 mg/kg po qid x 5 days (start within 24 hrs of rash).	Acyclovir slowed development and ↓ number of new lesions and ↓ duration of disease in children: 9 to 7.6 days (PIDJ 21:739, 2002). Oral dose of acyclovir in children should not exceed 80 mg per kg per day or 3200 mg per day.
Adolescents, young adults	**Acyclovir** 800 mg po 5x/day x 5–7 days (start within 24 hrs of rash) or **valacyclovir**[NFDA] 1000 mg po 3x/day x 5 days. **Famciclovir**[NAI] 500 mg po 3x/day probably effective but data lacking.	↓ duration of fever, time to healing, and symptoms (AnIM 130:922, 1999).
Pneumonia or chickenpox in 3rd trimester of pregnancy	**Acyclovir** 800 mg po 5 times per day or 10 mg per kg IV q8h times 5 days. Risks and benefits to fetus and mother still unknown. Many experts recommend rx, especially in 3rd trimester. Some would add VZIG (varicella-zoster immune globulin).	Varicella pneumonia associated with 41% mortality in pregnancy. Acyclovir ↓ incidence and severity (AJD 185:422, 2002). If varicella-susceptible mother exposed and respiratory symptoms develop within 10 days after exposure, start acyclovir.
Immunocompromised host	**Acyclovir** 10–12 mg per kg (500 mg per M²) IV (infused over 1 hr) q8h times 7 days	Disseminated 1° varicella infection reported during infliximab rx of rheumatoid arthritis (J Rheum 31:2517, 2004). Continuous infusion of high-dose acyclovir (2 mg per kg per hr) successful in 1 pt with severe hemorrhagic varicella (NEJM 336:732, 1997). Mortality high (43%) in AIDS pts (Int J Inf Dis 6:6, 2002).
Prevention—Postexposure prophylaxis Varicella deaths still occur in unvaccinated persons (MMWR 56 (RR-4) 1-40, 2007)	**CDC Recommendations for Prevention:** Since <5% of cases of varicella but >50% of varicella-related deaths occur in adults >20 yrs of age, the CDC recommends a more aggressive approach in this age group: **1st, varicella-zoster immune globulin** (VZIG) (125 units/10 kg (22 lbs) body weight IM up to a max. of 625 units; minimum dose is 125 units) is recommended for postexposure prophylaxis in susceptible persons at greater risk for complications (immunocompromised, pregnancy, preterm and newborn infants) as soon as possible after exposure (<96 hrs). If varicella develops, initiate treatment quickly (<24 hr of rash) with **acyclovir** as below. Some would rx. presumptively with acyclovir in high-risk pts. **2nd,** susceptible adults should be vaccinated. Check antibody in adults with negative or uncertain history of varicella (10–30% will be Ab-neg.) and vaccinate those who are Ab-neg. **3rd,** susceptible children should receive vaccination. Recommended routinely before age 12–18 mos. but OK at any age.	

* See page 2 for abbreviations. NOTE: All dosage recommendations are for adults (unless otherwise indicated) and assume normal renal function.

TABLE 14A (8)

VIRUS/DISEASE	DRUG/DOSAGE	SIDE EFFECTS/COMMENTS
Herpesvirus Infections/Varicella-Zoster Virus (VZV) *(continued)*		
Herpes zoster (shingles) *(See NEJM 342:635, 2000 & 347:340, 2002)*		
Normal host Effective therapy most evident in pts >50 yrs. (For treatment of post-herpetic neuralgia, see CID 36: 877, 2003) 25-fold ↓ in zoster after immunization (MMWR 48:R-6, 1999) New vaccine ↓ herpes zoster & post-herpetic neuralgia (NEJM 352: 2271, 2005; JAMA 292:157, 2006). Reviewed in J Am Acad Derm 58:361, 2008	**[NOTE: Trials showing benefit of therapy: only in pts treated within 3 days of onset of rash]** **Valacyclovir** 1000 mg po tid times 7 days (adjust dose for renal failure) (See Table 17) **OR** **Famciclovir** 500 mg tid x 7 days. Adjust for renal failure (see Table 17) **OR** **Acyclovir** 800 mg po 5 times per day times 7–10 days Add **Prednisone** in pts over 50 yrs old to decrease discomfort during acute phase of zoster. Does not decrease incidence of post-herpetic neuralgia. Dose: 30 mg po bid days 1–7, 15 mg bid days 8–14 and 7.5 mg bid days 15–21.	Valacyclovir ↓ post-herpetic neuralgia more rapidly than acyclovir in pts >50 yrs of age; median duration of zoster-associated pain was 38 days with valacyclovir and 51 days on acyclovir (Arch Fam Med 9:863, 2000). Toxicity of both drugs similar (AAC 39:1546, 1995). Time to healing more rapid. Reduced post-herpetic neuralgia (PHN) vs placebo in pts >50 yrs of age; duration of PHN with famciclovir 63 days, placebo 163 days. Famciclovir similar to acyclovir in reduction of acute pain and PHN (J Micro Immun 37:75, 2004). A meta-analysis of 4 placebo-controlled trials (691 pts) demonstrated that acyclovir accelerated by approx. 2-fold pain resolution by all measures employed and reduced post-herpetic neuralgia at 3 & 6 mos (CID 22:341, 1996); med. time to resolution of pain 41 days vs 101 days in those >50 yrs. Prednisone added to acyclovir reduced quality of life measurements (↓ acute pain, sleep, and return to normal activity) (AnIM 125:376, 1996). In post-herpetic neuralgia, controlled trials demonstrated effectiveness of gabapentin, the lidocaine patch (5%) & opioid analgesic in controlling pain (Drugs 64:937, 2004; J Clin Virol 29:248, 2004). Nortriptyline & amitriptyline are equally effective but nortriptyline is better tolerated (CID 36:877, 2003). Role of antiviral drugs in rx of PHN unproven (Neurol 64:21, 2005) but 8 of 15 pt improved with IV acyclovir 10 mg per kg q 8 hrs x 14 days followed by oral valacyclovir 1 gm 3x a day for 1 month (Arch Neur 63:940, 2006).
Immunocompromised host Not severe	**Acyclovir** 800 mg po 5 times per day times 7 days. (Options: **Famciclovir** 750 mg po q24h or 500 mg bid or 250 mg 3 times per day times 7 days **OR valacyclovir** 1000 mg po tid times 7 days, though both are not FDA-approved for this indication)	If progression, switch to IV. RA pts on TNF-alpha inhibitors at high risk for VZV. Zoster more severe, but less post-herpetic neuralgia (JAMA 301:737, 2009).
Severe: ≥1 dermatome, trigeminal nerve or disseminated	**Acyclovir** 10–12 mg per kg (1 hr infusion over 1 hr) q8h times 7–14 days. In older children, ↓ to 7.5 mg per kg. ↓ if nephrotoxicity and pt improving, ↓ to 5 mg per kg q8h.	A common manifestation of immune reconstitution following HAART in HIV-infected children (J Ad Clin Immun 113:742, 2004). Rx must be begun within 72 hrs. Acyclovir-resistant VZV occurs in HIV+ pts previously treated with acyclovir. **Foscarnet** (40 mg per kg IV q8h for 14–26 days) successful in 4/5 pts but 2 relapsed in 7 and 14 days (AnIM 115:19, 1991).

* See page 2 for abbreviations. NOTE: All dosage recommendations are for adults (unless otherwise indicated) and assume normal renal function.

TABLE 14A (9)

Influenza (A & B)

- Refs: http://www.cdc.gov/flu/weekly; http://www.cdc.gov/flu/professionals/antivirals/recommendations.htm
- Guidelines: ACIP (MMWR 60 (RR-1): Jan 21, 2011); IDSA (CID 48:1003-1032, 2009).
- **Novel A H1N1 Swine Flu emerged in Spring 2009** (Science 325:197, 2009). **Rapid Test for Influenza may be falsely negative in over 50% of cases of Swine Flu. During epidemic, treatment should be started based on symptoms alone.** Antiviral therapy cost-effective without viral testing in febrile pt with typical symptoms (CID 49:1090, 2009).
- Vaccine info (http://www.cdc.gov/h1n1flu/recommendations/htm).
- **Oseltamivir: Caution: potential for confusion in dosing oral suspension** (NEJM 361:1912, 2009).
- **Pathogenic avian influenza (H5N1)** emerged in poultry (mainly chickens & ducks) in East & Southeast Asia. As of August 30, 2006, 246 laboratory confirmed cases reported in 10 countries with 144 deaths (see www.cdc.gov/flu/avian/). Human-to-human transmission reported; most have had direct contact with poultry. Mortality highest in young age 10-19 (73%) vs. 56% overall and associated with high viral load and cytokine storm (Nature Medicine 12:1203, 2006). **Human isolates resistant to amantadine/rimantadine.** Oseltamivir therapy recommended if avian H5N1 suspected. ↑ dose & duration of oseltamivir necessary for maximum effect in mouse model (JID 192:665, 2005; Nature 435:419 2005).

Virus/Disease	Susceptible to (Recommended Drug/Dosage):	Resistant to:	Side Effects/Comments
Novel A/H1N1 (Swine)	**Oseltamivir** 75 mg po bid times 5 days (also approved for rx of children age 1–12 yrs, dose 2 mg per kg up to a total of 75 mg bid times 5 days)* **or** **Zanamivir** 2 inhalations (5 mg each) bid for 5 days. *In morbidly obese patient, increase dose of oseltamivir to 150 mg po bid. For patients who are severely ill with influenza, consideration may be given to use of oseltamivir at higher doses (150 mg bid) and for extended courses (eg, ≥10 days) (MMWR 58:749, 2009). Safety at high doses not established in pregnancy (http://www.who.int/csr/resources/publications/swineflu/clinical_management_h1n1.pdf).	Amantadine and rimantadine (100%)	**Caution:** do not reconstitute zanamivir powder for use in nebulizers or mechanical ventilators (MedWatch report of death). **For severe, life-threatening disease consider compassionate use IV Peramivir** (Biocryst/Shionogi: investigational) 600 mg IV daily for a minimum of 5 days. For access to compassionate use call 205-989-3262 or website: http://www.biocryst.com/ve_ind. Peramivir is an investigational IV neuraminidase inhibitor with activity against influenza A and B, including H1N1 Swine. In phase III studies a single IV dose (300 or 600 mg) was non-inferior to oseltamivir (75 mg bid x 5 days), time to symptom resolution was 78, 81 and 81.8 hrs, compared to oseltamivir at 81.8 hrs. In a second non-comparative study of pts at high risk for complications of influenza, using daily IV peramivir, the median time to alleviation of symptoms in all 37 pts was 68.6 hrs. In a placebo controlled study, peramivir was significantly better than placebo for both clinical symptoms (fever) and virologic shedding (Antimicrob Agents Chemother 54:4568, 2010).
A/H1N1 (Seasonal) The 2011–12 U.S. seasonal influenza vaccine virus strains are identical to those contained in the 2010–11 vaccine. These include A/California/7/2009 (H1N1)-like, A/Perth/16/2009 (H3N2)-like, and B/Brisbane/60/2008-like antigens. The influenza A (H1N1) vaccine virus strain is derived from a 2009 pandemic influenza A (H1N1) virus	**Oseltamivir** 75 mg po bid times 5 days (also approved for rx of children age 1–12 yrs, dose 2 mg per kg up to a total of 75 mg bid times 5 days) **or** **Zanamivir** 2 inhalations (5 mg each) bid for 5 days.	Amantadine/ rimantadine (>95% resistant)	**Peramivir IV** alternative agent for serious infection. (see above) Pts with COPD or asthma, **potential risk of bronchospasm with zanamivir.** All ↓ duration of symptoms if given within 30–36 hrs after onset of symptoms. Benefit influenced by duration of symptoms before rx: initiation of oseltamivir within 1st 12 hrs after fever onset ↓ total median illness duration by 74.6 hrs (JAC 51:123, 2003). ↓ risk of pneumonia (Curr Med Res Opin 21:761, 2005).

*See page 2 for abbreviations; NOTE: All dosage recommendations are for adults (unless otherwise indicated) and assume normal renal function.

TABLE 14A (10)

Virus/Disease	Susceptible to (Recommended Drug/Dosage):	Resistant to:	Side Effects/Comments
Influenza (A & B) (continued)			
A/H3N2	Oseltamivir or Zanamivir (as above)	Amantadine/ rimantadine (100% resistant)	**Peramivir** alternative agent for serious infection (as above).
A/H3N2v (swine variant)	Oseltamivir or Zanamivir (as above)		**Peramivir** alternative agent for serious infection (as above). New A/H3N2v variant reported in late 2011 (MMWR 60: 1-4, 2011). Transmission from pigs to humans. Most cases in children < 10 yrs old. Responds to neuraminidase inhibitors.
B	Oseltamivir or Zanamivir (as above)	No data	**Peramivir** alternative agent for serious infection (as above).
H5N1 (Avian)	Oseltamivir or Zanamivir (as above)	Amantadine/ rimantadine	Report of increasing resistance in up to 18% of children with H5N1 treated with oseltamivir and less responsive H5N1 virus in several patients. Less resistance to zanamivir so far.
Prevention: Influenza A & B	Give vaccine and if ≥13 yrs age, consider **oseltamivir** 75 mg po q24h or **zanamivir** 2 inhalations (5 mg each) once daily for 5 days for the two weeks following vaccination or for the duration of peak influenza in community or for outbreak control in high-risk populations if vaccination cannot be administered (CID 2009; 48:1003–1032). Avoid Oseltamivir if seasonal H1N1 infection predominates with Oseltamivir resistant strain. (Consider for similar populations as immunization recommendations.)		Immunization contraindicated if hypersensitive to chicken eggs.

VIRUS/DISEASE	DRUG/DOSAGE	SIDE EFFECTS/COMMENTS
Measles While measles is at the lowest rates ever (55/100,000) much higher rates reported in developing countries (CID 42:322, 2006). Imported measles in US on the rise (MMWR 57: 169, 2008). High attack rates in the unvaccinated (CID 47:1143, 2008). Concern about lack of vaccine effectiveness in developing countries (Lancet 373:1543, 2009).		
Children	No therapy, or **vitamin A** 200,000 units po daily times 2 days	Vitamin A may ↓ severity of measles.
Adults	No rx or **ribavirin** IV 20-35 mg per kg per day times 7 days	↓ severity of illness in adults (CID 20:454, 1994).
Metapneumovirus (hMPV) A paramyxovirus isolated from pts of all ages, with mild bronchiolitis/bronchospasm to pneumonia. Can cause lethal pneumonia in HSCT pts (Ann Intern Med 144:344, 2006)	**No proven antiviral therapy** (intravenous ribavirin used anecdotally with variable results)	Human metapneumovirus isolated from 6-21% of children with RTIs (NEJM 350:443, 2004). Dual infection with RSV assoc. with severe bronchiolitis (JID 191:382, 2005). Nucleic acid test now approved to detect 12 respiratory viruses (xTAG Respiratory Viral Panel, Luminex Molecular Diagnostics).
Monkey pox (orthopox virus) (see LnID 4:17, 2004) Outbreak from contact with ill prairie dogs. Source likely imported Gambian giant rats (MMWR 42:642, 2003).	**No proven antiviral therapy.** Cidofovir is active in vitro & in mouse model (AAC 66:1329, 2002; Antiviral Res 57:13, 2003) (Potential new drugs Virol J 4:8, 2007)	Incubation period of 12 days, then fever, headache, cough, adenopathy, & a vesicular papular rash that pustulates, umbilicates, & crusts on the head, trunk, & extremities. Transmission in healthcare setting rare (CID 40:789, 2005; CID 41:1742, 2005; CID 41:1765, 2005)
Norovirus (Norwalk-like virus, or NLV) Vast majority of outbreaks of non-bacterial gastroenteritis.	**No antiviral therapy.** Replete volume. Transmission by contaminated food, fecal-oral contact with contaminated surfaces, or fomites.	Sudden onset of nausea, vomiting, and/or watery diarrhea lasting 12-60 hours. Ethanol-based hand rubs effective (J Hosp Infect 60:144, 2005).

* See page 2 for abbreviations. NOTE: All dosage recommendations are for adults (unless otherwise indicated) and assume normal renal function.

TABLE 14A (11)

VIRUS/DISEASE	DRUG/DOSAGE	SIDE EFFECTS/COMMENTS
Papillomaviruses: Warts **External Genital Warts**	**Patient applied:** **Podofilox** (0.5% solution or gel): apply 2x/day x 3 days, 4th day no therapy, repeat cycle 4x; OR **Imiquimod** 5% cream: apply once daily hs 3x/wk for up to 16 wks. **Provider administered:** Cryotherapy with liquid nitrogen; repeat q1-2 wks; OR **Podophyllin resin** 10-25% in tincture of benzoin. Repeat weekly as needed; OR **Trichloroacetic acid (TCA)**: repeat weekly as needed; OR surgical removal.	**Podofilox:** Inexpensive and safe (pregnancy safety not established). Mild irritation after treatment. **Imiquimod:** Mild to moderate redness & irritation. Topical imiquimod effective for treatment of vulvar intraepithelial neoplasms (NEJM 358:1465, 2008). Safety in pregnancy not established. **Cryotherapy:** Blistering and skin necrosis common. **Podophyllin resin:** Must air dry before treated area contacts clothing. Can irritate adjacent skin. **TCA:** Caustic. Can cause severe pain on adjacent normal skin. Neutralize with soap or sodium bicarbonate.
Warts on cervix	Need evaluation for evolving neoplasia	Gynecological consult advised.
Vaginal warts	Cryotherapy with liquid nitrogen or **TCA**	
Urethral warts	Cryotherapy with liquid nitrogen or **Podophyllin resin** 10-25% in tincture of benzoin	
Anal warts	Cryotherapy with liquid nitrogen or **TCA** or surgical removal	Advise anoscopy to look for rectal warts.
Skin papillomas	Topical α-lactalbumin. **Oleic acid** (from human milk) applied 1x/day for 3 wks	lesion size & recurrence vs placebo (p <0.001) (NEJM 350:2663, 2004). Further studies warranted.
Parvo B19 Virus (Erythrovirus B19). Review: NEJM 350:586, 2004. Wide range of manifestation. **Treatment options for common symptomatic infections.** Erythema infectiosum Arthritis/arthralgia Transient aplastic crisis Fetal hydrops Chronic infection with anemia Chronic infection without anemia	Symptomatic treatment only Nonsteroidal anti-inflammatory drugs (NSAID) Transfusions and oxygen Intrauterine blood transfusion **IVIG** and transfusion Perhaps **IVIG**	Diagnostic tools: IgM and IgG antibody titers. Perhaps better: blood parvovirus PCR. Dose of IVIG not standardized: suggest 400 mg/kg IV of commercial IVIG for 5 or 10 days or 1000 mg/kg IV for 3 days. Most dramatic anemias in pts with pre-existing hemolytic anemia. Bone marrow shown erythrocyte maturation arrest with giant pronormoblasts.
Papovavirus/Polyomavirus **Progressive multifocal leukoencephalopathy (PML)** Serious demyelinating disease due to JC virus in immunocompromised pts.	No specific therapy for JC virus. Two general approaches: 1. In HIV pts: HAART. Cidofovir may be effective. 2. Stop or decrease immunosuppressive therapy.	Failure of treatment with interferon alfa-2b, cytarabine and topotecan. Immunosuppressive natalizumab temporarily removed from market due to reported associations with PML. Mixed reports on cidofovir. Most likely effective in pts with HAART experience.
BK Virus induced nephropathy in immunocompromised pts and hemorrhagic cystitis	Decrease immunosuppression if possible. Suggested antiviral therapy based on anecdotal data. If progressive renal dysfunction: 1. **Fluoroquinolone** first. 2. **IVIG** 0.5 gm/kg IV 3. **Leflunomide** 100 mg po daily x 3 days, then 10-20 mg po daily; 4. **Cidofovir** only if refractory to all of the above (see Table 14B for dose).	Use PCR to monitor viral "load" in urine and/or plasma. Report of cidofovir as potentially effective for BK hemorrhagic cystitis (CID 49:233, 2009).

* See page 2 for abbreviations. NOTE: All dosage recommendations are for adults (unless otherwise indicated) and assume normal renal function.

TABLE 14A (12)

VIRUS/DISEASE	DRUG/DOSAGE	SIDE EFFECTS/COMMENTS
Rabies (see Table 20B, page 215; see MMWR 54: RR-3:1, 2005, CDC Guidelines for Prevention and Control 2006, MMWR/55/RR-5, 2006) Rabid dogs account for 50,000 cases per yr worldwide. Most cases in the U.S. are cryptic, i.e., no documented evidence of bite or contact with a rabid animal (CID 35:738, 2003). 70% assoc. with 2 rare bat species (EID 9:151, 2003). An organ donor with early rabies infected 4 recipients (2 kidneys, liver & artery) who all died of rabies avg. 13 days after transplant (NEJM 352:1103, 2005).	**Mortality 100% with survivors those who receive rabies vaccine before the onset of illness/symptoms** (CID 36:61, 2003). A 15-year-old female who developed rabies 1 month post-bat bite survived after drug induction of coma (+ other rx) for 7 days; did not receive immunoprophylaxis (NEJM 352:2508, 2005).	Corticosteroids ↑ mortality rate and ↓ incubation time in mice. Therapies that have failed after symptoms develop include rabies vaccine, rabies immuno-globulin, rabies virus neutralizing antibody, ribavirin, alfa interferon, & ketamine.
Respiratory Syncytial Virus (RSV) Major cause of morbidity in neonates/infants. Nucleic acid test now approved to detect 12 respiratory viruses (xTAG Respiratory Viral Panel, Luminex Molecular Diagnostics). Ref: CID 56:258, 2013 (immunocompromised host)	Hydration, supplemental oxygen. Routine use of ribavirin not recommended. Ribavirin therapy, associated with small increases in O₂ saturation. No consistent decrease in need for mech. ventilation or ICU stays. High cost, aerosol administration & potential toxicity (Red Book of Pediatrics, 2006). RNA interference with ALN-RSV01 impedes the expression of nucleocapsid protein of RSV. Study of 85 healthy volunteers showed a significant reduction in RSV infection vs. placebo (Proc Nat Acad Sci U.S.A 107:8800, 2010).	In adults, RSV accounted for 10.6% of hospitalizations for pneumonia, 11.4% for COPD, 7.2% for asthma & 5.4% for CHF in pts >65 yrs of age (NEJM 352:1749, 2005). RSV caused 11% of clinically important respiratory illnesses in military recruits (CID 41:311, 2005). Palivizumab (Synagis) 15 mg/kg IM once per month November-April. Timing of coverage may need to be adjusted in some regions based on reported cases in the region, as opposed to using fixed dosing schedules (Pediatrics 126:e116, 2010).
Prevention of RSV in: (1) Children <24 mos. old with chronic lung disease (i.e., prematurity and/or bronchopulmonary dysplasia) requiring supplemental O₂ or (2) Premature infants (<32 wks gestation) and <6 mos. old at start of RSV season or (3) Children with selected congenital heart	Palivizumab (Synagis) 15 mg per kg IM q month Nov-April. Ref: Red Book of Pediatrics, 2006.	Expense argues against its use, but in 2004 approx. 100,000 infants received (Ped Ann 34:1177, 2005) [sic] reviewed (PIDJ 23:1051, 2004). Significant reduction in RSV hospitalization in children with congenital heart disease (Expert Opin Biol Ther. 7:1471-80, 2007)
Rhinovirus Colds See LN 361:51, 2003 Found in 1/2 of children with community-acquired pneumonia; role in pathogenesis unclear (CID 39:681, 2004) High rate of rhinovirus identified in children with significant lower resp tract infections (Ped Inf Dis 28:337, 2009)	No antiviral rx indicated (Ped Ann 34:53, 2005). Symptomatic rx: • Ipratropium bromide nasal (2 sprays per nostril tid) • Clemastine 1.34 mg 1-2 tab po bid-tid (OTC) Avoid zinc products (see Comment).	Sx relief: ipratropium nasal spray, ↓ rhinorrhea and sneezing vs placebo (AnIM 125:89, 1996). Clemastine (an antihistamine) ↓ sneezing, rhinorrhea but associated with dry nose, mouth & throat in 6-19% (CID 22:656, 1996). Oral pleconaril given within 1.34 mg of onset reduced duration (1 day) & severity of "cold symptoms" in DBPCT (p <.001) (CID 36:1523, 2003) – put to rest! Public health advisory working that three over-the-counter cold remedy products containing zinc (e.g., Zicam) should not be used because of multiple reports of permanent anosmia (www.fda.gov/Safety/MedWatch/SafetyInformation/SafetyAlertsforHumanMedicalProducts/ucm166696.htm).
Rotavirus: Leading recognized cause of diarrhea-related illness among infants and children world-wide and kills ½ million children annually.	No antiviral rx available: oral hydration life-saving. In one study, Nitazoxanide **7.5 mg/kg 2x/d x 3 days** reduced duration of illness from 75 to 31 hrs in Egyptian children, impact on rotavirus or other parameters not measured. (Lancet 368:100 & 124, 2006). Too early to recommend routine use (Lancet 368:100, 2006).	Two live-attenuated vaccines highly effective (85 and 98%) and safe in preventing rotavirus diarrhea and hospitalization (NEJM 354:1 & 23, 2006). ACIP recommends either of the two vaccines, RV1 or RV5, for infants (MMWR 58(RR02):1, 2009).
SARS-CoV: See page 156		
Smallpox (NEJM 346:1300, 2002)	Smallpox vaccine (if within 4 days of exposure) + cidofovir (dosage uncertain but likely similar to CMV (5 mg/kg IV once weekly for 2 weeks followed by once weekly dosing. Must be used with hydration and Probenecid; contact CDC: 770-488-7100)	
Contact vaccinia (JAMA 288:1901, 2002)	From vaccination: Progressive vaccinia—Vaccinia immune globulin may be of benefit. To obtain immune globulin, contact CDC: 770-488-7100. (CID 37:259, 776 & 819, 2004)	
West Nile virus: See page 157		

* See page 2 for abbreviations. NOTE: All dosage recommendations are for adults (unless otherwise indicated) and assume normal renal function.

TABLE 14B – ANTIVIRAL DRUGS (NON-HIV)

DRUG NAME(S) GENERIC (TRADE)	DOSAGE/ROUTE IN ADULTS*	COMMENTS/ADVERSE EFFECTS
CMV (See SANFORD GUIDE TO HIV/AIDS THERAPY)		
Cidofovir (Vistide)	5 mg/kg IV once weekly for 2 weeks, then once every other week. **Probenecid and IV prehydration with normal saline & Probenecid must be used with each cidofovir infusion:** 2 gm po 3 hrs before each dose and further 1 gm doses 2 & 8 hrs after completion of the cidofovir infusion. Renal function (serum creatinine and urine protein) must be monitored prior to each dose (see pkg insert for details). Contraindicated if creatinine > 1.5 mg/dL, CrCl ≤55 mL/min or urine protein ≥ 100 mg/dL	**Adverse effects:** Nephrotoxicity; dose-dependent proximal tubular injury (Fanconi-like syndrome); proteinuria, glycosuria, bicarbonaturia, phosphaturia, aminoaciduria (nephrogenic diabetes insipidus, Ln 350:413, 1997), acidosis, ↑ creatinine. Concomitant saline prehydration (probenecid, extends 1/2 life serum levels allow use but still highly nephrotoxic. Other toxicities: nausea 69%, fever 58%, alopecia 27%, myalgia 16%, probenecid hypersensitivity 16%, neutropenia 29%, iritis and uveitis reported; also ↓ intraocular pressure. **Black Box warning:** Renal impairment can occur after ≤2 doses. Contraindicated in pts receiving concomitant nephrotoxic agents. Monitor for ↓ WBC. In animals, carcinogenic, teratogenic, causes ↓ sperm and ↓ fertility. FDA indication only for CMV retinitis in HIV pts. **Comment:** Normal maintenance dose. If renal function changes during or after infusion, dose must be reduced or discontinued if changes in renal function occur during rx. For ↑ of 0.3–0.4 mg per dL in serum creatinine, cidofovir dose must be ↓ from 5 to 3 mg per kg; discontinue cidofovir if ↑ of 0.5 mg per dL above baseline or 3+ proteinuria develops (for 2+ proteinuria, observe pts carefully and consider discontinuation).
Foscarnet (Foscavir)	**Induction:** 90 mg per kg IV, over 1.5–2 hours, q12h **OR** 60 mg per kg, over 1 hour, q8h **Maintenance:** 90–120 mg per kg IV, over 2 hours, q24h Dosage adjustment with renal dysfunction (see Table 17).	Use infusion pump to control rate of administration. **Adverse effects: Major toxicity is renal impairment (1/3 of patients)** – ↑ creatinine, proteinuria, nephrogenic diabetes insipidus, ↓K+, ↓Ca++, ↓ Mg ++. Toxicity ↑ with other nephrotoxic drugs [ampho B, aminoglycosides or pentamidine (especially severe ↓ Ca++)]. Adequate hydration may ↓ toxicity. Other: headache, mild (10%), fatigue (10%), nausea (60%), fever (25%). CNS: seizures. Hematol: ↓ WBC, ↓ Hgb. Hepatic: liver function tests ↑. Neuropathy. Penile and oral ulcers.
Ganciclovir (Cytovene)	IV: 5 mg per kg q12h times 14 days (induction) 5 mg per kg IV q24h or 6 mg per kg 5 times per wk (maintenance) Dosage adjust. with renal dysfunction (see Table 17)	**Adverse effects: Black Box warnings:** cytopenias, carcinogenicity/teratogenicity & aspermia in animals. Absolute neutrophil count dropped below 500 per mm³ in 15%, thrombocytopenia 21%, anemia 6%. Fever 48%. GI 50%: nausea, vomiting, diarrhea, abdominal pain 19%, rash 10%. Retinal detachment 11% (likely due to underlying disease). Confusion, headache, psychiatric disturbances and seizures. Neutropenia may respond to granulocyte colony stimulating factor (G-CSF or GM-CSF). Severe myelosuppression may be ↑ with coadministration of zidovudine or azathioprine. 32% dc/interrupted rx, principally for neutropenia. Anemia/leukopenia.
Ganciclovir (Vitrasert)	Oral: 1.0 gm tid with food (fatty meal) (250 mg & 500 mg cap) Intraocular implant, 4.5 μg	Hematologic toxicity equal to that with IV. Granulocytopenia 18%, anemia 12%, thrombocytopenia 6%, skin same as with IV. Retinal detachment 7/30. **Adverse effects:** Late retinal detachment (7/30 eyes). Does not prevent CMV retinitis in good eye or visceral dissemination. **Comment:** Replacement every 6 months recommended.
Valganciclovir (Valcyte)	900 mg po bid (two 450 mg tabs) po bid times 21 days for induction, followed by 900 mg po q24h. Take with food. Dosage adjustment for renal dysfunction (See Table 17A).	A prodrug of ganciclovir with better bioavailability than oral ganciclovir: 60% with food. **Adverse effects:** Similar to ganciclovir.
Herpesvirus (non-CMV)		
Acyclovir (Zovirax or generic)	Doses: see Table 14A for various indications 400 mg or 800 mg tab 200 mg cap Suspension 200 mg per 5 mL Ointment or cream 5% IV injection Dosage adjustment for renal dysfunction (See Table 17A).	**po:** Generally well-tolerated with occ. diarrhea, vertigo, arthralgia. Less frequent rash, fatigue, insomnia, fever, menstrual abnormalities, acne, sore throat, nausea, lymphadenopathy. **IV:** Phlebitis, caustic with vesicular lesions with IV infiltration, CNS (1%): lethargy, tremors, confusion, hallucinations, seizures, coma; all reversible. Renal (5%): ↑ creatinine, hematuria. With high doses may crystallize in renal tubules → obstructive uropathy (rapid infusion, dehydration, renal insufficiency risk). Adequate pre-hydration may prevent such nephrotoxicity. Hepatic: ↑ ALT, AST. Uncommon: neutropenia, rash, diaphoresis, hypotension, headache, nausea.

*See page 2 for abbreviations. NOTE: All dosage recommendations are for adults (unless otherwise indicated) and assume normal renal function.

TABLE 14B (2)

DRUG NAME(S) GENERIC (TRADE)	DOSAGE/ROUTE IN ADULTS*	COMMENTS/ADVERSE EFFECTS
Herpesvirus (non-CMV) *(continued)*		
Famciclovir (Famvir)	125 mg, 250 mg, 500 mg tabs. Dosage depends on indication. *(see label and Table 14A).*	Metabolized to penciclovir. **Adverse effects:** similar to acyclovir, included headache, nausea, diarrhea, and dizziness but incidence does not differ from placebo. May be taken with or without regard to meals. Dose should be reduced if CrCl <60 mL per min (see package insert & Table 14A, page 160 & Table 17, page 211). May be taken with or without food.
Penciclovir (Denavir)	Topical 1% cream	Apply to area of recurrence of herpes labialis with start of sx, then q2h while awake times 4 days. Well tolerated.
Trifluridine (Viroptic)	Topical 1% solution: 1 drop q2h (max. 9 drops/day) until corneal re-epithelialization, then dose is ↓ for 7 more days (one drop q4h for at least 5 drops/day), not to exceed 21 days total rx.	Mild burning (5%), palpebral edema (3%), punctate keratopathy, stromal edema. For HSV keratoconjunctivitis or recurrent epithelial keratitis.
Valacyclovir (Valtrex)	500 mg, 1 gm tabs. Dosage depends on indication and renal function *(see label, Table 14A & Table 17A)*	An ester pro-drug of acyclovir that is well-absorbed, bioavailability 3-5 times greater than acyclovir. **Adverse effects** similar to acyclovir (see *JID 186:540, 2002*). Thrombotic thrombocytopenic purpura/hemolytic uremic syndrome reported in pts with advanced HIV disease and transplant recipients participating in clinical trials at doses of 8 gm per day.
Hepatitis		
Adefovir dipivoxil (Hepsera)	10 mg po q24h (with normal CrCl); see Table 17A if renal impairment. 10 mg tab	Adefovir dipivoxil is a prodrug of adefovir. It is an acyclic nucleotide analog with activity against hepatitis B (HBV) at 0.2-2.5 mM (IC₅₀). See Table 9 for Cmax & T½. Active against YMDD mutant lamivudine-resistant strains and in vitro vs. entecavir-resistant strains. To minimize resistance, package insert recommends using in combination with lamivudine for lamivudine-resistant virus; consider alternative therapy if viral load remains > 1,000 copies/mL with treatment. Primarily renal excretion—adjust dose. No food interactions. Generally few side effects, but **Black Box warning** regarding lactic acidosis/hepatic steatosis with nucleoside analogs and severe exacerbation of hepB on discontinuing therapy, monitor closely with frequent lab follow-up. At 10 mg per day, potential for renal toxicity and nephrotoxicity, esp. in pts with pre-existing or other risk for renal impairment. Pregnancy Category C. Hepatitis may exacerbate when treatment discontinued. Up to 25% of pts developed ALT ≥ 10 times normal within 12 wks; usually responds to re-treatment or self-limited, but hepatic decompensation has occurred.
Boceprevir (Victrelis)	For HCV genotype 1 800 mg po TID (with food) in combination with pegIFN + RBV*	*Initiate boceprevir 4 weeks after starting pegIFN + RBV. Use response guided therapy (see table 14A for details)* Most Common AEs: Fatigue, anemia, nausea, headache, and dysgeusia. Difficult to distinguish between AEs caused by pegIFN or RBV
Entecavir (Baraclude)	0.5 mg q24h. If refractory or resistant to lamivudine or telbivudine: 1 mg per day. Tabs: 0.5 mg & 1 mg. Oral solution: 0.05 mg/mL Administer on an empty stomach.	A nucleoside analog active against HBV including lamivudine-resistant mutants. Minimal adverse effects reported: headache, fatigue, dizziness, & nausea reported in 2-4% of pts. Allergic/anaphylactoid reactions reported. Potential for lactic acidosis and exacerbation of hepB at discontinuation (**Black Box warning**) as above. Do not use as single anti-retroviral agent in HIV co-infected pts; M184 mutation can emerge (*NEJM 356:2614, 2007*). Adjust dosage in renal impairment (see Table 17, page 211).

* See page 2 for abbreviations. NOTE: All dosage recommendations are for adults (unless otherwise indicated) and assume normal/renal function.

TABLE 14B (3)

DRUG NAME(S) GENERIC (TRADE)	DOSAGE/ROUTE IN ADULTS*	COMMENTS/ADVERSE EFFECTS
Hepatitis (continued)		
Interferon alfa is available as Roferon-A and Intron-A, alfa-2a (Roferon-A), alfa-2b (Intron-A)	For hepC, usual Roferon-A and Intron-A doses are 3 million international units 3x weekly subQ	Depending on agent, available in pre-filled syringes, vials of solution, or powder. **Black Box warnings:** include possibility of causing or aggravating serious neuropsychiatric disorders, ischemic events, infection. Withdraw therapy if any of these suspected. **Adverse effects:** Flu-like syndrome is common, esp. during 1st wk of rx: fever 98%, myalgia 73%, headache 71%, fatigue 89%, chills 54%, diarrhea 29%, N/V, dizziness 21%. Hemorrhagic or ischemic stroke. Rash 18%, may progress to Stevens Johnson Syndrome. Suicidal behavior, incl. completed suicide (N Engl J Med 354:6708, 2003) (depression, anxiety, emotional lability & agitation); consider prophylactic antidepressant in pts with h/o it. ↓ TSH, autoimmune thyroid disorders with ↓ or ↑ thyroidism. Hemato: ↓ WBC 49%, ↓ Hgb 27%, ↓ platelets 35%. Post-marketing reports of antibody-mediated pure red cell aplasia in patients receiving interferon/ribavirin with erythropoiesis-stimulating agents. Acute reversible hearing loss &/or tinnitus in up to 1/3 (Ln 343:1134, 1994). Optic neuropathy (retinal hemorrhage, cotton wool spots, ↓ in color vision) reported (AIDS 18:1805, 2004). Doses may require adjustment (or dc) based on individual response or adverse events, and can vary by product, indication (eg, HCV or HBV) and mode of use (mono- or combination-rx). (Refer to labels of individual products and to ribavirin if used in combination for details of use.)
PEG Interferon alfa-2b (PEG-Intron)	0.5–1.5 mcg/kg subQ q wk	
Pegylated-40k, interferon alfa-2a (Pegasys)	180 mcg subQ q wk	
Lamivudine (3TC) (Epivir-HBV)	Hepatitis B dose: 100 mg po q24h Dosage adjustment with renal dysfunction (see label).	**Black Box warnings:** caution, dose is lower than HIV doses so must exclude co-infection with HIV before using this formulation; lactic acidosis/hepatic steatosis; severe exacerbation of liver disease can occur on dc. YMDD-mutants resistant to lamivudine may emerge on treatment.
Ribavirin (Rebetol, Copegus)	Tabs 100 mg and oral solution 5 mg/mL. For use with an interferon for hepatitis C. Available as 200 mg caps and 40 and 40 mg tabs (Rebetol) or 200 mg and 400 mg tabs (Copegus) (See Comments regarding dosage)	**Adverse effects:** See Table 14D. **Black Box warnings:** ribavirin monotherapy of HCV is ineffective; hemolytic anemia may precipitate cardiac events; teratogenic/embryocidal (**Preg Category X**). Drug may persist for 6 mos., avoid pregnancy for at least 6 mos after end of rx of women or their partners. Only approved for pts with Ccr ≥ 50 mL/min. Also should not be used in pts with severe heart disease or some hemoglobinopathies. ARDS reported (Chest 124:406, 2003). **Adverse effects:** Hemolytic anemia (may require dose reduction or dc), dental/periodontal disorders, and all adverse effects of interferon (oral and dental problems include dry mouth, tooth and gum damage, bleeding, hypersensitivity reactions. See Table 14A for specific regimens, but dosing depends on interferon used, HCV genotype, and is modified (or dc) based on side effects (especially degree of hemolysis), with different criteria in those with/without cardiac disease). For example, initial Rebetol dose with Intron A (interferon alfa-2b) is wt-based: 400 mg am & 400 mg pm with meals. Doses and duration of Copegus with peg-interferon alfa-2a are less in pts with genotype 2 or 3 (800 mg per day divided into 2 doses, for 24 wks) than with genotypes 1 or 4 (HIV/HCV co-infected pts, dose is 800 mg per day regardless of genotype. (See individual labels for details, including initial dosing and criteria for dose modification in those with/without cardiac disease.)
Telaprevir (Incivek)	For HCV genotype 1 750 mg q8h (with food) in combination with INF+RBV	Must be used in combination with PegIFN/RBV. **Black Box Warning:** Rash (inc rare Stevens Johnson reaction, DRESS, and TEN, each of which may be fatal). D/c telaprevir after 12 weeks of Rx. Use response guided therapy (see table 14A for details). Most common AEs: Rash (inc rare Stevens Johnson reaction, DRESS, and TEN, each of which may be fatal), pruritis, nausea, anorexia, diarrhea, fatigue, anemia, insomnia, and dysgeusia. Difficult to dissect telaprevir AEs from IFN/ribavirin.
Telbivudine (Tyzeka)	600 mg orally q24h, without regard to food. Dosage adjustment with renal dysfunction. Ccr ≤ 50 mL/min (see label). 600 mg tabs; 100 mg per 5 mL solution.	An oral nucleoside analog approved for Rx of Hep B. It has ↑ rates of response and superior viral suppression than lamivudine (Ann Pharmacother 40:472, 2006; Medical Letter 49:11, 2007). **Black Box warnings** regarding lactic acidosis/hepatic steatosis with nucleosides and potential for severe exacerbation of HepB on dc. Generally well-tolerated wtih dc: 1 mitochondrial toxicity vs other nucleosides, and no dose limiting toxicity observed (Ann Pharmacother 40:472, 2006; Medical Letter 49:11, 2007). Myalgias, myopathy and rhabdomyolysis reported. Peripheral neuropathy. Genotypic resistance rate was 4.4% by one yr, 1 to 21.5% by 2 yrs of rx of e Ag+ pts. Selects for YMDD mutants. Less potent than lamivudine. Combination with lamivudine was inferior to monotherapy (Hepatology 45:507, 2007).

*See page 2 for abbreviations. NOTE: All dosage recommendations are for adults (unless otherwise indicated) and assume normal renal function.

TABLE 14B (4)

DRUG NAME(S) GENERIC (TRADE)	DOSAGE/ROUTE IN ADULTS*	COMMENTS/ADVERSE EFFECTS
Influenza A. Treatment and prophylaxis of influenza has become more complicated. Many circulating strains are resistant to adamantanes (amantadine & rimantadine), while others are resistant to the neuraminidase inhibitor, oseltamivir, but susceptible to adamantadine. Resistance to the neuraminidase inhibitor, zanamivir, is very rare, but there are limitations to the use of this inhalation agent. In this rapidly evolving area, close attention to guidance from public health authorities is warranted. In patients severely ill with influenza, combination therapy, higher than usual doses of oseltamivir and/or oseltamivir and/or longer than usual treatment courses may be considered in appropriate circumstances (MMWR 58: 749-752, 2009; NEJM 358:261-273, 2008).		
Amantadine (Symmetrel) or **Rimantadine** (Flumadine)	**Amantadine** 100 mg caps, tabs; 50 mg/mL oral solution & syrup. Treatment or prophylaxis: 100 mg bid; or 100 mg daily if age ≥65, dose reductions with CCr starting at ≤50 mL/min. **Rimantadine** 100 mg tabs, 50 mg/5 mL syrup. Treatment or prophylaxis: 100 mg bid, or 100 mg daily in elderly nursing home pts, or severe hepatic disease, or CCr ≤10 mL/min. For children, rimantadine only approved for prophylaxis.	**Side-effects/toxicity:** CNS (nervousness, anxiety, difficulty concentrating, and lightheadedness). Symptoms occurred in 6% on rimantadine vs 14% on amantadine. They usually 1st week and disappear when drug stopped. GI (nausea, anorexia). Some serious side-effects—delirium, hallucinations, and seizures—are associated with high plasma drug levels resulting from renal insufficiency, esp. in older pts, those with prior seizure disorders, or psychiatric disorders. Activity restricted to influenza A viruses.
Influenza A and B—For both drugs, initiate within 48 hrs of symptom onset		
Zanamivir (Relenza) For pts ≥ 7 yrs of age (treatment) or ≥ 5 yrs (prophylaxis)	Powder is inhaled by specially-designed inhalation device. Each blister contains 5 mg zanamivir. **Treatment:** oral inhalation of 2 blisters (10 mg) bid for 5 days. **Prophylaxis:** oral inhalation of 2 blisters (10 mg) once daily for 10 days (household outbreak) to 28 days (community outbreak).	Active by inhalation against neuraminidase of both influenza A and B and inhibits release of virus from epithelial cells of respiratory tract. Approx. 4–17% of inhaled dose absorbed into plasma. Excreted by kidney but with low absorption, dose reduction not necessary in renal impairment. Minimal side-effects: <3% cough, sinusitis, diarrhea, nausea and vomiting. **Reports of respiratory adverse events in pts with or without h/o airways disease, should be avoided in pts with underlying respiratory disease.** Allergic reactions and neuropsychiatric events have been reported. **Caution: do not reconstitute zanamivir powder for use in nebulizers or mechanical ventilators** (MedWatch report of death). Zanamivir for iv administration is available for compassionate use through an investigational IND application that can be accessed at: http://www.fda.gov/Drugs/DevelopmentApprovalProcess/HowDrugsareDevelopedandApproved/ApprovalApplications/InvestigationalNewDrugINDApplication/default.htm
Oseltamivir (Tamiflu) For pts ≥ 1 yr (treatment or prophylaxis)	For adults: **Treatment**, 75 mg po bid for 5 days; 150 mg po bid has been used for critically ill or morbidly obese patients but this dose is not FDA-approved. **Prophylaxis**, 75 mg po once daily for 10 days to 6 wks. (See label for pediatric weight-based dosing.) Adjust doses for CrCl ≤30 mL/min. 30 mg, 45 mg, 75 mg caps; powder for oral suspension.	Well absorbed (80% bioavailable) from GI tract as ethyl ester of active compound GS 4071. T½ 6-10 hrs; excreted unchanged by kidney. Adverse effects include diarrhea, nausea, vomiting, headache. Nausea ↓ with food. Rarely, severe skin reactions (toxic epidermal necrolysis), Stevens-Johnson syndrome, erythema multiforme]. **Delirium** & abnormal behavior reported (CID 48:1003, 2009).
Respiratory Syncytial Virus (RSV)		
Palivizumab (Synagis) Used for prevention of RSV infection in high-risk children	15 mg per kg IM a month throughout RSV season Single dose 100 mg vial	A monoclonal antibody directed against the F glycoprotein on surface of virus; side-effects are uncommon, occ. ↑ ALT. Anaphylaxis <1/100 pts; acute hypersensitivity reaction <1/1000. Postmarketing reports: URI, otitis media, fever, ↓ plts, injection site reactions. Preferred over polyclonal immune globulin IV in high risk infants & children.

See page 2 for abbreviations. NOTE: All dosage recommendations are for adults (unless otherwise indicated) and assume normal renal function.

TABLE 14B (5)

DRUG NAME(S) GENERIC (TRADE)	DOSAGE/ROUTE IN ADULTS*	COMMENTS/ADVERSE EFFECTS
Warts (See CID 28:S37, 1999)	Regimens are from drug labels specific for external genital and/or	perianal condylomata acuminata only (see specific labels for indications, regimens, age limits).
Interferon alfa-2b (IntronA)	Injection of 1 million international units into base of lesion, thrice weekly on alternate days for up to 3 wks. Maximum 5 lesions per course.	Interferons may cause "flu-like" illness and other systemic effects. 88% had at least one adverse effect. **Black box warning:** alpha interferons may cause or aggravate neuropsychiatric, autoimmune, ischemic or infectious disorders.
Interferon alfa-N3 (Alferon N)	Injection of 0.05 mL into base of each wart, up to 0.5 mL total per session, twice weekly for up to 8 weeks.	Flu-like syndrome and hypersensitivity reactions. Contraindicated with allergy to mouse IgG, egg proteins, or neomycin.
Imiquimod (Aldara)	5% cream. Thin layer applied at bedtime, washing off after 6-10 hr, three weekly to maximum of 16 wks.	Erythema, itching & burning, erosions. Flu-like syndrome, increased susceptibility to sunburn (avoid UV).
Podofilox (Condylox)	0.5% gel or solution twice daily for 3 days, no therapy for 4 days; can use up to 4 such cycles.	Local reactions—pain, burning, inflammation in 50%. Can ulcerate. Limit surface area treated as per label.
Sinecatechins (Veregen)	15% ointment. Apply 0.5 cm strand to each wart three times per day until healing but not more than 16 weeks.	Application site reactions, which may result in ulcerations, phimosis, meatal stenosis, superinfection.

* See page 2 for abbreviations; NOTE: All dosage recommendations are for adults (unless otherwise indicated) and assume normal renal function.

TABLE 14C – AT A GLANCE SUMMARY OF SUGGESTED ANTIVIRAL AGENTS AGAINST TREATABLE PATHOGENIC VIRUSES

Virus	Acyclovir	Amantadine	Adefovir Entecavir Lamivudine Tenofovir	Boceprevir Telaprevir	Cidofovir	Famciclovir	Foscarnet	Ganciclovir	αInterferon Or PEG INF	Oseltamivir	Ribavirin	Rimantadine	Valacyclovir	Valganciclovir	Zanamivir
Adenovirus	·	·	·	·	+	·	·	·	·	·	·	·	·	±	·
BK virus	·	·	·	·	+	·	·	·	·	·	·	·	·	·	·
Cytomegalovirus	±	·	·	·	+++	±	+++	+++	·	·	·	·	±	+++	·
Hepatitis B	·	·	+++	·	·	·	·	·	++	·	±	·	·	·	·
Hepatitis C	·	·	·	++++*	·	·	·	·	++*	·	++**	·	·	·	·
Herpes simplex virus	+++	·	·	·	++	+++	++	++	·	·	·	·	+++	·	·
Influenza A Influenza B	·	±**	·	·	·	·	·	·	·	+++*** ++	·	±**	·	·	+++ ++
JC Virus	·	·	·	·	+	·	·	·	·	·	+	·	·	·	·
Respiratory Syncytial Virus	·	·	·	·	·	·	·	·	·	·	+	·	·	·	·
Varicella-zoster virus	+++	·	·	·	+	++	++	·	·	·	·	·	+++	±	·

* 1st line rx = an IFN + Ribavirin plus either Boceprevir or Telaprevir if Genotype 1
*** High level resistance H1N1 (non-swine) in 2008; Swine H1N1 susceptible.
** not CDC recommended due to high prevalence of resistance

· = no activity; ± = possible activity; + = active, 3rd line therapy (least active clinically)
++ = Active, 2nd line therapy (less active clinically); +++ = Active, 1st line therapy (usually active clinically)

TABLE 14D – ANTIRETROVIRAL THERAPY (ART) IN TREATMENT-NAÏVE ADULTS (HIV/AIDS)

(See the SANFORD GUIDE TO HIV/AIDS THERAPY 2013 for additional information)

The U.S. Dept of Health & Human Svcs (DHHS) provides updated guidelines on a regular basis; the most recent update of the HHS Guidelines was September 2012. These, as well as recommendations for anti-retroviral therapy (ART) in pregnant women and in children, are available at www.aidsinfo.nih.gov. These documents provide detailed recommendations and explanations, drug characteristics, and additional alternatives concerning the use of ART. The new Guidelines include: (1) recommendations to start therapy at any CD4 count for asymptomatic patients unless there is a reason to defer treatment; the strength of the recommendation increases with lower CD4 count values; (2) Addition of new sections on HIV and Aging patients and Cost of ART (now included as Table 6II). (3) New recommendations for starting ART for those patients presenting with TB. For patients with CD4 counts <50 cells/mm³, ART should be initiated within 2 weeks of starting TB treatment (**AI**).

- For patients with CD4 counts ≥50 cells/mm³ with clinical disease of major severity as indicated by clinical evaluation (including low Karnofsky score, low body mass index [BMI], low hemoglobin, low albumin, organ system dysfunction, or extent of disease), the Panel recommends initiation of ART within 2 to 4 weeks of starting TB treatment (**BI** for CD4 count 50-200 cells/mm³ and **BIII** for CD4 count >200 cells/mm³).
- For other patients with CD4 counts ≥50 cells/mm³, ART can be delayed beyond 2 to 4 weeks but should be initiated by 8 to 12 weeks of TB therapy (**AI** for CD4 count 50-500 cells/mm³ **BIII** for CD4 count >500 cells/mm³). Note that immune reconstitution syndromes (IRS or IRIS) may result from initiation of any ART, and may require medical intervention.

The following principles and concepts guide therapy:
- **The goal of rx is to inhibit maximally viral replication, allowing re-establishment & persistence of an effective immune response that will prevent or delay HIV-related morbidity.**
- **Fully undetectable levels of virus is the target of therapy for ALL patients, regardless of stage of disease or number/type of prior regimens.**
- **The lower the viral RNA can be driven, the lower the rate of accumulation of drug resistance mutations & the longer the therapeutic effect will last.**
- **To achieve maximal & durable suppression of viral RNA, combinations of potent antiretroviral agents are required, as is a high degree of adherence to the chosen regimens.**
- **Virologic failure is defined as confirmed virus > 200 c/mL.**
- **Treatment regimens must be tailored to the individual as well as to the virus.**
- **Resistance testing (genotype) should be performed prior to the initiation of ARV therapy.** Antiretroviral drug toxicities can compromise adherence in the short term & can cause significant negative health effects over time. Carefully check for specific risks to the individual, for interactions between the antiretrovirals selected & between those & concurrent drugs, & adjust doses as necessary for body weight, for renal or hepatic dysfunction, & for possible pharmacokinetic interactions.

A. When to start therapy? (www.aidsinfo.nih.gov)

Guidelines	Any symptoms or CD4 <200/μL	CD4 200-350/μL	CD4 350-500/μL	CD4 >500/μL
IAS-USA: JAMA 308: 387, 2012	Treat	Treat	Treat	Consider Treatment* *No Apparent Harm in treating earlier
DHHS: www.aidsinfo.nih.gov	Treat	Treat	Treat	Treat* * Strength of rating increases as CD4 count decreases

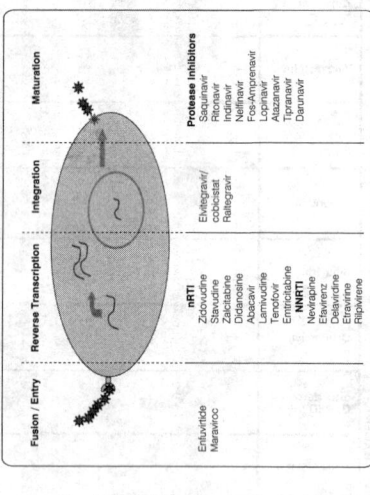

Life Cycle of HIV With Sites of Action of Antiretrovirals

Fusion / Entry	Reverse Transcription	Integration	Maturation
Enfuvirtide Maraviroc	**nRTI** Zidovudine Stavudine Zalcitabine Didanosine Abacavir Lamivudine Tenofovir Emtricitabine **NNRTI** Nevirapine Efavirenz Delavirdine Etravirine Rilpivirene	Elvitegravir/ cobicistat Raltegravir	**Protease Inhibitors** Saquinavir Ritonavir Indinavir Nelfinavir Fos-Amprenavir Lopinavir Atazanavir Tipranavir Darunavir

TABLE 14D (2)

B. **Approach to constructing ART regimens for treatment naive adults.** (See Guidelines for the Use of Antiretroviral Agents in HIV-1-Infected Adults and Adolescents at www.aidsinfo.nih.gov. for updates and further alternatives.)

- See Section D for specific regimens and tables which follow for drug characteristics, usual doses, adverse effects and additional details.
- Selection of components will be influenced by many factors, such as:
  - Co-morbidities (e.g., lipid effects of PIs, liver or renal disease, etc)
  - Pregnancy (e.g., avoid efavirenz, particularly in the first trimester when the neural tube is forming —pregnancy class D)
  - HIV status (e.g., avoid nevirapine in women with CD4 >250 and men with CD4 >400)
  - Results of viral resistance testing (recommended for all patients prior to initiation of ART)
  - Potential drug interactions or adverse drug effects; special focus on tolerability (even low grade side effects can profoundly effect adherence)
  - Convenience of dosing

Select 1 drug in column A + 1 NRTI combination in column B

	A	Initial Combination Regimen for ARV Naive Patients — B	COMMENTS
Preferred	**NNRTI** • Efavirenz (600 mg/qhs) **Ritonavir-Boosted PI** • Atazanavir/rit (300/100 qd) • Darunavir/rit (800/100 qd) **Integrase Inhibitor** • Raltegravir (400 BID) • Elvitegravir / Cobicistat (150/150 qd)	Tenofovir / FTC (300/200 qd) FTC = **Emtricitabine** FTC + Tenofovir = **Truvada** FTC + Tenofovir + Efavirenz = **Atripla** FTC + Tenofovir + Elvitegravir/Cobi = **Stribild**	Co-formulations increase convenience, but sometimes prescribing the two components individually is preferred, as when dose adjustments are needed for renal disease. **ATV/r** should not be used in patients who require >20 mg omeprazole equivalent per day. No / little data on Raltegravir + any other nRTI regimens. RTG 800 mg once daily not quite as effective as 400 mg bid. No data on Elvitegravir / cobicistat with other nucleosides.
Alternative	**NNRTI** • Rilpivirine (25 qd) • Etravirine (200 mg bid or 400 qd) **Ritonavir-Boosted PI** • Fosamprenavir (1400/100 qd) • Lopinavir/rit (400/100 qd) • Saquinavir/rit (1000/100 bid)	(In order of preference) Tenofovir / FTC (300/200 qd) Abacavir / 3TC (600/300 qd) Zidovudine/ 3TC (300/150 bid) FTC + TDF + RPV = **Complera/Eviplera**	Viramune XR 400 mg preferred formulation Rilpivirine is best used for patients with VL< 100K. Rilpivirine should not be used with any PPI therapy. Lopinavir Ritonavir should not be used once daily in pregnant women (should only be used twice daily) Etravirine and Rilpivirine are options for some patients who have NNRTI resistance mutations (e.g., K103N) at baseline. Expert consultation is recommended.
Acceptable	**NNRTI** • Nevirapine (400 qd) **Non-boosted PI** • Fosamprenavir (1400 bid) • Atazanavir (400 qd) **Boosted PI** • Nelfinavir* (1250 bid) **CCR5 INHIBITOR** • Saquinavir/rit (1000/100 bid) • Maraviroc (300 bid)**	(In order of preference) Tenofovir/ FTC (300/200 qd) Abacavir / 3TC (600/300 qd) Zidovudine / 3TC (300/150 bid) ddl (300) + 3TC (300) or FTC (200)	Nevirapine should be used with caution with ABC owing to possible overlap of idiosyncratic hypersensitivity Saquinavir associated with prolonged QTc. Boosted PIs can be administered once or twice daily. Non-boosted PIs are typically less preferred than boosted PIs. *Nelfinavir is used most often in pregnant women as an alternative PI. It has inferior virologic responses. No data on MVC and any NRTIs other than ZDV/3TC.

** Dosing effected by drug-drug interactions

C. **During pregnancy:** Expert consultation mandatory. Timing of rx initiation & drug choice must be individualized. Viral resistance testing should be strongly considered. Long-term effects of agents unknown. Certain drugs hazardous or contraindicated. (See Table 8A). For additional information & alternative options, see www.aidsinfo.nih.gov.

TABLE 14D (3)

D. Antiretroviral Therapies That Should NOT Be Offered (Modified from www.aidsinfo.nih.gov)

1. Regimens not recommended

	Regimen	Logic	Exception
a.	Monotherapy with NRTI	Rapid development of resistance & inferior antiviral activity	Perhaps ZDV to reduce peripartum mother-to-child transmission. See Perinatal Guidelines at www.aidsinfo.nih.gov and Table 8B, Sanford Guide to HIV/AIDS Therapy
b.	Dual NRTI combinations	Resistance and Inferior antiretroviral activity compared with standard drug combinations	Perhaps ZDV to reduce peripartum mother-to-child transmission. See Perinatal Guidelines at www.aidsinfo.nih.gov and Table 8B, Sanford Guide to HIV/AIDS Therapy
c.	Triple-NRTI combinations	Resistance-NRTI regimens have shown inferior virologic efficacy in clinical trials: (tenofovir + lamivudine + abacavir) & (didanosine + lamivudine + tenofovir) & others	ZIdovudine + lamivudine + abacavir) or (zidovudine + lamivudine + tenofovir) might be used if no alternative exists.
d.	Double Boosted PIs	Using 2 or more PI agents boosted with ritonavir adds nothing in terms of anti-HIV activity but can add extra toxicity	No exceptions
e.	2 NNRTI agents	Increased rate of side effects. Drug-drug interaction between etravirine and nevirapine and etravirine and efavirenz	No exceptions

2. Drug, or drugs, not recommended as part of antiretroviral regimen

		Logic	Exception
a.	Saquinavir hard gel cap or tab (Invirase), darunavir, or tipranavir as single (unboosted) PI	Bioavailability only 4%; inferior antiretroviral activity	No exceptions
b.	Stavudine + didanosine	High frequency of toxicity: peripheral neuropathy, pancreatitis & mitochondrial toxicity (lactic acidosis). In pregnancy: lactic acid acidosis, hepatic steatosis, ± pancreatitis	Toxicity partially offset by potent antiretroviral activity of the combination. Use only when potential benefits outweigh the sizeable risks.
c.	Efavirenz in pregnancy or in women who might become pregnant	Teratogenic in non-human primates. Pregnancy Category D—may cause fetal harm	Only if no other option available; major risk would be 1st trimester (first 4-6 weeks as neural tube is forming in fetus). Note that oral contraceptives alone may not be reliable for prevention of pregnancy in women on ART or other medications (see Safety & Toxicity of Individual Agents in Pregnancy at www.aidsinfo.nih.gov).
d.	Stavudine + zidovudine	Antagonistic	No exceptions
e.	Atazanavir + indinavir	Additive risk of hyperbilirubinemia	No exceptions
f.	Emtricitabine + lamivudine	Same target and resistance profile	No exceptions
g.	Abacavir + tenofovir	Rapid development of K65R mutation, loss of effect	Can avoid if zidovudine also used in the regimen; might be an option for salvage therapy but not earlier lines of therapy.
h.	Tenofovir + didanosine	Reduced CD4 cell count increase; concern for K 65R development	Use with caution. Likely increases ddI concentrations and serious ddI toxicities.
i.	Abacavir + didanosine	Insufficient data in naive patients	Use with caution

E. **Selected Characteristics of Antiretroviral Drugs** (CPE = CSF penetration effectiveness)

1. **Selected Characteristics of Nucleoside or Nucleotide Reverse Transcriptase Inhibitors (NRTIs)**

   All agents have Black Box warning: Risk of lactic acidosis/hepatic steatosis. Also, labels note risk of fat redistribution/accumulation with ARV therapy. For combinations, see warnings for component agents.

   * CPE (CNS Penetration Effectiveness) value: 1 = Low Penetration, 2 - 3 = Intermediate Penetration, 4 = Highest Penetration into CNS (Letendre, et al, CROI 2010, abs #430)

TABLE 14D (4)

Generic/ Trade Name	Pharmaceutical Prep.	Usual Adult Dosage & Food Effect	% Absorbed, po	Serum T½, hrs	Intracellular T½, hrs	CPE*	Elimination	Major Adverse Events/Comments (See Table 14E)
Abacavir (ABC; Ziagen)	300 mg tabs or 20 mg/mL oral solution	300 mg po bid or 600 mg po q24h. Food OK	83	1.5	20	1	Liver metab, renal excretion of metabolites, 82%	**Hypersensitivity reaction:** fever, rash, N/V, malaise, diarrhea, abdominal pain, respiratory symptoms. (Severe reactions may be ↑ with 600 mg dose. **Do not rechallenge!** Report to 800-270-0425. **Test HLA-B*5701 before use.** See Comment Table 14E. Studies raise concerns re ABC/3TC regimens in pts with VL ≥ 100,000 (www.niaid.nih.gov/news/newsreleases/2008/actg5202bulletin.htm). Recent report suggests possible ↑ risk of cardiac event in pts with other risk factors (D:A:D study group Lancet 2008; updated CROI 2009, LB abst 44).
Abacavir (ABC)/ lamivudine (Epzicom or Kivexa)	Film coated tabs: ABC 600 mg + 3TC 300 mg	1 tab once daily (not recommended)						(See Comments for individual components) Note: **Black Box warnings** for ABC hypersensitivity reaction & others. Should only be used for regimens intended to include these 3 agents. Black Box warning— limited data for VL >100,000 copies/mL. Not recommended as initial therapy because of inferior virologic efficacy.
Abacavir (ABC)/ lamivudine (3TC)/ zidovudine (AZT) (Trizivir)	Film-coated tabs: ABC 300 mg + 3TC 150 mg + ZDV 300 mg	1 tab po bid (not recommended for wt <40 kg or CrCl <50 mL/min or impaired hepatic function)			(See individual components)			
Didanosine (ddI; Videx or Videx EC)	125, 200, 250, 400 enteric-coated caps; 100, 167, 250 mg powder for oral solution.	≥60 kg Usually 400 mg enteric-coated po q24h 0.5 hr before or 2 hrs after meal. Do not crush. <60 kg: 250 mg EC po q24h. Food ↓ levels. See Comment	30–40	1.6	25–40	2	Renal excretion, 50%	**Pancreatitis,** peripheral neuropathy, lactic acidosis & hepatic steatosis (rare but life-threatening, esp. combined with stavudine in pregnancy). Retinal, optic nerve changes. **The combination ddI + TDF is generally avoided, but if used** reduce dose of ddI EC (from 400 mg to 250 mg EC q24h (or 200 mg EC to 250 mg EC q24h for adults <60 kg). **Monitor for ↑ toxicity & possible ↓ in efficacy of this combination; may result in ↓ CD4.** Possibly associated with noncirrhotic portal hypertension.

TABLE 14D (5)

E. Selected Characteristics of Antiretroviral Drugs (CPE = CSF penetration effectiveness)

1. Selected Characteristics of Nucleoside or Nucleotide Reverse Transcriptase Inhibitors (NRTIs) *(continued)*

Generic/ Trade Name	Pharmaceutical Prep.	Usual Adult Dosage & Food Effect	% Absorbed, po	Serum T½, hrs	Intracellular T½, hrs	CPE*	Elimination	Major Adverse Events/Comments (See Table 14E)
Emtricitabine (FTC, Emtriva)	200 mg caps; 10 mg per mL oral solution.	200 mg po q24h. Food OK.	93 (caps), 75 (oral sol'n)	Approx. 10	39	3	Renal excretion 86%, minor biotransformation, 14% excretion in feces	Well tolerated: headache, nausea, vomiting & diarrhea occasionally. Skin rash rarely. Skin hyperpigmentation. Differs only slightly in structure from lamivudine (5-fluoro substitution). **Exacerbation of Hep B reported in pts after stopping FTC.** Monitor at least several months after stopping FTC in Hep B pts; some may need anti-HBV therapy.
Emtricitabine/ tenofovir disoproxil fumarate (TRUVADA)	Film-coated tabs: FTC 200 mg + TDF 300 mg	1 tab po q24h for CrCl ≥50 mL/min. Food OK.	92/25	10/17	—	*(See individual components)*	Primarily renal/renal	See *Comments for individual agents* **Black Box warning—Exacerbation of HepB after stopping FTC**; but preferred therapy for those with Hep B.
Emtricitabine/ tenofovir/efavirenz (ATRIPLA)	Film-coated tabs: FTC 200 mg + TDF 300 mg + efavirenz 600 mg	1 tab po q24h on an empty stomach, preferably at bedtime. Do not use if CrCl <50 mL/min		*(See individual components)*				Not recommended for pts <18 yrs. (See *warnings for individual components*). **Exacerbation of Hep B reported in pts discontinuing component drugs**; some may need anti-HBV therapy (preferred anti-Hep B therapy). **Pregnancy Category D**: may cause fetal harm. Avoid in pregnancy or in women who may become pregnant.
Emtricitabine/ tenofovir/rilpivirine (COMPLERA)/ EVIPLERA)	Film-coated tabs: FTC 200 mg + TDF 300 mg + RPL 25 mg	1 tab po q24h with food		*(See individual components)*				See *individual components*. Preferred use in pts with HIV RNA level < 100,000 c/ml. Should not be used with PPI agents.
Lamivudine (3TC, Epivir)	150, 300 mg tabs; 10 mg/mL oral solution	150 mg po bid or 300 mg po q24h. Food OK	86	5–7	18	2	Renal excretion, minimal metabolism	**Use HIV dose, not Hep B dose.** Usually well-tolerated. **Risk of exacerbation of Hep B after stopping 3TC.** Monitor at least several months after stopping 3TC in Hep B pts; some may need anti-HBV therapy.
Lamivudine/ abacavir (Epzicom)	Film-coated tabs: 3TC 300 mg + abacavir 600 mg	1 tab po q24h. Food OK. Not recommended for CrCl <50 mL/min or impaired hepatic function	86/86	5–7/1.5	16/20	*(See individual components)*	Primarily renal metabolism	See *Comments for individual agents*. **Note abacavir hypersensitivity Black Box warnings** (severe reactions may be somewhat more frequent with 600 mg dose) and 3TC Hep B warnings. Test HLA-B*5701 before use.
Lamivudine/ zidovudine (Combivir)	Film-coated tabs: 3TC 150 mg + ZDV 300 mg	1 tab po bid. Not recommended for CrCl <50 mL/min or impaired hepatic function Food OK	86/64	5–7/ 0.5–3	—	*(See individual components)*	Primarily renal/ renal metabolism with renal excretion of glucuronide	See *Comments for individual agents* **Black Box warning**—exacerbation of Hep B in pts stopping 3TC

TABLE 14D (6)

Generic/ Trade Name	Pharmaceutical Prep.	Usual Adult Dosage & Food Effect	% Absorbed, po	Serum T½, hrs	Intracellular T½, hrs	CPE*	Elimination	Major Adverse Events/Comments (See Table 14E)
E. Selected Characteristics of Antiretroviral Drugs (CPE = CSF penetration effectiveness)								
1. Selected Characteristics of Nucleoside or Nucleotide Reverse Transcriptase Inhibitors (NRTIs) *(continued)*								
Stavudine (d4T; Zerit)	15, 20, 30, 40 mg capsules; 1 mg per mL oral solution	≥60 kg: 40 mg po bid <60 kg: 30 mg po bid Food OK	86	1.2–1.6	3.5	2	Renal excretion, 40%	Not recommended by DHHS as initial therapy because of adverse reactions. **Highest incidence of lipoatrophy, hyperlipidemia, & lactic acidosis of all NRTIs.** Pancreatitis. Peripheral neuropathy. (See *didanosine* comments.)
Tenofovir disoproxil fumarate (TDF; Viread)—a nucleotide	300 mg tabs	CrCl ≥50 mL/min: 300 mg po q24h. Food OK; high-fat meal ↑ absorption	39 (with food) 25 (fasted)	17	>60	1	Renal excretion	Headache. N/V. **Cases of renal dysfunction reported:** check renal function before using (dose reductions necessary if CrCl <50 cc/min); avoid concomitant nephrotoxic agents. One study found ↑ renal function at 48-wks in pts receiving TDF with a PI (mostly lopinavir/ritonavir) than with a NNRTI (*JID 197*:102, 2008). Must adjust dose of ddI (↓) if used concomitantly but best to avoid this combination (*see ddI Comments*). Atazanavir & lopinavir/ritonavir ↑ tenofovir concentrations: monitor for adverse effects. **Black Box warning— exacerbations of Hep B reported after stopping tenofovir.** Monitor several months after stopping TDF in Hep B pts; some may need anti-HBV Rx.
Zidovudine (ZDV, AZT; Retrovir)	100 mg caps, 300 mg tabs; 10 mg per mL IV solution; 10 mg/mL oral syrup	300 mg po q12h. Food OK	64	1.1	11	4	Metabolized to glucuronide & excreted in urine	Bone marrow suppression. GI intolerance, headache, insomnia, malaise, myopathy.
2. Selected Characteristics of Non-Nucleoside Reverse Transcriptase Inhibitors (NNRTIs)								
Delavirdine (Rescriptor)	100, 200 mg tabs	400 mg po three times daily. Food OK	85	5.8	3		Cytochrome P450 (3A inhibitor); 51% excreted in urine (<5% uncharged), 44% in feces	Rash severe enough to stop drug in 4.3%, ↑ AST/ALT, headaches. **Use of this agent is not recommended.**

179

TABLE 14D (7)

E. Selected Characteristics of Antiretroviral Drugs (CPE = CSF penetration effectiveness)
2. Selected Characteristics of Non-Nucleoside Reverse Transcriptase Inhibitors (NNRTIs) (continued)

Generic/ Trade Name	Pharmaceutical Prep.	Usual Adult Dosage & Food Effect	% Absorbed, po	Serum T½, hrs	Intracellular T½, hrs	CPE*	Elimination	Major Adverse Events/Comments (See Table 14E)
Efavirenz (Sustiva) **(Pregnancy Category D)**	50, 100, 200 mg capsules; 600 mg tablet	600 mg po q24h at bedtime, without food. Food may ↑ serum conc., which can lead to ↑ in risk of adverse events.	42	40–55 See Comment	3		Cytochrome P450 266 (3A mixed inducer/ inhibitor); 14–34% of dose excreted in urine as glucuroni- dated metabolites. 16–61% in feces	Rash severe enough to d/c use of drug in 1.7%. High frequency of diverse CNS AEs: somnolence, dreams, confusion, agitation. Serious psychiatric symptoms reported. Polymorphisms may predict exposure (CID 45:1230, 2007). False-pos. cannabinoid screen (CID 45:1230, 2007). **Pregnancy Category D—may cause fetal harm—avoid in pregnant women or those who might become pregnant.** (Note: No single method of contraception is 100% reliable). Very long tissue T½. **If rx is to be discontinued, stop efavirenz 1–2 wks before stopping companion drugs.** Otherwise, risk of developing efavirenz resistance as after 1–2 days only efavirenz in blood &/or tissue. Some authorities bridge this gap by adding a PI to the NRTI backbone, if feasible after efavirenz is discontinued. (CID 42:401, 2006)
Etravirine (Intelence)	100 mg tabs	200 mg twice daily after a meal	Unknown (↓ systemic exposure if taken fasting)	41	2		Metabolized by CYP 3A4 (inducer) & 2C9, 2C19 (inhibitor). Excreted into feces (>90%), mostly unchanged drug.	For pts with HIV-1 resistant to NNRTIs & others. Active in vitro against most such isolates. Rash common, but rarely can be severe. Potential for multiple drug interactions. Generally, multiple mutations are required for high-level resistance. See Table 3C, page 16, Sanford Guide to HIV/AIDS Therapy, for specific mutations and effects. Because of interactions, do not use with boosted atazanavir, boosted tipranavir, unboosted PIs or other NNRTIs.
Nevirapine (Viramune) Viramune XR	200 mg tabs; 50 mg per 5 mL oral suspension; XR 400 mg tabs	200 mg po q24h x 14 days & then 200 mg po bid (see comments & *Black Box warning*) Food: OK. If using Viramune XR, Still need the lead in dosing of 200 mg q24h prior to using 400 mg/d	>90	25–30	4		Cytochrome P450 (3A4, 2B6) inducer; 80% of dose excreted in urine as glu- curonidated metabolites, 10% in feces	**Black Box warning—fatal hepatotoxicity.** Women with CD4 >250 esp. vulnerable, inc. pregnant women. Avoid in this group unless benefits clearly > risks (www.fda.gov/cder/drug/advisory/nevirapine.htm). If used, intensive monitoring required. Men with CD4 >400 also at ↑ risk. Rash severe enough to stop drug in 7%, serious **life-threatening skin reactions** in 2%. Do not restart if any suspicion of such reactions. 2 wks dose escalation period may ↓ skin reactions. As with efavirenz, because of long T½, consider continuing companion agents for several days if nevirapine is discontinued.

TABLE 14D (8)

E. Selected Characteristics of Antiretroviral Drugs CPE = CSF penetration effectiveness)

2. Selected Characteristics of Non-Nucleoside Reverse Transcriptase Inhibitors (NNRTIs) *(continued)*

Generic/Trade Name	Pharmaceutical Prep.	Usual Adult Dosage & Food Effect	% Absorbed, po	Serum T½, hrs	Intracellular T½, hrs	CPE*	Elimination	Major Adverse Events/Comments (See Table 14E)
Rilpivirine (Edurant)	25 mg tabs	25 mg daily with food	absolute bioavailability unknown; 40% lower Cmax in fasted state	50	unknown		Metabolized by Cyp3A4 majority of drug metabolized by liver; 25% of dose excreted unchanged in feces.	QTc prolongation with doses higher than 50 mg per day. Most common side effects are depression, insomnia, headache, and rash. Rilpivirine should not be co-administered with carbamazepine, phenobarbital, phenytoin, rifabutin, rifampin, rifapentine, proton pump inhibitors, or multiple doses of dexamethasone. A fixed dose combination of rilpivirine + TDF/FTC (Complera/Eviplera) is approved. **Needs stomach acid for absorption. Do not administer with PPI.**

3. Selected Characteristics of Protease Inhibitors (PIs).

All PIs: Glucose metabolism: new diabetes mellitus or deterioration of glucose control; fat redistribution; possible hemophilia bleeding; hypertriglyceridemia. Exercise caution re: potential drug interactions & contraindications. QTc prolongation has been reported in a few pts taking PIs; some PIs can block HERG channels in vitro *(Lancet 365:682, 2005)*.

Generic/Trade Name	Pharmaceutical Prep.	Usual Adult Dosage & Food Effect	% Absorbed, po	Serum T½, hrs	CPE*	Elimination	Major Adverse Events/Comments (See Table 14E)
Atazanavir (Reyataz)	100, 150, 200, 300 mg capsules	400 mg q 24h with food. Ritonavir-boosted dose (atazanavir 300 mg po q24h + ritonavir 100 mg po q24h), with food, is recommended for ART-experienced pts. The boosted dose is also used when combined with either efavirenz 600 mg po q24h or TDF 300 mg po q24h. If used with buffered ddI, take with food 2 hrs pre or 1 hr post ddI.	Good oral bioavailability; food enhances bioavailability & ↓ pharmacokinetic variability. Absorption ↓ by antacids, H₂-blockers, proton pump inhibitors. Avoid unboosted drug with PPIs/H2-blockers. Boosted drug can be used with or > 10 hr after H2-blockers, or > 12 hr after a PI; as long as limited doses of the acid agents are used (see 2008 drug label changes).	Approx. 7	2	Cytochrome P450 (3A4, 1A2 & 2C9 inhibitor) & UGT1A1 inhibitor. 13% excreted in urine (7% unchanged), 79% excreted in feces (20% unchanged)	Lower potential for ↑ lipids. Asymptomatic unconjugated hyperbilirubinemia common; jaundice especially likely in Gilbert's syndrome (*JID 192:1381, 2005*). Headache, rash, GI symptoms. Prolongation of PR interval (1st degree AV block) reported. Caution in pre-existing conduction system disease. Efavirenz & tenofovir ↓ atazanavir exposure: use atazanavir/ritonavir regimen, also, atazanavir ↑ tenofovir concentrations—watch for adverse events. In rx-experienced pts taking TDF and needing H2-blockers, atazanavir 400 mg with ritonavir 100 mg can be given; do not use PPIs. Compared to PIs, increased risk of renal stones, p<0.001 (*CID 55:1262, 2012*)
Darunavir (Prezista)	400 mg, 600 mg tablets	600 mg darunavir + 100 mg ritonavir po bid, with food **or** [800 mg darunavir (two 400 mg tabs) + 100 mg ritonavir] po once daily with food (Preferred regimen in ART naive pts)	82% absorbed (taken with ritonavir). Food ↑ absorption.	Approx 15 hr (with ritonavir)	3	Metabolized by CYP3A and is a CYP3A inhibitor	Once daily dosing regimen mostly in 1st line therapy. Contains sulfa moiety. Rash, nausea, headaches seen. Coadmin of certain drugs cleared by CYP3A is contraindicated (see label). Use with caution in pts with hepatic dysfunction. (Recent FDA warning about occasional hepatic dysfunction early in the course of treatment). Monitor carefully, esp. first several months and with pre-existing liver disease. May cause hormonal contraception failure.

TABLE 14D (9)

E. Selected Characteristics of Antiretroviral Drugs (CPE = CSF penetration effectiveness)
3. Selected Characteristics of Protease Inhibitors (PIs), (continued)

Generic/ Trade Name	Pharmaceutical Prep.	Usual Adult Dosage & Food Effect	% Absorbed, po	Serum T½, hrs	CPE*	Elimination	Major Adverse Events/Comments (See Table 14E)
Fosamprenavir (Lexiva)	700 mg tablet, 50 mg/mL oral suspension	1400 mg (two 700 mg tabs) with ritonavir: [1400 mg fosamprenavir (2 tabs) + ritonavir 200 mg] po q24h **OR** [1400 mg fosamprenavir (2 tabs) + ritonavir 100 mg] po q24h **OR** [700 mg fosamprenavir (1 tab) + ritonavir 100 mg] po bid	Bioavailability not established. Food OK.	7.7 Amprenavir	3	Hydrolyzed to amprenavir, then acts as cytochrome P450 (3A4 substrate, inhibitor, inducer)	Amprenavir prodrug. Contains sulfa moiety. Potential for serious drug interactions (see label). Rash, including Stevens-Johnson syndrome. Once daily dosing (1) is not recommended for PI-experienced pts, (2) additional ritonavir needed if given with efavirenz (see label). Boosted twice daily regimen is recommended for PI-experienced pts. Potential for PI cross-resistance with darunavir.
Indinavir (Crixivan)	100, 200, 400 mg capsules Store in original container with desiccant	Two 400 mg caps (800 mg) po q8h, without food or with light meal. Can take with enteric-coated Videx. (If taken with ritonavir (e.g., 800 mg indinavir + 100 mg ritonavir po q12h) no food restrictions)	65	1.2–2	4	Cytochrome P450 (3A4 inhibitor)	**Maintain hydration. Nephrolithiasis,** nausea, inconsequential ↑ of indirect bilirubin (jaundice in Gilbert syndrome), ↑ AST/ALT, headache, asthenia, blurred vision, metallic taste, hemolysis, ↑ urine WBC (>10/hpf) has been assoc. with nephritis/ medullary calcification, cortical atrophy
Lopinavir + ritonavir (Kaletra)	(200 mg lopinavir + 50 mg ritonavir, and (100 mg lopinavir + 25 mg ritonavir) tablets Tabs do not need refrigeration. Oral solution: (80 mg lopinavir + 20 mg ritonavir) per mL. Refrigerate, but can be kept at room temp. (≤77°F) x 2 mos.	(400 mg lopinavir + 100 mg ritonavir)—2 tabs po bid. Higher dose may be needed in non-rx-naive pts when used with efavirenz, nevirapine, or unboosted fosamprenavir. [Dose adjustment in concomitant drugs may be necessary, see Table 17A]	No food effect with tablets.	5–6	3	Cytochrome P450 (3A4 inhibitor)	Nausea/vomiting/diarrhea (worse when administered with zidovudine), ↑ AST/ALT, pancreatitis. Oral solution 42% alcohol. Lopinavir + ritonavir can be taken as a single daily dose of 4 tabs (total 800 mg lopinavir + 200 mg ritonavir), except in treatment-experienced pts or those taking concomitant efavirenz, nevirapine, amprenavir, or nelfinavir. Possible PR and QT prolongation. Use with caution in those with cardiac conduction abnormalities or when used with drugs with similar effects
Nelfinavir (Viracept)	625, 250 mg tabs 50 mg/mg oral powder	Two 625 mg tabs (1250 mg) po bid, with food	20–80 Food ↑ exposure & ↓ variability	3.5–5	1	Cytochrome P450 (3A4 inhibitor)	Diarrhea. Coadministration of drugs with life-threatening toxicities & which are cleared by CYP3A4 is contraindicated. Not recommended in initial regimens because of inferior efficacy; prior concerns about EMs now resolved. Acceptable choice in pregnant women although it has inferior virologic efficacy than most other ARV anchor drugs.

TABLE 14D (10)

E. Selected Characteristics of Antiretroviral Drugs (CPE = CSF penetration effectiveness)

3. Selected Characteristics of Protease Inhibitors (PIs), (continued)

Generic/ Trade Name	Pharmaceutical Prep.	Usual Adult Dosage & Food Effect	% Absorbed, po	Serum T½, hrs	CPE*	Elimination	Major Adverse Events/Comments (See Table 14E)
Ritonavir (Norvir)	100 mg capsules; 600 mg per 7.5 mL solution. Refrigerate caps but not room temperature for 1 mo. is OK.	Full dose not recommended (see comments). **With rare exceptions, used exclusively to enhance pharmacokinetics of other PIs, using lower ritonavir doses.**	Food ↑ absorption	3–5	1	Cytochrome P450 & potent inhibitor 3A4 & d6	Nausea/vomiting/diarrhea, extremity & circumoral paresthesias, hepatitis, pancreatitis, taste perversion; ↑ CPK, ↑ AST, uric acid. **Black Box warning**—potentially fatal drug interactions. Many drug interactions—see Table 22A–Table 22B.
Saquinavir (Invirase—hard gel caps or tabs) + ritonavir	Saquinavir 200 mg caps, 500 mg film-coated tabs; ritonavir 100 mg caps	Saquinavir (1000 mg) + 1 cap ritonavir (100 mg) po bid with food [2 tabs saquinavir (1000 mg) + 1 cap ritonavir (100 mg)]	Erratic. ↓ (saquinavir alone). Much more reliably absorbed when boosted with ritonavir.	1–2	1	Cytochrome P450 (3A4 inhibitor)	Nausea, diarrhea, headache, ↑ AST/ALT. Avoid rifampin with saquinavir + ritonavir: ↑ hepatitis risk. **Black Box warning**—Invirase to be used only with ritonavir. Possible QT prolongation. Use with caution in those with cardiac conduction abnormalities or when used with drugs with similar effects.
Tipranavir (Aptivus)	250 mg caps. Refrigerate unopened bottles. Use opened bottles within 2 mos. 100 mg/mL solution	[500 mg (two 250 mg caps) + ritonavir 200 mg caps] po bid with food.	Absorption low. ↑ with high fat meal, ↓ with Al^{++} & Mg^{++} antacids.	5.5–6	1	Cytochrome 3A4 but with ritonavir, most of drug is eliminated in feces.	Contains sulfa moiety. **Black Box warning—reports of fatal/nonfatal intracranial hemorrhage, hepatitis, fatal and non-fatal. Use cautiously in pts with hep B, hep C, contraindicated in Child-Pugh class B-C. Monitor LFTs. Coadministration of certain drugs contraindicated (see label). For highly ART-experienced pts or for multiple-PI resistant virus.** Do not use tipranavir and etravirine together owing to 76% reduction in etravirine levels.

4. Selected Characteristics of Fusion Inhibitors

Generic/ Trade Name	Pharmaceutical Prep.	Usual Adult Dosage	% Absorbed	Serum T½, hrs	CPE*	Elimination	Major Adverse Events/Comments (See Table 14E)
Enfuvirtide (T20, Fuzeon)	Single-use vials of 90 mg/mL when reconstituted. Vials should be stored at room temperature. Reconstituted vials can be refrigerated for 24 hrs only.	90 mg (1 mL) subcut. bid. Rotate injection sites, avoiding those currently inflamed.	84	3.8	1	Catabolism to its constituent amino acids with subsequent recycling of the amino acids in the body pool. Elimination pathway(s) have not been performed in humans. Does not alter the metabolism of CYP3A4, CYP2 d6, CYP1A2, CYP2C19 or CYP2E1 substrates.	Local reaction site reactions 98%, 4% discontinue; erythema/induration ~80-90%, nodules/cysts ~80%. **Hypersensitivity reactions reported** (fever, rash, chills, N/V, ↓ BP, & /or ↑ AST/ALT)—do not restart if occur. Including background regimen, peripheral neuropathy 8.9%, insomnia 11.3%, ↓ appetite 6.3%, myalgia 5%, lymphadenopathy 2.3%, eosinophilia ~10%, ↑ incidence of bacterial pneumonias. Alone offers little benefit to a failing regimen (NEJM 348:2249, 2003).

183

TABLE 14D (11)

Generic/Trade Name	Pharmaceutical Prep.	Usual Adult Dosage	% Absorbed	Serum T½, hrs	CPE*	Elimination	Major Adverse Events/Comments (See Table 14E)
E. Selected Characteristics of Antiretroviral Drugs (CPE = CSF penetration effectiveness) *(continued)*							
5. Selected Characteristics of CCR-5 Co-receptor Antagonists							
Maraviroc (Selzentry)	150 mg, 300 mg film-coated tabs	Without regard to food: - 150 mg bid if concomitant meds include CYP3A inhibitors including PIs (except tipranavir/ritonavir) and delavirdine (with/without CYP3A inducers) - 300 mg bid without significantly interacting meds including NRTIs, tipranavir/ritonavir, nevirapine - 600 mg bid if concomitant meds include CYP3A inducers, including efavirenz (without strong CYP3A inhibitors)	Est. 33% with 300 mg dosage	14-18	3	CYP3A and P-glycoprotein substrate. Metabolites (via CYP3A) excreted feces > urine	**Black Box Warning–Hepatotoxicity,** may be preceded by rash, ↑ eos or IgE. NB: no hepatotoxicity was noted in MVC trials. Black box inserted owing to concern about potential OCR6 class effect. Data lacking in hepatic/renal insufficiency. ↑ concern with either could ↑ risk of ↓BP. Currently for treatment-experienced patients with multi-resistant strains. **Document CCR-5-tropic virus before use, as treatment failures assoc. with appearance of CXCR-4 or mixed-tropic virus.**
6. Selected Characteristics of Integrase Inhibitors							
Raltegravir (Isentress)	400 mg film-coated tabs	400 mg bid, without regard to food	Unknown	~9	3	Glucuronidation via UGT1A1, with excretion into feces and urine. (Therefore does NOT require ritonavir boosting)	For both treatment naive patients and treatment experienced pts with multiply-resistant virus. Generally well-tolerated. Nausea, diarrhea, headache, fever similar to placebo. CK↑ & rhabdomyolysis reported, with unclear relationship to drug. Watch for increased depression in those with a history of depression. Low genetic barrier to resistance. Increase in CPK, myositis, rhabdomyolysis have been reported. Rare Stevens Johnson Syndrome.
Elvitegravir/cobicistat/FTC/TDF (Stribild)	150 mg ELV + 150 mg Cobi + 200 mg FTC + 300 mg TDF	one tab daily with or without food	<10%	12.9 (Cobi), 3.5 (ELV)	Un-known	The majority of **elvitegravir** metabolism is mediated by CYP3A enzymes. Elvitegravir also undergoes glucuronidation via UGT1A1/3 enzymes. **Cobicistat** is metabolized by CYP3A and to a minor extent by CYP2D6	For both treatment naive patients and treatment experienced pts with multiply-resistant virus. Generally well-tolerated. Use of cobicistat increases serum creatinine by ~ 0.1 mg/dl via inhibition of proximal tubular enzyme; this does not result in reduction in true GFR but will result in erroneous apparent reduction in eGFR by MDRD or Cockcroft Gault calculations. Usual AEs are similar to those observed with ritonavir (Cobi) and tenofovir/FTC. (*Letendre, et al, CROI 2010, abs #430*)

* CPE (CNS Penetration Effectiveness) value: 1 = Low Penetration; 2 - 3 = Intermediate Penetration; 4 = Highest Penetration into CNS

TABLE 14E- ANTIRETROVIRAL DRUGS & ADVERSE EFFECTS
(www.aidsinfo.nih.gov)

See also www.aidsinfo.nih.gov; for combinations, see individual components

DRUG NAME(S): GENERIC (TRADE)	MOST COMMON ADVERSE EFFECTS	MOST SIGNIFICANT ADVERSE EFFECTS
Nucleoside Reverse Transcriptase Inhibitors (NRTI) Black Box warning for all nucleoside/nucleotide RTIs: **lactic acidosis/hepatic steatosis, potentially fatal.** Also carry Warnings that fat redistribution and immune reconstitution syndromes (including autoimmune syndromes with delayed onset) have been observed		
Abacavir (Ziagen)	Headache 7–13%, nausea 7–19%, diarrhea 7%, malaise 7–12%	Black Box warning: **hypersensitivity reaction (HR)** in 8% with malaise, fever, GI upset, rash, lethargy & respiratory symptoms most commonly reported; myalgia, arthralgia, edema, paresthesia less common. **Discontinue immediately if HR suspected. Rechallenge contraindicated; may be life-threatening.** Severe HR may be more common with once-daily dosing. **HLA-B*5701 allele** predicts ↑ risk of HR in Caucasian pop.; excluding pts with B*5701 ↓'d HR incidence (*NEJM 358:568, 2008; CID 46:1111-1118, 2008*). DHHS guidelines recommend testing for B*5701 and use of abacavir-containing regimens only if HLA-B*5701 negative; Vigilance essential in all groups. Possible increased risk of MI with use of abacavir had been suggested (*JID 201:318, 2010*). Other studies found no increased risk of MI (*CID 52: 929, 2011*). A meta-analysis of randomized trials by FDA also did not show increased risk of MI factors when abacavir is used. (www.fda.gov/drugs/drugsafety/ucm245164.htm). Nevertheless, care is advised to optimize potentially modifiable risk
Didanosine (ddI) (Videx)	Diarrhea 28%, nausea 6%, rash 9%, headache 7%, fever 12%, hyperuricemia 2%	**Pancreatitis 1–9%**. Black Box warning—Cases of fatal & nonfatal pancreatitis have occurred in pts receiving ddI, especially when used in combination with d4T or d4T + hydroxyurea. Fatal lactic acidosis in pregnancy with ddI + d4T. Peripheral neuropathy in 20%, ↓ by dose reduction. ↑ toxicity if used with tenofovir. Use with TDF generally avoided but would require dose reduction of ddI because of ↑ toxicity and possible ↓ efficacy; may result in ↓CD4. Rarely, retinal changes or optic neuritis. Diabetes mellitus and rhabdomyolysis reported in post-marketing surveillance. Possible increased rate of MI under study (www.fda.gov/CDER; *JID 201:318, 2010*). Non-cirrhotic portal hypertension with ascites, varices, splenomegaly reported in post-marketing surveillance. See *Clin Infect Dis 49:626, 2009; Amer J Gastroenterol 104:1707, 2009*.
Emtricitabine (FTC) (Emtriva)	Well tolerated. Headache, diarrhea, nausea, rash, skin hyperpigmentation	Potential for lactic acidosis (as with other NRTIs). Also in Black Box warning—**severe exacerbation of hepatitis B on stopping drug reported—monitor clinical/labs for several months on stopping in pts with hepB.** Anti-HBV rx may be warranted if FTC stopped.
Lamivudine (3TC) (Epivir)	Well tolerated. Headache 35%, nausea 33%, diarrhea 18%, abdominal pain 9%, insomnia 11% (all in combination with ZDV). Pancreatitis more common in pediatrics.	Black Box warning. Make sure to use HIV dosage, not Hep B dosage. **Exacerbation of hepatitis B on stopping drug. Patients with hepB who stop lamivudine require close clinical/lab monitoring for several months.** Anti-HBV rx may be warranted if 3TC stopped.
Stavudine (d4T) (Zerit)	Diarrhea, nausea, vomiting, headache	**Peripheral neuropathy 15–20%.** Pancreatitis 1%. Appears to produce lactic acidosis, hepatic steatosis and lipoatrophy/lipodystrophy more commonly than other NRTIs. Black Box warning—**Fatal & nonfatal pancreatitis with d4T + ddI.** Use with TDF generally avoided (but would require dose reduction of ddI because of ↑ toxicity and possible ↓ efficacy; may result in ↓ CD4. Rarely, retinal changes or optic neuritis). Diabetes mellitus and rhabdomyolysis reported in post-marketing surveillance. **Fatal lactic acidosis/steatosis in pregnant women receiving d4T + ddI.** Use with caution and non-fatal lactic acidosis and severe hepatic steatosis can occur in others receiving d4T. Use with particular caution in patients with risk factors for liver disease, but lactic acidosis can occur even in those without known risk factors. Possible ↑ toxicity if used with ribavirin. Motor weakness in the setting of lactic acidosis mimicking the clinical presentation of Guillain-Barré syndrome (including respiratory failure). (rare)
Zidovudine (ZDV, AZT) (Retrovir)	Nausea 50%, anorexia 20%, vomiting 17%, **headache 62%**. Also reported: asthenia, insomnia, myalgias, nail pigmentation. Macrocytosis expected with all dosage regimens.	Black Box warning—**hematologic toxicity, myopathy. Anemia** (<8 gm, 1%), granulocytopenia (<750, 1.8%). Anemia may respond to epoetin alfa if endogenous serum erythropoietin levels are ≤500 milliUnits/mL. Possible ↑ toxicity if used with ribavirin. Co-administration with Ribavirin not advised. Hepatic decompensation may occur in HIV/HCV co-infected patients receiving zidovudine with interferon alfa ± ribavirin.

185

TABLE 14E (2)

DRUG NAME(S): GENERIC (TRADE)	MOST COMMON ADVERSE EFFECTS	MOST SIGNIFICANT ADVERSE EFFECTS
Nucleoside/Nucleotide Reverse Transcriptase Inhibitor (NRTI) Black Box warning for all nucleoside/nucleotide RTIs: lactic acidosis/hepatic steatosis, potentially fatal. Also carry Warnings that fat redistribution and immune reconstitution syndromes (including autoimmune syndromes with delayed onset) have been observed (continued)		
Tenofovir disoproxil fumarate (TDF) (Viread)	Diarrhea 11%, nausea 8%, vomiting 5%, flatulence 4% (generally well tolerated)	**Black Box Warning—Severe exacerbations of hepatitis B reported in pts who stop tenofovir.** Monitor carefully if drug is stopped, anti-HBV rx may be warranted if TDF stopped. Reports of renal injury from TDF, including Fanconi syndrome (CID (DF e174, 2003; JAIDS 35:269,204; CID 42:283, 2006). Fanconi syndrome and diabetes insipidus reported with TDF + ddl (AIDS Reader 19:114, 2009). Modest decline in renal function appears greater with TDF than with NRTIs (CID 51:1296, 2010) and may be greater in those receiving TDF with a PI instead of an NNRTI (JID 197:102, 2008; AIDS 26:567, 2012). In a VA study that followed >10,000 HIV-infected individuals, TDF exposure was significantly associated with increased risk of proteinuria, a more rapid decline in renal function and chronic kidney disease (AIDS 26:867, 2012). Monitor Ccr, serum phosphate and urinalysis, especially carefully in those with pre-existing renal dysfunction or nephrotoxic medications. TDF also appears to be associated with increased risk of bone loss. In a substudy of an ACTG comparative treatment trial, those randomized to TDF-FTC experienced greater decreases in spine and hip bone mineral density (BMD) at 96 weeks compared with those treated with ABC-3TC (JID 203:1791, 2011). Consider monitoring BMD in those with history of pathologic fractures, or who have risks for osteoporosis or bone loss.
Non-Nucleoside Reverse Transcriptase Inhibitors (NNRTI). Labels caution that fat redistribution and immune reconstitution can occur with ART.		
Delavirdine (Rescriptor)	Nausea, diarrhea, vomiting, headache	Skin rash has occurred in 18%, can continue or restart drug in most cases. Stevens-Johnson syndrome & erythema multiforme have been reported rarely. Elevation in liver enzymes in <5% of patients.
Efavirenz (Sustiva)	**CNS side effects 52%;** symptoms include dizziness, insomnia, somnolence, impaired concentration, psychiatric sx, & abnormal dreams; symptoms are worse after 1st or 2nd dose & improve over 2-4 weeks; discontinuation rate 2.6%. Rash 26% (vs. 17% in comparators), often improves with oral antihistamines, discontinuation rate 1.7%. Can cause false-positive urine test results for cannabinoid with CEDIA DAU multi-level THC assay. Metabolite can cause false-positive urine screening test for benzodiazepines (CID 48:1787, 2009).	**Caution:** CNS effects may impair driving and other hazardous activities. Serious neuropsychiatric symptoms reported, including severe depression (2.4%) & suicidal ideation (0.7%). Elevation in liver enzymes. Fulminant hepatic failure has been reported (see FDA label). **Teratogenicity reported in primates; pregnancy category D—may cause fetal harm,** avoid in pregnant women or those who might become pregnant. NOTE: No single method of contraception advised. Barrier + 2° method of contraception advised, continued 12 weeks after stopping efavirenz. Contraindicated with certain drugs metabolized by CYP3A4. Slow metabolism in those homozygous for the CYP-2B6 G516T allele can result in exaggerated toxicity and intolerance. This allele much more common in blacks and Asians (CID 42:408, 2006). Stevens-Johnson syndrome and erythema multiforme reported in post-marketing surveillance.
Etravirine (Intelence)		Severe rash (erythema multiforme, toxic epidermal necrolysis, Stevens-Johnson syndrome) has been reported. Hypersensitivity reactions can occur with rash, constitutional symptoms and organ dysfunction, including hepatic failure (see FDA label). Potential for CYP450-mediated drug interactions. Rhabdomyolysis has been reported in post-marketing surveillance.
Nevirapine (Viramune)	**Rash 37%:** usually occurs during 1st 6 wks of therapy. Follow recommendations for 14-day lead-in period to ↓ risk of rash (see Table 14D). Women experience 7-fold ↑ in risk of severe rash. CID 32:124, 2001. 50% resolve within 2 wks of dc drug; 80% by 1 month; 6.7% discontinuation rate.	Black Box warning: Severe life-threatening skin reactions reported: Stevens-Johnson syndrome, toxic epidermal necrolysis, & hypersensitivity reaction of drug rash with eosinophilia & systemic symptoms (DRESS) (AIM 161:2501, 2001). For severe rashes, dc drug immediately & do not restart. In a clinical trial, the use of prednisone ↑ the risk of rash. **Black Box warning—Life-threatening hepatotoxicity reported,** 2/3 during the first 12 wks of rx. Overall 1% develops hepatitis. Pts with pre-existing ↑ in ALT or AST &/or history of chronic Hep B or C↑ susceptible (Hepato 35:182, 2002). Women with CD4 > 250, including pregnant women, at ↑ risk. Avoid in this group unless no other option. Men with CD4 >400 also at ↑ risk. Monitor for pts intensively (clinical & LFTs), esp. during the first 12 wks of rx. If clinical hepatotoxicity, severe skin or hypersensitivity reactions occur, dc drug & never rechallenge.

TABLE 14E (3)

DRUG NAME(S): GENERIC (TRADE)	MOST COMMON ADVERSE EFFECTS (continued)	MOST SIGNIFICANT ADVERSE EFFECTS
Non-Nucleoside Reverse Transcriptase Inhibitors (NNRTI) (continued)		
Rilpivirine (Edurant)	Headache (3%), rash (3%; led to discontinuation in 0.1%), insomnia (3%), depressive disorders (4%). Psychiatric disorders led to discontinuation in 1%. Increased liver enzymes observed.	Drugs that induce CYP3A or increase gastric pH may decrease plasma concentration of rilpivirine and co-administration with rilpivirine should be avoided. Among these are certain anticonvulsants, rifamycins, PPIs, dexamethasone and St. John's wort. At supra-therapeutic doses, rilpivirine can increase QTc interval; use with caution with other drugs known to prolong QTc interval. May cause depression including suicide attempts or suicidal ideation. Overall, appears to cause fewer neuropsychiatric side effects than efavirenz (JAIDS 60:33, 2012).
Protease Inhibitors (PI)		

Abnormalities in glucose metabolism, dyslipidemias, fat redistribution syndromes are potential problems. Pts taking PI may be at increased risk for developing osteopenia/osteoporosis. Spontaneous bleeding episodes have been reported in HIV+ pts with hemophilia being treated with PIs. Rheumatic complications have been reported with use of PIs (An Rheum Dis 61:82, 2002). Potential of some PIs for QTc prolongation has been noted (Lancet 365:682, 2005). **Caution for all PIs**—Coadministration with certain drugs dependent on CYP3A or other enzymes for elimination & for which PI levels can cause serious toxicity may be contraindicated. As with other classes, rx may result in immune reconstitution syndromes, which may include early or late presentations of autoimmune syndromes. Taking into account both spontaneous and induced deliveries, a French cohort study demonstrated increased premature births among women receiving ritonavir-boosted PIs as compared with those receiving other antiretroviral therapy, even after accounting for other potential risk factors (CID 54:1348, 2012).

Atazanavir (Reyataz)	Asymptomatic unconjugated hyperbilirubinemia in up to 60% of pts, jaundice in 7-9% [especially in HIV pts with Gilbert syndrome (JID 192: 1381, 2005)]. Moderate to severe events: Diarrhea 1-3%, nausea 6-14%, abdominal pain 4%, headache 6%, rash 20%.	Prolongation of PR interval (1st degree AV block in 5-6%) reported; rarely 2° AV block. QTc increase and torsades reported (CID 44:e67, 2007). Acute interstitial nephritis (Am J Kid Dis 44:E81, 2004) and urolithiasis (atazanavir stones) reported (AIDS 20:2131, 2006; NEJM 355:2158, 2006). Potential ↑ transaminases in pts co-infected with HBV or HCV. Severe skin eruptions (Stevens-Johnson syndrome, erythema multiforme, and toxic eruptions, or DRESS syndrome) have been reported.
Darunavir (Prezista)	With background regimens, headache 15%, nausea 18%, diarrhea 20%, ↑ amylase 17%. Rash in 10% of treated; 0.5% discontinuation.	Hepatitis in 0.5%, some with fatal outcome. Use caution in pts with HBV or HCV co-infections or other hepatic dysfunction. Monitor for clinical symptoms and LFTs. Stevens-Johnson syndrome, toxic epidermal necrolysis, erythema multiforme. Contains sulfa moiety. Potential for hormonal contraceptive May cause failure of hormonal contraceptives.
Fosamprenavir (Lexiva)	Skin rash — 20% (moderate or worse in 3-8%), nausea, headache, diarrhea.	Rarely Stevens-Johnson syndrome, hemolytic anemia. Pro-drug of amprenavir. Contains sulfa moiety. Angioedema, and paresthesias, myocardial infarction and nephrolithiasis reported in post-marketing experience. Elevated LFTs seen with higher than recommended doses; increased risk in those with pre-existing liver abnormalities. Acute hemolytic anemia reported with amprenavir.
Indinavir (Crixivan)	↑ in indirect bilirubin 10-15% (≥ 2.5 mg/dl), with overt jaundice especially likely in those with Gilbert syndrome (JID 192: 1381, 2005). Nausea 12%, vomiting 4%, diarrhea 5%. Metallic taste. Paronychia and ingrown toenails reported (CID 32:140, 2001).	**Kidney stones.** Due to indinavir crystals in collecting system. Nephrolithiasis in 12% of adults, higher in pediatrics. Minimize risk with good hydration (at least 48 oz. water/day) (AAC 42:332, 1998). Tubulointerstitial nephritis/renal cortical atrophy reported in association with asymptomatic ↑ urine WBC. Severe hepatitis reported in 3 cases (Ln 349:924, 1997). Hemolytic anemia reported.
Lopinavir/Ritonavir (Kaletra)	GI: **diarrhea** 14-24%, nausea 2-16%. More diarrhea with q24h dosing.	Lipid abnormalities in up to 20-40%. Possible interaction of MI with cumulative exposure (JID 201:318, 2010). ↑ PR interval, 2° or 3° heart block described. Post-marketing reports of ↑ QTc and torsades: avoid use in congenital QTc prolongation or in other circumstances that prolong QTc or increase susceptibility to torsades. Hepatitis, with hepatic decompensation; caution especially in those with pre-existing liver disease. Pancreatitis. Inflammatory edema of legs reported (AIDS 16:673, 2002). Stevens-Johnson syndrome & erythema multiforme. Note high drug concentration in oral solution. Toxic potential of oral solution (contains ethanol and propylene glycol) in neonates.
Nelfinavir (Viracept)	Mild to moderate **diarrhea** 20%. Oat bran tabs, calcium, or oral anti-diarrheal agents (e.g., loperamide, diphenoxylate/atropine sulfate) can be used to manage diarrhea.	Potential for drug interactions. Powder contains phenylalanine.

TABLE 14E (4)

DRUG NAME(S): GENERIC (TRADE)	MOST COMMON ADVERSE EFFECTS	MOST SIGNIFICANT ADVERSE EFFECTS
Protease Inhibitors (PI) *(continued)*		
Ritonavir (Norvir) (Currently, primary use is to enhance levels of other anti-retrovirals, because of toxicity, interactions with full-dose ritonavir)	GI: bitter aftertaste ↓ by taking with chocolate milk, Ensure, or Advera. nausea 23%, ↓ by initial dose esc. (titration) regimen; vomiting 13%, diarrhea 15%. Circumoral paresthesias 5-6%. Dose >100 mg bid assoc. with ↑ GI side effects & ↑ in lipid abnormalities.	**Black Box** warning relates to many important drug-drug interactions—inhibits P450 CYP3A & CYP2 D6 system—may be life-threatening (see Table 22A). Several cases of iatrogenic Cushing's syndrome reported with concomitant use of ritonavir and corticosteroids, including dosing of the latter by inhalation, epidural injection, or IM injection. Rarely Stevens-Johnson syndrome, toxic epidermal necrolysis anaphylaxis. Primary A-V block (and higher) and pancreatitis have been reported. Hepatic reactions, including fatalities. Monitor LFTs carefully during therapy, especially in those with pre-existing liver disease, including HBV and HCV.
Saquinavir (Invirase) hard cap, tablet	**Diarrhea**, abdominal discomfort, nausea, headache	**Warning—Use Invirase only with ritonavir**. Avoid garlic capsules (may reduce SQV levels) and use cautiously with proton-pump inhibitors (increased SQV levels significant. Use of saquinavir/ritonavir can prolong QTc interval or may rarely cause 2° or 3° heart block; torsades reported. Contraindicated in patients with prolonged QTc or those taking drugs or who have other conditions (e.g., low K+ or Mg++) that pose a risk with prolonged QTc (http://www.fda.gov/drugs/DrugSafety/ucm230096.htm, accessed May 25, 2011). Contraindicated in patients with complete AV block, or those at risk, who do not have pacemaker. Hepatic toxicity encountered in patients with pre-existing liver disease or in individuals receiving concomitant rifampin. Rarely, Stevens-Johnson syndrome.
Tipranavir (Aptivus)	Nausea & vomiting, diarrhea, abdominal pain. Rash in 8-14%, more common in women. & 33% in women taking ethinyl estradiol. Major lipid effects.	**Black Box Warning—associated with hepatitis & fatal hepatic failure.** Risk of hepatotoxicity increased in hepB or hepC co-infection. Possible photosensitivity skin reactions. Contraindicated in Child-Pugh Class B or C hepatic impairment. **Associated with fatal/nonfatal intracranial hemorrhage (can inhibit platelet aggregation).** Caution in those with bleeding risks. Potential for major drug interactions. Contains sulfa moiety and vitamin E.
Fusion Inhibitor		
Enfuvirtide (T20, Fuzeon)	Local injection site reactions (98% at least 1 local ISR, 4% dc because of ISR) (pain & discomfort, induration, erythema, nodules & cysts, pruritus, & ecchymosis). ↑ Risk of URI, nausea 23%, fatigue 20%.	Rate of bacterial pneumonia (3.2 pneumonia events/100 pt yrs). **hypersensitivity reactions** <1% (rash, fever, nausea & vomiting, chills, rigors, hypotension, & ↑ serum liver transaminases); can occur with reexposure. Cutaneous amyloidosis deposits containing enfuvirtide peptide reported in skin plaques persisting after discontinuation of drug (*J Cutan Pathol 39:220, 2012*).
CCR5 Co-receptor Antagonists		
Maraviroc (Selzentry)	With ARV background: Cough 13%, fever 12%, rash 10%, abdominal pain 8%. Also, dizziness, myalgia, arthralgias. ↑ Risk of URI, HSV infection.	**Black box warning–Hepatotoxicity.** May be preceded by allergic features (rash, ↑ eosinophils or ↑ IgE levels). Use with caution in pt with HepB or C. Cardiac ischemia/infarction in 1.3%. May cause ↓BP, orthostatic syncope, especially in patients with renal dysfunction. Significant interactions with CYP3A inducers/inhibitors. Long-term risk of malignancy unknown. Stevens-Johnson syndrome reported post-marketing. Generally favorable safety profile during trial of ART-naive individuals (*JID 201: 803, 2010*).
Integrase Inhibitors		
Raltegravir (Isentress)	Diarrhea, headache, insomnia, nausea. LFT ↑ may be more common in pts co-infected with HBV or HCV.	Hypersensitivity reactions can occur. Rash, Stevens-Johnson syndrome, toxic epidermal necrolysis reported. Hepatic failure reported. ↑CK, myopathy and rhabdomyolysis reported (*AIDS 22:1382, 2008*). ↑ of preexisting depression reported in 4 pts; all could continue raltegravir after adjustment of psych. meds (*AIDS 22:1890, 2008*). Chewable tablets contain phenylalanine.
Elvitegravir (Stribild)	Nausea and diarrhea are the two most common AEs. An increase in serum creatinine of 0.1 - 0.15 mg/dl with use of cobicistat (related to inhibition of prox. tubular enzymes, not a true reduction in GFR).	Same Black Box warnings as ritonavir and tenofovir. Rare lactic acidosis syndrome. Owing to renal toxicity, should not initiate Rx when pre-Rx eGFR is < 70 cc/min. Follow serial serum creatinine and urinary protein and glucose. Discontinue drug if serum Cr rises > 0.4 mg/dl above baseline value.

TABLE 14F– HEPATITIS A & HBV TREATMENT

Hepatitis A *(Ln 351:1643, 1998)*

1. **Drug/Dosage:** No therapy recommended. If within 2 wks of exposure, IVIG 0.02 mL per kg IM times 1 protective. Hep A vaccine equally effective as IVIG in randomized trial and is emerging as preferred Rx *(NEJM 357:1685, 2007)*.
2. **Side Effects/Comments:** 40% of pts with chronic Hep C who developed superinfection with Hep A developed fulminant hepatic failure *(NEJM 338:286, 1998)*.

HBV Treatment

When to Treat HBV

HBeAg status	HBV DNA: "viral load"	ALT	Fibrosis*	Treatment** IFN = interferon; NUC = nucleoside/tide analogue	Comments
+	> 20,000	< 2xULN	F0–F2	Observe	Low efficacy with current Rx; biopsy helpful in determining whether to Rx. Lean toward Rx if older age or + Family Hx HCC
+	> 20,000	< 2x ULN	F3-F4	Treat: IFN or NUC	**No IFN if decompensated cirrhosis**
+	>20,000	> 2x ULN	Any	Treat: IFN or NUC	INF has higher chance of seroconversion to HBeAg Negative and HBsAg Negative status.
-	< 2000	< 1xULN	Any	Observe	Might Treat if F4; **No IFN if decompensated cirrhosis.**
-	2000-20,000	< 2x ULN	F0 – F2	Observe	
-	2000-20,000	< 2x ULN	F3 – F4	Treat: NUC or (IFN)	NUCs favored if HBeAg negative; Treatment duration ill-defined. Certainly > 1 year, likely chronic Rx (indefinitely)
-	> 20,000	> 2xULN	Any	Treat: NUC or IFN	NUCs favored if HBeAg negative; Treatment duration chronic / indefinite

Modified from *AASLD HBV Treatment Guidelines* (www.aasld.org); Lok/ McMahon, Hepatology .2009; 50. p. 1-36
* Liver Biopsy or fibrosure assay is helpful in determining when and how to treat
** Treatment options listed below

Treatment Regimens. Single drug therapy is usually sufficient; combination therapy used with HIV co-infection.

	Drug/Dose	Comments
Preferred Regimens	**Pegylated-Interferon-alpha 2a** 180 µg sc once weekly OR **Entecavir** 0.5 mg po once daily OR **Tenofovir** 300 mg po once daily	PEG-IFN: Treat for 48 weeks Entecavir: Do not use Entecavir if Lamivudine resistance present. Entecavir/Tenofovir: Treat for at least 24-48 weeks after seroconversion from HBeAg to anti-HBe. Indefinite chronic therapy for HBeAg negative patients. Renal impairment dose adjustments necessary.
Alternative Regimens	**Lamivudine** 100 mg po once daily OR **Telbivudine** 600 mg po once daily OR **Emtricitabine** 200 mg po once daily (investigational) OR **Adefovir** 10 mg po once daily	These alternative agents are rarely used except in combination. When used, restrict to short term therapy owing to high rates of development of resistance. Not recommended as first-line therapy. Use of Adefovir has mostly been replaced by Tenofovir.
Preferred Regimen for HIV-HBV Co-Infected Patient	**Truvada** (Tenofovir 300 mg + Emtricitabine 200 mg) po once daily + another anti-HIV drug	ALL patients if possible as part of a fully suppressive anti-HIV/anti-HBV regimen. Continue therapy indefinitely.

TABLE 14G– HCV TREATMENT REGIMENS AND RESPONSE

1. **Hepatitis C (HCV) Treatment Setting.** Indications for treatment of HCV must take into account both relative and absolute contraindications. Response to therapy reflects defined terms. Duration of therapy is response guided based on Genotype. Recommended follow-up during and post-treatment.
2. **Indications for Treatment.** Assuming use of Pegylated Interferon (Peg-IFN) + Ribavirin in the regimen: motivated patient, acute HCV infection, biopsy: chronic hepatitis and significant fibrosis, cryoglobulinemic vasculitis, cryoglobulinemic glomerulonephritis, stable HIV infection, compensated liver disease, acceptable hematologic parameters, creatinine < 1.5 (GFR > 50).

TABLE 14G (2)

3. **Contraindications for Treatment.** Contraindications (both relative and absolute) also assume use of Pegylated Interferon (Peg-IFN) + Ribavirin in the regimen.
   a. **Relative Contraindications.** Hgb < 10, ANC < 1000, PTLs < 50K, hemodialysis and/or GFR < 50, active substance and alcohol use, anticipated poor compliance, untreated mental health disorder, e.g. depression, stable auto-immune disease, Thalassemia and sickle cell anemia, sarcoidosis, HIV co-infection (CD4 < 200, concurrent zidovudine)
   b. **Absolute Contraindications.** Uncontrolled, active, major psychiatric illness, especially depression; hepatic decompensation (encephalopathy, coagulopathy, ascites); severe uncontrolled medical disease (DM, CHF, CAD, HTN, TB, cancer); untreated thyroid disease; pregnancy, nursing, child-bearing potential (anticipated pregnancy, no birth control); active untreated autoimmune disease; HIV co-infection (CD4 < 100, concurrent ddI)

4. **Response to Therapy.** Predictors of successful response to therapy include: recent infection with HCV, Genotype 2 or 3 infection, favorable IL-28B haplotype, less severe liver disease on biopsy, HCV viral load < 800,000.

5. **Definitions of Response to Therapy.**

Null	Failure to decrease HCV VL by >2 log at week 12.
Non-Responder	Failure to clear HCV RNA by week 24.
Partial Response	>2 log ↓ HIV RNA by week 12 but not undetectable at week 24.
Early Virologic Response (EVR)	>2 log ↓ at week 12 and undetectable at week 24; **Complete EVR =** undetectable at both week 12 and 24.
Rapid Virologic Response (RVR)	Undetectable by week 4 and sustained through course of Rx
Extended Rapid Virologic Response (eRVR)	New terminology with Direct Acting Agents (DAAs). Undetectable after 4 weeks of DAA treatment (e.g., week 4 for telaprevir or week 8 for boceprevir), with sustained undetectable HCV RNA at weeks 12 and 24.
End of Treatment Response (ETR)	Undetectable at end of treatment.
Relapse	Undetectable at end of therapy (ETR) but rebound (detectable) virus within 24 weeks after therapy stopped.
Sustained Virologic Response (SVR)	CURE! Still undetectable at end of therapy and beyond 24 weeks after therapy is stopped.

6. **HCV Treatment Regimens**
   - Biopsy is a 'gold standard' for staging HCV infection and is helpful in some settings to determine the ideal timing of HCV treatment. When bx not obtained, "non-invasive" tests are often employed to assess the relative probability of advanced fibrosis or cirrhosis.
   - Resistance tests: Genotypic resistance assays are available that can determine polymorphisms associated with reduction in susceptibility to some DAAs (Direct Acting Agents, e.g., protease inhibitors). **However, resistance tests are not routinely recommended in pts naive to Rx and are reserved for selective use in patients who have received treatment previously unsuccessful treatment with a DAA.**
   - **IMPORTANT NOTE REGARDING TREATMENT DECISION-MAKING:** Newer drugs are in development. **Emerging data suggest a high probability that newer regimens that spare the use of pegylated Interferon (peg-IFN) and/or Ribavirin (RBV) will be successful and available in the next 1-2 years (or sooner).** Therefore, the timing of the decision to initiate HCV therapy needs to be individualized based on: the patients current clinical status, the viral genotype, the pt's ability to tolerate peg-IFN/RBV based therapies, and the likelihood of disease progression over the next 5 years while newer treatments are developed. The Ultimate Goal for treatment of HCV: no Interferon or Ribavirin, only Direct Acting Agents (DAA).

Genotype	Regimen
All	• Either **Pegylated Interferon (PEG-IFN) alfa 2a** (Pegasys) 180 mcg SQ weekly OR • **PEG-IFN Alfa 2b** (PEG-Intron) 1.5 mcg/kg SQ weekly
	PLUS
2, 3	• **Ribavirin** 400 mg bid (if using response guided Rx, dose Ribavirin as for Genotype 1, 4)
1, 4	• **Ribavirin** 600 mg bid (wt > 75 kg) OR • **Ribavirin** 400 mg qAM + 600 mg qPM (wt < 75 kg)
	PLUS

1 Only	• **Telaprevir** (Incivek) 750 mg (2 tabs) po tid (with food–not low fat) for 12 wks only
	  ▪ Start immediately with PEG-IFN + Ribavirin at recommended doses
	  ▪ Must stop Telaprevir at week 12 and continue PEG-IFN + Ribavirin for remainder of duration of therapy

	OR

1 Only	• **Boceprevir** (Victrelis) 800 mg (4 caps) po tid (with food–meal or light snack)
	  ▪ Start 4 weeks after starting PEG-IFN + Ribavirin at recommended doses
	  ▪ Continue along with PEG-IFN + Ribavirin for full duration of therapy

WARNINGS:	• Never use Telaprevir or Boceprevir as monotherapy • Never Dose Reduce Either Telaprevir or Boceprevir • Never Combine Telaprevir or Boceprevir • Never use either drug in sequence owing to shared resistance profiles

TABLE 14G (3)

7. **Duration of HCV Therapy.** Predictors of SVR: *CID 56:118, 2013*.

Genotype	Response Guided Therapy

2, 3	• If RVR: Treat for 16-24 weeks of total therapy*
	  ▪ Check for SVR at week 40 or 48 depending on duration of therapy (16 or 24 weeks)
	• If EVR: Treat for 24 weeks of total therapy
	  ▪ Check for SVR at week 48
	• If Partial or Null Response: Discontinue therapy at week 12 (treatment failure)

4	• If eRVR or EVR: Treat for 48 weeks of total therapy ▪ Check for SVR at week 72 • If Partial or Null Response: Discontinue at weeks 24 and 12, respectively.

1**	• If eRVR: Continue therapy for 24 weeks (28 for boceprevir)
	  ▪ Check for SVR at week 48 (week 52 for boceprevir)
	• IF EVR: Continue therapy for 48 weeks
	  ▪ Check for SVR at week 72
	• If Null, Partial Response, or **NOT complete EVR:** Discontinue therapy at week 12 therapy at week 12

* Similar SVR rates for 16 vs. 24 wks but higher relapse with 16 wks of therapy. Re-treatment in such settings usually results in SVR with longer (24 wks) duration.

** Assuming use of Direct Acting Agents (DAA), e.g., Telaprevir or Boceprevir. If DAAs are not being used, treatment duration is the same as for Genotype 4.

TABLE 15A – ANTIMICROBIAL PROPHYLAXIS FOR SELECTED BACTERIAL INFECTIONS*

CLASS OF ETIOLOGIC AGENT/DISEASE/CONDITION	PROPHYLAXIS AGENT/DOSE/ROUTE/DURATION	COMMENTS
Group B streptococcal disease (GBS), neonatal: Approaches to management [CDC Guidelines, *MMWR* 59 *(RR-10):1, 2010]:*		

Pregnant women—intrapartum antimicrobial prophylaxis procedures:
1. Screen all pregnant women with vaginal & rectal swab for GBS at 35–37 wks gestation (unless other indications for prophylaxis exist: GBS bacteriuria during this pregnancy or previously delivered infant with invasive GBS disease, even when cultures may be useful for susceptibility testing). Use transport medium; GBS survive at room temp. up to 96 hrs. **Rx during labor if swab culture positive.**
2. Rx during labor if previously delivered infant with invasive GBS infection, or if any GBS bacteriuria during this pregnancy.
3. Rx if GBS status unknown but if any of the following are present: (a) delivery at <37 wks gestation [see *MMWR* 59 *(RR-10):1, 2010* algorithms for preterm labor and preterm premature rupture of membranes]; or (b) duration of ruptured membranes ≥18 hrs; or (c) intrapartum temp. ≥100.4°F (≥38.0°C). If amnionitis suspected, broad-spectrum antibiotic coverage should include an agent active vs. group b streptococci.
4. Rx if positive intra-partum NAAT for GBS.
5. Rx not indicated if: negative vaginal/rectal cultures at 35–37 wks gestation or C-section performed before onset of labor with intact amniotic membranes (use standard surgical prophylaxis).
	Regimens for prophylaxis against early-onset group B streptococcal disease in neonate used during labor:
	Penicillin G 5 million Units IV (initial dose) then 2.5 to 3 million Units IV q4h until delivery
	Alternative: **Ampicillin** 2 gm IV (initial dose) then 1 gm IV q4h until delivery
	Penicillin-allergic patient:
	• Patient not at high risk for anaphylaxis from β-lactams: **Cefazolin** 2 gm IV (initial dose) then 1 gm IV q8h until delivery
	• Patient at high risk for anaphylaxis from β-lactams:
	  ◻ If organism is both clindamycin- and erythromycin-susceptible, **or** is erythromycin-resistant, but clindamycin-susceptible confirmed by D-zone test (or equivalent) showing lack of inducible resistance: **Clindamycin** 900 mg IV q8h until delivery
	  ◻ If susceptibility of organism unknown, lack of inducible resistance to clindamycin has not been excluded, or patient is allergic to clindamycin: **Vancomycin** 1 gm IV q12h until delivery.	

Neonate of mother given prophylaxis		
Preterm, premature rupture of the membranes in Group B strep-negative women	(IV **ampicillin** 2 gm q6h + IV **erythromycin** 250 mg q6h) for 48 hrs followed by po **amoxicillin** 250 mg + po **erythromycin** base 333 mg q8h for 5 days. Decreases infant morbidity. (*JAMA* 278:989, 1997) (*Note:* May require additional antibiotics for therapy of specific existing infections)	Antibiotic rx reduced infant respiratory distress syndrome (50.6% to 40.8%, p = 0.03), necrotizing enterocolitis (5.8% to 2.3%, p = 0.03) and prolonged pregnancy (2.9 to 6.1 days. In 1 large study (4809 pts), po erythromycin rx improved neonatal outcomes vs placebo (11.2% vs 14.4% composite score, p = 0.02 single births) but no co-AM-CL or both + tags in contrast to drugs in controlled assoc. with necrotizing enterocolitis) (*Ln* 357:979, 2001). (See ACOG discussion, *Ob Gyn* 102:875, 2003; *Practice Bulletin* in *Ob Gyn* 109:1007, 2007; *Rev Obstet Gynecol Can* 31:863 & 868, 2009).
Post-splenectomy bacteremia. Likely agents: Pneumococci (90%), meningococci, H. influenzae type b. Bacteremia due to Enterobacteriaceae, S. aureus, Capnocytophaga spp. and rarely P. aeruginosa described. Also at ↑ risk for fatal malaria, severe babesiosis. Ref: *Redbook Online, 2009. Amer Acad Pediatrics.*	**Immunizations:** Ensure admin. of pneumococcal vaccine, H. influenzae B, & quadrivalent meningococcal vaccines at recommended times. In addition, asplenic children with sickle cell anemia, thalassemia, & perhaps others, daily antimicrobial prophylaxis until at least age 5—see Comments and *Redbook Online, 2009*. Sepsis due to susceptible organisms may occur despite daily prophylaxis (*J Clin Path* 54:214, 2001).	Antimicrobial prophylaxis until age 5: **Amox.** 20 mg/kg/day or Pen V-K 125 mg bid. Over age 5: Consider Pen V-K 250 mg bid for at least 1 yr in children post-splenectomy. Some recommend prophylaxis for a minimum of 3 yrs or until at least age 18. Maintain immunizations plus self-administered AM-CL with any febrile illness while seeking physician assistance for self-administered therapy, other oral alternatives if penicillin-allergic, oral cephalosporins; alternatively, respiratory FQ can be considered in beta lactam-allergic pt in appropriate situations. Pen. allergy: TMP-SMX, or clarithro are options, but resistance in *S. pneumo* may be significant in some areas, particularly among pen-resistant isolates.

TABLE 15A (2)

CLASS OF ETIOLOGIC AGENT/DISEASE/CONDITION	PROPHYLAXIS AGENT/DOSE/ROUTE/DURATION	COMMENTS
Sexual Exposure Sexual assault survivor [likely agents and risks, see *MMWR* 59 (RR-12):1, 2010]. For review of overall care: *NEJM* 365:834, 2011.	[(**Ceftriaxone** 250 mg IM) + (**Metronidazole** 2 gm po as single dose) + [(**Azithromycin** 1 gm po once) or (**Doxycycline** 100 mg po bid for 7 days)]	• Obtain expert advice re: forensic exam & specimens, pregnancy, physical trauma, psychological support. • Test for gonococci and chlamydia (NAAT) at appropriate sites. Check wet mount for T. vaginalis (and culture), check specimen for bacterial vaginosis and Candida if appropriate. • Serologic evaluation for syphilis, HIV, HBV; HCV not easily transmitted from sexual activity, but consider test in high-risk circumstances (*MMWR* 60:945, 2011). • Initiate post-exposure protocols for HBV vaccine, HIV post-exposure prophylaxis as appropriate (see Table 15D). • Follow-up exam for STDs in 1-2 weeks; retest if prophylaxis not given initially or if symptomatic. • Follow-up serologies for syphilis, HIV, HBV (and HCV if done) at 6 wks, 3 mos and 6 mos. **Notes:** Ceftriaxone is preferred over cefixime for treatment of gonorrhoea; the latter is less effective for pharyngeal infection and strains with decreased susceptibility to cephalosporins are beginning to appear; those with decreased susceptibility to cefixime are more prevalent than those with decreased susceptibility to ceftriaxone (*MMWR* 60:873, 2011). Cefixime 400 mg po once can be used in place of ceftriaxone, if the latter is unavailable (*Derived from CDC STD treatment update MMWR* 61:590, 2012). Azithromycin is preferred to doxycycline because it also provides activity against some GC with reduced susceptibility to cephalosporins, azithromycin 2 gm po once can be used in place of ceftriaxone.
Contact with specific sexually transmitted diseases	See comprehensive guidelines for specific pathogens in *MMWR* 59 (RR-10):1, 2010.	
Syphilis exposure		Presumptive rx for exposure within 3 mos., as tests may be negative. See Table 1, page 24. If exposure occurred > 90 days prior, establish dx or treat empirically (*MMWR* 59 (RR-12):1, 2010).
Sickle-cell disease. Likely agent: S. pneumoniae (see post-splenectomy, page 170). Ref.: 2009 Red Book Online, Amer Acad Pediatrics	Children <5 yrs: **Penicillin V** 125 mg po bid ≥5 yrs: **Penicillin V** 250 mg po bid. (Alternative in children: Amoxicillin 20 mg per kg per day)	Start prophylaxis by 2 mos. (*Pediatrics* 106:367, 2000); continue until at least age 5. When to d/c must be individualized. Age-appropriate vaccines, including pneumococcal, Hib, influenza, meningococcal. Treating infections, consider possibility of penicillin non-susceptible pneumococci.

TABLE 15B – ANTIBIOTIC PROPHYLAXIS TO PREVENT SURGICAL SITE INFECTIONS IN ADULTS*
(*CID* 38:1706, 2004; *Am J Surg* 189:395, 2005; *Med Lett* 10:73, 2012)

General Comments:
- To be maximally effective, antibiotics must be started within 2 hrs before surgical incision (*NEJM* 326:281, 1992), preferably ≤ 1 hr before incision for most agents except vancomycin and quinolones (*JAC* 58:645, 2006; *CID* 38:1706, 2004).
- Most applications employ a single preoperative dose (*Treat Guide Med Lett* 7:47, 2009).
- For procedures lasting > 2 half-lives of prophylactic agent, intraoperative dose(s) may be required (see *CID* 38:1706, 2004 for schedule).
- Standard regimens may give relatively low tissue levels in pts with high BMI, but implications of this are not clear (see *Surgery* 136:738, 2004 for cefazolin; *Eur J Clin Pharm* 54:632, 1998 for vancomycin; *CID* 38:1706, 2004 for wt-based dosing).
- In most cases, prophylaxis is not extended beyond 24 hrs (*CID* 38:1706, 2004).
- Prolonging does can ↑ risk, e.g., C. difficile colitis (*CID* 46:1838, 2008).
- Active screening for S. aureus nasal colonization and application of chlorhexidine washes and intranasal mupirocin has been reported as a strategy that decreases surgical site infection in an area of low MRSA prevalence (*NEJM* 362:9, 2010). Avoid contact of chlorhexidine soap with eyes.

Use of Vancomycin:
- For many common prophylaxis indications, vancomycin is considered an alternative to β-lactams in pts allergic to or intolerant of the latter.
- Vancomycin use may be justifiable in centers where rates of post-operative infection with methicillin-resistant staphylococci are high or in pts at high risk for these.

TABLE 15B (2)

- Unlike β-lactams in common use, vancomycin has no activity against gram-negative organisms. **When gram-negative bacteria are a concern following specific procedures, it may be necessary or desirable to add a second agent with appropriate in vitro activity.** This can be done using cefazolin with vancomycin in the non-allergic pt, or to pts intolerant of β-lactams using vancomycin with another gram-negative agent (e.g., aminoglycoside, fluoroquinolone, possibly aztreonam; if not allergic; local resistance patterns and pt factors would influence choice).
- Infusion of vancomycin, especially too rapidly, may result in hypotension or other manifestations of histamine release syndrome (J Cardiothor Vasc Anesth 5:574, 1991).

TYPE OF SURGERY	PROPHYLAXIS	COMMENTS
Cardiovascular Surgery Antibiotic prophylaxis in cardiovascular surgery has been proven beneficial in the following procedures: • Reconstruction of abdominal aorta • Procedures on the leg that involve a groin incision • Any vascular procedure that inserts prosthesis/foreign body • Lower extremity amputation for ischemia • Cardiac surgery • Permanent Pacemakers (Circulation 121:458, 2010)	**Cefazolin** 1-2 gm IV as a single dose or q8h for 1-2 days or **cefuroxime** 1.5 gm IV as a single dose or q12h for total of 6 gm or **vancomycin** 1 gm IV as single dose or q12h for 1-2 days. For pts weighing > 90 kg, use vanco 1.5 gm IV as a single dose or q12h for 1-2 days. Consider **intranasal mupirocin** evening before, day of surgery & bid for 5 days post-op in pts with pos. nasal culture for S. aureus. Mupirocin resistance has been encountered (CID 49:935, 2009).	Single infusion just before surgery probably as effective as multiple doses. Not needed for cardiac catheterization. For prosthetic heart valves, customary to stop prophylaxis either after removal of retrosternal drainage catheters or just a 2nd dose after coming off bypass. Vancomycin may be preferable in hospitals with ↑ freq of MRSA or in high-risk pts (CID 38: 1555, 2004), or those colonized with MRSA (CID 38:1706, 2004); however, does not give gm-neg. bacilli, therefore would add cefazolin. Meta-analysis failed to demonstrate overall superiority of vancomycin over β-lactam prophylaxis for cardiac surgery (CID 38: 1357, 2004). Intranasal mupirocin ↓ sternal wound infections from S. aureus in 1950 pts; used historical controls (An Thor Surg 71:1572, 2001). In another trial, it ↓ nosocomial S. aureus infections only in nasal carriers (NEJM 346:1871, 2002). One study of 0.12% chlorhexidine gluconate gel to naris and oral rinse showed ↓ deep surg site and lower resp infections (JAMA 296:2460, 2006).
Gastric, Biliary and Colonic Surgery **Gastroduodenal/Biliary** Gastroduodenal, includes percutaneous endoscopic gastrostomy (high-risk only; see Comments).	**Cefazolin** (1-2 gm IV) or **cefoxitin** (1-2 gm IV) or **cefotetan** (1-2 gm IV) or **cefuroxime** (1.5 gm IV) as a single dose (some give additional doses q12h for 2-3 days).	Gastroduodenal: High-risk includes marked obesity, obstruction, ↓ gastric acid or ↓ motility. Meta-analysis supports use in percutaneous endoscopic gastrostomy (Am J Gastro 95:3133, 2000).
Biliary, includes laparoscopic cholecystectomy (high-risk only; see Comments).	No rx without obstruction. If obstruction: **Ciprofloxacin** 500-750 mg po 2 hrs prior to procedure or **PIP-TZ** 4.5 gm IV 1 hr prior to procedure	Biliary high-risk: age >70, acute cholecystitis, non-functioning gallbladder, obstructive jaundice or common duct stones. With cholangitis, treat as infection, not prophylaxis (See Table 1, page 17). For guidelines of American Soc of Gastrointestinal Endoscopy, see Gastroint Endosc 67:791, 2008).
Endoscopic retrograde cholangiopancreatography Controversial: No benefit from single dose piperacillin in randomized placebo-controlled trial. AJHM 125:442, 1996		Most studies show that **achieving adequate drainage** will prevent post-procedural cholangitis or sepsis and no further benefit from prophylactic antibiotics; greatest benefit likely when complete drainage cannot be achieved. Meta-analysis suggested antibiotics may ↓ bacteremia, but not sepsis/cholangitis (Endoscopy 31:718, 1999). Oral flora (strep, enterococci) in 2 studies & less expensive but quinolone resistance increasing (CID 23:380, 1996). See Table 1, page 17, and Amer Soc Gastroint Endosc recommendations.
Colorectal	Oral antibiotics for elective surgery (see Comments) **Parenteral regimens** (emergency or elective): [**Cefazolin** 1-2 gm IV + **metronidazole** 0.5 gm IV (see Comment)] or **cefoxitin** or **cefotetan** 1-2 gm IV (if available) or **AM-SB** 3 gm IV or **ERTA** 1 gm IV (NEJM 355:2640, 2006 study found ertapenem more effective than cefotetan, but associated with non-significant ↑ risk of C. difficile)	Oral regimens: **Neomycin** + **erythromycin**. Pre-op day. (1) 10 am 4L polyethylene glycol electrolyte solution (Colyte, GoLYTELY) po over 2 hr. (2) Clear liquid diet only. (3) 1 pm, 2 pm & 11 pm, neomycin 1 gm + erythro base 1 gm po & 11 pm. NPO after midnight. Alternative regimens have been less well studied: GoLYTELY 1-6 pm, then neomycin 2 gm po + metronidazole 2 gm po at 7 pm & 11 pm. Oral regimen as effective as parenteral; parenteral in addition to oral not required but often used (Am J Surg 189:395, 2005). Many used both parenteral + oral regimens for elective procedures (Am J Surg 189:395, 2005), but recent ↓ enthusiasm for mechanical bowel preparation. Meta-analysis did not support mech bowel prep in preventing anastomotic leaks with elective colorectal surg (Coch Database Syst Rev 1:CD001544, 2009). Cefazolin dosing: Some experts recommend 2 gm for all and 3 gm if patient weight > 120 kg. Repeat dose 4 hours after 1st dose if patient still in surgery

Ruptured viscus: See Peritoneum/Peritonitis, Secondary; Table 1, page 47.

TABLE 15B (3)

TYPE OF SURGERY	PROPHYLAXIS	COMMENTS
Head and Neck Surgery (Ann Otol Rhinol Laryngol 101 Suppl: 16, 1992)		
Cefazolin 2 gm IV (Single dose) (some add **metronidazole** 500 mg IV (Treat Guide Med Lett 7:47, 2009)) OR **Clindamycin** 600–900 mg IV (single dose) ± **gentamicin** 1.5 mg/kg IV (single dose) (See Table 10D for weight-based dose calculation).		Antimicrobial prophylaxis in head & neck surg appears efficacious only for procedures involving oral/pharyngeal mucosa (e.g., laryngeal or pharyngeal tumor) but even with prophylaxis, wound infection rate can be high (Head Neck 23:447, 2001). Uncontaminated head & neck surg does not require prophylaxis.
Neurosurgical Procedures [Prophylaxis not effective in 1 infection rate with intracranial pressure monitors in retrospective analysis of 215 pts (J Neurol Neurosurg Psych 69:381, 2000)]		
Clean, non-implant; e.g., craniotomy	**Cefazolin** 1–2 gm IV once. Alternative: **vanco** 1 gm IV once; for pts weighing > 90 kg, use vanco 1.5 gm IV as single dose. **Clindamycin** 900 mg IV (single dose)	Reference: Ln 344:1547, 1994
Clean, contaminated (cross sinuses, or naso/oropharynx)	**Clindamycin** 900 mg IV (single dose)	British recommend amoxicillin-clavulanate 1.2 gm IV[a,b] or metronidazole 0.5 gm IV.
CSF shunt surgery	**Cefazolin** 1–2 gm IV once. Alternative: **vanco** 1 gm IV once; for pts weighing > 90 kg, use vanco 1.5 gm IV as single dose.	Meta-analysis suggests benefit (Cochrane Database 3: CD 005365). Randomized study in a hospital with high prevalence of infection due to methicillin-resistant staphylococci showed vancomycin was more effective than cefazolin in preventing CSF shunt infections (J Hosp Infect 69:337, 2008).
Obstetric/Gynecologic Surgery (See ACOG Practice Bulletin in Obstet & Gyn 113:1180, 2009 for additional procedures and alternatives).		
Vaginal or abdominal hysterectomy	**Cefazolin** 1–2 gm or **cefoxitin** 1–2 gm or **cefotetan** 1–2 gm or **cefuroxime** 1.5 gm all IV 30 min. before surgery.	1 study found cefotetan superior to cefazolin (CID 20:677, 1995). For prolonged procedures, doses can be repeated q4–8h for duration of procedure. Ampicillin-sulbactam is considered an acceptable alternative (CID 43:322, 2006). Treat pts with bacterial vaginosis pre-op.
Cesarean section for premature rupture of membranes or active labor	**Cefazolin** 1–2 gm IV. (See Comments).	Prophylaxis decreases risk of endometritis and wound infection. Traditional approach had been to administer antibiotics after cord is clamped to avoid exposing infant to antibiotic. However, recent studies suggest that administering prophylaxis before the skin incision results in fewer surgical site infections (Obstet Gynecol 115:1787, 2010; Amer J Obstet Gynecol 199:301.e1 and 310.e1, 2008) and endometritis (Amer J Obstet Gynecol 196:455.e1, 2007). Meta-analysis showed benefit of antibiotic prophylaxis in all risk groups. (Ob Gyn 87:884, 1996).
Surgical Abortion (1st trimester)	1st trimester: **Doxycycline** 300 mg po, as 100 mg 1 hr before procedure + 200 mg post-procedure.	One regimen was doxy 100 mg orally 1 hr before procedure, then 200 mg after procedure (CID 38:1706, 2004).
Orthopedic Surgery		
Hip arthroplasty, spinal fusion	Same as cardiac	Customarily stopped after "Hemovac" removed. NSIPP workgroup recommends stopping prophylaxis within 24 hrs of surgery (CID 38:1706, 2004).
Total joint replacement (other than hip)	**Cefazolin** 1–2 gm IV pre-op (± 2nd dose) or **vancomycin** 1 gm IV. For pts weighing > 90 kg, use vanco 1.5 gm IV as single dose.	NSIPP workgroup recommends stopping prophylaxis within 24 hrs of surgery (CID 38:1706, 2004). Usual to administer before tourniquet inflation, but a recent study in total knee arthroplasty found dosing ceftriaxone 1.5 gm (just prior to tourniquet release (+ 2nd dose 6 hr after surgery) was not inferior to dosing before inflation (+ 2nd dose) (CID 46:1009, 2008).
Open reduction of closed fracture with internal fixation	**Ceftriaxone** 2 gm IV or IM once	3.6% (ceftriaxone) vs 8.3% (for placebo) infection found in Dutch trauma trial (Ln 347:1133, 1996). Several alternative antimicrobials can ↓ risk of infection (Cochrane Database Syst Rev 2010: CD 000244).

195

TABLE 15B (4)

TYPE OF SURGERY	PROPHYLAXIS	COMMENTS
Prophylaxis to protect prosthetic joints from hematogenous infection related to distant procedures (patients with plates, pins and screws only are not considered to be at risk)		• In 2003, the American Academy of Orthopedic Surgeons (AAOS), in conjunction with the American Dental Association and the American Urological Association, developed *Advisory Statements* on the use of antibiotic prophylaxis to prevent infection of implanted joint prostheses for procedures that may cause bacteremia. (*J Am Dental Assn 134:895, 2003; J Urol 169:1796, 2003*). These documents stratified procedures for risk of bacteremia, described patient factors that might place joints at ↑ risk of infection (incl. all pts in first 2 years after insertion), and offered antibiotic options. (See also *Med Lett 47:59, 2005* and review in *Infect Dis Clin N Amer 19:931, 2005*). • A February 2009 *Information Statement* from the AOS listed patient factors that may ↑ risk of infection, but recommended that antibiotic prophylaxis be considered for any invasive procedure that may cause bacteremia in all patients with a joint replacement (http://aaos.org/about/papers/advistmt/1033.asp). • The editors believe that the latter approach is excessively broad and exposes many to the risks of antibiotics without definite evidence of benefit. As pointed out in guidelines for prevention of endocarditis, transient bacteremias occur with routine daily activities (*Circulation 2007; 116:1736*). • **A recent prospective, case-control study concluded that antibiotic prophylaxis for dental procedures *did not* decrease the risk of hip or knee prosthesis infection (*Clin Infect Dis 50:8, 2010*).** • For patients with prosthetic joints, infections involving tissue to be manipulated surgically should be treated before surgery whenever possible. Prophylaxis with an anti-staphylococcal β-lactam or vancomycin (according to susceptibility of the organism) for procedures involving tissues colonized by staphylococci would be appropriate, as these organisms are common causes of prosthetic joint infections. In other circumstances, decisions must be based on individual judgment; for now, the 2003 documents cited above appear to provide the best information on which to base such decisions.
	Vancomycin single 1 gm IV dose 12 hrs prior to procedure	Effectively reduced peritonitis during 14 days post-placement in 221 pts: vanco 1%, cefazolin 7%, placebo 12% (p=0.02) (*Am J Kidney Dis 36:1014, 2000*).
Peritoneal Dialysis Catheter Placement		
Urologic Surgery/Procedures		
See Best Practice Policy Statement of Amer. Urological Assoc. (*J Urol 179:1379, 2008*) for detailed recommendations on specific procedures/circumstances. • Selection of agents targeting urinary pathogens may require modification based on local resistance patterns; ↑ TMP-SMX and/or fluoroquinolone (FQ) resistance among enteric gram-negative bacteria is a concern.		
Cystoscopy		• Prophylaxis generally not necessary if urine is sterile (however, AUA recommends FQ or TMP-SMX for those with several potentially adverse host factors (e.g., advanced age, immunocompromised state, anatomic abnormalities, etc.) • Treat patients with UTI prior to procedure using an antimicrobial active against pathogen isolated
Cystoscopy with manipulation	**Ciprofloxacin** 500 mg po (TMP-SMX 1 DS tablet po may be an alternative in populations with low rates of resistance)	Targeted therapy include ureteroscopy, biopsy, fulguration, TURP, etc. Treat UTI with targeted therapy before procedure if possible.
Transrectal prostate biopsy	**Ciprofloxacin** 500 mg po 12 hrs prior to biopsy and repeated 12 hrs after 1st dose. See *Comment*.	Bacteremia 7% with CIP vs 37% with gentamicin (*JAC 39:115, 1997*). Levofloxacin 500 mg 30-60 min before procedure was effective in low risk pts; additional doses were given for risk ↑ (*J Urol 168:1021, 2002*). Serious bacteremias due to FQ-resistant organisms have been reported in patients receiving FQ prophylaxis. Clinicians should advise patients to immediately report symptoms suggesting infection. Pre-operative prophylaxis should be determined on an institutional basis based on susceptibility profiles of prevailing organisms. Although 2nd or 3rd generation Cephalosporins or addition of single-dose gentamicin has been suggested, infections due to ESBL-producing and gent-resistant organisms have been encountered (*J Urol 74:332, 2009*).
Other		
Breast surgery, herniorrhaphy	**Cefazolin** 1-2 gm IV pre-op	Benefits of prophylaxis for clean surgical procedures not clear (*Treat Guide Med Lett 7:47, 2009*). Antibiotics may reduce risk of surgical site infection in breast cancer surgery (studies not examining immediate reconstruction), but great variability in regimens selected (*Cochrane Database Syst Rev 2006; (2): CD 005360*). For inguinal hernia repair, one analysis found prophylaxis to be beneficial in repairs with mesh (*J Hosp Infect 62: 427, 2006*), while another concluded that antibiotics may reduce risk of infection in pooled population of those repaired with prosthetic material (mesh), but that the data were not sufficiently strong to make firm recommendations for or against their use universally (*Cochrane Database Syst Rev 2007; (3): CD 003769*).

TABLE 15C – ANTIMICROBIAL PROPHYLAXIS FOR THE PREVENTION OF BACTERIAL ENDOCARDITIS IN PATIENTS WITH UNDERLYING CARDIAC CONDITIONS*

In 2007, the American Heart Association guidelines for the prevention of bacterial endocarditis were updated. The resulting document (*Circulation 2007; 116:1736-1754* and http://circ.ahajournals.org/cgi/reprint/116/15/1736), which was also endorsed by the Infectious Diseases Society of America, represents a significant departure from earlier recommendations.
- Antibiotic prophylaxis for dental procedures is now directed at individuals who are likely to suffer the most devastating consequences should they develop endocarditis.
- Prophylaxis to prevent endocarditis is no longer specified for gastrointestinal or genitourinary procedures. The following is adapted from and reflects the new AHA recommendations.
See original publication for explanation and precise details.

SELECTION OF PATIENTS FOR ENDOCARDITIS PROPHYLAXIS

FOR PATIENTS WITH ANY OF THESE HIGH-RISK CARDIAC CONDITIONS ASSOCIATED WITH ENDOCARDITIS:	WHO UNDERGO DENTAL PROCEDURES INVOLVING:	WHO UNDERGO INVASIVE RESPIRATORY PROCEDURES INVOLVING:	WHO UNDERGO INVASIVE PROCEDURES OF THE GI OR GU TRACTS:	WHO UNDERGO PROCEDURES INVOLVING INFECTED SKIN AND SOFT TISSUES:
Prosthetic heart valves Previous infective endocarditis Congenital heart disease with any of the following: • Completely repaired cardiac defect using prosthetic material (Only for 1st 6 months) • Partially corrected but with residual defect near prosthetic material • Unrepaired cyanotic congenital heart disease • Surgically constructed shunts and conduits Valvuloplasty following heart transplant	Any manipulation of gingival tissue, dental periapical regions, or perforating the oral mucosa. **PROPHYLAXIS IS RECOMMENDED‡** (See *Dental Procedures Regimens* table below) (Prophylaxis is *not* recommended for routine anesthetic injections (unless through infected tissue), dental x-rays, shedding of primary teeth, adjustment of orthodontic appliances or placement of orthodontic brackets or removable appliances).	Incision or biopsy of respiratory tract mucosa **CONSIDER PROPHYLAXIS** (See *Dental Procedures Regimens* table) Or For treatment of established infection **PROPHYLAXIS RECOMMENDED** (see *Dental Procedures Regimens* table for oral flora, but include anti-staphylococcal coverage when *S. aureus* is of concern)	PROPHYLAXIS is no longer recommended solely to prevent endocarditis, **but the following approach is reasonable:** For patients with enterococcal UTIs treat before elective GU procedures • include enterococcal coverage in perioperative regimen for non-elective procedures For patients with existing GU or GI infections or those who receive peri-operative antibiotics to prevent surgical site infections or sepsis • it is reasonable to include agents with anti-enterococcal activity in perioperative coverage†	Include coverage against staphylococci and β-hemolytic streptococci in treatment regimens

† Agents with anti-enterococcal activity include penicillin, ampicillin, amoxicillin, piperacillin, vancomycin and others. Check susceptibility if available. (See *Table 5 for highly resistant organisms.*)
‡ 2008 AHA/ACC focused update of guidelines on valvular heart disease use term "it is reasonable to reflect level of evidence (*Circulation 118:887, 2008*).

PROPHYLACTIC REGIMENS FOR DENTAL PROCEDURES

SITUATION	AGENT	REGIMEN[1]
Usual oral prophylaxis	Amoxicillin	Adults 2 gm, children 50 mg per kg; IV or IM, within 30 min before procedure
Unable to take oral medications	Ampicillin[2]	Adults 2 gm, children 50 mg per kg; IV or IM, within 30 min before procedure
Allergic to penicillins	Cephalexin[3] OR	Adults 2 gm, children 50 mg per kg; orally, 1 hour before procedure
	Clindamycin OR	Adults 600 mg, children 20 mg per kg; orally, 1 hour before procedure
	Azithromycin or clarithromycin	Adults 500 mg, children 15 mg per kg; orally, 1 hour before procedure
Allergic to penicillins and unable to take oral medications	Cefazolin[3] OR	Adults 1 gm, children 50 mg per kg; IV or IM, within 30 min before procedure
	Clindamycin	Adults 600 mg, children 20 mg per kg; IV or IM, within 30 min before procedure

[1] Children's dose should not exceed adult dose. AHA document lists all doses as 30-60 min before procedure.
[2] AHA lists cefazolin or ceftriaxone (at appropriate doses here.
[3] Cephalosporins should not be used in individuals with immediate-type hypersensitivity reaction (urticaria, angioedema, or anaphylaxis) to penicillins or other β-lactams. AHA proposes ceftriaxone as potential alternative to cefazolin; and other 1st or 2nd generation cephalosporin in equivalent doses as potential alternatives to cephalexin.

TABLE 15D – MANAGEMENT OF EXPOSURE TO HIV-1 AND HEPATITIS B AND C*

OCCUPATIONAL EXPOSURE TO BLOOD, PENILE/VAGINAL SECRETIONS OR OTHER POTENTIALLY INFECTIOUS BODY FLUIDS OR TISSUES WITH RISK OF TRANSMISSION OF HEPATITIS B/C AND/OR HIV-1 (E.G. NEEDLESTICK INJURY)

Free consultation for occupational exposures, call (PEPline) 1-888-448-4911. *[Information also available at www.aidsinfo.nih.gov]*

General steps in management:
1. Wash clean wounds/flush mucous membranes immediately (use of caustic agents or squeezing the wound is discouraged, data lacking regarding antiseptics).
2. Assess risk by doing the following: (a) Characterize exposure; (b) Determine/evaluate source of exposure by medical history, risk behavior, & testing for hepatitis B/C, HIV; (c) Evaluate and test exposed individual for hepatitis B/C & HIV.

Hepatitis B Occupational Exposure

Exposed Person[1]	Exposure Source		
	HBs Ag+	HBs Ag−	Status Unknown or Unavailable for Testing[1]
Unvaccinated	Give HBIG 0.06 mL per kg IM & initiate HB vaccine	Initiate HB vaccine	Initiate HB vaccine
Vaccinated (antibody status unknown)	Do anti-HBs on exposed person: If titer ≥10 milli-International units per mL, no rx If titer <10 milli-International units per mL, give HBIG + 1 dose HB vaccine**	No rx necessary	Do anti-HBs on exposed person: If titer ≥10 milli-International units per mL, no rx If titer <10 milli-International units per mL, give 1 dose of HB vaccine**

[1] Persons previously infected with HBV are immune to reinfection and do not require postexposure prophylaxis.

For known vaccine series responder (titer ≥10 milli-International units per mL), monitoring of levels or booster doses not currently recommended. Known non-responder (<10 milli-International units per mL) to 1° series HB vaccine & exposed to either HBsAg+ source or suspected high-risk source—rx with HBIG & re-initiate vaccine series **or** give 2 doses HBIG 1 month apart. For non-responders after a 2nd vaccine series, 2 doses HBIG 1 month apart is preferred approach to new exposure.

** Follow-up to assess vaccine response or address completion of vaccine series.

Hepatitis B Non-Occupational Exposure (see *MMWR 54 (RR11)*, 2006; *MMWR 59 (RR-10):1*, 2010)

Postexposure prophylaxis is recommended for persons with discrete nonoccupational exposure to blood or body fluids. Exposures include percutaneous (e.g., bite, needlestick or mucous membrane exposure to HBsAg-positive blood or sterile body fluids), sexual or needle-sharing contact of an HBsAg-positive person, or a victim of sexual assault or sexual abuse by a perpetrator who is HBsAg-positive. If immunoprophylaxis is indicated, it should be initiated ideally within 24 h of exposure. Postexposure prophylaxis is unlikely to be effective if administered more than 7 days after a parenteral exposure or 14 days after a sexual exposure. The hepatitis B vaccine series should be completed regardless. The same guidelines for management of occupational exposures can also be used for nonoccupational exposures. For a previously vaccinated person (i.e., written documentation of being vaccinated) and no documentation of postvaccination titers with a discrete exposure to an HBsAg-positive source, it is acceptable to administer a booster dose of hepatitis B vaccine without checking titers. No treatment is required for a vaccinated person exposed to a source of unknown HBsAg status.

Hepatitis C Exposure

Determine antibody to hepatitis C for both exposed person &, if possible, exposure source. If source + or unknown and exposed person negative, follow-up HCV testing for HCV RNA (detectable in blood within 1-2 wks post exposure) at 4-6 wks and HCV antibody testing at 3 months). If acute HCV infection develops, Monitor for spontaneous resolution of acute infection, as therapy may raise risk of progression to chronic hepatitis. Persons with chronic HCV infection treated with a course of pegylated interferon (*Gastro 130:632, 2006* and *Hot 43:923, 2006*). See Table 14G. Case-control study suggested risk factors for occupational HCV transmission include percutaneous exposure to needle that had been in artery or vein, deep injury, male sex of HCW, & was more likely when source VL >6 log10 copies/mL.

TABLE 15D (2)

HIV: Occupational exposure management [Adapted from CDC recommendations, MMWR 54 (RR9), 2005, available at www.cdc.gov/mmwr/indrr_2005.html]

The decision to initiate postexposure prophylaxis (PEP) for HIV is a clinical judgment that should be made in concert with the exposed health-care worker (HCW). It is based on:
1. Likelihood of the source patient having HIV infection: 1. with history of high-risk activity (injection drug use, sexual activity with multiple partners (either hetero- or homosexual), receipt of blood products 1978–1985), with clinical signs suggestive of advanced HIV (unexplained wasting, night sweats, thrush, seborrheic dermatitis, etc.).
2. Type of exposure (approx. 1 in 300–400 needlesticks from infected source will transmit HIV).
3. Limited data regarding efficacy of PEP (Cochrane Database Syst Rev. Jan 24; (1):CD002835, 2007).
4. Significant adverse effects of PEP drugs & potential for drug interactions.

Substances considered potentially infectious include: blood, tissues, semen, vaginal secretions, CSF, synovial, pleural, peritoneal, pericardial and amniotic fluids; and other visibly bloody fluids.
Fluids normally considered low risk for transmission, unless visibly bloody, include: urine, vomitus, stool, sweat, saliva, nasal secretions, tears and sputum.

- If source person is **known positive for HIV or likely to be infected** and **status of exposure warrants PEP**, antiretroviral drugs should be started **immediately**. If source person is HIV antibody negative, drugs can be stopped **unless source is suspected of having acute HIV infection**. The HCW should be re-tested at **3–4 weeks, 3 & 6 months whether PEP is used or not** (the vast majority of seroconversions will occur by 3 months; delayed conversions after 6 months are exceedingly rare). Tests for HIV RNA should not be used for dx of HIV infection in HCW because of false-positives (esp. at low titers) & these tests are only approved for established HIV infection [a possible exception is if pt develops signs of acute HIV (mononucleosis-like) syndrome within the 1st 4–6 wks of exposure when antibody tests might still be negative.]
- PEP for HIV is usually given for **4 wks** and monitoring of adverse effects recommended: baseline **complete blood count, renal and hepatic panel** to be repeated at 2 weeks, 50–75% of HCW on PEP demonstrates mild side-effects (nausea, diarrhea, myalgias, headache, etc.) but in up to ⅓ severe enough to discontinue PEP. Consultation with infectious diseases/ HIV specialist valuable when questions regarding PEP arise. **Seek expert help in special situations, such as pregnancy, renal impairment, treatment-experienced source.**

3 Steps to HIV Postexposure Prophylaxis (PEP) After Occupational Exposure: [Latest CDC recommendations available at www.aidsinfo.nih.gov]

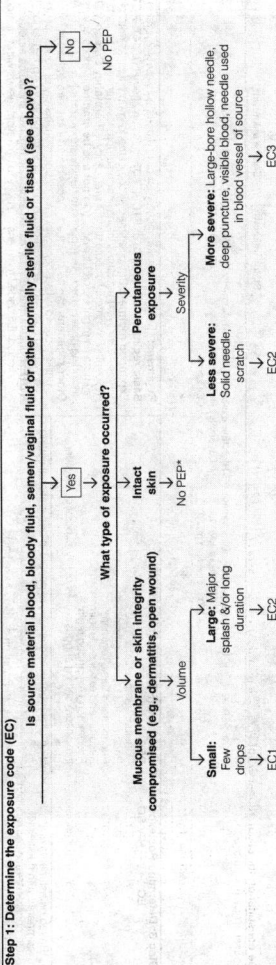

Step 1: Determine the exposure code (EC)

Is source material blood, bloody fluid, semen/vaginal fluid or other normally sterile fluid or tissue (see above)?

→ Yes → What type of exposure occurred?

- **Mucous membrane or skin integrity compromised** (e.g., dermatitis, open wound)
  - Volume
    - **Small:** Few drops → EC1
    - **Large:** Major splash &/or long duration → EC2
- **Intact skin** → No PEP*
- **Percutaneous exposure**
  - Severity
    - **Less severe:** Solid needle, scratch → EC2
    - **More severe:** Large-bore hollow needle, deep puncture, visible blood, needle used in blood vessel of source → EC3

→ No → No PEP

*Exceptions can be considered when there has been prolonged, high-volume contact.

TABLE 15D (3)

3 Steps to HIV Postexposure Prophylaxis (PEP) After Occupational Exposure (continued)

Step 2: Determine the HIV Status Code (HIV SC)

What is the HIV status of the exposure source?

- HIV negative → No PEP
- HIV positive
  - Low titer exposure: asymptomatic & high CD4 count, low VL (<1500 copies per mL) → HIV SC 1
  - High titer exposure: advanced AIDS, primary HIV, high viral load or low CD4 count → HIV SC 2
- Status unknown → HIV SC unknown
- Source unknown → HIV SC unknown

Step 3: Determine Postexposure Prophylaxis (PEP) Recommendation

EC	HIV SC	PEP
1	1	Consider basic regimen[a]
1	2	Recommend basic regimen[a,b]
2	1	Recommend basic regimen[b]
2	2	Recommend expanded regimen
3	1,2	Recommend expanded regimen
1,2,3	Unknown	If exposure setting suggests risks of HIV exposure, consider basic regimen[c]

Regimens: (Treat for 4 weeks; monitor for drug side-effects every 2 weeks):
Basic regimen: ZDV + 3TC; or FTC + TDF, or as an alternative d4T + 3TC.
Expanded regimen: Basic regimen + one of the following: lopinavir/ritonavir (preferred), or (as alternatives) atazanavir/ritonavir or fosamprenavir/ritonavir. Efavirenz can be considered (except in pregnancy or potential for pregnancy—**Pregnancy Category D**), but CNS symptoms might be problematic. **Do not use nevirapine:** serious adverse reactions including hepatic necrosis reported in healthcare workers.]

Other regimens can be designed. If possible, use antiretroviral drugs for which resistance is unlikely based on susceptibility data or treatment history of source pt (if known). Seek expert consultation of ART-experienced source pt in pregnancy or potential for pregnancy.
NOTE: Although the basic 2-drug regimen is considered sufficient for most exposures, PEP is indicated. Expanded regimens are likely to be advantageous with ↑ numbers of ART-experienced source pts or when there is doubt about exact extent of exposures in decision algorithm. Mathematical model suggests that under some conditions, completion of full course basic regimen is better than prematurely discontinued expanded regimen. However, while expanded PEP regimens have ↑ adverse effects, there is not necessarily ↑ discontinuation.

[a] Based on estimates of ↓ risk of infection after mucous membrane exposure in occupational setting compared with needlestick.
[b] Or, expanded regimen[b].
[c] In high risk circumstances, consider expanded regimen[c] on case-by-case basis.

Around the clock, urgent expert consultation available from: National Clinicians' Postexposure Prophylaxis Hotline (PEPline) at 1-888-448-4911 (1-888-HIV-4911) and on-line at http://www.ucsf.edu/hivcntr

---

POSTEXPOSURE PROPHYLAXIS FOR NON-OCCUPATIONAL EXPOSURES TO HIV-1
(Adapted from CDC recommendations, MMWR 54 (RR2), 2005, available at www.cdc.gov/mmwr/indrr_2005.html)

Because the risk of transmission of HIV via sexual contact or sharing needles may reach or exceed that of occupational needlestick exposure, it is reasonable to consider PEP in persons who have had a non-occupational exposure to blood or other potentially infected fluids (e.g., genital/rectal secretions, breast milk) from an HIV+ source. Risk of HIV acquisition per exposure varies with the act (for needle sharing and receptive anal intercourse, ≥0.5%; approximately 10-fold lower with insertive vaginal or anal intercourse, 0.05–0.07%). Overt or occult traumatic lesions may ↑ risk in survivors of sexual assault.

For pts at risk of HIV acquisition through non-occupational exposure to HIV+ source material having occurred ≤72 hours before evaluation, DHHS recommendation is to treat for 28 days with an antiretroviral **expanded regimen**, using preferred regimens: [efavirenz (not in pregnancy/*Pregnancy Category D*) + (3TC or FTC) + (ZDV or TDF)] **or** [lopinavir/ritonavir + (3TC or FTC) + ZDV] or one of several alternative regimens (see *Occupational PEP above*, and *MMWR 54(RR-2):11, 2005*). Failures of prophylaxis have been reported, and may be associated with longer interval from exposure to start of PEP; this supports prompt initiation of PEP if it is to be used.

Areas of uncertainty: (1) expanded regimens are not proven to be superior to 2-drug regimens, (2) while PEP not recommended for exposures >72 hours before evaluation, it may possibly be effective in some cases, (3) when HIV status of source patient is unknown, decision to treat and regimen selection must be individualized based on assessment of specific circumstances.

Evaluate for exposures to Hep B, Hep C (see *Table 15A*) and treat as indicated. DHHS recommendations for sexual exposures to HepB and bacterial pathogens are available in *MMWR 55(RR-11), 2006*. Persons who are unvaccinated or who have not responded to full HepB vaccine series should receive hepB immune globulin preferably within 24-hours of percutaneous or mucosal exposure to blood or body fluids of an HbsAg-positive person, along with hepB vaccine, with follow-up to complete vaccine series. Unvaccinated or non-fully-vaccinated persons exposed to a source with unknown HepBsAg-status should receive vaccine and complete vaccine series. See *MMWR 55(RR-11), 2006* for details and recommendations in other circumstances.

TABLE 15E – PREVENTION OF SELECTED OPPORTUNISTIC INFECTIONS IN HUMAN HEMATOPOIETIC CELL TRANSPLANTATION (HCT) OR SOLID ORGAN TRANSPLANTATION (SOT) IN ADULTS WITH NORMAL RENAL FUNCTION.

General comments: Medical centers performing transplants will have detailed protocols for the prevention of opportunistic infections. Due to the infections encountered, patients represented and resources available at those sites. Regimens continue to evolve and protocols adopted by an institution may differ from those at other centers. Care of transplant patients should be guided by physicians with expertise in this area.

References:
For HCT: Expert guidelines endorsed by the IDSA, updating earlier guidelines (*MMWR* 49 (RR-10):1, 2000) in: *Biol Blood Marrow Transpl* 15:1143, 2009. These guidelines provide recommendations for prevention of additional infections not discussed in this table and provide more detailed information on the infections included here.
For SOT: Recommendations of an expert panel of The Transplantation Society for management of CMV in solid organ transplant recipients in: *Transplantation* 89:779, 2010. Timeline of infections following SOT in: *Amer J Transpl* 9 (suppl 4):S3, 2009.

OPPORTUNISTIC INFECTION	TYPE OF TRANSPLANT	PROPHYLACTIC REGIMENS
CMV (Recipient + or Donor +/Recipient –)	SOT	**Prophylaxis approach:** • **Kidney, kidney/pancreas:** Valganciclovir 900 mg po q24h or 450 mg po q24h for 3-6 months. Ref for low dose: *Pharm Ther* 35:676, 2010; *CID* 52:313, 2011. However, concern has been expressed about possibly greater chance of failure and resistance emerging on low-dose prophylaxis, particularly in D+/R-(*CID* 52: 322, 2011). Hence, low-dose NOT recommended for D+/R- patients. Alternative: Ganciclovir iv or po-treat accordingly. • **Liver:** Ganciclovir 5 mg/kg iv q24h or Ganciclovir 1 gm po tid for 3-6 months. Valganciclovir^{NFDA} 900 mg po q24h for 3-6 months not FDA approved for this indication, but is widely used and recommended as an alternative. • **Lung:** Ganciclovir 5 mg/kg iv q24h (some give this dose bid for 5-7 days initially, before switching to q24h) or Valganciclovir 900 mg po q24h for ≥ 6 months. Some add CMV immune globulin in selected cases. • **Heart:** Ganciclovir 5 mg/kg iv q24h or Ganciclovir 1 gm po tid or Valganciclovir 900 mg po q24h for 3-6 months. Some add CMV immune globulin in selected cases. • **Intestine:** Ganciclovir 5 mg/kg iv q24h or Ganciclovir 1 gm po tid or Valganciclovir 900 mg po q24h for ≥ 6 months. Some add CMV immune globulin in selected cases. **Pre-emptive therapy:** for kidney, liver, pancreas, heart, monitor weekly for viremia (by PCR or antigenemia) for at least 3 months post-transplant. If viremia detected, begin treatment doses of Ganciclovir 5 mg/kg iv bid or Valganciclovir 900 mg po bid. Continue treatment until clearing of test for viremia, but for not less than 2 weeks. At that point, either switch to secondary prophylaxis or resume pre-emptive approach. **Comments:** • Expert panel recommendations from which the above are adopted favor prophylaxis approach in highest risk recipients of SOT (*Transplantation* 89:779, 2010). • With 14-wk viral prophylaxis, onset of CMV disease appearing later maintain viral vigilance for possible late-onset CMV disease and treat accordingly. • Anti-lymphocyte therapies increase risk of CMV and may require extension or re-institution of prophylaxis or pre-emptive approach. • CMV immune globulin regimens for lung, heart, liver or pancreas SOT: 150 mg/kg within 72 h of transplant and at 2, 4, 6 and 8 weeks; then 100 mg/kg at weeks 12 and 16.
	HCT	**Pre-emptive therapy:** monitor ≥ once weekly from day 10 to 100 for CMV viremia by PCR or CMV-antigenemia, and start treatment if positive. **Allogeneic:** Ganciclovir 5 mg/kg iv bid for 7-14 days (induction), then once daily (maintenance) until negative viral tests (minimum treatment 3 weeks total course of induction + maintenance). **Autologous:** Ganciclovir 5 mg/kg iv bid 7 days (induction), then 900 mg po bid induction, then 900 mg po once daily for maintenance) has been used in place of iv Ganciclovir, but is not approved for this indication. • Continue screening after completion of each course. **OR, alternatively:** **Prophylaxis approach:** from engraftment through day 100, Ganciclovir 5 mg/kg iv bid for 5-7 days (induction); then 5 mg/kg once daily (maintenance). **Late CMV reactivation:** certain HCT recipients require screening for CMV reactivation (and pre-emptive treatment) beyond 100 days (for details, see *Biol Blood Marrow Transpl* 15:1143, 2009).

201

TABLE 15E (2)

PROPHYLACTIC REGIMENS

OPPORTUNISTIC INFECTION	TYPE OF TRANSPLANT	PROPHYLACTIC REGIMENS
Hepatitis B	SOT	For anti-viral agents with activity against HBV, see Table 14B, page 169 to 170. For discussion of HBV hyperimmune globulin in liver transplantation, see *J Viral Hepatitis (Suppl 1):37, 2007*. Regimens to prevent re-infection after transplantation are evolving (*Liver Transplantation 14 (Suppl 2):S23, 2008*).
	HCT	Patients who are anti-HBc positive and anti-HBs positive, but without evidence of acute viral replication, can be monitored for ALTs and presence of HBV DNA, and given pre-emptive therapy at that time. Alternatively, prophylactic anti-viral therapy can be given, commencing before transplant. (See guidelines for other specific situations: *Biol Blood Marrow Transpl 15:1143, 2009*). These guidelines recommend Lamivudine 100 mg po q24h as an anti-viral.
Herpes simplex	SOT	Acyclovir 400 mg po bid, starting early post-transplant (*Clin Microbiol Rev 10:86, 1997*).
	HCT	Acyclovir 250 mg per meter-squared iv q12h **or** Acyclovir 400 mg to 800 mg po bid, from conditioning to engraftment or resolution of mucositis. For those requiring prolonged suppression of HSV, the higher dose (Acyclovir 800 mg po bid) is recommended to minimize the risk of emerging resistance.
Aspergillus spp.	SOT	Lung/heart-lung transplant: optimal mgmt unknown. Aerosolized lipid Ampho B + oral anti-aspergillus agent used (*Amer J Transpl 4 (Suppl 10):110, 2004; Am J Transpl 9 (Suppl 4):S244, 2009*).
	HCT	Posaconazole 200 mg po tid approved for prophylaxis of invasive infection due to Aspergillus spp. and Candida spp. in high-risk, severely immunocompromised patients (eg, HCT with GVHD). In comparative trial in patients with GVHD, Posaconazole was similar to Fluconazole in preventing invasive fungal infections, but was more effective in preventing invasive Aspergillus infection (*NEJM 356:335, 2007*). Retrospective analysis suggests that Voriconazole[14] would have efficacy in steroid-treated patients with GVHD (*Bone Marrow Transpl 45:662, 2010*), but is not approved for this indication.
Candida spp.	SOT	Liver: Fluconazole 400 mg po q24h x 3 mos. High risk pts (re-transplants, dialysis, SBP) (*Transpl 75:2023, 2003*). Fluconazole resistance (*Liver Transpl 12:850, 2006*).
	HCT	Fluconazole 400 mg po or iv once daily from day 0 to engraftment or when ANC consistently >1000, or Posaconazole 200 mg po tid approved for high-risk patients (e.g., with GVHD) or prolonged neutropenia), or Micafungin 50 mg iv once daily.
Coccidioides immitis	Any	Fluconazole 200-400 mg po q24h (*Transpl Inf Dis 5:3, 2003; Am J Transpl 6:340, 2006*). See *CCID 21:45, 2008* for approach at one center in endemic area; e.g., for seropositive serology without evidence of active infection. Fluconazole 400 mg q24h for first year post-transplant, then 200 mg q24h thereafter.
Pneumocystis jiroveci	SOT	TMP-SMX 1 single-strength tab po q24h or 1 double-strength tab po once daily for 3 to 7 days per week. Duration: kidney: 6 mos to 1 year (*Amer J Transpl 9 (suppl 3): S59, 2009*); heart, lung, liver: 3-12 months, life-long (*Amer J Transpl 4 (suppl 10): 135, 2004*).
	HCT	TMP-SMX 1 single-strength tab po q24h or 1 double-strength tab po once daily or once a day for 3 days per week, from engraftment to 6 mos post-transplant
Toxoplasma gondii	SOT	TMP-SMX (1 SS tab po q24h or 1 DS tab po once daily) x 3-7 days/wk for 6 mos post-transplant. (See *Clin Micro Infect 14:1089, 2008*).
	HCT	TMP-SMX 1 single-strength tab po q24h or 1 double-strength tab po once daily or once a day for 3 days per week, from engraftment to 6 mos post-transplant for seropositive allogeneic transplant recipients.
Trypanosoma cruzi	Heart	May be transmitted from organs of transplantation (*CID 48:1534, 2009*). Inspect peripheral blood of suspected cases for parasites (*MMWR 55:1534, 2006*). Risk of reactivation during immunosuppression is variable (*JAMA 298:2171, 2007; JAMA 299:1134, 2008; J Cardiac Fail 15:249, 2009*). If known Chagas disease in donor or recipient, contact CDC for treatment options (phone 770-488-7775 or in emergency 770-488-7100).

TABLE 16 – PEDIATRIC DOSAGES OF SELECTED ANTIBACTERIAL AGENTS*
*Adapted from: (1) Nelson's Pocket Book of Pediatric Antimicrobial Therapy 2009,
J. Bradley & J. Nelson, eds., American Academy of Pediatrics, 2009.*

DRUG	BODY WEIGHT <2000 gm 0-7 days	BODY WEIGHT <2000 gm 8-28 days	BODY WEIGHT >2000 gm 0-7 days	BODY WEIGHT >2000 gm 8-28 days	>28 DAYS OLD
Aminoglycosides, IV or IM (check levels; some dose by gestational age + wks of life; *see Nelson's Pocket Book, p. 25*)					
Amikacin	7.5 q18-24h	7.5 q12h	10 q12h	10 q12h	10 q8h
Gent/tobra	2.5 q18-24h	2.5 q12h	2.5 q12h	2.5 q12h	2.5 q8h
Aztreonam, IV	30 q12h	30 q8h	30 q8h	30 q6h	30 q6h
Cephalosporins					
Cefaclor					20-40 div q8h
Cefadroxil					30 div q12h (max 2 gm per day)
Cefazolin	25 q12h	25 q12h	25 q12h	25 q8h	25 q8h
Cefdinir					7 q12h or 14 q24h
Cefepime	30 q12h	30 q12h	30 q12h	30 q12h	150 div q8h
Cefixime					8 as q24h or div bid
Cefotaxime	50 q12h	50 q8h	50 q12h	50 q8h	50 q8h (75 q6h for meningitis)
Cefoxitin			20 q12h		80-160 div q6h
Cefpodoxime					10 div bid (max 400 mg per day)
Cefprozil					15-30 div bid (max 1 gm per day)
Ceftazidime	50 q12h	50 q8h	50 q8h	50 q8h	50 q8h
Ceftibuten					4.5 bid
Ceftizoxime					33-66 q8h
Ceftriaxone	25 q24h	50 q24h	25 q24h	50 q24h	50 q24h (meningitis 100)
Cefuroxime IV	50 q12h	50 q8h	50 q8h	50 q8h	50 q8h (80 q8h for meningitis)
po					10-15 bid (max 1 gm per day)
Cephalexin					25-50 div q6h (max 4 gm per day)
Loracarbef					15-30 div q12h (max 0.8 gm per day)
Chloramphenicol IV	25 q24h	25 q12h	25 q12h	15 q12h	12.5-25 q6h (max 2-4 gm per day)
Clindamycin IV	5 q12h	5 q8h	5 q8h	5 q6h	7.5 q6h
po					
Ciprofloxacin[2]					20-30 div q12h (max 1.5 gm per day)
Ertapenem IV	No data	No data	No data	No data	15 q12h (max. 1g/day)
Imipenem[3] IV			25 q12h	25 q8h	15-25 q6h (max 2-4 gm per day)
Linezolid	10 q12h	10 q8h	10 q8h	10 q8h	10 q8h to age 12
Macrolides					
Erythro IV & po	10 q12h	10 q8h	10 q12h	13 q8h	10 q6h
Azithro po/IV	5 q24h	10 q24h	5 q24h	10 q24h	10 q24h
Clarithro po					7.5 q12h (max. 1 gm per day)
Meropenem IV	20 q12h	20 q8h	20 q8h	20 q8h	60-120 div q8h (120 for meningitis)
Metro IV & po	7.5 q24h	7.5 q12h	7.5 q12h	15 q12h	7.5 q6h
Penicillins					
Ampicillin	50 q12h	50 q8h	50 q8h	50 q6h	50 q6h
AMP-sulbactam					100-300 div q6h
Amoxicillin po				30 div tid	25-50 div tid
Amox-Clav po			30 div bid	30 div bid	45 or 90 (AM/CL-HD) div bid if over 12wks
Dicloxacillin					12-25 div q6h
Mezlocillin	75 q12h	75 q8h	75 q8h	75 q12h	75 q6h
Nafcillin, oxacillin IV	25 q12h	25 q8h	25 q8h	37 q6h	37 q6h (to max. 8-12 gm per day)
Piperacillin, PIP-tazo IV	50 q12h	100 q12h	100 q12h	100 q8h	100 q6h
Ticarcillin, TC/CL IV	75 q12h	75 q8h	75 q8h	75 q6h	75 q6h
Tinidazole					> Age 3: 50 mg/kg for 1 dose
Penicillin G, U/kg IV	50,000 q12h	75,000 q8h	50,000 q8h	50,000 q6h	50,000 units/kg per day
Penicillin V					25-50 mg per kg per day div q6-8h
Rifampin IV, po	10 q24h	10 q12h	10 q24h	10 q12h	10 q12h
Sulfisoxazole po					120-150 mg/kg per day div q4-6h
TMP-SMX po, IV; UTI: 8-12 TMP component div bid; Pneumocystis: 20 TMP component div q6h					
Tetracycline po (age 8 or older)					25-50 div q6h (>7yr old)
Doxycycline po, IV (age 8 or older)					2-4 div bid to max of 200 (>7yr old)
Vancomycin IV	12.5 q12h	15 q12h	18 q12h	22 q12h	40 div q6-8h [some start with 15 mg/kg IV q6h (normal renal function)]; 60 for meningitis.

[1] May need higher doses in patients with meningitis: see *CID* 39:1267, 2004.
[2] With exception of cystic fibrosis, anthrax, and complicated UTI, not approved for use under age 18.
[3] Not recommended in children with CNS infections due to risk of seizures.
* See page 2 for abbreviations

TABLE 17A – DOSAGE OF ANTIMICROBIAL DRUGS IN ADULT PATIENTS WITH RENAL IMPAIRMENT

- For listing of drugs with NO need for adjustment for renal failure, see *Table 17B*.
- Adjustments for renal failure are based on an estimate of creatinine clearance (CrCl) which reflects the glomerular filtration rate.
- **Different methods for calculating estimated CrCl are suggested for non-obese and obese patients.**
  - Calculations for ideal body weight (IBW) in kg:
    - Men: 50 kg plus 2.3 kg/inch over 60 inches height.
    - Women: 45 kg plus 2.3 kg/inch over 60 inches height.
  - Obese is defined as 20% over ideal body weight or body mass index (BMI) >30

- Calculations of estimated CrCl (References, see (NEJM 354:2473, 2006 (non-obese), AJM 84:1053, 1988 (obese)):
  - **Non-obese patient**—
    - Calculate ideal body weight (IBW) in kg (as above)
    - Use the following formula to determine estimated CrCl

    (140 minus age)(IBW in kg)   CrCl in mL/min for men.
    ───────────────────────── = Multiply answer by 0.85
          72 x serum creatinine   for women (estimated)

  - **Obese patient**—
    - Weight ≥20% over IBW or BMI >30
    - Use the following formulas to determine estimated CrCl

    $$\frac{(137 \text{ minus age}) \times [(0.285 \times \text{wt in kg}) + (12.1 \times \text{ht in meters}^2)]}{51 \times \text{serum creatinine}} = \text{CrCl (obese male)}$$

    $$\frac{(146 \text{ minus age}) \times [(0.287 \times \text{wt in kg}) + (9.74 \times \text{ht in meters}^2)]}{60 \times \text{serum creatinine}} = \text{CrCl (obese female)}$$

- If estimated CrCl ≥90 mL/min, see *Tables 10C and 10D for dosing.*
- What weight should be used to calculate dosage on a mg/kg basis?
  - If less than 20% over IBW, use the patient's actual weight for all drugs.
  - **For obese patients** (≥20% over IBW or BMI >30):
    - **Aminoglycosides**: IBW plus 0.4(actual weight minus IBW) = adjusted weight.
    - **Vancomycin**: actual body weight whether non-obese or obese.
    - **All other drugs**: insufficient data (*Pharmacotherapy 27:1081, 2007*).

- For slow or sustained extended daily dialysis **(SLEDD)** over 6-12 hours, adjust does as for CRRT. For details, see *CID 49:433, 2009; CCM 39:560, 2011.*
- General reference: Drug Prescribing in Renal Failure, 5th ed., Aronoff, et al. (eds) (*Amer College Physicians, 2007 and drug package inserts*).

TABLE 17A (2)

ANTIMICROBIAL	HALF-LIFE (NORMAL/ ESRD) hr	DOSE FOR NORMAL RENAL FUNCTION	METHOD (see footer)	ADJUSTMENT FOR RENAL FAILURE Estimated creatinine clearance (CrCl), mL/min				HEMODIALYSIS, CAPD	COMMENTS & DOSAGE FOR CRRT
		>50		>50-90	10-50	<10			
ANTIBACTERIAL ANTIBIOTICS										
Aminoglycoside Antibiotics: traditional multiple daily doses—adjustment for renal disease										
Amikacin	1.4–2.3/17–150	7.5 mg/kg q12h or 15 mg/kg once daily (see below)	I	7.5 mg/kg q24h	30–50: 7.5 mg/kg q24h 10–30: 7.5 mg/kg q48h **Same dose for CRRT**	7.5 mg/kg q72h	HEMO: 7.5 mg/kg AD CAPD: 15–20 mg lost per L dialysate per day (see *Comment*)	**High flux hemodialysis** membranes lead to unpredictable aminoglycoside clearance, measure post-dialysis drug levels for efficacy and toxicity. With **CAPD**, pharmacokinetics highly variable—**check serum levels**. Usual method for CAPD: 2 liters of dialysis fluid placed qid or 8 liters per day (give 8L/20 mg lost per L = 160 mg of amikacin supplement IV per day)
Gentamicin, Tobramycin (Monitor levels)	2–3/20–60	1.7 mg per kg q8h. Once daily dosing below	I	5–7 mg/kg once daily or 1.7, 2.3 mg/kg q8h	1.7 mg/kg q12-48h **Same dose for CRRT** See *Gent SLEDD dose*	1.7 mg/kg q48-72h	HEMO: 3 mg/kg AD. Monitor levels. CAPD: 3–4 mg lost per L dialysate per day	
Netilmicin[NUS]	2–3/35–72	2 mg per kg q8h. Once daily dosing below	I	2 mg/kg q12-24h or 6.5 mg/kg once daily	2 mg/kg q12-24h **Same dose for CRRT**	2 mg/kg q48h	HEMO: 3 mg/kg AD CAPD: 3–4 mg lost per L dialysate per day	Adjust dosing weight for obesity. (ideal body weight + 0.4 (actual body weight – ideal body weight))
Streptomycin	2–3/30–80	15 mg per kg (max. of 1 gm) q24h. Once daily dosing below	I	15 mg/kg q24h **Same dose for CRRT**	15 mg/kg q24-72h **Same dose for CRRT**	15 mg/kg q72-96h	HEMO: 7.5 mg/kg AD CAPD: 20–40 mg lost per L dialysate per day	**Gent SLEDD dose** in critically ill: 6 mg/kg IV q48h starting 30 min before start of SLEDD (daily SLEDD; q48h Gent). (*AAC:54:3635, 2010*).

ONCE-DAILY AMINOGLYCOSIDE THERAPY: ADJUSTMENT IN RENAL INSUFFICIENCY (*see Table 10D for OD dosing/normal renal function*)

Creatinine Clearance (mL per min.)	60-80	40-60	20-30	10-20	<10-0
Drug	Dose q24h (mg per kg)			Dose q48h (mg per kg)	Dose q72h and AD
Gentamicin/Tobramycin	5.1	3.5	2.5	4	2
Amikacin/Kanamycin/streptomycin	15	12	7.5	7.5	3
Isepamicin	8	8	8 q48h	8 q72h	8 q96h
Netilmicin[NUS]	6.5	4	2	3	2.5

Carbapenem Antibiotics								
Doripenem	1/18	500 mg IV q8h	D&I	500 mg IV q8h	≥30 – ≤50: 250 mg IV q8h >10 – <30: 250 mg IV q12h	No data	No data. CRRT ref: *AAC 55:1187, 2011*.	
Ertapenem	4/>4	1 gm q24h	D	1 gm q24h	0.5 gm q24h (CrCl <30)	0.5 gm q24h	HEMO: Dose as for CrCl <10; if dosed <6 hrs prior to HD, give 150 mg supplement AD	
Imipenem (see *Comment*)	1/4	0.5 gm q6h	D&I	250–500 mg q6–8h	250–500 mg q6–12h **Dose for CRRT:** 0.5–1 gm q12h (*AAC 49:2421, 2005*)	125–250 mg q12h	HEMO: Dose AD CAPD: Dose for CrCl <10	1 potential for seizures if recommended doses exceeded in pts with CrCl <20 mL per min. See pkg insert, esp. for pts <70 kg
Meropenem	1/6–8	1 gm q8h	D&I	1 gm q8h	1 gm q12h **Same dose for CRRT**	0.5 gm q24h	HEMO: Dose AD CAPD: Dose for CrCl <10	

Abbreviation Key: Adjustment Method: **D** = dose adjustment; **I** = interval adjustment; **CAPD** = continuous ambulatory peritoneal dialysis; **CRRT** = continuous renal replacement therapy; **HEMO** = hemodialysis; **AD** = after dialysis; "**Supplement**" or "**Extra**" is to replace drug lost during dialysis—additional drug beyond continuation of regimen for CrCl < 10 mL/min.

TABLE 17A (3)

ANTIMICROBIAL	HALF-LIFE (NORMAL/ESRD) hr	DOSE FOR NORMAL RENAL FUNCTION	METHOD (see footer)	ADJUSTMENT FOR RENAL FAILURE Estimated creatinine clearance (CrCl), mL/min			HEMODIALYSIS, CAPD	COMMENTS & DOSAGE FOR CRRT
				>90-50	10-50	<10		
ANTIBACTERIAL ANTIBIOTICS *(continued)*								
Cephalosporin Antibiotics: DATA ON SELECTED **PARENTERAL** CEPHALOSPORINS								
Cefazolin	1.9/40-70	1-2 gm q8h		q8h	q12h **Same dose for CRRT**	q24-48h	HEMO: Extra 0.5-1 gm AD CAPD: 0.5 gm q12h	
Cefepime	2.2/18	2 gm q8h (max. dose)	D&I	2 gm q8h	2 gm q12-24h **Same dose for CRRT**	1 gm q24h	HEMO: Extra 1 gm AD CAPD: 1-2 gm q48h	
Cefotaxime, Ceftizoxime	1.7/15-35	2 gm q8h		q8-12h	2 gm q12-24h **Same dose for CRRT**	q24h	HEMO: Extra 1 gm AD CAPD: 0.5-1 gm q24h	Active metabolite of cefotaxime in ESRD, ↓ dose further for hepatic & renal failure.
Cefotetan	3.5/13-25	1-2 gm q12h	D	100%	1-2 gm q24h **Same dose for CRRT**	1-2 gm q48h	HEMO: Extra 1 gm AD CAPD: 1 gm q24h	CRRT dose: 750 mg q12h
Cefoxitin	0.8/13-23	2 gm q8h		q8h	q8-12h **Same dose for CRRT**	q24-48h	HEMO: Extra 1 gm AD CAPD: 1 gm q24h	May falsely increase serum creatinine by interference with assay.
Ceftaroline	1.6/—	600 mg IV q12h	D	600 mg q12h	30-50: 400 mg q12h 15-30: 300 mg q12h	< 15: 200 mg q12h	HEMO: 200 mg q12h	1-hr infusion for all doses
Ceftazidime	1.2/13-25	2 gm q8h		q8-12h	Q12-24h **Same dose for CRRT**	q24-48h	HEMO: Extra 1 gm AD CAPD: 0.5 gm q24h	Since 1/2 dose is dialyzed, post-dialysis dose is max. of 3 gm.
Ceftobiprole	2.9-3.3/21	500 mg IV q8-12h		500 mg IV q8-12h	≥30 & ≤50: 500 mg q12h over 2 hrs ≥10 & <30: 250 mg q12h over 2 hrs	No data	No data	
Cefuroxime sodium	1.2/17	0.75-1.5 gm q8h	I	q8h	q8-12h **Same dose for CRRT**	q24h	HEMO: Dose AD CAPD: Dose for CrCl <10	
Fluoroquinolone Antibiotics								
Ciprofloxacin	3-6/6-9	500-750 mg po (or 400 mg IV) q12h	D	100%	50-75% CRRT 400 mg IV q24h	50%	HEMO: 250 mg or 200 mg IV q12h CAPD: 250 mg po or 200 mg IV q8h	
Gatifloxacin[NUS]	7-14/11-40	400 mg po/IV q24h	D	400 mg q24h	400 mg, then 200 mg q24h **Same dose for CRRT**	400 mg, then 200 mg q24h	HEMO: 200 mg q24h AD CAPD: 200 mg q24h	
Gemifloxacin	7/>7	320 mg po q24h	D	320 mg q24h	160 mg q24h	160 mg q24h	HEMO: 160 mg q24h AD CAPD: 160 mg q24h	
Levofloxacin	6-8/76	750 mg q24h IV, PO	D&I	750 mg q24h	**20-49:** 750 q48h	**<20:** 750 mg once, then 500 mg q48h	**<20:** 750 mg once, then 500 mg q48h	CRRT 750 mg once, then 500 mg q8h, although not FDA-approved.
Ofloxacin	7/28-37	200-400 mg q12h	D	200-400 mg q12h	200-400 mg q24h **Same dose for CRRT**	200 mg q24h	HEMO: Dose for CrCl <10, AD CAPD: 300 mg q24h	
Macrolide Antibiotics								
Clarithromycin	5-7/22	0.5-1 gm q12h	D	100%	75%	50-75%	HEMO: Dose AD CAPD: None	CRRT as for CrCl 10-50
Erythromycin	1.4/5-6	250-500 mg q6h	D	100%	100%	50-75%	HEMO/CAPD/CRRT: None	Ototoxicity with high doses in ESRD

Abbreviation Key; Adjustment Method: **D** = dose adjustment; **I** = interval adjustment; **AD** = after dialysis; "**Supplement**" or "**Extra**" is to replace drug lost during dialysis – additional dosage of regimen for CrCl < 10 mL/min.
HEMO = hemodialysis; **CAPD** = continuous ambulatory peritoneal dialysis; **CRRT** = continuous renal replacement therapy;

TABLE 17A (4)

ANTIMICROBIAL	HALF-LIFE (NORMAL/ESRD) hr	DOSE FOR NORMAL RENAL FUNCTION	METHOD (see footer)	ADJUSTMENT FOR RENAL FAILURE Estimated creatinine clearance (CrCl), mL/min >50-90	10-50	<10	HEMODIALYSIS, CAPD	COMMENTS & DOSAGE FOR CRRT
ANTIBACTERIAL ANTIBIOTICS (continued)								
Miscellaneous Antibacterial Antibiotics								
Colistin (Polymyxin E) Based on 105 pts (AAC 55:3284, 2011) All doses refer to Colistin "base" in mg	<6/≥48	See Table 10A, page 101 for loading dose and maintenance dose	D & I	$3.5 \times [(1.5 \times CrCln) = 30] \times$ (pt BSA in m2/1.73m²) = total daily dose of Colistin base. Divide and give q12h **CrCln** = normalized CrCl based on body surface area (BSA); Pt BSA in m²/1.73m².	4-6 mg/kg per day	CrCl <30, 4-6 mg per kg q48h CRRT: 8 mg/kg q48h (CCM 39:19, 2011)	**Intermittent Hemodialysis:** • Calculation of dose: 3.5 (30) =105 mg (CrCl is zero). On days with no hemodialysis, give total daily dose of 105 mg divided bid. • On dialysis days, need to supplement the dose by 50% due to colistimethate filtration by the dialysis membrane. • So, on dialysis days the total dose is 150 mg; divide and give half the dose during the last hr of hemodialysis and the second half 12 hours later	**CAPD:** • 160 mg q24h (unable to locate modern CAPD data) **CRRT:** • For average serum steady state concentration of 3.5 µg/mL, the total daily dose is 672 mg; the dose is divided and given q12h. **The dose is necessarily high due to removal of drug by the dialysis membranes.** Rationale: 3.5 µg/mL as the targeted serum level X 192 mg for each 1 µg/mL of targeted serum level = total daily dose, i.e., 3.5 x 192 = 672. See AAC 55: 3284, 2011 for data.
Daptomycin	9.4/30	4-6 mg per kg per day	I	4-6 mg per kg per day		600 mg q12h AD	HEMO & CAPD: 6 mg per kg q48h (during or after q48h dialysis if possible). If next planned dialysis is 72 hrs away, give 9 mg/kg (AAC 55:1677, 2011)	
Linezolid	5-6/6-8	600 mg po/IV q12h	None	600 mg q12h **Same dose for CRRT**			HEMO: As for CrCl <10 AD CAPD & CRRT: No dose adjustment	Accumulation of 2 metabolites—risk unknown (JAC 56:172, 2005)
Metronidazole	6-14/7-21	7.5 mg per kg q6h	D	100% **Same dose for CRRT**	100%	50%	HEMO: Dose as for CrCl <10 AD CAPD: Dose for CrCl <10	
Nitrofurantoin	0.5/1	50-100 mg	D	100%	Avoid	Avoid	Not applicable	
Sulfamethoxazole (SMX)	10/20-50	1 gm q8h	I	q12h	q18h Same dose for CAVH	q24h	HEMO: Extra 1 gm AD CAPD: 1 gm q24h	
Teicoplanin[NUS]	45/62-230	6 mg per kg per day	I	q24h	q48h	q72h	HEMO: Dose for CrCl <10 CAPD: Dose for CrCl <10	**Same dose for CRRT**
Telithromycin	10/15	800 mg q24h	D	800 mg q24h	600 mg q24h (<30, 600 mg q24h)	600 mg q24h	HEMO: 600 mg q24h AD CAPD: No data	If CrCl <30, reduce dose to 600 mg once daily. If both liver and renal failure, dose is 400 mg once daily
Telavancin	7.8/17.9	10 mg/kg q24h	D&I	10 mg/kg q24h	**30-50:** 7.5 mg/kg q24h	**<30:** 10 mg/kg q48h	No data	
Temocillin		1-2 gm q12h	I	1-2 gm q12h	1 gm q24h	1 gm q48h	HEMO: 1 gm q48h AD CAPD: 1 gm q48h	

Abbreviation Key: Adjustment Method: **D** = dose adjustment, **I** = interval adjustment; **CAPD** = continuous ambulatory peritoneal dialysis; **CRRT** = continuous renal replacement therapy; **HEMO** = hemodialysis, **AD** = after dialysis; "**Supplement**" or "**Extra**" is to replace drug lost during dialysis – additional drug beyond continuation of regimen for CrCl < 10 mL/min.

TABLE 17A (5)

ANTIMICROBIAL	HALF-LIFE (NORMAL/ESRD) hr	DOSE FOR NORMAL RENAL FUNCTION	METHOD (see footer)	ADJUSTMENT FOR RENAL FAILURE Estimated creatinine clearance (CrCl), mL/min >50-90	10-50	<10	HEMODIALYSIS, CAPD	COMMENTS & DOSAGE FOR CRRT
ANTIBACTERIAL ANTIBIOTICS (continued)								
Trimethoprim (TMP)	11/20-49	100-200 mg q12h	I	q12h	>30: q12h; 10-30: q18h Same dose for CRRT	q24h	HEMO: Dose AD CAPD: q24h	CRRT dose: q18h
Trimethoprim-sulfamethoxazole-DS (Doses based on TMP component)								
Treatment (based on TMP component)	As for TMP	5-20 mg/kg/day divided q6-12h	D	No dose adjustment	30-50: No dose adjustment 10-29: Reduce dose by 50%	Not recommended; but if used: 5-10 mg/kg q24h	Not recommended; but if used: 5-10 mg/kg AD CRRT: 5-7.5 mg/kg q8h	
TMP-SMX Prophylaxis	As for TMP	1 tab po q24h or 3 times per week	No change	100%	100%	100%		
Vancomycin[a]	6/200-250	1 gm q12h	D&I	1 gm q12h	1 gm q24-96h	1 gm q4-7 days	HEMO: For trough conc of 15-20 μg/mL, give 15 mg/kg if next dialysis in 1 day; give 25 mg/kg if next dialysis in 2 days; give 35 mg/kg if next dialysis in 3 days (CID 53:124, 2011).	CAVH/CVVH: 500 mg q24-48h. New hemodialysis membranes ↑ clear. of vanco; **check levels**
Penicillins								
Amoxicillin	1/5-20	250-500 mg q8h	I	q8h	q8-12h	q24h	HEMO: Dose AD CAPD: 250 mg q12h	IV amoxicillin not available in the U.S. CRRT: dose for CrCl 10-50
Ampicillin	1/7-20	250 mg-2 gm q6h		q6h	q6-12h	q12-24h		
Amoxicillin/Clavulanate[2]	1.3 AM/1, 5-20/4	500/125 mg q8h (see Comments)	D&I	500/125 mg q8h	250-500 mg AM component q12h	250-500 mg AM component q24h	HEMO: As for CrCl <10; extra dose after dialysis	**If CrCl <30 per mL, do not use 875/125 or 1000/62.5 AM/CL**
Amoxicillin ext. rel. tabs	1.5/?	775 mg once daily		Once daily	CrCl <30, no data, avoid usage			
Ampicillin (AM)/Sulbactam (SB)	1 (AM)/1 (SB), 9 (AM)/10 (SB)	2 gm AM + 1 gm SB q6h		q6h	q8-12h	q24h	HEMO: Dose AD CAPD: 2 gm AM/1 gm SB q24h	CRRT dose: 1.5 AM/0.75 SB q12h
Aztreonam	2/6-8	2 gm q8h	D	100%	50-75% Same dose for CRRT	25%	HEMO: Extra 0.5 gm AD CAPD: Dose for CrCl <10	Technically is a β-lactam antibiotic.
Penicillin G	0.5/6-20	0.5-4 million U q4h		100%	75% Same dose for CRRT	20-50%	HEMO: Dose AD CAPD: Dose for CrCl <10	1.7 mEq potassium per million units. ↑s potential of seizure. 10 million units per day max. dose in ESRD.
Piperacillin	1/3.3-5.1	3-4 gm q4-6h		q4-6h	q6-8h Same dose for CRRT	q8h	HEMO: 2 gm q8h plus 1 gm extra AD CAPD: Dose for CrCl <10	1.9 mEq sodium per gm

[1] If renal failure, use EMIT assay to measure levels; levels overestimated by RIA or fluorescent immunoassay.
[2] Clavulanate cleared by liver, not kidney. Hence as dose of combination decreased, a deficiency of clavulanate may occur (JAMA 285:386, 2001).

Abbreviation Key, Adjustment Method: **D** = dose adjustment; **I** = interval adjustment; **CAPD** = continuous ambulatory peritoneal dialysis; **CRRT** = continuous renal replacement therapy; **HEMO** = hemodialysis; **AD** = after dialysis; "**Supplement**" or "**Extra**" is to replace drug lost during dialysis – additional continuation of regimen for CrCl < 10 mL/min.

TABLE 17A (6)

ANTIMICROBIAL	HALF-LIFE (NORMAL/ ESRD) hr	DOSE FOR NORMAL RENAL FUNCTION	METHOD (see footer)	ADJUSTMENT FOR RENAL FAILURE Estimated creatinine clearance (CrCl) mL/min >50–90	10–50	<10	HEMODIALYSIS, CAPD	COMMENTS & DOSAGE FOR CRRT
ANTIBACTERIAL ANTIBIOTICS (continued)								
Pip (P)/tazo(t)	0.71-1.2 (both)/2-6	3.375 – 4.5 gm q6-8h	D&I		2.25 gm q6h <20: q8h Same dose for CRRT	2.25 gm q8h	HEMO: Dose for CrCl <10 + extra 0.75 gm AD CAPD: 4.5 gm q12h; CRRT: 2.25 gm q6h	
Ticarcillin	1.2/13	3 gm q4h	D&I	1-2 gm q4h	1-2 gm q8h Same dose for CRRT	1-2 gm q12h	HEMO: Extra 3.0 gm AD CAPD: Dose for CrCl <10	5.2 mEq sodium per gm
Ticarcillin/ Clavulanate²	1.2/1-16	3.1 gm q4h	D&I	3.1 gm q4h	3.1 gm q8-12h Same dose for CRRT	2 gm q12h	HEMO: Extra 3.1 gm AD CAPD: 3.1 gm q12h	See footnote²
Tetracycline Antibiotics								
Tetracycline	6-10/57-108	250-500 mg qid	I	q8-12h	q12-24h Same dose for CRRT	q24h	HEMO/CAPD/CAVH: None	Avoid in ESRD
ANTIFUNGAL ANTIBIOTICS								
Amphotericin B & Lipid-based ampho B	24h–15 days/unchanged	Non-lipid: 0.4–1 mg/kg/day ABLC: 5 mg/kg/day LAB: 3-5 mg/kg/day	I	q24h	q24h Same dose for CRRT	q24h	HEMO/CAPD/CRRT: No dose adjustment	For ampho B, toxicity lessened by saline loading; risk amplified by concomitant cyclosporine A, aminoglycosides, or pentamidine
Fluconazole	37/100	100-400 mg q24h	D	100%	50%	50%	HEMO: 100% of recommended dose AD CAPD: Dose for CrCl <10	CRRT: 200-400 mg q24h
Flucytosine	3-6/75-200	37.5 mg per kg q6h	I	q12h	q12-24h Same dose for CRRT	q24h	HEMO: Dose AD CAPD: 0.5-1 gm q24h	Goal is peak serum level >25 mcg per mL and <100 mcg per mL
Itraconazole, po soln	21/25	100–200 mg q12h	D	100%	100% Same dose for CRRT	50%	HEMO/CAPD oral solution: 100 mg q12-24h	
Itraconazole, IV	21/25	200 mg IV q12h	I	200 mg IV bid	Do not use IV if CrCl <30 due to accumulation of carrier: cyclodextrin			
Terbinafine	36-200/?	250 mg po per day	I	q24h	Use has not been studied. Recommend avoidance of drug.			
Voriconazole, IV	Non-linear kinetics	6 mg per kg IV q12h times 2, then 4 mg per kg q12h	I	No change	If CrCl <50 mL per min, accum. of IV vehicle (cyclodextrin). Switch to po or DC For CRRT: 4 mg/kg po q12h			
ANTIPARASITIC ANTIBIOTICS								
Pentamidine	3-12/73-18	4 mg per kg per day	I	q24h	q24h Same dose for CRRT	q24-36h	HEMO: 4 mg/kg q48h AD CAPD: Dose for CrCl <10	
Quinine	5-16/5-16	650 mg q8h	I	650 mg q8h	650 mg q24h Same dose for CRRT	650 mg q24h	HEMO: Dose AD CAPD: Dose for CrCl <10	Marked tissue accumulation

Abbreviation Key: Adjustment Method: **D** = dose adjustment; **I** = interval adjustment; **AD** = after dialysis; "**Supplement**" or "**Extra**" is to replace drug lost during dialysis – additional drug beyond continuation of regimen; **CAPD** = continuous ambulatory peritoneal dialysis; **CRRT** = continuous renal replacement therapy. **HEMO** = hemodialysis; **AD** = after dialysis; for CrCl < 10 mL/min.

TABLE 17A (7)

ANTIMICROBIAL	HALF-LIFE NORMAL/ESRD) hr	DOSE FOR NORMAL RENAL FUNCTION	METHOD (See footer)	ADJUSTMENT FOR RENAL FAILURE Estimated creatinine clearance (CrCl), mL/min			HEMODIALYSIS, CAPD	COMMENTS & DOSAGE FOR CRRT
				>50-90	10-50	<10		
ANTITUBERCULOUS ANTIBIOTICS (See http://i11ntcc.ucsd.edu/TB)									
Amikacin/Streptomycin (see page 205)								
Bedaquiline	24-30	ND		400 mg po qd × 2 wks, then 200 mg tiw × 22 wks	No adjustment for mild-moderate renal impairment; use with caution if severe renal impairment or ESRD			
Capreomycin		15 mg/kg q24h		15 mg/kg q24h	CrCl <30: 15 mg/kg	15 mg/kg AD 3x/wk	HEMO: 15 mg/kg AD 3x/wk	
Cycloserine		10-15 mg/kg/day in 2 div doses		10-15 mg/kg/day in 2 div doses	CrCl 10-20: 10-15 mg/kg q12-24h	10-15 mg/kg q24h	HEMO: 10-15 mg/kg AD 3x/wk	
Ethambutol	4/7-15	15-25 mg per kg q24h		15-25 mg/kg q24h	15 mg/kg q24-36h **Same dose for CRRT For CrCl 10-20:** 15-25 mg/kg q24-48h	15-25 mg/kg q48h	HEMO: 20 mg/kg 3x/wk AD CAPD: 25 mg/kg q48h	If possible, do serum levels on dialysis pts.
Ethionamide	2.1/?	250-500 mg q12h	D	100%	100%	50%	HEMO/CAPD/CRRT: No dosage adjustment	
Isoniazid	0.7-4/8-17	5 mg per kg per day (max. 300 mg)	D	100%	100%	100%	HEMO: Dose AD CAPD: Dose for CrCl < 10	
Pyrazinamide	9/26	25 mg per kg q24h (max. dose 2.5 gm q24h)	D	25 mg/kg q24h	25 mg/kg q24h **Same dose for CRRT For CrCl 10-20:** 25 mg/kg q48h	30 mg per kg 3x/wk **Same dose for CRRT**	HEMO: 25 mg/kg 3x/wk AD CAPD: No reduction	Biologically active metabolite
Rifampin	1.5-5/1.8-11	600 mg per day	D	600 mg q24h	600 mg q24h	300-600 mg q24h	HEMO: No adjustment CAPD: Dose for CrCl <10	
ANTIVIRAL AGENTS For ANTIRETROVIRALS (See CID 40:1559, 2005)									
Acyclovir, IV	2-4/20	5-12.4 mg per kg q8h	D&I	100% q8h	100% q12-24h	50% q24h	HEMO: Dose AD CAPD: Dose for CrCl <10	Rapid IV infusion can cause ↑ Cr. CRRT dose: 5-10 mg/kg q24h
Adefovir	7.5/15	10 mg po q24h	I	10 mg q24h	10 mg q48-72h[3]	10 mg q72h[3]	HEMO: 10 mg q week AD	CAPD: No data; CRRT: Dose?
Amantadine	12/500	100 mg po bid	I	q12h	q24-48h	q 7 days	HEMO/CAPD: Dose for CrCl<10/	CRRT: Dose for CrCl 10-50
Atripla	See each drug	200 mg emtricitabine + 300 mg tenofovir + 600 mg efavirenz	I	Do not use if CrCl <50				
Cidofovir: **Complicated dosing**—see package insert									

[3] Ref: Transplantation 80:1086, 2005

Abbreviation Key. Adjustment Method: **D** = dose adjustment; **I** = interval adjustment; **CAPD** = continuous ambulatory peritoneal dialysis; **CRRT** = continuous renal replacement therapy; **HEMO** = hemodialysis; **AD** = after dialysis; "**Supplement**" or "**Extra**" is to replace drug lost during dialysis – additional continuation of regimen for CrCl < 10 mL/min.

TABLE 17A (8)

ANTIMICROBIAL	HALF-LIFE (NORMAL/ESRD) hr	DOSE FOR NORMAL RENAL FUNCTION	METHOD (see footer)	ADJUSTMENT FOR RENAL FAILURE Estimated creatinine clearance (CrCl), mL/min			HEMODIALYSIS, CAPD	COMMENTS & DOSAGE FOR CRRT
				>90	50-90	10-50	<10		
ANTIVIRAL AGENTS For ANTIRETROVIRALS *(continued)*									
Induction	2.5/unknown	5 mg per kg once per wk, for 2 wks	I	5 mg per kg once per wk		Contraindicated in pts with CrCl ≤ 55 mL/min.			Major toxicity is renal. No efficacy, safety, or pharmacokinetic data in pts with moderate/severe renal disease.
Maintenance	2.5/unknown	5 mg per kg q2wks	I	5 mg per kg q2wks		Contraindicated in pts with CrCl ≤ 55 mL/min.			
Didanosine tablets[a]	0.6-1.6/4.5	125-200 mg q12h buffered tabs	D		200 mg q24h	125-200 mg q24h	<60 kg: 150 mg q24h >60 kg: 100 mg q24h	HEMO: Dose AD CAPD/CRRT: Dose for CrCl <10	Based on incomplete data. Data are estimates.
		400 mg q24h enteric-coated tabs	D		400 mg q24h	30-49: 200 mg q48h 10-29: 200 mg q72h	Do not use EC tabs	HEMO/CAPD: Dose for CrCl <10	If <60 kg & CrCl <10 mL per min, do not use EC tabs
Emtricitabine (CAPS)	10/>10	200 mg q24h	I		200 mg q24h	30-50: 1 tab q48h	200 mg q96h	HEMO: Dose for CrCl <10	See package insert for oral solution.
Emtricitabine + Tenofovir	See each drug		I		No change		CrCl <30: Do not use		
Entecavir	128-149/?	0.5 mg q24h	D		0.5 mg q24h	0.15-0.25 mg q24h	0.05 mg q24h	HEMO/CAPD: 0.05 mg q24h	Give after dialysis on dialysis days
Famciclovir	2.3-3/10-22	500 mg q8h	D&I		500 mg q8h	500 mg q12-24h	250 mg q24h	HEMO: Dose AD CAPD: No data	CRRT: Not applicable
Foscarnet (CMV dosage). Dosage adjustment based on est. CrCl divided by wt (kg)	Normal half-life (T½) 3 hrs with terminal T½ of 18-88 hrs. T½ very long with ESRD	Induction: 60 mg/kg IV q8h × 2-3 wks		CrCl (mL/min per kg body weight—only for Foscarnet)					See package insert for further details
				>1.4	>1-1.4	>0.8-1	>0.6-0.8	>0.5-0.6	>0.4-0.5	<0.4		
				60 q6h	45 q6h	50 q12h	40 q12h	50 q24h	Do not use		
		Maintenance 90-120 mg/kg/day IV		120 q24h	90 q24h	65 q24h	105 q48h	80 q48h	65 q48h	Do not use		
Ganciclovir	3.6/30	IV: Induction 5 mg per kg q12h IV	D&I	70-90: 5 mg per kg q12h 50-60: 2.5-5.0 mg per kg q12h	25-49: 2.5 mg per kg q24h 10-24: 1.25 mg/kg q24h		1.25 mg per kg 3 times per wk	HEMO: Dose AD CAPD: Dose for CrCl <10	
		Maintenance 5 mg per kg q24h IV	D&I	2.5-5.0 mg per kg q24h	0.6-1.25 mg per kg q24h	0.625 mg per kg 3 times per wk	0.625 mg per kg AD CAPD: Dose for CrCl <10	HEMO: 0.6 mg per kg AD CAPD: Dose for CrCl <10	
	po:	1 gm tid po	D&I	0.5-1 gm tid	0.5-1 gm q24h	0.5 gm 3 times per week	HEMO: 0.5 gm AD		
Maraviroc	14-18/No data	300 mg bid		300 mg bid					Risk of side effects increased if concomitant CYP3A inhibitor
Lamivudine	5-7/15-35	300 mg po q24h	D&I	300 mg po q24h	50-150 mg q24h	25-50 mg q24h	HEMO: Dose AD; CAPD: Dose for CrCl <10. CRRT: 100 mg 1st day, then 50 mg/day		

[a] Ref: for NRTIs and NNRTIs: *Kidney International* 60:821, 2001

Abbreviation Key. Adjustment Method: **D** = dose adjustment; **I** = interval adjustment; **CAPD** = continuous ambulatory peritoneal dialysis; **CRRT** = continuous renal replacement therapy; **HEMO** = hemodialysis; **AD** = after dialysis; "**supplement**" or "**Extra**" is to replace drug lost during dialysis – additional drug beyond continuation of regimen for CrCl < 10 mL/min.

TABLE 17A (9)

ANTIMICROBIAL	HALF-LIFE (NORMAL/ ESRD) hr	DOSE FOR NORMAL RENAL FUNCTION	METHOD (See footer)	ADJUSTMENT FOR RENAL FAILURE Estimated creatinine clearance (CrCl), mL/min			HEMODIALYSIS, CAPD	COMMENTS & DOSAGE FOR CRRT
				>50–90	10–50	<10		
ANTIVIRAL AGENTS For ANTIRETROVIRALS (continued)									
Oseltamivir, therapy	6-10/>20	75 mg bid – treatment		75 mg q12h	**30-49:** 75 mg bid **<30:** 75 mg once daily	No data	HEMO: 30 mg non-dialysis days[a]; CAPD: 30 mg once per week	Dose for prophylaxis if CrCl <30: 75 mg once daily CRRT: 75 mg po bid
Peramivir		600 mg once daily	P&I	600 mg once daily	**31-49:** 150 mg q24h **10-30:** 100 mg q24h	100 mg (single dose) then 15 mg q24h	HEMO: 100 mg (single dose) then 100 mg 2 hrs AD (dialysis days only)	CRRT: http://www.cdc.gov/h1n1flu/eva/peramivir.htm
Ribavirin	Use with caution in patients with creatinine clearance <50 mL per min.							
Rimantadine	13–65/Prolonged	100 mg bid po	I	100 mg bid	100 mg q24h-bid	100 mg q24h	HEMO/CAPD: No data	Use with caution, little data
Stavudine, po	1-1.4/5-8	30-40 mg q12h	D&I	100%	50% q12–24h	≥60 kg: 20 mg per day <60 kg: 15 mg per day	HEMO: Dose as for CrCl <10 AD CAPD: No data CRRT: Full dose	
Stribild		1 tab daily		If CrCl <70: contraindicated	If CrCl <50: discontinue			
Telbivudine	40-49/No data	600 mg daily	I	600 mg q48h	**30-49:** 600 mg q48H **<30:** 600 mg q72h	600 mg q96h	HEMO: As for CrCl <10 AD	
Tenofovir, po	17/?	300 mg q24h	I	300 mg q24h	**30-49:** 300 mg q48h **10-29:** 300 mg q72-96h	No data	HEMO: 300 mg q7d or after 12 hrs of HEMO.[a]	
Valacyclovir	2.5-3.3/14	1 gm q8h	D&I	1 gm q8h	1 gm q12-24h **Same dose for CRRT**	0.5 gm q24h	HEMO: Dose AD CAPD: Dose for CrCl <10	CAVH dose: As for CrCl 10-50
Valganciclovir	4/67	900 mg po bid	D&I	900 mg po bid	450 mg q24h to 450 mg every other day	DO NOT USE	See package insert	
Zalcitabine	2/>8	0.75 mg q8h	D&I	0.75 mg q8h	0.75 mg q12h **Same dose for CRRT**	0.75 mg q24h	HEMO: Dose AD CAPD: No data	CRRT dose: As for CrCl 10-50
Zidovudine	1.1-1.4/1.4-3	300 mg q12h	D&I	300 mg q12h	300 mg q12h **Same dose for CRRT**	100 mg q8h	HEMO: Dose for CrCl <10 AD CAPD: Dose for CrCl <10	

[a] HEMO wt-based dose adjustments for children age >1 yr (dose after each HEMO): ≤15 kg: 7.5 mg; 16-23 kg: 10 mg; 24-40 kg: 15 mg; >40 kg: 30 mg (CID 50:127, 2010).
[b] Acute renal failure and Fanconi syndrome reported.

Abbreviation Key; Adjustment Method: **D** = dose adjustment, **I** = interval adjustment; **CAPD** = continuous ambulatory peritoneal dialysis; **CRRT** = continuous renal replacement therapy; **HEMO** = hemodialysis; **AD** = after dialysis; "**Supplement**" or "**Extra**" is to replace drug lost during dialysis – additional continuation of regimen for CrCl <10 mL/min.

213

TABLE 17B – NO DOSAGE ADJUSTMENT WITH RENAL INSUFFICIENCY BY CATEGORY*

Antibacterials		Antifungals	Anti-TBc	Antivirals	
Azithromycin	Minocycline	Anidulafungin	Ethionamide	Abacavir	Lopinavir
Ceftriaxone	Moxifloxacin	Caspofungin	Isoniazid	Atazanavir	Nelfinavir
Chloramphenicol	Nafcillin	Itraconazole oral solution	Rifampin	Darunavir	Nevirapine
Ciprofloxacin XL	Polymyxin B	Ketoconazole	Rifabutin	Delavirdine	Raltegravir
Clindamycin	Pyrimethamine	Micafungin	Rifapentine	Efavirenz	Ribavirin
Doxycycline	Rifaximin	Voriconazole, **po only**		Enfuvirtide[1]	Saquinavir
Linezolid	Tigecycline			Fosamprenavir	Tipranavir
				Indinavir	

[1] Enfuvirtide: Not studied in patients with CrCl <35 mL/min. DO NOT USE

TABLE 18 – ANTIMICROBIALS AND HEPATIC DISEASE: DOSAGE ADJUSTMENT*

The following alphabetical list indicates antibacterials excreted/metabolized by the liver **wherein a dosage adjustment may be indicated** in the presence of hepatic disease. Space precludes details; consult the PDR or package inserts for details. List is **not** all-inclusive:

Antibacterials		Antifungals	Antivirals[§]	
Ceftriaxone	Nafcillin	Caspofungin	Abacavir	Indinavir
Chloramphenicol	Rifabutin	Itraconazole	Atazanavir	Lopinavir/ritonavir
Clindamycin	Rifampin	Voriconazole	Darunavir	Nelfinavir
Fusidic acid	Synercid**		Delavirdine	Nevirapine
Isoniazid	Telithromycin**		Efavirenz	Rimantadine
Metronidazole	Tigecycline		Enfuvirtide	Ritonavir
	Tinidazole		Fosamprenavir	Stribild

[§] Ref. on antiretrovirals: *CID* 40:174, 2005   ** Quinupristin/dalfopristin   ** Telithro: reduce dose in renal & hepatic failure

---

TABLE 19 – TREATMENT OF CAPD PERITONITIS IN ADULTS*
(Periton Dial Intl 30:393, 2010)[2]

EMPIRIC Intraperitoneal Therapy: Culture Results Pending *(For MRSA see footnote[3])*

Drug		Residual Urine Output	
		<100 mL per day	>100 mL per day
(Cefazolin or Vanco) +	Can mix in same bag	1 gm per bag, q24h	20 mg per kg BW per bag, q24h
Ceftazidime		1 gm per bag, q24h	20 mg per kg BW per bag, q24h

Drug Doses for SPECIFIC Intraperitoneal Therapy—Culture Results Known. NOTE: Few po drugs indicated

Drug	Intermittent Dosing (once per day)		Continuous Dosing (per liter exchange)	
	Anuric	Non-Anuric	Anuric	Non-Anuric
Amphotericin B	NA	NA	MD 1.5 mg	NA
Ampicillin	250–500 mg po bid	ND	No LD, MD 125 mg	ND
Amp-sulbactam	2 gm q12h	ND	LD 1 gm, MD 100 mg	LD 1 gm, MD ↑ 25%
Cefazolin	15 mg per kg	20 mg per kg	LD 500 mg, MD 125 mg	LD 500 mg, ↑ MD 25%
Cefepime	1 gm in one exchange/day	1.25 gm	LD 500 mg, MD 125 mg	LD 500 mg, ↑ MD 25%
Ceftazidime	1000–1500 mg	ND	LD 500 mg, MD 125 mg	LD 500 mg; ↑ MD 25%
Ciprofloxacin	500 mg po bid		LD 50 mg, MD 25 mg	ND
Daptomycin			LD 100 mg, MD 20 mg	LD 500 mg, ↑ MD 25%
Fluconazole	200 mg q24h	ND	200 mg q24h	ND
Gentamicin	0.6 mg per kg	↑ dose 25%	Not recommended	Not recommended
Imipenem	1 gm in one exchange q12h		LD 250 mg, MD 50 mg	LD 250 mg, ↑ MD 25%
Itraconazole	100 mg q12h	100 mg q12h	100 mg q12h	100 mg q12h
Metronidazole	250 mg po bid	ND	250 mg po bid	ND
TMP-SMX	160/800 mg po bid	ND	LD 320/1600 mg po, MD 80/400 mg po q24h	ND
Vancomycin	15–30 mg per kg q3–7 days	↑ dose 25%	LD 1 gm; MD 25 mg	LD 1 gm, ↑ MD 25%

CAPD = continuous ambulatory peritoneal dialysis
Indications for catheter removal: 1) Relapse with same organism within 1 mo; 2) Failure to respond clinically within 5 days;
3) Exit site and tunnel infection; 4) Fungal peritonitis; 5) Fecal flora peritonitis (suggests bowel perforation).
[1] Ref. for NRTIs and NNRTIs: *Kidney International* 60:821, 2001
[2] **All doses IP unless indicated otherwise.**
LD = loading dose, **MD** = maintenance dose, **ND** = no data; **NA** = not applicable—dose as normal renal function.
Anuric = <100 mL per day, **non-anuric** = >100 mL per day
[3] **Does not provide treatment for MRSA.** If gram-pos cocci on gram stain, include vanco.
* See page 2 for other abbreviations

TABLE 20A – ANTI-TETANUS PROPHYLAXIS, WOUND CLASSIFICATION, IMMUNIZATION

WOUND CLASSIFICATION

Clinical Features	Tetanus Prone	Non-Tetanus Prone
Age of wound	> 6 hours	≤ 6 hours
Configuration	Stellate, avulsion	Linear
Depth	> 1 cm	≤ 1 cm
Mechanism of injury	Missile, crush, burn, frostbite	Sharp surface (glass, knife)
Devitalized tissue	Present	Absent
Contaminants (dirt, saliva, etc.)	Present	Absent

(From ACS Bull. 69:22,23, 1984, No. 10)

IMMUNIZATION SCHEDULE

History of Tetanus Immunization	Dirty, Tetanus-Prone Wound Td[1,3]	Dirty, Tetanus-Prone Wound Tetanus Immune Globulin	Clean, non-Tetanus-Prone Wound Td[1,2]	Clean, non-Tetanus-Prone Wound Tetanus Immune Globulin
Unknown or < 3 doses[3]	Yes	Yes	Yes	No
3 or more doses	No[4]	No	No[5]	No

References: MMWR 39:37, 1990; MMWR 46 (SS-2):15, 1997; MMWR 61:1-468, 2012; general vaccine considerations; MMWR 60 (RR-2):1, 2011; and general immunization schedule, MMWR 61:1, 2012.

[1] Td = Tetanus & diphtheria toxoids, adsorbed (adult). For adult who has not received Tdap previously, substitute one dose of Tdap for Td when immunization is indicated (MMWR 61:::-468, 2012).
[2] For children < 7 years, use DTaP unless contraindicated; for persons ≥ 7 years, Td is preferred to tetanus toxoid alone, but single dose of Tdap can be used if required for catch-up series.
[3] Individuals who have not completed vaccine series should do so.
[4] Yes, if > 5 years since last booster
[5] Yes, if > 10 years since last booster

TABLE 20B – RABIES POSTEXPOSURE PROPHYLAXIS

All wounds should be cleaned immediately & thoroughly with soap & water. This has been shown to protect 90% of experimental animals![1]

Postexposure Prophylaxis Guide, United States, 2012

(MMWR 57 (RR-3): 1, 2008; http://wwwnc.cdc.gov/travel/yellowbook/2012/chapter-3-infectious-diseases-related-to-travel/rabies.htm)

Animal Type	Evaluation & Disposition of Animal	Recommendations for Prophylaxis
Dogs, cats, ferrets	Healthy & available for 10-day observation	Don't start unless animal develops sx, then immediately begin HRIG + vaccine
	Rabid or suspected rabid	Immediate HRIG + vaccine
	Unknown (escaped)	Consult public health officials
Skunks, raccoons, bats,* foxes, coyotes, most carnivores	Regard as rabid	Immediate vaccination
Livestock, horses, rodents, rabbits; includes hares, squirrels, hamsters, guinea pigs, gerbils, chipmunks, rats, mice, woodchucks	Consider case-by-case	Consult public health officials. Bites of squirrels, hamsters, guinea pigs, gerbils, chipmunks, rats, mice, other small rodents, rabbits, and hares **almost never** require rabies post-exposure prophylaxis

* Most recent cases of human rabies in U.S. due to contact (not bites) with silver-haired bats or rarely big brown bats but risk of acquiring rabies from non-contact bat exposure is exceedingly low *(CID 48:1493, 2009)*. For more detail, see *CID 30:4, 2000; JAVMA 219:1687, 2001; CID 37:96, 2003 (travel medicine advisory); Ln 363:959, 2004; EID 11:1921, 2005; MMWR 55 (RR-5), 2006.*

Postexposure Rabies Immunization Schedule

IF NOT PREVIOUSLY VACCINATED

Treatment	Regimen[2]
Local wound cleaning	**All postexposure treatment should begin with immediate, thorough cleaning of all wounds with soap & water.**
Human rabies immune globulin (HRIG)	20 units per kg body weight given once on day 0. If anatomically feasible, the full dose should be infiltrated around the wound(s), the rest should be administered IM in the gluteal area. If the calculated dose of HRIG is insufficient to inject all the wounds, it should be diluted with normal saline to allow infiltration around additional wound areas. HRIG should **not** be administered in the **same syringe**, **or** into the **same anatomical site** as vaccine, or more than 7 days after the initiation of vaccine. Because HRIG may partially suppress active production of antibody, no more than the recommended dose should be given.[3]
Vaccine	Human diploid cell vaccine (HDCV), rabies vaccine adsorbed (RVA), or purified chick embryo cell vaccine (PCECV) 1 mL **IM (deltoid area**[4]**)**, one each days 0, 3, 7, 14[5].

IF PREVIOUSLY VACCINATED[6]

Treatment	Regimen[2]
Local wound cleaning	All postexposure treatment should begin with immediate, thorough cleaning of all wounds with soap & water.
HRIG	HRIG should **not** be administered
Vaccine	HDCV or PCEC, 1 mL **IM (deltoid area**[4]**)**, one each on days 0 & 3

CORRECT VACCINE ADMINISTRATION SITES

Age Group	Administration Site
Children & adults	**DELTOID**[4] only (**NEVER** in gluteus)
Infants & young children	Outer aspect of thigh (anterolateral thigh) may be used (**NEVER** in gluteus)

---

[1] From *MMWR 48:RR-1, 1999; CID 30:4, 2000;* B. T. Matyas, Mass. Dept. of Public Health.

[2] These regimens are applicable for all age groups, including children.

[3] In most reported post-exposure treatment failures, only identified deficiency was failure to infiltrate wound(s) with HRIG *(CID 22:228, 1996)*. However, several failures reported from SE Asia in patients in whom WHO protocol followed *(CID 28:143, 1999)*.

[4] The **deltoid** area is the **only** acceptable site of vaccination for adults & older children. For infants & young children, outer aspect of the thigh (anterolateral thigh) may be used. Vaccine should **NEVER** be administered in gluteal area.

[5] Note that this is a change from previous recommendation of 5 doses (days 0, 3, 7, 14 & 28) based on new data & recommendations from ACIP. Note that the number of doses for persons with altered immunocompetence remains unchanged (5 doses on days 0, 3, 7, 14 & 28) and recommendations for pre-exposure prophylaxis remain 3 doses administered on days 0, 7 and 21 or 28 *(MMWR 59 (RR-2), 2010).*

[6] Any person with a history of pre-exposure vaccination with HDCV, RVA, PCECV; prior post-exposure prophylaxis with HDCV, PCEC or rabies vaccine adsorbed (RVA); or previous vaccination with any other type of rabies vaccine & a documented history of antibody response to the prior vaccination.

TABLE 21 SELECTED DIRECTORY OF RESOURCES

ORGANIZATION	PHONE/FAX	WEBSITE(S)
ANTIPARASITIC DRUGS & PARASITOLOGY INFORMATION (CID 37:694, 2003)		
CDC Drug Line	Weekdays: 404-639-3670	http://www.cdc.gov/ncidod/srp/drugs/drug-service.html
	Evenings, weekends, holidays: 404-639-2888	
DPDx: Lab ID of parasites		www.dpd.cdc.gov/dpdx/default.htm
Gorgas Course Tropical Medicine		http://info.dom.uab.edu/gorgas
Malaria	daytime: 770-488-7788	www.cdc.gov/malaria
	other: 770-488-7100	
	US toll free: 855-856-4713	
Expert Compound. Pharm.	800-247-9767/818-787-7256	www.uniquerx.com
World Health Organization (WHO)		www.who.int
Parasites & Health		www.dpd.cdc.gov/dpdx/HTML/Para_Health.htm
BIOTERRORISM		
Centers for Disease Control & Prevention	770-488-7100	www.bt.cdc.gov
Infectious Diseases Society of America	703-299-0200	www.idsociety.org
Johns Hopkins Center Civilian Biodefense		www.jhsph.edu
Center for Biosecurity of the Univ. of Pittsburgh Med. Center		www.upmc-biosecurity.org
US Army Medical Research Institute of Inf. Dis.		www.usamriid.army.mil
HEPATITIS B		
Hepatitis B Foundation		www.hepb.org, www.natap.org
HEPATITIS C (CID 35:754, 2002)		
CDC		www.cdc.gov/ncidod/diseases/hepatitis/C
Individual		http://hepatitis-central.com
		www.natap.org
Medscape		www.medscape.com
HIV		
General		
HIV InSite		http://hivinsite.ucsf.edu
Johns Hopkins AIDS Service		www.hopkins-aids.edu
		www.natap.org
Drug Interactions		
Johns Hopkins AIDS Service		www.hopkins-aids.edu
Liverpool HIV Pharm. Group		www.hiv-druginteractions.org
Other		http://AIDS.medscape.com
Prophylaxis/Treatment of Opportunistic Infections; HIV Treatment		www.aidsinfo.nih.gov
IMMUNIZATIONS (CID 36:355, 2003)		
CDC, Natl. Immunization Program	404-639-8200	www.cdc.gov/vaccines/
FDA, Vaccine Adverse Events	800-822-7967	www.fda.gov/cber/vaers/vaers.htm
National Network Immunization Info.	877-341-6644	www.immunizationinfo.org
Influenza vaccine, CDC	404-639-8200	www.cdc.gov/vaccines/
Institute for Vaccine Safety		www.vaccinesafety.edu
OCCUPATIONAL EXPOSURE, BLOOD-BORNE PATHOGENS (HIV, HEPATITIS B & C)		
National Clinicians' Post-Exposure Hotline	888-448-4911	www.ucsf.edu/hivcntr
Q-T$_c$ INTERVAL PROLONGATION BY DRUGS		www.qtdrugs.org
SEXUALLY TRANSMITTED DISEASES		www.cdc.gov/std/treatment/TOC2002TG.htm
	Slides: http://www.phac-aspc.gc.ca/slm-maa/slides/index.html	
TRAVELERS' INFO: Immunizations, Malaria Prophylaxis, More		
Amer. Soc. Trop. Med. & Hyg.		www.astmh.org
CDC, general	877-394-8747/888-232-3299	http://wwwn.cdc.gov/travel/default.asp
CDC, Malaria:		www.cdc.gov/malaria
Prophylaxis		http://wwwn.cdc.gov/travel/default.asp
Treatment	770-488-7788	www.who.int/health_topics/malaria
MD Travel Health		www.mdtravelhealth.com
Pan American Health Organization		www.paho.org
World Health Organization (WHO)		www.who.int/home-page
VACCINE & IMMUNIZATION RESOURCES (CID 36:355, 2003)		
American Academy of Pediatrics		www.cispimmunize.org
CDC, National Immunization Program		www.cdc.gov/vaccines/
National Network for Immunization Information		www.immunizationinfo.org

TABLE 22A – ANTI-INFECTIVE DRUG-DRUG INTERACTIONS

Importance: ± = theory/anecdotal; + = of probable importance; ++ = of definite importance
To check for interactions between more than 2 drugs, see: http://www.drugs.com/drug_interactions.html
and http://www.healthline.com/druginteractions

ANTI-INFECTIVE AGENT (A)	OTHER DRUG (B)	EFFECT	IMPORT
Abacavir	Methadone	↓ levels of B	++
Amantadine (Symmetrel)	Alcohol	↑ CNS effects	+
	Anticholinergic and anti-Parkinson agents (ex. Artane, scopolamine)	↑ effect of B: dry mouth, ataxia, blurred vision, slurred speech, toxic psychosis	+
	Trimethoprim	↑ levels of A & B	+
	Digoxin	↑ levels of B	±
Aminoglycosides— parenteral (amikacin, gentamicin, kanamycin, netilmicin, sisomicin, streptomycin, tobramycin)	Amphotericin B	↑ nephrotoxicity	++
	Cis platinum (Platinol)	↑ nephro & ototoxicity	+
	Cyclosporine	↑ nephrotoxicity	+
	Neuromuscular blocking agents	↑ apnea or respiratory paralysis	+
	Loop diuretics (e.g., furosemide)	↑ ototoxicity	++
	NSAIDs	↑ nephrotoxicity	+
	Non-polarizing muscle relaxants	↑ apnea	+
	Radiographic contrast	↑ nephrotoxicity	+
	Vancomycin	↑ nephrotoxicity	+
Aminoglycosides— oral (kanamycin, neomycin)	Oral anticoagulants (dicumarol, phenindione, warfarin)	↑ prothrombin time	+
Amphotericin B and ampho B lipid formulations	Antineoplastic drugs	↑ nephrotoxicity risk	+
	Digitalis	↑ toxicity of B if K⁺ ↓	+
	Nephrotoxic drugs: aminoglycosides, cidofovir, cyclosporine, foscarnet, pentamidine	↑ nephrotoxicity of A	++
Ampicillin, amoxicillin	Allopurinol	↑ frequency of rash	++
Artemether-lumefantrine	CYP3A inhibitors: amiodarone, atazanavir, itraconazole, ritonavir, voriconazole	↑ levels of A; ↑ QTc interval	++
	CYP2D6 substrates: flecainide, imipramine, amitriptyline	↑ levels of B; ↑ QTc interval	++
Atazanavir	See protease inhibitors and Table 22B		
Atovaquone	Rifampin (perhaps rifabutin)	↓ serum levels of A; ↑ levels of B	+
	Metoclopramide	↓ levels of A	+
	Tetracycline	↓ levels of A	++

Azole Antifungal Agents [**Flu** = fluconazole; **Itr** = itraconazole; **Ket** = ketoconazole; **Posa** = posaconazole; **Vor** = voriconazole; + = occurs; **blank space** = either studied & no interaction OR no data found (may be in pharm. co. databases)]

Flu	Itr	Ket	Posa	Vor		EFFECT	IMPORT
+	+				Amitriptyline	↑ levels of B	+
+	+	+		+	Calcium channel blockers	↑ levels of B	++
	+			+	Carbamazepine (vori contraindicated)	↓ levels of A	++
+	+	+	+	+	Cyclosporine	↑ levels of B, ↑ risk of nephrotoxicity	+
	+	+			Didanosine	↓ absorption of A	+
+	+	+	+	+	Efavirenz	↓ levels of A, ↑ levels of B	++ (avoid)
	+	+	+		H₂ blockers, antacids, sucralfate	↓ absorption of A	+
+	+	+		+	Hydantoins (phenytoin, Dilantin)	↑ levels of B, ↓ levels of A	++
+	+	+			Isoniazid	↓ levels of A	+
+	+	+	+	+	Lovastatin/simvastatin	Rhabdomyolysis reported; ↑ levels of B	++
				+	Methadone	↑ levels of B	+
+	+	+	+	+	Midazolam/triazolam, po	↑ levels of B	++
+	+			+	Oral anticoagulants	↑ effect of B	++
+	+				Oral hypoglycemics	↑ levels of B	++
			+	+	Pimozide	↑ levels of B—**avoid**	++
	+	+		+	Protease inhibitors	↑ levels of B	++
+	+	+	+	+	Proton pump inhibitors	↓ levels of A, ↑ levels of B	++
+	+	+	+	+	Rifampin/rifabutin (vori contraindicated)	↑ levels of B, ↓ serum levels of A	++
	+				Rituximab	Inhibits action of B	++
		−	+	+	Sirolimus (vori and posa contraindicated)	↑ levels of B	++
+		+	+	+	Tacrolimus	↑ levels of B with toxicity	++
+					Theophyllines	↑ levels of B	+
		+			Trazodone	↑ levels of B	++
+					Zidovudine	↑ levels of B	+

TABLE 22A (2)

ANTI-INFECTIVE AGENT (A)	OTHER DRUG (B)	EFFECT	IMPORT
Bedaquiline	Rifampin	↓ levels of A	++
	Ketoconazole	↑ levels of A	
Caspofungin	Cyclosporine	↑ levels of A	++
	Tacrolimus	↓ levels of B	++
	Carbamazepine, dexamethasone, efavirenz, nevirapine, phenytoin, rifampin	↓ levels of A; ↑ dose of caspofungin to 70 mg/d	++
Chloramphenicol	Hydantoins	↑ toxicity of B, nystagmus, ataxia	++
	Iron salts, Vitamin B12	↓ response to B	++
	Protease inhibitors—HIV	↑ levels of A & B	++
Clindamycin (Cleocin)	Kaolin	↓ absorption of A	++
	Muscle relaxants, e.g., atracurium, baclofen, diazepam	↑ frequency/duration of respiratory paralysis	++
	St John's wort	↓ levels of A	++
Cobicistat	See Stribild, below		
Cycloserine	Ethanol	↑ frequency of seizures	+
	INH, ethionamide	↑ frequency of drowsiness/dizziness	+
Dapsone	Atazanavir	↑ levels of A - Avoid	++
	Didanosine	↓ absorption of A	+
	Oral contraceptives	↓ effectiveness of B	+
	Pyrimethamine	↑ in marrow toxicity	+
	Rifampin/Rifabutin	↓ serum levels of A	+
	Trimethoprim	↑ levels of A & B (methemoglobinemia)	+
	Zidovudine	May ↑ marrow toxicity	+
Daptomycin	HMG-CoA inhibitors (statins)	Consider DC statin while on dapto	++
Delavirdine (Rescriptor)	See Non-nucleoside reverse transcriptase inhibitors (NNRTIs) and Table 22B		
Didanosine (ddI) (Videx)	Allopurinol	↑ levels of A—**AVOID**	++
	Cisplatin, dapsone, INH, metronidazole, nitrofurantoin, stavudine, vincristine, zalcitabine	↑ risk of peripheral neuropathy	+
	Ethanol, lamivudine, pentamidine	↑ risk of pancreatitis	+
	Fluoroquinolones	↓ absorption 2° to chelation	+
	Drugs that need low pH for absorption: dapsone, indinavir, itra-/ketoconazole, pyrimethamine, rifampin, trimethoprim	↓ absorption	+
	Methadone	↓ levels of A	++
	Ribavirin	↑ levels ddI metabolite—**avoid**	++
	Tenofovir	↑ levels of A **(reduce dose of A)**	++
Doripenem	Probenecid	↑ levels of A	++
	Valproic acid	↓ levels of B	++
Doxycycline	Aluminum, bismuth, iron, Mg++	↓ absorption of A	+
	Barbiturates, hydantoins	↓ serum t½ of A	+
	Carbamazepine (Tegretol)	↓ serum t½ of A	+
	Digoxin	↑ serum levels of B	+
	Warfarin	↑ activity of B	++
Efavirenz (Sustiva)	See non-nucleoside reverse transcriptase inhibitors (NNRTIs) and Table 22B		
Elvitegravir	See Stribild, below		
Ertapenem (Invanz)	Probenecid	↑ levels of A	++
	Valproic acid	↓ levels of B	++
Ethambutol (Myambutol)	Aluminum salts (includes didanosine buffer)	↓ absorption of A & B	+
Etravirine	See non-nucleoside reverse transcriptase inhibitors (NNRTIs) and Table 22B		
Fluoroquinolones	(**Cipro** = ciprofloxacin; **Gati** = gatifloxacin; **Gemi** = gemifloxacin; **Levo** = levofloxacin; **Moxi** = moxifloxacin; **Oflox** = ofloxacin)		

Cipro	Gati	Gemi	Levo	Moxi	Oflox	NOTE: Blank space = either studied and no interaction OR no data found		
	+		+	+	+	Antiarrhythmics (procainamide, amiodarone)	↑ Q-T interval (torsade)	++
+	+		+	+	+	Insulin, oral hypoglycemics	↑ & ↓ blood sugar	++
+						Caffeine	↑ levels of B	+
+				+		Cimetidine	↑ levels of A	+
+						Cyclosporine	↑ levels of B	±
+	+		+	+	+	Didanosine	↓ absorption of A	++

TABLE 22A (3)

Fluoroquinolones (continued)

ANTI-INFECTIVE AGENT (A)	OTHER DRUG (B)	EFFECT	IMPORT
Cipro / Gati / Gemi / Levo / Moxi / Oflox	NOTE: Blank space = either studied and no interaction OR no data found		
+ + + + + +	**Cations: Al+++, Ca++, Fe++, Mg++, Zn++ (antacids, vitamins, dairy products), citrate/citric acid**	↓ absorption of A (some variability between drugs)	++
+	Methadone	↑ levels of B	++
+ + +	NSAIDs	↑ risk CNS stimulation/seizures	++
+ +	Phenytoin	↑ or ↓ levels of B	+
+ + +	Probenecid	↓ renal clearance of A	+
+ +	Rasagiline	↑ levels of B	++
+	Rifampin	↓ levels of A *(CID 45:1001, 2007)*	++
+ + + + +	**Sucralfate**	**↓ absorption of A**	++
+ + + +	Theophylline	↑ levels of B	++
+	Thyroid hormone	↓ levels of B	++
+ +	Tizanidine	↑ levels of B	++
+ + + +	Warfarin	↑ prothrombin time	+

Ganciclovir (Cytovene) & **Valganciclovir** (Valcyte)	Imipenem	↑ risk of seizures reported	+
	Probenecid	↑ levels of A	+
	Zidovudine	↓ levels of A, ↑ levels of B	+

| **Gentamicin** | *See Aminoglycosides—parenteral* | | |

Imipenem & Meropenem	BCG	↓ effectiveness of B – avoid combination	++
	Divalproex	↓ levels of B	++
	Ganciclovir	seizure risk	++
	Probenecid	↑ levels of A	++
	Valproic acid	↓ levels of B	++

| **Indinavir** | *See protease inhibitors and Table 22B* | | |

Isoniazid	**Alcohol, rifampin**	**↑ risk of hepatic injury**	++
	Aluminum salts	↓ absorption (take fasting)	++
	Carbamazepine, phenytoin	↑ levels of B with nausea, vomiting, nystagmus, ataxia	++
	Itraconazole, ketoconazole	↓ levels of B	+
	Oral hypoglycemics	↓ effects of B	+

| **Lamivudine** | Zalcitabine | **Mutual interference—do not combine** | ++ |

Linezolid (Zyvox)	Adrenergic agents	Risk of hypertension	++
	Aged, fermented, pickled or smoked foods —↑ tyramine	Risk of hypertension	+
	Clarithromycin	↑ levels of A	++
	Rasagiline (MAO inhibitor)	Risk of serotonin syndrome	+
	Rifampin	↓ levels of A	++
	Serotonergic drugs (SSRIs)	Risk of serotonin syndrome	++

| **Lopinavir** | *See protease inhibitors* | | |

Macrolides [**Ery** = erythromycin; **Azi** = azithromycin; **Clr** = clarithromycin; + = occurs; **blank space** = either studied and no interaction OR no data]

Ery	Azi	Clr			
+		+	Carbamazepine	↑ serum levels of B, nystagmus, nausea, vomiting, ataxia	++ (avoid w/ erythro)
+		+	Cimetidine, **ritonavir**	↑ levels of B	+
+		+	Clozapine	↑ serum levels of B, CNS toxicity	+
		+	**Colchicine**	**↑ levels of B (potent, fatal)**	++ (avoid)
+		+	Corticosteroids	↑ effects of B	+
+	+	+	Cyclosporine	↑ serum levels of B with toxicity	+
+		+	Digoxin, digitoxin	↑ serum levels of B (10% of cases)	+
		+	Efavirenz	↓ levels of A	++
+		+	Ergot alkaloids	↑ levels of B	++
		+	Linezolid	↑ levels of B	++
+		+	Lovastatin/simvastatin	↑ levels of B; rhabdomyolysis	++
+		+	Midazolam, triazolam	↑ levels of B, ↑ sedative effects	+
+		+	Phenytoin	↑ levels of B	+
+	+	+	Pimozide	**Q-T interval**	++
+		+	Rifampin, rifabutin	↓ levels of A	+
+		+	Tacrolimus	↑ levels of B	++
+		+	Theophylline	↑ serum levels of B with nausea, vomiting, seizures, apnea	++
		+	Valproic acid	↑ levels of B	+
+		+	Warfarin	May ↑ prothrombin time	+
		+	Zidovudine	↓ levels of B	+

TABLE 22A (4)

ANTI-INFECTIVE AGENT (A)	OTHER DRUG (B)	EFFECT	IMPORT
Maraviroc	Clarithromycin	↑ serum levels of A	++
	Delavirdine	↑ levels of A	++
	Itraconazole/ketoconazole	↑ levels of A	++
	Nefazodone	↑ levels of A	++
	Protease Inhibitors (not tipranavir/ritonavir)	↑ levels of A	++
	Anticonvulsants: carbamazepine, phenobarbital, phenytoin	↓ levels of A	++
	Efavirenz	↓ levels of A	++
	Rifampin	↓ levels of A	++
Mefloquine	β-adrenergic blockers, calcium channel blockers, quinidine, quinine	↑ arrhythmias	+
	Divalproex, valproic acid	↓ level of B with seizures	++
	Halofantrine	Q-T prolongation	++ (avoid)
Meropenem	See Imipenem		
Methenamine mandelate or hippurate	Acetazolamide, sodium bicarbonate, thiazide diuretics	↓ antibacterial effect 2° to ↑ urine pH	++
Metronidazole Tinidazole	Alcohol	Disulfiram-like reaction	+
	Cyclosporin	↑ levels of B	++
	Disulfiram (Antabuse)	Acute toxic psychosis	+
	Lithium	↑ levels of B	+
	Oral anticoagulants	↑ anticoagulant effect	++
	Phenobarbital, hydantoins	↑ levels of B	++
Micafungin	Nifedipine	↑ levels of B	+
	Sirolimus	↑ levels of B	+
Nelfinavir	See protease inhibitors and Table 22B		
Nevirapine (Viramune)	See non-nucleoside reverse transcriptase inhibitors (NNRTIs) and Table 22B		
Nitrofurantoin	Antacids	↓ absorption of A	+

Non-nucleoside reverse transcriptase inhibitors (NNRTIs): For interactions with protease inhibitors, see Table 22B.
Del = delavirdine; **Efa** = efavirenz; **Etr** = etravirine; **Nev** = nevirapine

Del	Efa	Etr	Nev	Co-administration contraindicated (See package insert):		
+		+		Anticonvulsants: carbamazepine, phenobarbital, phenytoin		++
+		+		Antimycobacterials: rifabutin, rifampin		++
+		+		Antipsychotics: pimozide		++
+	+	+		Benzodiazepines: alprazolam, midazolam, triazolam		++
+	+			Ergotamine		++
+	+	+		HMG-CoA inhibitors (statins): lovastatin, simvastatin, atorvastatin, pravastatin		++
+	+	+		St. John's wort		++
				Dose change needed:		
+				Amphetamines	↑ levels of B—**caution**	++
		+	+	Antiarrhythmics: amiodarone, lidocaine, others	↑ or ↓ levels of B—**caution**	++
+	+	+	+	Anticonvulsants: carbamazepine, phenobarbital, phenytoin	↓ levels of A and/or B	++
+		+	+	Antifungals: itraconazole, ketoconazole, voriconazole, posaconazole	Potential ↓ levels of B, ↑ levels of A	++ (avoid)
+				Antirejection drugs: cyclosporine, rapamycin, sirolimus, tacrolimus	↑ levels of B	++
+				Calcium channel blockers	↑ levels of B	++
+		+	+	Clarithromycin	↑ levels of B metabolite, ↑ levels of A	++
+				Cyclosporine	↑ levels of B	++
+		+	+	Dexamethasone	↓ levels of B	++
+	+	+	+	Sildenafil, vardenafil, tadalafil	↑ levels of B	++
+		+	+	Fentanyl, methadone	↑ levels of B	++
+				Gastric acid suppression: antacids, H-2 blockers, proton pump inhibitors	↓ levels of A	++
	+	+	+	Methadone, fentanyl	↓ levels of B	++
	+	+	+	Oral contraceptives	↑ or ↓ levels of B	++
+	+	+	+	Protease inhibitors—see Table 22B		
+	+	+	+	**Rifabutin, rifampin**	↑ or ↓ levels of rifabutin; ↓ levels of A—**caution**	++
+	+	+	+	St. John's wort	↓ levels of B	++
+		+	+	Warfarin	↑ levels of B	++
Pentamidine, IV				Amphotericin B	↑ risk of nephrotoxicity	+
				Pancreatitis-assoc drugs, eg, alcohol, valproic acid	↑ risk of pancreatitis	+
Piperacillin				Cefoxitin	Antagonism vs pseudomonas	++
Pip-tazo				Methotrexate	↑ levels of B	++
Polymyxin B				Curare paralytics	Avoid: neuromuscular blockade	++

TABLE 22A (5)

ANTI-INFECTIVE AGENT (A)	OTHER DRUG (B)	EFFECT	IMPORT
Polymyxin E (Colistin)	Curare paralytics	Avoid: neuromuscular blockade	++
	Aminoglycosides, Ampho B, Vanco	↑ nephrotoxicity risk	++
Primaquine	Chloroquine, dapsone, INH, probenecid, quinine, sulfonamides, TMP/SMX, others	↑ risk of hemolysis in G6PD-deficient patients	++

Protease Inhibitors—Anti-HIV Drugs. (**Atazan** = atazanavir; **Darun** = darunavir; **Fosampren** = fosamprenavir; **Indin** = indinavir; **Lopin** = lopinavir; **Nelfin** = nelfinavir; **Saquin** = saquinavir; **Tipran** = tipranavir). For interactions with antiretrovirals, see Table 22B. Only a partial list—check package insert

Also see http://aidsinfo.nih.gov
To check for interactions between more than 2 drugs, see:
http://www.drugs.com/drug_interactions.html and http://www.healthline.com/druginteractions

Atazan	Fosampren	Indin	Lopin	Nelfin	Saquin	Tipran	OTHER DRUG (B)	EFFECT	IMPORT
						+	**Analgesics:** 1. Alfentanil, fentanyl, hydrocodone, tramadol	↑ levels of B	+
	+		+		+	+	2. Codeine, hydromorphone, morphine, methadone	↓ levels of B (JAIDS 41:563, 2006)	+
+	+	+	+	+	+		**Anti-arrhythmics: amiodarone, lidocaine, mexiletine, flecainide**	↑ levels of B; **do not co-administer or use caution** (See package insert)	++
	+		+		+	+	**Anticonvulsants: carbamazepine, clonazepam, phenobarbital**	↓ levels of A, ↑ levels of B	++
+		+	+				Antidepressants, all tricyclic	↑ levels of B	++
+	+						Antidepressants, all other	↑ levels of B; do not use pimozide	++
	+						Antidepressants, SSRIs	↓ levels of B - avoid	++
						+	Antihistamines	Do not use	++
+	+	+	+	+			Benzodiazepines, e.g., diazepam, midazolam, triazolam	↑ levels of B—do not use	++
+	+	+	+	+	+	+	Calcium channel blockers (all)	↑ levels of B	++
+	+		+			+	Clarithro, erythro	↑ levels of B if renal impairment	+
+	+		+	+	+	+	Contraceptives, oral	↓ levels of A & B	++
	+		+	+			Corticosteroids: prednisone, dexamethasone	↓ levels of A, ↑ levels of B	+
+	+	+	+	+	+	+	Cyclosporine	↑ levels of B, monitor levels	+
						+	Digoxin	↑ levels of B	++
+	+	+	+	+	+	+	Ergot derivatives	**↑ levels of B—do not use**	++
	+	+		+	+		Erythromycin, clarithromycin	↑ levels of A & B	+
		+		+	+		Grapefruit juice (>200 mL/day)	↓ indinavir & ↑ saquinavir levels	++
+	+	+	+	+	+	+	H2 receptor antagonists	↓ levels of A	++
+	+	+	+	+	+	+	**HMG-CoA reductase inhibitors (statins): lovastatin, simvastatin**	**↑ levels of B—do not use**	++
+							Irinotecan	↑ levels of B—do not use	++
+	+	+	+	+	+	+	Ketoconazole, itraconazole, ? vori.	↑ levels of A, ↓ levels of B	+
+	+	+	+	+	+	+	Posaconazole	↑ levels of A, no effect on B	++
			+				Metronidazole	Poss. disulfiram reaction, alcohol	+
			+				Phenytoin (JAIDS 36:1034, 2004)	↓ levels of A & B	++
+	+	+	+	+	+	+	**Pimozide**	**↑ levels of B—do not use**	++
+	+		+	+	+	+	Proton pump inhibitors	↓ levels of A	++
+	+	+	+	+	+	+	Rifampin, rifabutin	↓ levels of A, ↑ levels of B **(avoid)**	++ (avoid)
+	+	+	+	+	+	+	Sildenafil (Viagra), tadalafil, vardenafil	Varies, some ↑ & some ↓ levels of B	++
+	+	+	+	+	+	+	**St. John's wort**	**↓ levels of B—do not use**	++
+	+	+	+	+	+	+	Sirolimus, tacrolimus	↑ levels of B	++
+							Tenofovir	↓ levels of A—add ritonavir	++
	+		+	+			Theophylline	↓ levels of B	+
	+		+			+	Warfarin	↑ levels of B	+
Pyrazinamide							INH, rifampin	May ↑ risk of hepatotoxicity	±
Pyrimethamine							Lorazepam	↑ risk of hepatotoxicity	±
							Sulfonamides, TMP/SMX	↑ risk of marrow suppression	+
							Zidovudine	↑ risk of marrow suppression	±
Quinine							Digoxin	↑ digoxin levels; ↑ toxicity	++
							Mefloquine	↑ arrhythmias	+
							Oral anticoagulants	↑ prothrombin time	++
Quinupristin- dalfopristin (Synercid)							Anti-HIV drugs: NNRTIs & PIs	↑ levels of B	++
							Antineoplastic: vincristine, docetaxel, paclitaxel	↑ levels of B	++
							Calcium channel blockers	↑ levels of B	++
							Carbamazepine	↑ levels of B	++
							Cyclosporine, tacrolimus	↑ levels of B	++

TABLE 22A (6)

ANTI-INFECTIVE AGENT (A)	OTHER DRUG (B)	EFFECT	IMPORT
Quinupristin-dalfopristin (Synercid) *(continued)*	Lidocaine	↑ levels of B	++
	Methylprednisolone	↑ levels of B	++
	Midazolam, diazepam	↑ levels of B	++
	Statins	↑ levels of B	++
Raltegravir	**Rifampin**	**↓ levels of A**	++
Ribavirin	Didanosine	↑ levels of B → toxicity—**avoid**	++
	Stavudine	↓ levels of B	++
	Zidovudine	↓ levels of B	++
Rifamycins (rifampin, rifabutin) Ref.: *ArIM* 162:985, 2002 The following is a partial list of drugs with rifampin-induced ↑ metabolism and hence lower than anticipated serum levels: ACE inhibitors, dapsone, diazepam, digoxin, diltiazem, doxycycline, fluconazole, fluvastatin, haloperidol, moxifloxacin, nifedipine, progestins, triazolam, tricyclics, voriconazole, zidovudine *(Clin Pharmacokinetic 42:819, 2003).*	Al OH, ketoconazole, PZA	↓ levels of A	+
	Atovaquone	↑ levels of A, ↓ levels of B	+
	Beta adrenergic blockers (metoprolol, propranolol)	↓ effect of B	+
	Caspofungin	↓ levels of B—increase dose	++
	Clarithromycin	↑ levels of A, ↓ levels of B	++
	Corticosteroids	replacement requirement of B	++
	Cyclosporine	↓ effect of B	++
	Delavirdine	**↑ levels of A, ↓ levels of B—avoid**	++
	Digoxin	↓ levels of B	++
	Disopyramide	↓ levels of B	++
	Fluconazole	↑ levels of A	+
	Amprenavir, indinavir, nelfinavir, ritonavir	↑ levels of A (↓ dose of A), ↓ levels of B	++
	INH	Converts INH to toxic hydrazine	++
	Itraconazole, ketoconazole	↓ levels of B, ↑ levels of A	++
	Linezolid	↓ levels of B	++
	Methadone	serum levels (withdrawal)	+
	Nevirapine	**↓ levels of B—avoid**	++
	Oral anticoagulants	Suboptimal anticoagulation	++
	Oral contraceptives	↓ effectiveness; spotting, pregnancy	+
	Phenytoin	↓ levels of B	+
	Protease inhibitors	**↓ levels of A, ↑ levels of B—CAUTION**	++
	Quinidine	↓ effect of B	+
	Raltegravir	↓ levels of B	++
	Sulfonylureas	↓ hypoglycemic effect	+
	Tacrolimus	**↓ levels of B**	++
	Theophylline	↑ levels of B	+
	TMP/SMX	↓ levels of A	+
	Tocainide	↓ effect of B	+
Rimantadine	*See Amantadine*		
Ritonavir	*See protease inhibitors and Table 22B*		
Saquinavir	*See protease inhibitors and Table 22B*		
Stavudine	Dapsone, INH	May ↑ risk of peripheral neuropathy	±
	Ribavirin	↓ levels of A—**AVOID**	++
	Zidovudine	Mutual interference—do not combine	++
Stribild (Elvitegravir & Cobicistat components) *(See Emtricitabine & Tenofovir for other components)*			
Elvitegravir	Antacids	↓ levels of A	++
Cobicistat	Antiarrhythmics & digoxin	↑ levels of B	++
Cobicistat	Clarithromycin, telithromycin	↑ levels of B	++
Cobicistat & Elvitegravir	Carbamazepine, phenobarbital, phenytoin	↓ levels of A – **AVOID**	++
Cobicistat	SSRIs, TCAs, trazodone, antidepressants	↓ levels of A – **AVOID**	++
Cobicistat	Itraconazole, ketoconazole, voriconazole	↑ levels of B	++
Cobicistat	Colchicine	↑ levels of B – lower dose	++
Elvitegravir & Cobicistat	Rifabutin, rifapentine	↓ levels of A – **AVOID**	++
Cobicistat	Beta blockers	↑ levels of B	++
Cobicistat	Calcium channel blockers	↑ levels of B	++
Cobicistat & Elvitegravir	Dexamethasone	↓ levels of A	++
Cobicistat	Bosentan	↑ levels of B	++
Cobicistat	HMG-CoA reductase inhibitor, sirolimus	↑ levels of B	++
Cobicistat	Cyclosporine, tacrolimus	↑ levels of B	++
Cobicistat	Neuroleptics	↑ levels of B	++
Cobicistat	PDE5 inhibitors, e.g., Sildenafil, vardenafil, tadalafil	↑ levels of B – **AVOID**	++
Cobicistat	Benzodiazepines	↑ levels of B	++
Cobicistat	Ergot derivatives	↑ levels of B – **AVOID**	++
Cobicistat	Cisapride	↑ levels of B – **AVOID**	++
Cobicistat & Elvitegravir	St. John's wort	↑ levels of B – **AVOID**	++

TABLE 22A (7)

ANTI-INFECTIVE AGENT (A)	OTHER DRUG (B)	EFFECT	IMPORT
Sulfonamides	Beta blockers	↑ levels of B	++
	Cyclosporine	↓ cyclosporine levels	+
	Methotrexate	↑ antifolate activity	+
	Oral anticoagulants	↑ prothrombin time; bleeding	+
	Phenobarbital, rifampin	↓ levels of A	+
	Phenytoin	↑ levels of B; nystagmus, ataxia	+
	Sulfonylureas	↑ hypoglycemic effect	+
Telithromycin (Ketek)	Carbamazine	↓ levels of A	++
	Digoxin	↑ levels of B—do digoxin levels	++
	Ergot alkaloids	**↑ levels of B—avoid**	++
	Itraconazole; ketoconazole	↑ levels of A; no dose change	+
	Metoprolol	↑ levels of B	++
	Midazolam	↑ levels of B	++
	Oral anticoagulants	↑ prothrombin time	+
	Phenobarbital, phenytoin	↓ levels of A	++
	Pimozide	**↑ levels of B; QT prolongation—AVOID**	++
	Rifampin	**↓ levels of A—avoid**	++
	Simvastatin & other "statins"	↑ levels of B (↑ risk of myopathy)	++
	Sotalol	↓ levels of B	++
	Theophylline	↑ levels of B	++
Tenofovir	Atazanavir	↓ levels of B—add ritonavir	++
	Didanosine (ddI)	**↑ levels of B (reduce dose)**	++
Terbinafine	Cimetidine	↑ levels of A	+
	Phenobarbital, rifampin	↓ levels of A	+
Tetracyclines	See Doxycycline, plus:		
	Atovaquone	↓ levels of B	+
	Digoxin	↑ toxicity of B (may persist several months—up to 10% pts)	++
	Methoxyflurane	↑ toxicity; polyuria, renal failure	+
	Sucralfate	↓ absorption of A (separate by ≥2 hrs)	+
Thiabendazole	Theophyllines	↑ serum theophylline, nausea	+
Tigecycline	Oral contraceptives	↓ levels of B	++
Tinidazole (Tindamax)	See Metronidazole—similar entity, expect similar interactions		
Tobramycin	See Aminoglycosides		
Trimethoprim	Amantadine, dapsone, digoxin, methotrexate, procainamide, zidovudine	↑ serum levels of B	++
	Potassium-sparing diuretics	↑ serum K+	++
	Repaglinide	↑ levels of B (hypoglycemia)	++
	Thiazide diuretics	↓ serum Na+	+
Trimethoprim-Sulfamethoxazole	Ace inhibitors	↑ serum K+	++
	Amantadine	↑ levels of B (toxicity)	++
	Azathioprine	Reports of leukopenia	+
	Cyclosporine	↓ levels of B, ↑ serum creatinine	+
	Loperamide	↑ levels of B	+
	Methotrexate	Enhanced marrow suppression	++
	Oral contraceptives, pimozide, and 6-mercaptopurine	↓ effect of B	+
	Phenytoin	↑ levels of B	+
	Rifampin	↑ levels of B	+
	Warfarin	↑ activity of B	+
Valganciclovir (Valcyte)	See Ganciclovir		
Vancomycin	Aminoglycosides	↑ frequency of nephrotoxicity	++
Zalcitabine (ddC) (HIVID)	Valproic acid, pentamidine (IV), alcohol, lamivudine	↑ pancreatitis risk	+
	Cisplatin, INH, metronidazole, vincristine, nitrofurantoin, d4T, dapsone	↑ risk of peripheral neuropathy	+
Zidovudine (ZDV) (Retrovir)	Atovaquone, fluconazole, methadone	↑ levels of A	+
	Clarithromycin	↓ levels of A	±
	Indomethacin	↑ levels of ZDV toxic metabolite	+
	Nelfinavir	↓ levels of A	++
	Probenecid, TMP/SMX	↑ levels of A	+
	Rifampin/rifabutin	↓ levels of A	++
	Stavudine	**Interference—DO NOT COMBINE!**	++
	Valproic Acid	↑ levels of A	++

TABLE 22B – DRUG-DRUG INTERACTIONS BETWEEN NON-NUCLEOSIDE REVERSE TRANSCRIPTASE INHIBITORS (NNRTIS) AND PROTEASE INHIBITORS
(Adapted from Guidelines for the Use of Antiretroviral Agents in HIV-Infected Adults & Adolescents; see www.aidsinfo.nih.gov)

NAME (Abbreviation, Trade Name)	Atazanavir (ATV, Reyataz)	DARUNAVIR (DRV, Prezista)	Fosamprenavir (FOS-APV, Lexiva)	Indinavir (IDV, Crixivan)	Lopinavir/Ritonavir (LP/R, Kaletra)	Nelfinavir (NFV, Viracept)	Saquinavir (SQV, Invirase)	Tipranavir (TPV)
Delavirdine (DLV, Rescriptor)	No data	No data	Co-administration not recommended	IDV levels ↑ 40%. Dose: IDV 600 mg q8h; DLV standard	Expect LP/R levels ↑. No dose data	NFV levels ↑ 2X; DLV levels ↓ 50%. Dose: No data	SQV levels ↑ 5X. Dose: SQV 800 mg q8h; DLV standard	No data
Efavirenz (EFZ, Sustiva)	ATV AUC ↓ 74%. Dose: ATV/RTV 300/100 mg q24h with food	Standard doses of both drugs	FOS-APV levels ↓. Dose: EFZ standard; FOS-APV 1400 mg + RTV 300 mg q24h or 700 mg FOS-APV + 100 mg RTV q12h	Levels: IDV ↓ 31%. Dose: IDV 1000 mg q8h; EFZ standard	Level of LP ↓ 40%. Dose: LP/R 533/133 mg q12h, EFZ standard	Standard doses	Level: SQV ↓ 62%. Dose: SQV 400 mg + RTV 400 mg q12h	No dose change necessary
Etravirine (ETR, Intelence)	↑ ATV & ↓ ETR levels.	Standard doses of both drugs	↑ levels of FOS-APV	↓ level of IDV.	↑ levels of ETR. ↓ levels of LP/R.	↑ levels of NFV	↓ ETR levels 33%; SQV/R no change. Standard dose of both drugs.	↓ levels of ETR, ↑ levels of TPV & RTV. **Avoid combination.**
Nevirapine (NVP, Viramune)	Avoid combination. ATZ increases NVP concentrations > 25%. NVP decreases ATZ AUC by 42%	Standard doses of both drugs	Use with caution. NVP AUC increased 14% (700/100 Fos/rit); NVP AUC inc 29% (Fos 1400 mg bid)	IDV levels ↓ 28%. Dose: IDV 1000 mg q8h or combine with RTV; NVP standard	LP levels ↓ 53%. Dose: LP/R 533/133 mg q12h; NVP standard	Standard doses	Dose: SQV + RTV 400/400 mg, both q12h	Standard doses

TABLE 23 – LIST OF GENERIC AND COMMON TRADE NAMES

GENERIC NAME: TRADE NAMES	GENERIC NAME: TRADE NAMES	GENERIC NAME: TRADE NAMES
Abacavir: Ziagen	Efavirenz/Emtricitabine/Tenofovir: Atripla	Nitrofurantoin: Macrobid, Macrodantin
Abacavir + Lamivudine: Epzicom	Elvitegravir + Cobicistat + Emtricitabine	Nystatin: Mycostatin
Abacavir + Lamivudine + Zidovudine: Trizivir	+ Tenofovir: Stribild	Ofloxacin: Floxin
Acyclovir: Zovirax	Emtricitabine: Emtriva	Oseltamivir: Tamiflu
Adefovir: Hepsera	Emtricitabine + tenofovir: Truvada	Oxacillin: Prostaphlin
Albendazole: Albenza	Emtricitabine + tenofovir + rilpivirine: Complera	Palivizumab: Synagis
Amantadine: Symmetrel	Enfuvirtide (T-20): Fuzeon	Paromomycin: Humatin
Amikacin: Amikin	Entecavir: Baraclude	Pentamidine: NebuPent, Pentam 300
Amoxicillin: Amoxil, Polymox	Ertapenem: Invanz	Piperacillin: Pipracil
Amoxicillin extended release: Moxatag	Etravirine: Intelence	Piperacillin/tazobactam: Zosyn, Tazocin
Amox./clav.: Augmentin, Augmentin ES-600; Augmentin XR	Erythromycin(s): Ilotycin	Piperazine: Antepar
Amphotericin B: Fungizone	*Ethyl succinate*: Pediamycin	Podophyllotoxin: Condylox
Ampho B-liposomal: AmBisome	*Gluceptonate*: Erythrocin	Polymyxin B: Poly-Rx
Ampho B-lipid complex: Abelcet	*Estolate*: Ilosone	Posaconazole: Noxafil
Ampicillin: Omnipen, Polycillin	Erythro/sulfisoxazole: Pediazole	Praziquantel: Biltricide
Ampicillin/sulbactam: Unasyn	Ethambutol: Myambutol	Primaquine: Primachine
Artemether-Lumefantrine: Coartem	Ethionamide: Trecator	Proguanil: Paludrine
Atazanavir: Reyataz	Famciclovir: Famvir	Pyrantel pamoate: Antiminth
Atovaquone: Mepron	Fidaxomicin: Dificid	Pyrimethamine: Daraprim
Atovaquone + proguanil: Malarone	Fluconazole: Diflucan	Pyrimethamine/sulfadoxine: Fansidar
Azithromycin: Zithromax	Flucytosine: Ancobon	Quinupristin/dalfopristin: Synercid
Azithromycin ER: Zmax	Fosamprenavir: Lexiva	Raltegravir: Isentress
Aztreonam: Azactam, Cayston	Foscarnet: Foscavir	Retapamulin: Altabax
Bedaquiline: Sirturo	Fosfomycin: Monurol	Ribavirin: Virazole, Rebetol
Boceprevir: Victrelis	Fusidic acid: Taksta	Rifabutin: Mycobutin
Caspofungin: Cancidas	Ganciclovir: Cytovene	Rifampin: Rifadin, Rimactane
Cefaclor: Ceclor, Ceclor CD	Gatifloxacin: Tequin	Rifapentine: Priftin
Cefadroxil: Duricef	Gemifloxacin: Factive	Rifaximin: Xifaxan
Cefazolin: Ancef, Kefzol	Gentamicin: Garamycin	Rilpivirine: Edurant
Cefdinir: Omnicef	Griseofulvin: Fulvicin	Rimantadine: Flumadine
Cefditoren pivoxil: Spectracef	Halofantrine: Halfan	Ritonavir: Norvir
Cefepime: Maxipime	Idoxuridine: Dendrid, Stoxil	Saquinavir: Invirase
Cefixime[NUS]: Suprax	INH + RIF: Rifamate	Spectinomycin: Trobicin
Cefoperazone-sulbactam: Sulperazon[NUS]	INH + RIF + PZA: Rifater	Stavudine: Zerit
Cefotaxime: Claforan	Interferon alfa: Intron A	Stibogluconate: Pentostam
Cefotetan: Cefotan	Interferon, pegylated: PEG-Intron, Pegasys	Silver sulfadiazine: Silvadene
Cefoxitin: Mefoxin	Interferon + ribavirin: Rebetron	Sulfamethoxazole: Gantanol
Cefpodoxime proxetil: Vantin	Imipenem + cilastatin: Primaxin, Tienam	Sulfasalazine: Azulfidine
Cefprozil: Cefzil	Imiquimod: Aldara	Sulfisoxazole: Gantrisin
Ceftaroline: Teflaro	Indinavir: Crixivan	Telaprevir: Incivek
Ceftazidime: Fortaz, Tazicef, Tazidime	Itraconazole: Sporanox	Telavancin: Vibativ
Ceftibuten: Cedax	Iodoquinol: Yodoxin	Telbivudine: Tyzeka
Ceftizoxime: Cefizox	Ivermectin: Stromectol, Sklice	Telithromycin: Ketek
Ceftobiprole: Zeftera	Kanamycin: Kantrex	Temocillin: Negaban, Temopen
Ceftriaxone: Rocephin	Ketoconazole: Nizoral	Tenofovir: Viread
Cefuroxime: Zinacef, Ceftin	Lamivudine: Epivir, Epivir-HBV	Terbinafine: Lamisil
Cephalexin: Keflex	Lamivudine + abacavir: Epzicom	Thalidomide: Thalomid Thiabendazole: Mintezol
Cephradine: Anspor, Velosef	Levofloxacin: Levaquin	Ticarcillin: Ticar
Chloroquine: Aralen	Linezolid: Zyvox	Tigecycline: Tygacil
Cidofovir: Vistide	Lomefloxacin: Maxaquin	Tinidazole: Tindamax
Ciprofloxacin: Cipro, Cipro XR	Lopinavir/ritonavir: Kaletra	Tipranavir: Aptivus
Clarithromycin: Biaxin, Biaxin XL	Loracarbef: Lorabid	Tobramycin: Nebcin
Clindamycin: Cleocin	Mafenide: Sulfamylon	Tretinoin: Retin A
Clofazimine: Lamprene	Maraviroc: Selzentry	Trifluridine: Viroptic
Clotrimazole: Lotrimin, Mycelex	Mebendazole: Vermox	Trimethoprim: Primsol
Cloxacillin: Tegopen	Mefloquine: Lariam	Trimethoprim/sulfamethoxazole: Bactrim, Septra
Colistimethate: Coly-Mycin M	Meropenem: Merrem	Valacyclovir: Valtrex
Cycloserine: Seromycin	Mesalamine: Asacol, Pentasa	Valganciclovir: Valcyte
Daptomycin: Cubicin	Methenamine: Hiprex, Mandelamine	Vancomycin: Vancocin
Darunavir: Prezista	Metronidazole: Flagyl	Voriconazole: Vfend
Delavirdine: Rescriptor	Micafungin: Mycamine	Zalcitabine: HIVID
Dicloxacillin: Dynapen	Minocycline: Minocin	Zanamivir: Relenza
Didanosine: Videx	Moxifloxacin: Avelox	Zidovudine (ZDV): Retrovir
Diethylcarbamazine: Hetrazan	Mupirocin: Bactroban	Zidovudine + 3TC: Combivir
Diloxanide furoate: Furamide	Nafcillin: Unipen	Zidovudine + 3TC + abacavir: Trizivir
Doripenem: Doribax	Nelfinavir: Viracept	
Doxycycline: Vibramycin	Nevirapine: Viramune	
Efavirenz: Sustiva	Nitazoxanide: Alinia	

TABLE 23 (2)
LIST OF COMMON TRADE AND GENERIC NAMES

TRADE NAME: GENERIC NAME	TRADE NAME: GENERIC NAME	TRADE NAME: GENERIC NAME
Abelcet: Ampho B-lipid complex	Garamycin: Gentamicin	Rifadin: Rifampin
Albenza: Albendazole	Halfan: Halofantrine	Rifamate: INH + RIF
Aldara: Imiquimod	Hepsera: Adefovir	Rifater: INH + RIF + PZA
Alinia: Nitazoxanide	Herplex: Idoxuridine	Rimactane: Rifampin
Altabax: Retapamulin	Hiprex: Methenamine hippurate	Rocephin: Ceftriaxone
AmBisome: Ampho B-liposomal	HIVID: Zalcitabine	Selzentry: Maraviroc
Amikin: Amikacin	Humatin: Paromomycin	Septra: Trimethoprim/sulfa
Amoxil: Amoxicillin	Ilosone: Erythromycin estolate	Seromycin: Cycloserine
Ancef: Cefazolin	Ilotycin: Erythromycin	Silvadene: Silver sulfadiazine
Ancobon: Flucytosine	Incivek: Telaprevir	Sirturo: Bedaquiline
Anspor: Cephradine	Intelence: Etravirine	Sklice: Ivermectin lotion
Antepar: Piperazine	Intron A: Interferon alfa	Spectracef: Cefditoren pivoxil
Antiminth: Pyrantel pamoate	Invanz: Ertapenem	Sporanox: Itraconazole
Aptivus: Tipranavir	Invirase: Saquinavir	Stoxil: Idoxuridine
Aralen: Chloroquine	Isentress: Raltegravir	Stribild: Elvitegravir + Cobicistat + Emtricitabine + Tenofovir
Asacol: Mesalamine	Kaletra: Lopinavir/ritonavir	Stromectol: Ivermectin
Atripla: Efavirenz/emtricitabine/tenofovir	Kantrex: Kanamycin	Sulfamylon: Mafenide
Augmentin, Augmentin ES-600	Keflex: Cephalexin	Sulperazon[NUS]: Cefoperazone-sulbactam
Augmentin XR: Amox./clav.	Ketek: Telithromycin	Suprax: Cefixime[NUS]
Avelox: Moxifloxacin	Lamisil: Terbinafine	Sustiva: Efavirenz
Azactam: Aztreonam	Lamprene: Clofazimine	Symmetrel: Amantadine
Azulfidine: Sulfasalazine	Lariam: Mefloquine	Synagis: Palivizumab
Bactroban: Mupirocin	Levaquin: Levofloxacin	Synercid: Quinupristin/dalfopristin
Bactrim: Trimethoprim/sulfamethoxazole	Lexiva: Fosamprenavir	Taksta: Fusidic acid
Baraclude: Entecavir	Lorabid: Loracarbef	Tamiflu: Oseltamivir
Biaxin, Biaxin XL: Clarithromycin	Macrodantin, Macrobid: Nitrofurantoin	Tazicef: Ceftazidime
Biltricide: Praziquantel	Malarone: Atovaquone + proguanil	Teflaro: Ceftaroline
Cancidas: Caspofungin	Mandelamine: Methenamine mandel.	Tegopen: Cloxacillin
Cayston: Aztreonam (inhaled)	Maxaquin: Lomefloxacin	Tequin: Gatifloxacin
Ceclor, Ceclor CD: Cefaclor	Maxipime: Cefepime	Thalomid: Thalidomide
Cedax: Ceftibuten	Mefoxin: Cefoxitin	Ticar: Ticarcillin
Cefizox: Ceftizoxime	Mepron: Atovaquone	Tienam: Imipenem
Cefotan: Cefotetan	Merrem: Meropenem	Timentin: Ticarcillin-clavulanic acid
Ceftin: Cefuroxime axetil	Minocin: Minocycline	Tinactin: Tolnaftate
Cefzil: Cefprozil	Mintezol: Thiabendazole	Tindamax: Tinidazole
Cipro, Cipro XR: Ciprofloxacin & extended release	Monocid: Cefonicid	Trecator SC: Ethionamide
Claforan: Cefotaxime	Monurol: Fosfomycin	Trizivir: Abacavir + ZDV + 3TC
Coartem: Artemether-Lumefantrine	Moxatag: Amoxicillin extended release:	Trobicin: Spectinomycin
Coly-Mycin M: Colistimethate	Myambutol: Ethambutol	Truvada: Emtricitabine + tenofovir
Combivir: ZDV + 3TC	Mycamine: Micafungin	Tygacil: Tigecycline
Complera: Emtricitabine + tenofovir + rilpivirine	Mycobutin: Rifabutin	Tyzeka: Telbivudine
Crixivan: Indinavir	Mycostatin: Nystatin	Unasyn: Ampicillin/sulbactam
Cubicin: Daptomycin	Nafcil: Nafcillin	Unipen: Nafcillin
Cytovene: Ganciclovir	Nebcin: Tobramycin	Valcyte: Valganciclovir
Daraprim: Pyrimethamine	NebuPent: Pentamidine	Valtrex: Valacyclovir
Dificid: Fidaxomicin	Nizoral: Ketoconazole	Vancocin: Vancomycin
Diflucan: Fluconazole	Norvir: Ritonavir	Vantin: Cefpodoxime proxetil
Doribax: Doripenem	Noxafil: Posaconazole	Velosef: Cephradine
Duricef: Cefadroxil	Omnicef: Cefdinir	Vermox: Mebendazole
Dynapen: Dicloxacillin	Omnipen: Ampicillin	Vfend: Voriconazole
Edurant: Rilpivirine	Pediamycin: Erythro. ethyl succinate	Vibativ: Telavancin
Emtriva: Emtricitabine	Pediazole: Erythro. ethyl succinate + sulfisoxazole	Vibramycin: Doxycycline
Epivir, Epivir-HBV: Lamivudine	Pegasys, PEG-Intron: Interferon, pegylated	Victrelis: Boceprevir
Epzicom: Lamivudine + abacavir	Pentam 300: Pentamidine	Videx: Didanosine
Factive: Gemifloxacin	Pentasa: Mesalamine	Viracept: Nelfinavir
Famvir: Famciclovir	Pipracil: Piperacillin	Viramune: Nevirapine
Fansidar: Pyrimethamine + sulfadoxine	Polycillin: Ampicillin	Virazole: Ribavirin
Flagyl: Metronidazole	Polymox: Amoxicillin	Viread: Tenofovir
Floxin: Ofloxacin	Poly-Rx: Polymyxin B	Vistide: Cidofovir
Flumadine: Rimantadine	Prezista: Darunavir	Xifaxan: Rifaximin
Foscavir: Foscarnet	Priftin: Rifapentine	Yodoxin: Iodoquinol
Fortaz: Ceftazidime	Primaxin: Imipenem + cilastatin	Zerit: Stavudine
Fulvicin: Griseofulvin	Primsol: Trimethoprim	Zeftera: Ceftobiprole
Fungizone: Amphotericin B	Prostaphlin: Oxacillin	Ziagen: Abacavir
Furadantin: Nitrofurantoin	Rebetol: Ribavirin	Zinacef: Cefuroxime
Fuzeon: Enfuvirtide (T-20)	Rebetron: Interferon + ribavirin	Zithromax: Azithromycin
Gantanol: Sulfamethoxazole	Relenza: Zanamivir	Zmax: Azithromycin ER
Gantrisin: Sulfisoxazole	Rescriptor: Delavirdine	Zovirax: Acyclovir
	Retin A: Tretinoin Retrovir: Zidovudine (ZDV)	Zosyn: Piperacillin/tazobactam
	Reyataz: Atazanavir	Zyvox: Linezolid

227

INDEX OF MAJOR ENTITIES

PAGES (page numbers bold if major focus)

A

Abacavir 81, 90, 175, 176, 177, 185, 213, 217, 225, 226
Abortion, prophylaxis/septic 25, **195**
Acanthamoeba **14**, 142
Acinetobacter 22, 41, 47, 50, **67**, 72, 74, 76, 77, 94
Acne rosacea and vulgaris **51**, 152, 168
Actinomycosis 42, 67, 72, 74, 76
Acyclovir 7, 13, 15, 28, 49, 52, 54, 62, 81, 82, 89, 160, 161, 162, 163, **168**, 169, 173, 202, 210, 225, 226
Adalimumab 53
Adefovir 81, 89, 169, 173, 189, 210, 225, 226
Adenovirus 12, 36, 38, 45, 156, 173
Adverse reactions
  Antibacterials 104
  Antifungals 124
  Antimycobacterials 138
  Antiparasitic drugs 152, 155
  Antiviral drugs 168
Aeromonas hydrophila 17, 55, 67, 72, 74, 75
Aggregatibacter aphrophilus 68
AIDS 6, **10**, 15, **20**, 21, 24, 27, 36, **44**, 46, 51, 57, 62, 70, **118**, 119, 126, 129, 132, 134, 135, 138, 141, 142, 145, 146, 151, 158, 161, 162, 163, 168, 200, 216
Albendazole 81, 88, 141, 142, 147, 148, 149, 150, **152**, **154**, 225, 226
Allergic bronchopulmonary aspergillosis 111
Amantadine 81, **171**, 173, 210, 217, 222, 223, 225, 226
Amebiasis 17, 20, 36, **141**
Amebic meningoencephalitis 142
Amikacin 7, 45, 53, 68, 75, 81, 85, 104, **109**, 135, 136, 137, 203, 205, 212, 217, 225, 226
Amikacin/Streptomycin 210
Amniotitis, septic abortion 25
Amoxicillin 11, 21, 23, 35, 37, 38, 39, 41, 42, 43, 50, 51, 58, 58, 69, 71, 83, 84, 93, 104, 192, 195, 203, 208, 217, 225, 226
Amoxicillin extended release 83, 93, 208, 225, 226
Amoxicillin-clavulanate 7, 11, 14, 22, 34, 37, 38, 39, 41, 42, 46, 48, 50, 52, 55, 63, 67, 68, 69, 83, 93, 104, 119, 137, 192, 195, 203
Amphotericin B, ampho B 14, 15, 56, 63, 65, 81, 87, 109, 111, 112, 118, 119, 122, **124**, 125, 142, 209, 217, 220, 225, 226
  lipid ampho B preps 63, 87, 111, 118, 122, **124**, 209, 217
Ampicillin 7, 8, 9, 17, 18, 22, 25, 28, 29, 30, 33, 35, 38, 41, 42, 47, 60, 61, 67, 68, 69, 71, 83, **93**, **94**, 104, 192, 203, 208, 213, 217, 225, 226
Ampicillin-sulbactam 16, 17, 22, 25, 26, 27, 30, 35, 36, 41, 42, 43, 44, 52, 67, 71, 83, **94**, 104, 203, 213
Anaerobic lung infection 41
Anaplasma (Ehrlichia) 58, 68
Ancylostoma caninum 148
Anemia 185
Angiostrongylus cantonensis (Angiostrongyliasis) 10, 148, 155
Anidulafungin 31, 63, 81, 87, 125, 213
Anisakiasis 147
Antacids 222
Anthrax 39, **43**, 51, 52, 56, 67
Antibacterials, Prolonged/Continuous Dosing 110
Antifungals 111
ANTIMICROBIAL DOSING IN OBESITY 82
Antimony compounds 152
Antiretroviral Drugs & Therapy/Antiviral Drugs 156
Aphthous stomatitis 46, 61, 139
Appendicitis 20, **47**

Arcanobacterium haemolyticum 67
Artemether 81, 88, 152
Artemether-Lumefantrine 144, 145, 152, 217, 225, 226
Artesunate 145, 152
Arthritis, septic 17, 23, **31**, **32**, 33, 58, 61, 70, 97, 153, 162
  reactive (Reiter's) 27, **31**
Ascariasis **147**
Aspergilloma 111
Aspergillosis 14, 15, 31, 41, 50, 63, 65, 66, **111**, 125, 126, 127, 202
Aspergillus flavus 127
Aspergillus fumigatus 127
Aspergillus terreus 127
Asplenia 52, 63, 142, 192
Atabrine 152
Atazanavir 81, 90, 92, 175, 176, 179, 181, 187, 200, 213, 217, 218, 221, 223, 224, 225, 226
Athlete's foot (Tinea pedis) 120
Atovaquone, atovaquone + proguanil 57, 81, 88, 91, 142, 143, 145, 146, 147, **152**, 217, 222, 223, 225, 226
Atripla 178, 210
Azithromycin 10, 11, 12, 13, 17, 19, 20, 23, 24, 34, 37, 38, 39, 40, 41, 42, 43, 44, 45, 48, 50, 51, 52, 54, 55, 57, 58, 59, 61, 67, 68, 69, 70, 75, 81, 85, 92, 98, 107, 134, 135, 142, 193, 203, 213, 219, 225, 226
Azole antifungals 102, **111**
AZT (zidovudine) 81, 91, 168, 200, 212, 217, 218, 219, 221, 222, 223, 225, 226
Aztreonam 4, 9, 16, 17, 22, 42, 43, 47, 48, 62, 63, 66, 71, 81, 85, **95**, 96, 104, 203, 208, 225, 226

B

Babesia, babesiosis **57**, 58, **142**, 192
Bacillary angiomatosis 51, **57**
Bacillus anthracis (anthrax) 39, 43, 51, 52, 56, 67
Bacillus cereus, subtilis **15**, 67
Bacitracin 67, 103
Bacterial endocarditis 21, 28, 29, 30, 31, 56, 70, 97, 197
Bacterial peritonitis 17, 22, 26, 36, 47, 55, 56, 62, 124, 194, 196
Bacterial vaginosis **26**, 68
Bacteriuria, asymptomatic **35**, 70, 192
Bacteroides species 6, 17, **22**, 25, 26, 36, 44, 47, 52, 55, 56, 66, 67, 72, 74, 76
Balanitis **26**, **27**, 31
Balantidium coli 141
Bartonella henselae, quintana 30, 36, 45, 51, **57**, 67
Baylisascariasis 148
BCG 128, **134**
Bedaquiline 87, **139**, 210, 218, 225
Bell's palsy **160**
Benzathine penicillin, Bicillin 24, 25, 48, 58, 61, 67, 83, 93
Benznidazole 147, **153**
Biliary sepsis **17**, 22, 62
Biloma, post-transplant 36
Biological weapons 216
Bites 28, **52**, 55, 161, 167, 215
Bithionol 149, **154**
BK virus, post-renal transplant 173
Blastocystis hominis 141
Blastomyces dermatitidis 112, 122
Blastomycosis 56, **112**, 122
Blepharitis **12**
Boceprevir 89, 169, 173, 225, 226
Boils (furunculosis) **53**, **54**, 78
Bordetella pertussis (whooping cough) **37**, 67

Bold numbers indicate major considerations. Antibiotic selection often depends on modifying circumstances and alternative agents.

PAGES (page numbers bold if major focus)	
Borrelia burgdorferi, B. garinii, B. afzelii	32, **58**, 67
Bosentan	222
Botulism (food-borne, infant, wound)	**64**
Brain abscess	**6**, **7**, 12, 50, 122, 123, 146
Breast infection (mastitis, abscess)	6
Bronchitis, bronchiolitis	36, 37, 38, 39, 98, 165
Bronchopneumonia	38
Brucellosis	32, **60**, 67, 70, 76
Brugia malayi	148
Buccal cellulitis	46
Burkholderia (Pseudomonas) cepacia	**44**, 67, 72, 74, 76
Burkholderia pseudomallei (melioidosis)	**41**, 56, 67
Burns	**53**, 64, 65, 214
Bursitis, septic	33
Buruli ulcer	136
C	
Calymmatobacterium granulomatis	24
Campylobacter jejuni, fetus	17, 20, 31, 67
Canaliculitis	14
Candida albicans, glabrata, krusei, lusitaniae	21, 26, 124, 126, 127
Candida Stomatitis, Thrush	46
Candidemia, candidiasis	14, 15, 17, 21, 26, 27, 28, 31, 36, 46, 53, 54, 56, 62, 63, 65, **113**, 124, 125, 126, 127, 202
Candidiasis	
Bloodstream - Neutropenic patient	**114**
Bloodstream - Non-neutropenic patient	**113**
Candida esophagitis	**115**
CNS Infection	**116**
Cutaneous	**116**
Cystitis	**117**
Endocarditis	**114**
Endophthalmitis	**116**
Myocarditis	**114**
Neonatal candidiasis	**117**
Oropharyngeal candidiasis	**115**
Osteomyelitis	**114**
Pericarditis	**115**
Peritonitis	**117**
Pyelonephritis	**117**
Septic arthritis	**114**
Vulvovaginitis	**116**
Canimorsus	52
CAPD peritonitis	48, 213
Capillariasis	147
Capnocytophaga ochracea, canimorsus	**52**, 63, 67
Capreomycin	81, 87, 130, **139**, 210
Carbamazepine	222
Carbapenems	66, 67, 68, 69, 77, 84, 94, 95, 104
Caspofungin	56, 63, 65, 81, 87, 111, 122, **124**, 146, 213, 218, 225, 226
Cat bite	52
Catfish sting	52
Cat-scratch disease	36, 45, 51, 52, 57
Cayetanensis	141
CD4 cell count	176
CDC Drug Service	141
Cefaclor, Cefaclor-ER	11, 73, 84, **96**, 105, 203, 225, 226
Cefadroxil	73, 83, **96**, 105, 203, 225, 226
Cefazolin	4, 14, 15, 29, 33, 46, 54, 64, 67, 73, 82, 83, **95**, 105, 194, 195, 196, 203, 213, 225, 226
Cefdinir	11, 39, 48, 50, 73, 84, 96, 105, 203, 225, 226
Cefditoren pivoxil	39, 73, 84, **96**, 105, 225, 226
Cefepime	4, 5, 8, 9, 10, 11, 31, 33, 35, 41, 47, 48, 50, 56, 62, 63, 66, 68, 73, 77, 82, 84, 96, 105, 110, 203, 206, 213, 225, 226
Cefixime	19, 23, 27, 69, 73, 84, 96, 105, 203
Cefmetazole	135
Cefoperazone-sulbactam	95

PAGES (page numbers bold if major focus)	
Cefotaxime	6, 7, 8, 9, 12, 15, 19, 23, 32, 38, 39, 44, 47, 49, 54, 58, 61, 62, 68, 73, 84, **95**, 96, 105, 203, 206, 225, 226
Cefotetan	22, 26, 47, 66, 67, 73, 84, **95**, 105, 194, 195, 206, 225, 226
Cefoxitin	22, 23, 25, 26, 36, 44, 47, 66, 67, 73, 84, **95**, 96, 105, 135, 194, 195, 203, 206, 220, 225, 226
Cefpirome	**96**
Cefpodoxime	23
Cefpodoxime proxetil	11, 39, 48, 50, 68, 84, 203, 225, 226
Cefprozil	11, 39, 50, 73, 84, **96**, 105, 203, 225, 226
Ceftaroline	56, 69, 73, 77, 78, 84, **97**, 105, 206, 225
Ceftaroline fosamil	96
Ceftazidime	4, 5, 8, 9, 10, 11, 14, 15, 20, 35, 41, 43, 44, 48, 50, 54, 56, 63, 67, 69, 73, 84, 95, 96, 105, 110, 203, 206, 213, 225, 226
Ceftibuten	11, 73, 84, **96**, 105, 203, 225, 226
Ceftizoxime	23, 32, 73, 84, **95**, 105, 194, 203, 206, 225, 226
Ceftobiprole	16, 74, 84, 96, 105, 206, 225, 226
Ceftriaxone	4, 6, 8, 9, 10, 11, 15, 19, 20, 21, 23, 24, 25, 26, 27, 28, 30, 32, 33, 35, 39, 40, 42, 43, 44, 46, 47, 48, 49, 52, 57, 58, 60, 61, 62, 63, 64, 66, 67, 68, 69, 70, 73, 77, 84, **95**, 105, 193, 195, 203, 213, 225, 226
desensitization	80
Cefuroxime	11, 15, 39, 46, 52, 58, 68, 73, 84, **95**, 96, 105, 192, 194, 195, 203, 206, 225, 226
Cefuroxime axetil	11, 52, 58, 73, 84, **96**, 105, 226
Cellulitis (erysipelas)	15, 46, 52, 54, 64, 70
Cephalexin	6, 52, 55, 68, 73, 83, **96**, 105, 203, 225, 226
Cephalosporin	48
Cephalosporins	68, 69, 81, 96
Cephalosporins, overall/generations	73, 83, 84, 95, 96
Cephradine	225, 226
Certolizumab	33
Cervicitis	**23**, **25**, 70
Cestodes (tapeworms)	**150**, **151**, 154
Chagas disease	147
Chancroid	**23**, 45, 68
Chickenpox	13, 15, 64, 159, 162, 163
Chlamydia trachomatis	12, 13, 23, 24, 25, 27, 31, 34, 38, 67
Chlamydophila pneumoniae (Chlamydia)	36, 37, 39, 67, 72, 76
Chloramphenicol	9, 19, 24, 44, 59, 61, 67, 68, 69, 75, 81, 86, 92, **98**, 107, 203, 213, 218
Chlorhexidine	14, 53
Chloroquine	81, 143, 144, 145, **153**, 154, 221, 225, 226
Cholangitis	**17**, 36, 194
Cholecystitis	17, 194
Cholera	17, **19**, 69
Chromoblastomycosis	**117**, 126
Cidofovir	81, 89, 156, 159, 165, 166, **168**, 173, 210, 217, 225, 226
Ciprofloxacin	4, 5, 9, 10, 11, 14, 16, 17, 19, 20, 22, 23, 24, 27, 31, 32, 33, 34, 35, 36, 41, 43, 45, 47, 48, 51, 52, 54, 55, 56, 59, 60, 61, 62, 63, 66, 67, 68, 69, 70, 71, 81, 85, 92, **100**, 107, 130, 131, 135, 136, **139**, 141, 142, 194, 196, 203, 206, 213, 218, 225, 226
Cisapride	222
Citrobacter	67, 72, 74
Clarithromycin	11, 21, 37, 39, 41, 43, 48, 50, 51, 54, 55, 59, 67, 68, 75, 81, 85, 92, **98**, 107, 134, 135, 136, 137, 140, 142, 192, 203, 206, 219, 220, 221, 222, 223, 225, 226

PAGES (page numbers bold if major focus)

Clindamycin	4, 11, 15, 20, 22, 25, 26, 30, 38, 42, 43, 44, 46, 47, 48, 49, 51, 52, 53, 55, 56, 57, 61, 64, 66, 67, 68, 69, 75, 78, 81, 86, 92, **98**, 107, 142, 144, 145, 146, 147, 195, 203, 213, 218, 225
Clofazimine	81, 122, 135, 136, 137, **139**, 225, 226
Clonorchis sinensis	149
Clostridial myonecrosis	46, 55, 70
Clostridium difficile colitis	17, **18**, 67, 72, 74, 76, 95, 96, 98
Clostridium perfringens	25, 46, 55, 67, 72, 74
Clotrimazole	26, 28, 225
Cloxacillin	71, 83, 93, 225, 226
Cobicistat	81, 92, 175, 184, 218, 222, 225, 226
Coccidioides immitis	118, 127, 202
Coccidioidomycosis	10, 43, 54, **118**, 126
Colchicine	222
Colistin	41, 67, 68, 75, 77, 81, 107
Colistin, Polymyxin E	86, 207
Colitis, antibiotic-associated	*See C. difficile colitis*
Combivir	178
Complera/Eviplera	175, 178, 181
Conjunctivitis (all types)	7, **12, 13**, 23, 31, 61, 160
Contaminated traumatic wound	**46**
Continuous Dosing, Antibacterials	110
Coronavirus	45, **156**
Corticosteroids and meningitis	**8, 9, 10**
Corynebacterium diphtheriae	67
Corynebacterium jeikeium	65, 67, 71, 73, 75
Corynebacterium minutissimum	67
Coxiella burnetii	30, 31, **39**, **67**
"Crabs" (Phthirus pubis)	24, 151
Creeping eruption	148
Cryptococcosis	10, 27, **118, 119**, 122, 126, 127
Cryptococcus neoformans	**10**, 27, 127
Cryptosporidium	17, 20, 109, **141**
C-Section	25
CSF	7, 8, 9, 10, 21, 43, 58, 91, 93, 121, 125, 132, 139, 146, 156, 157, 159, 160, 168, 195
Cyclosporine	81, 87, 130, 136, 137, 139, 210, 218, 225, 226
Cyclospora	17, 20, **141**
Cyclosporiasis	**141**
Cyclosporine	99, 109, 124, 209, 217, 218, 219, 220, 221, 222, 223
Cystic fibrosis	39, 40, **43**, 109
Cysticercosis	**154**
Cystitis	**34**, 70, 93, 156
Cystoisospora belli	**142**
Cystoscopy	196
Cystoscopy with manipulation	196
Cytochrome P450 Interactions	92
Cytomegalovirus (CMV)	15, 21, 38, 158, 168, 169, 173
retinitis	15, 159, 168

D

d4T (stavudine)	81, 91, 200, 212, 218, 222, 223, 225, 226
Dacryocystitis	14
Dandruff (seborrheic dermatitis)	**54**, 199
Dapsone	52, 81, 88, 92, 137, **139**, 145, 146, **153**, 218, 221, 222, 223
Daptomycin	30, 31, 54, 55, 56, 65, 66, 69, 75, 77, 78, 81, 82, 86, 92, 97, 107, 207, 213, 218, 225, 226
Darunavir	81, 90, 92, 175, 181, 187, 213, 221, 224, 225, 226
ddC (zalcitabine)	81, 212, 218, 219, 223, 225, 226
ddI (didanosine)	81, 90, 175, 177, 185, 211, 217, 218, 222, 223, 225, 226
Delavirdine	81, 90, 92, 179, 186, 213, 218, 220, 222, 224, 225, 226

PAGES (page numbers bold if major focus)

Dematiaceous molds	127
Dengue	61, **157**
Dermatophytosis	**120**
Desensitization	
Ceftriaxone	80
Penicillin	80
TMP-SMX	80
Dexamethasone	8, 9, 61, 222
Diabetic foot	5, **16**, 54
Dialysis: Hemo- and peritoneal	**207, 208, 211**
Diarrhea	17, **19, 20**, 70, 93, 94, 95, 96, 98, 101, 102, 104, 106, 107, 124, 125, 126, 136, 139, 141, 142, 152, 153, 154, 156, 165, 167, 168, 169, 171, 182, 185, 186, 187, 188, 199
Dicloxacillin	6, 10, 33, 52, 55, 68, 71, 83, **93**, 193, 203, 225, 226
Didanosine (ddI)	81, 90, 175, 177, 185, 211, 217, 218, 222, 223, 225, 226
Dientamoeba fragilis	141
Diethylcarbamazine	148, **154**, 225
Digoxin	221, 222
Diloxanide	141, 152, 225
Diphtheria; C. diphtheriae	49, 70
Dipylidium caninum	150
Dirofilariasis (heartworms)	149
Disulfiram reactions	98, 125, 138, 152, 220, 221
Diverticulitis	17, 22, 47
Dog bite (also see Rabies)	**52**
Donovanosis	24
Doripenem	16, 17, 22, 25, 35, 36, 40, 47, 54, 55, 56, 67, 68, 71, 77, 81, 84, 94, 104, 105, 110, 205, 218, 225, 226
Doxycycline	7, 12, 13, 16, 19, 20, 23, 24, 25, 26, 27, 31, 34, 37, 39, 41, 42, 43, 45, 47, 50, 51, 52, 53, 54, 57, 58, 59, 60, 67, 68, 69, 70, 75, 78, 86, **99**, 107, 135, 136, 143, 144, 145, 148, 193, 195, 203, 213, 218, 223, 225, 226
Doxycylcne	48
Dracunculus (guinea worm)	148
Drug-drug interactions	39, 98, 99, 105, 106, 108, 124, 125, 126, 134, 138, 152, 169, 216, 217, 218, 219, 220, 221, 223, 224
Duodenal ulcer (Helicobacter pylori)	21, 68, 70
Dysentery, bacillary	70, 141

E

Ear Infections	**10**, 11, 70
Ebola/Marburg virus	156
EBV (Epstein-Barr virus)	**45, 159**
Echinocandin antifungals	127
Echinococcosis	150
Efavirenz	175, 176, 180, 181, 186, 224, 225, 226
Efavirenz (Sustiva)	81, 90, 92, 132, 200, 213, 217, 218, 219, 220, 222, 226
Eflornithine	81, 147, **153**
Ehrlichiosis, monocytic & granulocytic	57, 58, 59, 68
Eikenella	30, 49, 52, **68**
Elephantiasis (filariasis)	148
Elizabethkingae	68
Elvitegravir	81, 90, 92, 175, 184, 188, 218, 222, 225, 226
Empyema, lung	44
Empyema, subdural	**7**
Emtricitabine	81, 90, 178, 184, 185, 189, 211, 225, 226
Emtricitabine/lamivudine	176
Emtricitabine/tenofovir	186
Emtricitabine/tenofovir/efavirenz	178
Emtricitabine/tenofovir/rilpivirine	178
Encephalitis	**7**, 45, 57, 58, 147, **160**, 161
Encephalitozoon	142

	PAGES (page numbers bold if major focus)
Endocarditis	
Native valve	28, 29, 30, 31, 70
Prosthetic valve	30, 31
Endomyometritis	22, **25**
Endophthalmitis	**15**
Endotoxin shock (septic shock)	63
Enfuvirtide	183, 188
Enfuvirtide (T20, fusion inhibitor)	81, 90, 213, 225, 226
Entamoeba histolytica	17, 20, 36, **141**
Entecavir	81, 89, 169, 173, 189, 211, 225, 226
Enteric fever (typhoid fever)	61
Enterobacter	11, 53, 61, 68, 71, 73, 75, 96
Enterobius vermicularis	**147**
Enterococci	8, 15, 17, 22, **27**, **28**, **29**, 30, 31, 34, 35, 36, 46, 47, 56, 62, 68, 70, 71, 73, 75, 95
Drug-resistant	**29**, 71, 95
Vancomycin-resistant	**29**, 36, 75, 76
Enterococcus faecalis	**29**, 34, 53, 68, 71, 73, 75
Enterococcus faecium	29, 68, 71, 75, 95
Enterococcus sp.	77
Enterocolitis, pseudomembranous or neutropenic	17, **20**, 70, 96
Enterocytozoon bieneusi	20, 142
Enterovirus	7, 46, **156**
Eosinophilic meningitis	149
Epididymitis	**27**
Epiglottitis	49, 68
Epstein-Barr virus (infectious mono)	**45**, **159**
Epzicom	178
Ertapenem	16, 22, 33, 35, 40, 46, 47, **71**, 81, 84, **94**, **104**, 203, 205, 218, 225, 226
Erysipelas	15, 54, 64
Erysipelothrix	**68**
Erythema multiforme	**54**, 96
Erythema nodosum	**54**, 137, 139, 140
Erythrasma	**54**, 67, 120
Erythromycin	12, 13, 17, 19, 23, 24, 25, 37, 38, 39, 42, 43, 46, 49, 51, 52, 54, 55, 56, 57, 58, 59, 61, 67, 68, 69, 75, 81, 86, 92, **98**, 107, 109, 136, 194, 203, 206, 219, 221, 225, 226
Erythrovirus B19	166
Escherichia coli	6, 8, 9, 17, 18, **20**, **34**, 35, 47, 50, 53, 61, 68, 71, 73, 75, 77, 141
0157 H7	17, 18
enterotoxigenic (traveler's diarrhea)	17
Etanercept	33
Ethambutol	81, 87, 129, 130, 131, 132, 133, 134, 135, 136, **138**, 210, 218, 225, 226
Ethionamide	81, 88, 92, 130, 132, 137, **139**, 210, 213, 218, 225, 226
Etravirine	81, 90, 92, 175, 180, 186, 218, 220, 224, 225, 226
Eviplera (Complera)	175, 178, 181
Extended-spectrum β-lactamases (ESBL)	41, 47, **77**
Eye worm (Onchocerca volvulus)	148
F	
F. moniliforme	120
F. oxysporum	120
F. verticillioides	120
Famciclovir	13, 28, 81, 89, 160, 161, 162, 163, **169**, 173, 211, 225, 226
Fansidar (pyrimethamine sulfadoxine)	153, 154, 225, 226
Fasciola buski, gigantica	149
Fasciola buski, hepatica	**149**
Fever blisters (cold sores)	**161**
Fever in Returning Travelers	61
Fidaxomicin	81, 98, 225, 226
Filariasis	**148**, **149**, 164
Fitzhugh-Curtis syndrome	25
Flavivirus	61

	PAGES (page numbers bold if major focus)
Flucloxacillin	**93**
Fluconazole	26, 27, 31, 36, 46, 48, 50, 56, 62, 65, 81, 87, 92, 111, 112, 118, 119, 120, 124, 125, 127, 142, 202, 209, 213, 217, 222, 223, 225, 226
Flucytosine	81, 82, 87, 118, **119**, **125**, 142, 209, 225, 226
Fluke infestation (Trematodes)	149, 150
Fluoroquinolones	11, 13, 17, 19, 20, 23, 24, 27, 31, 34, 35, 37, 39, 41, 42, 43, 44, 47, 50, 51, 52, 61, 63, 67, 68, 69, 70, 71, 91, 98, **100**, 131, 135, 138, 139, 218, 219
Folliculitis; hot tub folliculitis	54, 56
Fomivirsen	159
Foot, diabetic	5, 16, 54
Fosamprenavir	81, 90, 92, 175, 182, 187, 200, 213, 221, 224, 225, 226
Foscarnet	81, 89, **168**, 211, 217, 225, 226
Foscavir	225, 226
Fosfomycin	34, 69, 75, 81, 86, **101**, 225, 226
Fournier's gangrene	**56**
Francisella tularensis	39, 43, **45**, 56, **59**, 68, 70, 76
Fumagillin	142, 153
Furunculosis	**53**, **54**
Fusariosis	120, 126
Fusarium solani	120
Fusarium sp.	126, 127
Fusidic acid	4, 55, 69, 75, 78, 81, 86, 103, 213, 225, 226
Fusobacterium necrophorum	14, 36, 49, 51, 52, 72, 74, 76
G	
G6PD deficiency	34, 52, 102, 139, 140, 143, 144, 145, 152, 153, 221
Ganciclovir	13, 62, 81, 89, 158, 159, 161, **168**, 173, 201, 211, 219, 223, 225, 226
Gardnerella vaginalis	**26**, 68
Gas gangrene	**46**, 55, 56, 63, 70
Gastric ulcer, gastritis (H. pylori)	**21**, 68, 70
Gastroenteritis	17, 18, 19, 20, 165
Gatifloxacin	9, 13, 15, 35, 39, 40, 43, 50, 71, 81, **100**, 107, 134, 136, 206, 218, 219, 225, 226
Gemifloxacin	37, 39, 42, 50, 71, 81, 85, **100**, 107, 206, 218, 219, 225, 226
Genital herpes	7, 28, 160, 161
Gentamicin	8, 9, 13, 14, 17, 20, 26, 28, 29, 30, 31, 35, 38, 45, 48, 57, 59, 60, 63, 67, 68, 69, 70, 75, 81, 82, 85, 104, **109**, 195, 203, 205, 213, 217, 219, 225, 226
Giardiasis	17, 20, **141**
Gnathostoma	10, 149
Golimumab	33
Gongylonemiasis	**147**
Gonococcal arthritis, disseminated GC	**32**, 70
Gonococcal ophthalmia	**12**
Gonorrhea	12, 13, **23**, 25, 26, 27, 32, 68, 71, 73, 75
Granuloma inguinale	**24**
Griseofulvin	120, **125**, 225, 226
Group B strep, including neonatal	4, 8, 25, 27, 32, 38, **61**, **192**
Guillain-Barré syndrome	185
H	
HABCEK acronym; infective endocarditis	**30**
Haemophilus aphrophilus, H. ducreyi	23, **30**, 68
Haemophilus influenzae	**8**, **9**, **10**, **11**, 12, 13, 14, 15, 32, 35, 37, 38, 39, 41, 43, 44, 46, 49, 50, 61, 62, 63, 66, 68, 70
Hantavirus pulmonary syndrome	45, 149, 156
Headache	179, 181, 185
Heartworms (dirofilariasis)	149
Helicobacter pylori	21, 68, 70
Hemodialysis (drug dosages)	65, **205**, **208**
Hemolytic uremic syndrome	**17**, 18, 169
Hemophilus aphrophilus, H. ducreyi	72, 74, 76

PAGES (page numbers bold if major focus)

Hemophilus influenzae	71, 73, 75, **192**
Hemorrhagic bullae (Vibrio skin infection)	54
Hemorrhagic fevers	156, 157
Hepatic abscess	**36**, **141**
Hepatic disease/drug dosage adjustment	213
Hepatitis	187
Hepatitis A	189
Hepatitis A, B & C	32, 36, 57, 138, 169, 170, 173, 198, 200, 202, 216, 225, 226
Hepatitis B	178, 179, 185, 186, 189
Hepatitis B occupational exposure	198
Hepatitis B prophylaxis	**198**, 216
Hepatitis C	189
Response to Therapy	190
Treatment Contraindications	190
Treatment Duration	191
Treatment Regimens	190
Herpes infections	7, 12, 13, 15, 20, 23, 24, 28, 34, 46, 54, 62, 158, 159, 160, 161, 163, 169, 173, 202
mucocutaneous	**161**
Herpes simiae	52, **161**
Herpes simplex	7, 12, 13, 15, 21, 24, 28, 45, 46, **160**, **161**, 173, 202
Herpes zoster	54, 163
Heterophyes (intestinal fluke)	149
HHV-6, HHV-7, HHV-8 infections	159
Hidradenitis suppurativa	53
Histoplasma capsulatum	121, 127
Histoplasmosis	10, 43, 44, **121**, 126, 127
HIV	**6**, **7**, 10, 15, 20, 21, 23, 24, 43, 44, 45, 46, 51, 57, 89, 90, 91, 118, 119, 122, 125, 128, 129, 132, 133, 134, 135, 136, 137, 138, 141, 142, 146, 158, 159, 161, 162, 163, 168, 169, 198, 199, 216, 218, 221, 224
Prophylaxis: needlestick & sexual	**199**, **200**
Hookworm	147, 148
Hordeolum (stye)	12
Hot tub folliculitis	**56**
Hymenolepsis diminuta	150
Hyperalimentation, sepsis	65

I

Imidazoles, topical	**125**
Imipenem	7, 10, 11, 12, 16, 17, 22, 29, 35, 36, 41, 44, 45, 46, 47, 50, 52, 54, 55, 56, 62, 63, 65, 66, 67, 68, 69, 71, 77, 81, 84, 94, **95**, 104, 135, 203, 205, 213, 219, 225, 226
Imipenem-Cilastatin	46
Imiquimod	172, 225, 226
Immune globulin, IV (IVIG)	7, 61, 64, 157, 189
Impetigo	55
Inclusion conjunctivitis	13
Indinavir	81, 90, 92, 132, 182, 187, 213, 218, 219, 221, 222, 224, 225, 226
Infectious mononucleosis (see EBV)	159, 199
Inflammatory bowel disease	54, 152
Infliximab	33, 162
Influenza A	118, **164**, **165**, 171, 173, 216
INH (isoniazid)	81, 88, 92, 128, 129, 130, 131, 132, 133, 134, 136, **138**, 140, 210, 213, 217, 218, 219, 221, 222, 223, 225, 226
Interferon alfa	170
Interferons	118, 134, 156, 157, 161, 172, 173, 225, 226
Iodoquinol	141, **152**, 225, 226
Isentress	184, 188
Isepamicin	81, **109**, 205
Isoniazid	213
Isospora belli	20
Isotretinoin	**51**
Itraconazole	26, 27, 81, 87, 92, 111, 112, 118, 119, 120, 122, 123, **125**, 127, 142, 209, 213, 217, 218, 219, 220, 221, 222, 223, 225, 226

PAGES (page numbers bold if major focus)

IV line infection & prophylaxis	15, 65, 66
Ivermectin	81, 88, 147, 148, 149, 151, **154**, 225, 226

J

JC Virus	173
Jock itch (T. cruris)	120

K

Kala-azar	153
Kaletra	182, 187, 224
Kanamycin	85, 104, 109, 130, 131, 136, 205, 217, 225, 226
Kaposi's sarcoma	44, 159
Katayama fever	150
Kawasaki syndrome	**61**, 156
Keratitis	12, 13, 14, 15, 142, 160
Ketoconazole	10, 54, 81, 87, 92, 120, **122**, **125**, 142, 213, 217, 218, 219, 220, 221, 222, 223, 225, 226
Kikuchi-Fujimoto (necrotizing lymphadenitis)	45
Klebsiella species	11, 35, 36, 41, 43, 47, 61, 68, 71, 73, 75, **77**

L

Lactobacillus sp.	65, **68**
Lamivudine (3TC)	81, 90, 169, 170, 173, 177, 178, 185, 189, 200, 202, 211, 218, 219, 223, 225, 226
Larva migrans	**148**, **149**
Laryngitis	49
Lassa fever, Ebola	156
Legionnaire's disease/Legionella sp.	30, 39, 40, 41, 42, 44, 62, 68, 70, 72, 74, 76
Leishmaniasis	45, 56, **142**, 153
Lemierre's **syndrome** (jugular vein **suppurative** phlebitis)	49
Leprosy	**136**, 139, 148
Leptospirosis	7, 36, **60**, 68, 99
Leuconostoc	65, **68**
Leukemia	93, 129
Levofloxacin	4, 5, 13, 14, 15, 16, 17, 19, 20, 22, 23, 27, 31, 32, 33, 34, 35, 36, 37, 39, 40, 41, 42, 43, 44, 47, 49, 50, 51, 55, 56, 58, 60, 62, 63, 68, 69, 71, 82, **100**, 107, 130, 131, 136, 206, 218, 219, 225, 226
Lexiva	225
Lice	
body, head, pubic, & scabies	24, 30, 57, **151**, 154
Lincomycin	**98**
Lindane	151
Line sepsis	15, **65**, **66**
Linezolid	4, 5, 7, 9, 12, 16, 29, 33, 36, 38, 40, 42, 44, 45, 53, 54, 55, 56, 62, 64, 66, 68, 69, 75, 77, 78, 81, 86, 92, 97, **99**, 104, 131, 135, 136, 137, 203, 207, 213, 219, 225, 226
Listeria monocytogenes	7, 8, 9, 10, 14, 18, 38, 61, 68, 70, 71, 73, 75
Liver abscess	36, **141**
Liver disease/drug dosage adjustment	**213**
Loa loa	148
Lobomycosis	122
Lomefloxacin	219, 225, 226
Lopinavir/ritonavir & lopinavir	81, 90, 92, 132, 200, 213, 219, 221, 225, 226
Loracarbef	11, 73, 203, 225, 226
Ludwig's angina	46, **49**
Lumefantrine	81, 88, 152
Lung abscess	45
Lung abscess, putrid	70
Lyme disease	10, **31**, **32**, 45, 57, **58**, 70
Lymphadenitis	45, 51, 57
Lymphangitis, nodular	45
Lymphedema (congenital = Milroy's disease)	**54**
Lymphogranuloma venereum	**24**, 45

231

PAGES (page numbers bold if major focus)

M
MAC, MAI (Mycobacterium avium-intracellulare complex) **134, 135,** 136
Macrolide antibiotics 11, 39, 42, 54, **75,** 81, 85, 86, 98, 107, 136, 203, 206, 219
Madura foot **122,** 123
Malacoplakia (pyelonephritis variant) 35
Malaria 61, 91, 99, 141, **143, 145,** 153, 154, 192, 216
Malarone (atovaquone + proguanil) 143, 145, **152**
Malassezia furfur (Tinea versicolor) 54, 65, **120**
Malathion 151
Mansonella **148, 149**
Maraviroc 81, 90, 92, 175, 184, 188, 211, 220, 225, 226
Mastitis 6
Mastoiditis 12
Measles, measles vaccine 96, **165**
Mebendazole 81, 147, 149, **154,** 225, 226
Mefloquine 81, 88, 92, 143, 144, **153,** 220, 221, 225, 226
Meibomianitis 12
Melarsoprol 147, **153**
Meleney's gangrene 55, 56
Melioidosis (Burkholderia pseudomallei) **41,** 56, **67**
Membranous pharyngitis 49
Meningitis
 Aseptic 7, 10, 102, 156, 157
 Bacterial (acute and chronic) 7, **8, 9, 10,** 58, 68, 95, 132, 203
 eosinophilic 10, **147,** 148
Meningococcus 8, 9, 15, 32, 62, 63, 68, 70, 71, 73, 75, 99, 192
Meningococcus, meningitis 8, 9, 10, 15, 32, 63, 68, 70, 71, 73, 75
 Prophylaxis 10
Meropenem 7, 8, 9, 10, 11, 16, 17, 22, 25, 33, 35, 36, 41, 44, 46, 47, 50, 54, 55, 56, 62, 63, 66, 67, 68, 69, 71, 77, 81, 84, 94, **95,** 104, 110, 203, 205, 219, 225, 226
Mesalamine 225, 226
Metagonimus 149
Metapneumovirus 45, 165
Methenamine mandelate & hippurate **101,** 220, 225, 226
Methicillin 29, 30, 31, 68, 69, 71
Methicillin-resistant Staph. aureus (MRSA) 4, 5, 6, 8, 13, 14, 15, 16, 28, 29, 31, 32, 33, 35, 38, 40, 41, 42, 43, 44, 46, 47, 50, 52, 53, 54, 55, 56, 61, 62, 63, 64, 65, 69, 71, 73, 75, 194
Methotrexate 220
Metronidazole 6, 7, 15, 16, 17, 19, 21, 22, 23, 26, 27, 36, 43, 46, 47, 49, 51, 52, 55, 56, 62, 66, 67, 68, 75, 81, 86, 88, 92, **102,** 107, 141, 152, 193, 194, 195, 203, 207, 213, 218, 220, 221, 223, 225, 226
Micafungin 31, 63, 81, 87, 111, 124, 202, 213, 220, 225, 226
Miconazole 26, **125**
Microsporidia 20, 142
Miltefosine 81, 88, 153
Minocycline 45, 51, 53, 55, 56, 66, 67, 68, 69, 75, 77, 78, 86, 99, 135, 136, 137, 213, 225, 226
Mollaret's recurrent meningitis 160
Monkey bite **52,** 156, 161
Monobactams **95,** 104
Mononeuritis multiplex (CMV) 158
Moraxella 52
Moraxella catarrhalis 11, 15, 37, 39, 40, 42, 50, 68, 71, 73, 75
Morganella species 68, 72, 73
Moxifloxacin 9, 13, 15, 19, 22, 34, 37, 39, 40, 41, 42, 43, 44, 46, 47, 50, 51, 62, 63, 68, 69, 71, 81, 82, **100,** 107, 131, 134, 135, 136, 137, 139, 213, 218, 219, 225, 226

PAGES (page numbers bold if major focus)

MRSA 4, 5, 6, 8, 13, 14, 15, 16, 28, 29, 31, 32, 33, 35, 38, 40, 41, 42, 43, 44, 46, 48, 50, 52, 53, 54, 55, 56, 61, 62, 63, 64, 65, 69, 71, 73, 75, 95, 97, 194
MSSA 95
Mucormycosis 50, 66, **122,** 127
Multidrug-resistant TB 130, 131
Mumps 46
Mupirocin 53, 55, 103, 194, 225, 226
Mycobacteria 10, 32, 33, 43, 44, 45, 46, 56, 76, 99, 128, **129, 130, 131, 132, 134, 135, 136**
Mycobacterium abscessus, M. bovis, M. celatum, M.chelonae, M. genavense, M. gordonae, M. haemophilum, M. kansasii, M. marinum, M. scrofulaceum, M. simiae, M. ulcerans, M. xenopi, M. leprae **28, 29,** 33, 45, 52, 99, 134, **135, 136, 161**
Mycobacterium tuberculosis 10, 33, 43, 44, 45, 54, 128, 129, 130, 131, 132, 134
 Directly observed therapy (DOT) 129, **130,** 132
 Drug-resistant **134**
 Pulmonary 43, 44, **130, 131**
Mycoplasma
 genitalium 23
 pneumoniae 36, 37, 39, 68, 72, 76
Mycotic aneurysm **66**
Myiasis 151
Myositis 46, 64

N
Naegleria fowleri 142
Nafcillin 4, 6, 8, 12, 15, 28, 29, 30, 31, 33, 35, 42, 43, 44, 46, 54, 52, 54, 56, 64, 69, 71, 83, 92, 93, 104, 203, 213, 225, 226
Necrotizing enterocolitis **17,** 192
Necrotizing fasciitis 46, 54, 55, 56, 64
Needlestick, HIV, Hepatitis B & C **198,** 199, **200**
Neisseria
 gonorrhoeae 12, 13, 23, 25, 26, 27, 32, 68, 71, 73, 75
 meningitidis 9, 15, 32, 63, **68,** 70, 71, 73, 75
Nelfinavir 81, 90, 92, 130, 131, 182, 187, 213, 220, 221, 222, 223, 224, 225, 226
Nematodes (roundworms) **147,** 154
Neomycin 10, 103, **109,** 152, 194, 217
Neonatal sepsis 61, 192
Netilmicin 81, 104, 109, 205, 217
Neurocysticercosis 150
Neurosyphilis 24
Neutropenia 20, 40, 41, 50, 53, 62, 63, 65, 93, 99, **104, 106, 107,** 111, 124, 142, 153, 168
Nevirapine 81, 90, 92, 175, 180, 186, 200, 213, 218, 220, 222, 224, 225, 226
Niclosamide 150
Nifurtimox 147, **153**
Nitazoxanide 81, 88, 102, 141, 152, 167, 225, 226
Nitrofurantoin 34, 69, 75, 81, 101, **102,** 207, 218, 220, 223, 225, 226
Nocardia brasiliensis, asteroides 68, 99
Nocardiosis 6, 7, **45,** 68, 99, **122**
Norovirus (Norwalk-like virus) 17, 165
NRTIs 177, 178, 179, 180, 181, 185, 186, 187
Nursing (breast milk) & antibiotics 6, 25
Nystatin 14, 26, **125,** 225, 226

O
Ofloxacin 10, 20, 23, 34, 68, 71, 81, 85, **100,** 107, 130, 135, 136, 137, **139,** 206, 218, 219, 225, 226
Onchocerciasis 148, 154
Onychomycosis 16, 120, 125, 126
Ophthalmia neonatorum 12
Opisthorchis (liver fluke) 149
Orbital cellulitis 15
Orchitis **27**
Orthopedic Surgery 195

PAGES (page numbers bold if major focus)

Entry	Pages
Oseltamivir	45, 81, 82, 89, 91, **164, 165**, 171, 173, 212, 225, 226
Osteomyelitis	
Chronic	5, 70
Contiguous (post-operative, post-nail puncture)	**4, 5**
Foot	16
Hematogenous	5, 70
Osteonecrosis of the jaw	5
Vertebral	**4**, 57
Otitis externa—chronic, malignant, & swimmer's ear	**10**
Otitis media	7, **11, 12**, 70, 98
Oxacillin	4, 6, 12, 28, 29, 30, 31, 32, 33, 35, 42, 43, 44, 46, 52, 54, 55, 56, 62, 64, 69, 71, 83, **93**, 104, 203, 225, 226

P

Entry	Pages
P. knowlesi	144
Palivizumab	36, **171,** 225, 226
Pancreatitis	177, 179, 185, 187
pancreatic abscess	46, 61, 95, 99, 153, 218, 220, 223
Papillomavirus	**166**
Papovavirus/Polyoma virus	166
Paracoccidioidomycosis	122
Paragonimus	149
Parapharyngeal space infection	49
Parasitic infections	141–52
Paromomycin	109, 141, 142, 152, 225, 226
Paronychia	28
Parotitis	46
Parvovirus B19	32, **166**
PAS (para-aminosalicylic acid)	**88**, 140
Pasteurella canis	52
Pasteurella multocida	52, 68, 72, 74
Pefloxacin	71
Pegylated interferon	156, 170, 173, 225, 226
Pegylated-Interferon-alpha 2a	189
Peliosis hepatis	**36, 57**
Pelvic actinomycosis	25
Pelvic inflammatory disease (PID)	**25, 26,** 70
Pelvic suppurative phlebitis	25
Penciclovir	160, 161, 169
Penicillin	
desensitization	80
Penicillin allergy	8, 9, 24, 25, 28, 29, 30, 47, 50, 52, 54, 55, 58, 93, 94, 95, 96
Penicillin G	6, 7, 9, 14, 21, 24, 25, 28, 29, 33, 39, 42, 43, 46, 49, 52, 54, 56, 58, 60, 61, 64, 67, 68, 69, 71, 83, **93**, 104, 203, 208
Penicillin V	48, 52, 54, 61, 71, 83, **93**, 192, 193, 203
Penicillin VK	25, 42, 47, 54
Penicillins	81
Penicilliosis	**122**
Pentamidine	44, 81, 142, 146, 147, **153**, 209, 217, 218, 220, 223, 225, 226
Peptostreptococcus	6, 69, **72, 74**, 76
Peramivir	89, **164, 165**, 212
Pericarditis	**31**, 70, 132
Perinephric abscess	**35**
Perirectal abscess	20, **22**
Peritoneal dialysis, infection	48, 196, **213**
Peritonitis	
Bacterial/spontaneous	17, 22, 47
Spontaneous—prevention	47
Peritonsillar abscess	48, 49
Pertussis	**37**, 67
Phaeohyphomycosis	**122**
Pharmacodynamics	92
Pharmacokinetics, pharmacology	**92**
Pharyngitis	
Diffuse erythema	48

Entry	Pages
Exudative	48, 49
Membranous	49
Vesicular, ulcerative pharyngitis	49
Pharyngitis/tonsillitis	23, 31, 32, 61, 70
Phenobarbital	222
Phenytoin	222
Phlebitis, septic	12, 25, 53, **65**
Photosensitivity	51, 99, 100, 102, 104, 105, 107, 108, 125, 126, 138, 153, 154
PID	**25, 26,** 70
Pinworms	147, 154
Piperacillin	14, 44, 53, 71, **94**, 104, 194, 203, 208, 220, 225, 226
Piperacillin-tazobactam	12, 16, 17, 22, 25, 27, 35, 36, 41, 42, 44, 47, 49, 52, 53, 55, 56, 62, 63, 66, 67, 69, 71, 83, 94, 104, 110, 111, 203, 220
Plague	39, 43, 56, 69
Plasmodia sp.	61
Plesiomonas shigelloides	17, 68
PML (progressive multifocal leukoencephalopathy)	**166**
Pneumococci, drug-resistant	11, 42, 44, **69**
Pneumocystis (carinii) jiroveci	44, 70, 102, 145, 202, 203
Pneumonia	38–42
adult	38, 41, 42, 43, 44, 53, 59, 70, 78, 145, 156, 158, 162, 167, 171, 173
aspiration	43
chronic	43
community-acquired	**41, 62,** 167
community-associated	78
health care-associated	**40**
hospital-acquired	**41**
Infants, Children	38
neonatal/infants/children	**38**
ventilator-acquired	41, 78
Podofilox	166, **172**
Polyenes	127
Polymyxin B	10, 13, 81, 86, **101**, 103, 213, 220, 225, 226
Polymyxin E, Colistin	77, 101, 207, 221
Polyoma virus	166
Posaconazole	81, 87, 92, 111, 117, 118, 122, 123, 126, 127, 202, 217, 220, 221, 225, 226
Post Renal Transplant Obstructive Uropathy	**35**
PPD (TST)	128, 129
Praziquantel	81, 88, 92, 149, 150, **154**, 225, 226
Prednisone	146, 149
Pregnancy, antibiotics in	9, 23, 25, 26, 34, 35, 41, 43, 45, 51, 58, 99, 118, 124, 125, 129, 132, 138, 140, 141, 143, 144, 145, 146, 149, 153, 154, 162, 169, 170, 199, 200, 222
Pregnancy, risk from anti-infectives	**81**
Primaquine	44, 143, 144, 145, 146, **153**, 221, 225
Proctitis	20, 23
Progressive multifocal leukoencephalopathy (PML)	**166**
Proguanil	81, 92
Proguanil, atovaquone-proguanil	81, 143, 145, 152, 225, 226
Prolonged Dosing, Antibacterials	110
Prostatitis, prostatodynia	23, 27, 35, 70
Prosthetic joint infection/prophylaxis	5, 19, 33
Prosthetic valve endocarditis	30, 31, **194**
Protease inhibitors (PI)	132, 136, 176, 179, 180, 182, 183, 186, 187, 188, 217, 218, 219, 220, 221, 222
Protein binding (antimicrobials)	**83–91**
Providencia species	68
Pseudallescheria boydii (Scedosporium sp.)	122, **123**, 125, 126, 127
Pseudomembranous enterocolitis	70, 98
Pseudomonas aeruginosa	4, 5, 8, 9, 10, 12, 14, 16, 20, 22, 27, 31, 32, 33, 35, 36, 38, 40, 41, 42, 43, 44, 47, 51, 53, 54, 56, 68, 72, 74, 76, **77**, 94, 96

PAGES (page numbers bold if major focus)

Pseudotumor cerebri	99
Puncture wound	56
Pyelonephritis	34, 35, 62, 70, 101
Pyomyositis	46
Pyrantel pamoate	147, 148, 154, 225, 226
Pyrazinamide	81, 88, 129, **130**, **131**, **132**, **133**, 134, 136, **138**, 210, 221, 222, 225, 226
Pyridium	34
Pyridoxine	132, 136, 138, 139
Pyrimethamine	81, 88, 142, 146, 147, **153**, 154, 213, 218, 221, 225, 226

Q

Q fever	31, 67
QTc prolongation	**98**, **100**, 126, 145, 181, 187
Quinacrine HCl	141, 152
Quinidine gluconate	81, 145, 153, 220, 222
Quinine	57, 81, 142, 144, 145, 153, **154**, 209, 220, 221
Quinolones	92, 107
Quinupristin-dalfopristin	29, 65, 69, 75, 77, 78, 81, 92, **99**, 107, 213, 221, 222, 225, 226

R

Rabies, rabies vaccine	52, 153, 167, 215
Raltegravir	81, 90, 92, 175, 184, 188, 213, 222, 225, 226
Rape victim	193
Rat bite	**52**
Raxibacumab	43
Red neck syndrome & vancomycin	**97**
Reiter's syndrome	27, **31**
Relapsing fever	
Louse-borne	59
Tick-borne	59
Renal failure, dosing	205, 213
Resistance	
Acinetobacter	77
Carbapenemase	77
Enterococcus sp.	77
Escherichia coli	**77**
Gram Negative Bacilli	77
Gram Positive Bacteria	77
Klebsiella species	77
Pseudomonas aeruginosa	**77**
Staph. aureus	77
Stenotrophomonas maltophilia	77
Streptococcus pneumoniae	77
Resistant bacteria	71
Resource directory (phone numbers, websites)	216
Respiratory syncytial virus (RSV)	36, 38, 45, 165, 171, 173
Retapamulin	55, 103, 225, 226
Retinal necrosis, progressive outer	15
Retinitis	**15**, 45, 146, 158, 159
Rheumatic fever	31, 32, 48, 61
Rheumatoid arthritis, septic joint	**32**, 70
Rhinosinusitis	11, 50, 51
Rhinovirus	38, 50, **167**
Rhodococcus equi	69
Ribavirin	36, 81, 89, 156, 165, 167, 170, 173, 212, 213, 218, 222, 225, 226
Rickettsial diseases	**59**, 61, 69, 76
Rifabutin	81, 88, 92, 129, 130, 132, 134, 135, 136, **140**, 217, 218, 219, 220, 221, 222, 223, 225, 226
Rifampin	33, 60, 77, 213
Rifampin, Rifamate, Rifater	4, 5, 9, 10, 30, 31, 43, 51, 53, 57, 58, 59, 66, 67, 68, 69, 75, 78, 81, 86, 88, 92, 102, 107, 126, 128, 129, 130, 131, 132, 133, 134, 135, 136, 137, **138**, 140, 142, 203, 210, 213, 217, 218, 219, 220, 221, 222, 223, 225, 226
Rifamycins	132, 222

PAGES (page numbers bold if major focus)

Rifapentine	88, 92, 130, 132, 133, **140**, 213, 222, 225, 226
Rifaximin	20, 81, 86, 102, 213, 225, 226
Rilpivirine	81, 90, 175, 181, 187, 225, 226
Rimantadine	81, 89, **171**, 173, 212, 213, 222, 225, 226
Ringworm	120
Ritonavir	81, 90, 91, 92, 132, 181, 183, 187, 188, 200, 213, 219, 221, 222, 223, 224, 225, 226
Rocky Mountain spotted fever	62, 70
Rubella vaccine	32

S

Salmonella sp.	61
Salmonellosis, bacteremia	4, **17**, **19**, **20**, 31, 32, 60, **61**, 69, 72, 73, 75
Salpingitis	26
Saquinavir	81, 90, 92, 132, 175, 176, 183, 188, 213, 221, 222, 224, 225, 226
SARS (Severe Acute Resp. Syndrome)	45, 156, 167
SBE (subacute bacterial endocarditis)	28, 29, 30, 31
SBP (spontaneous bacterial peritonitis)	47
Scabies & Norwegian scabies	24, 151, 154
Scedosporium apiospermum (Pseudallescheria boydii)	127
Scedosporium sp. (Pseudallescheria boydii)	122, **123**, 125, 126, 127
Schistosomiasis	150, 155
Scrofula	26
Seborrheic dermatitis (dandruff)	54, 199
"Sepsis" and "septic shock"	17, 52, 53, 55, 61, 62, **63**, 64, 134, 194
Sepsis, abortion; amnionitis	**25**
Sepsis, neonatal	**61**
Septata intestinalis	20, 142
Serratia marcescens	69, 72, 73, 76, 96
Severe acute respiratory distress syndrome (SARS)	45, 156, 167
Severe fever with thrombocytopenia syndrome virus (SFTSV)	157
Sexual contacts/assaults	12, 13, **23**, 26, 45, 125, **193**, 199, 200
SFTSV (Severe fever with thrombocytopenia syndrome virus)	157
Shigellosis	**17**, **19**, **20**, 31, 69, 72, 73, 75
Shingles	54, 163
Sickle cell disease	4, 32, 192, 193
Sildenafil	222
Silver sulfadiazine	103
Sinecatechins	172
Sinusitis	7, 36, **50**, 70, 98, 111, 122, 171
Sirturo	226
Skin	178, 186, 187
Ulcerated	56
Smallpox	167
Snake bite, spider bite	52
Sparganosis	**151**
Spectinomycin	109, 225, 226
Spinal implant infection	5
Spiramycin	154
Spirochetosis	19
Splenectomy	52, 56, 63, 142, **192**
Splenic abscess	**56**
Sporotrichosis	45, 123
Spotted fevers	59, 62, 70
Staph. aureus	4, 5, 6, 8, 10, 11, 12, 13, 14, 15, 16, 28, 29, 30, 31, 32, 33, 35, 38, 39, 40, 41, 42, 43, 44, 45, 46, 49, 50, 51, 52, 53, 54, 55, 56, 61, 62, 64, 65, 66, 69, 70, 71, 73, 75, **77**, 96, 97, 194
Community-associated	56, 69
Endocarditis	29, 70, 97

PAGES (page numbers bold if major focus)

Staph. epidermidis	5, 8, 12, 14, 15, 17, 30, 31, 46, 48, 52, 53, 61, 65, 69, 71, 73, 75, 78
Staph. hemolyticus	35, **69**
Staph. lugdunensis	6, 69
Staph. saprophyticus	34, 69
Staph. scalded skin syndrome	**56**
Stavudine (d4T)	81, 91, 176, 179, 185, 200, 212, 218, 222, 223, 225, 226
Stenotrophomonas maltophilia	41, 42, 69, 72, 74, 76, 77, 94
Stevens-Johnson syndrome	182, 186, 187, 188
Stibogluconate	152, 225
Stomatitis	**46**, 61, 139, 160
Streptobacillus moniliformis	**52**, 69
Streptococcal toxic shock	53, 56, 64
Streptococci	4, 6, 8, 11, 12, 15, 25, 26, 27, 28, 29, 30, 31, 32, 36, 38, 42, 44, 45, 46, 49, 50, 51, 52, 53, 54, 55, 56, 61, 62, 63, 64, 66, 69, 70, 71, 73, 75, 95, 136, 192
Streptococcus	
anginosus group	69
bovis	**28**, **29**, 134
group B, prophylaxis	**192**
milleri complex	43, 44, 71
pneumoniae	8, 9, 11, 12, 13, 14, 15, 31, 38, 40, 42, 44, 49, 50, 62, 63, 69, 70, 71, 73, 75, **77**, 193
pyogenes	6, 8, 12, 14, 16, 32, 48, 49, 53, 54, 64, 69
Streptococcus sp.	54, 56, 66
Streptomycin	21, 29, 45, 68, 70, 81, 88, 109, 128, 130, 131, 132, 136, **138**, 205, 217
Stribild	90, 175, 184, 212, 213
Strongyloidiasis	**147**, 154
Subdural empyema	**7**
Sulfadiazine	53, 61, 66, 142, 146, 153, 154, 225, 226
Sulfadoxine + pyrimethamine	81, 153, 154, 225, 226
Sulfasalazine	225
Sulfisoxazole	11, 38, **45**, 61, **102**, 203, 225, 226
Sulfonamides	34, 45, 54, 69, 81, 102, 154, 207, 221, 223, 225, 226
Suppurative phlebitis	12
Suppurative Phlebitis	
Cavernous sinus thrombosis	**66**
Other	**66**
Suppurative Phlebitis	
Thrombophlebitis	**66**
Supraglottis	49
Suramin	**147**, **154**
Surgical procedures, prophylaxis	193, 195, 196
Synercid® (quinupristin-dalfopristin)	29, 65, 69, 77, 78, **99**, 107, 213, 221, 222, 225, 226
Syphilis	10, 20, **23**, **24**, **25**, 38, 45, 193
T	
Tacrolimus	222
Tadalafil	222
Tapeworms	
Taenia saginata, T. solium, D. latum, D. caninum	148, **150**
Teicoplanin	18, 29, 35, 69, 75, **97**, 207
Telaprevir	89, 170, 173, 225, 226
Telavancin	55, 56, 69, 75, 81, 86, **97**, 107, 207, 225, 226
Telbivudine	81, 89, 169, 170, 189, 212, 225, 226
Telithromycin	39, 50, 67, 69, 75, 81, 86, 92, **98**, 104, 207, 213, 222, 223, 225, 226
Temocillin	**94**, 207, 225
Tenofovir	81, 91, 175, 176, 177, 178, 179, 181, 184, 186, 189, 211, 212, 218, 221, 223, 225, 226
Terbinafine	81, 92, 117, 120, 122, 123, **126**, 209, 223, 225, 226
Tetanus prophylaxis	52, **214**
Tetanus, Clostridium tetani	16, 52, 55, 56, 65, 67, **214**

Tetracycline	12, 13, 19, 21, 23, 24, 25, 51, 52, 53, 58, 59, 64, 68, 69, 86, 99, 107, 141, 144, 145, 154, 203, 209, 217
Thalidomide	81, 137, 140, 225, 226
Thiabendazole	223, 225, 226
Thrombophlebitis	
Jugular vein suppurative phlebitis (Lemierre's syndrome)	**49**
Pelvic vein(s)	**25**
Septic (suppurative)	**53**, **65**
Thrush	199
Ticarcillin	14, 43, 71, **94**, 104, 203, 209, 225, 226
Ticarcillin-clavulanate	11, 12, 16, 17, 22, 25, 27, 35, 36, 42, 44, 47, 49, 52, 55, 56, 62, 63, 69, 71, 77, 83, **94**, 104, 203
Tigecycline	22, 47, 69, 75, 81, 87, 99, **109**, 135, 203, 205, 217, 223, 225, 226
Tinea capitis, corporis, cruris, pedis, versicolor	**120**, 151
Tinidazole	21, 26, 68, 81, 102, 140, 141, 152, 203, 213, 220, 223, 225, 226
Tipranavir	81, 91, 92, 183, 188, 213, 221, 224, 225, 226
TMP-SMX	80
desensitization	**80**
Tobramycin	10, 13, 14, 15, 20, 31, 33, 41, 42, 43, 45, 59, 63, 68, 75, 81, 82, 85, 104, **109**, 135, 203, 205, 217, 223, 225, 226
Tonsillitis	
Diffuse erythema	**48**
Exudative	48, 49
Torsades de pointes	98, 100
Toxic shock syndrome (strep., staph., clostridia)	53, 56, 64
Toxocariasis	149
Toxoplasma gondii, toxoplasmosis	6, 45, **146**, **147**, 202
Trachoma	**13**
Transplantation, infection	118
Transrectal prostate biopsy	196
Traveler's diarrhea	**20**, 70, 102
Trazodone	222
Trematodes (flukes)	**149**, **150**, 154
Trench fever	57
Trench mouth	46
Trichinellosis	**149**
Trichinosis	149
Trichomoniasis (vaginitis)	23, **26**, 141
Trichostrongylus	148
Trichuris	148
Triclabendazole	149, **154**
Tricuspid valve infection, S. aureus	30
Trifluridine	13, 160, **169**, 225
Trimethoprim	75, 92, 223, 226
Trimethoprim-sulfamethoxazole	4, 6, 7, 9, 11, 16, 17, 18, 20, 21, 22, 24, 27, 28, 33, 34, 35, 37, 38, 41, 42, 43, 44, 45, 46, 47, 50, 51, 52, 53, 54, 55, 56, 60, 62, 67, 68, 69, 75, 77, 78, 87, 92, 101, **102**, 107, 122, 135, 136, 141, 142, 145, 146, 153, 192, 196, 202, 203, 208, 213, 221, 222, 223, 225, 226
Truvada	178, **193**
Trypanosomiasis	**147**, 202
Tuberculosis	10, 33, 43, 44, 45, 54, 122, **128**, **129**, **130**, **131**, **132**, **133**, 134, 135, 136, 139, 213
Multidrug-resistant	**130**, **131**, 132
Tuberculin skin test (TST)	**128**, **129**
Tularemia (Francisella tularensis)	39, 43, **45**, 56, **59**, 68, 70, 76
Tumor Necrosis Factor	8, 33, 43, 118, 129, 163
Typhlitis—neutropenic enterocolitis—cecitis	**20**
Typhoid fever	17, 19, 61, 70
Typhus group (louse-borne, murine, scrub)	**59**, 99

PAGES (page numbers bold if major focus)

U
Ulcerative colitis	141
Ulcerative gingivitis	46
Uncomplicated/P. malariae	144
Urethral catheter, indwelling	**35**, 101
Urethritis, non-gonococcal	23, 25, 70
Urinary tract infection	34, 35, 64, 68, 69, 94, 102, 203

V
Vaccinia, contact	167
Vaginitis	34
Vaginosis, bacterial	26, 68
Valacyclovir	13, 28, 81, 89, 160, 161, 162, 163, **169**, 173, 212, 225, 226
Valganciclovir	81, 89, 158, 159, **168**, 173, 201, 212, 219, 223, 225, 226
Vancomycin	4, 5, 6, 8, 9, 11, 12, 14, 15, 16, 17, 18, 28, 29, 30, 31, 32, 33, 35, 38, 40, 41, 42, 43, 44, 46, 49, 50, 53, 54, 55, 56, 61, 62, 63, 64, 65, 66, 67, 68, 69, 75, 77, 78, 81, 82, 87, 92, 95, **97**, 99, 107, 109, 193, 194, 195, 196, 203, 208, 213, 217, 223, 225, 226
Vardenafil	222
Varicella zoster	13, 15, 64, 159, 162, 163, 173
Ventilator-associated pneumonia	41, 42
Vibrio cholerae, parahemolyticus, vulnificus	**19, 20**, 54, 69, 76
Vincent's angina	46
Viral infections	174
Visceral larval migrans	149

V (cont.)
Voriconazole	31, 63, 81, 82, 87, 92, 111, 112, 118, 122, 123, **126**, 127, 209, 213, 217, 220, 221, 222, 225, 226
VRE (vancomycin-resistant enterococci)	29, 36, 95

W
Warts	25, 172
West Nile virus	7, 64, 157, 167
Whipple's disease	10, **21**
Whipworm	148
Whirlpool	
Nail Salon	**56**
Whirlpool folliculitis (hot tub folliculitis)	**56**
Whitlow, herpetic	**28**, 161
Whooping cough	37, 67
Wound infection, post-op, post-trauma	46, 55, 56
Wuchereria bancrofti	148

X
Xanthomonas (Stenotrophomonas) maltophilia	42, 69, 72, 74, 76

Y
Yersinia enterocolitica & pestis	**20**, 31, 36, **45**, 54, 69, 72, 74, 76

Z
Zalcitabine (ddC)	81, 212, 218, 219, 223, 225, 226
Zanamivir	45, 81, **164, 165, 171**, 173, 225, 226
Zeftera	225
Zidovudine (ZDV, AZT)	81, 91, 168, 175, 176, 177, 178, 179, 185, 200, 212, 217, 218, 219, 221, 222, 223, 225, 226